Medical Titles in the Current Therapy Series

Bardin:
Current Therapy in Endocrinology and Metabolism
Bayless:
Current Management of Inflammatory Bowel Disease
Bayless:
Current Therapy in Gastroenterology and Liver Disease
Bayless, Brain, Cherniack:
Current Therapy in Internal Medicine
Brain, Carbone:
Current Therapy in Hematology–Oncology
Callaham:
Current Therapy in Emergency Medicine
Charles:
Current Therapy in Obstetrics
Cherniack:
Current Therapy of Respiratory Disease
Dubovsky, Shore:
Current Therapy in Psychiatry
Eichenwald, Ströder:
Current Therapy in Pediatrics
Foley, Payne:
Current Therapy of Pain
Fortuin:
Current Therapy in Cardiovascular Disease
Garcia, Mastroianni, Amelar, Dubin:
Current Therapy of Infertility
Glassock:
Current Therapy in Nephrology and Hypertension
Jeejeebhoy:
Current Therapy in Nutrition
Johnson:
Current Therapy in Neurologic Disease
Kacmarek, Stoller:
Current Respiratory Care
Kass, Platt:
Current Therapy in Infectious Disease
Lichtenstein, Fauci:
Current Therapy in Allergy, Immunology, and Rheumatology
Nelson:
Current Therapy in Neonatal–Perinatal Medicine
Nelson:
Current Therapy in Pediatric Infectious Disease
Parrillo:
Current Therapy in Critical Care Medicine
Peat:
Current Physical Therapy
Provost, Farmer:
Current Therapy in Dermatology
Rogers:
Current Practice in Anesthesiology
Torg, Welsh, Shephard:
Current Therapy in Sports Medicine

CURRENT THERAPY IN OBSTETRICS

CURRENT THERAPY IN OBSTETRICS

Editor

DAVID CHARLES, M.D.

Formerly, Professor and Chairman
Obstetrics and Gynecology
Marshall University School of Medicine
Huntington, West Virginia

Associate Editor

DOUGLAS D. GLOVER, M.D.

Professor of Obstetrics
West Virginia University School of Medicine
Associate Professor of Clinical Pharmacy
West Virginia University School of Pharmacy
Morgantown, West Virginia

1988

B.C. Decker Inc • Toronto • Philadelphia

Publisher

B.C. Decker Inc
3228 South Service Road
Burlington, Ontario L7N 3H8

B.C. Decker Inc
320 Walnut Street
Suite 400
Philadelphia, Pennsylvania 19106

Sales and Distribution

United States and Possessions
The C.V. Mosby Company
11830 Westline Industrial Drive
Saint Louis, Missouri 63146

Canada
The C.V. Mosby Company, Ltd.
5240 Finch Avenue East, Unit No. 1
Scarborough, Ontario M1S 5P2

United Kingdom, Europe and the Middle East
Blackwell Scientific Publications, Ltd.
Osney Mead, Oxford OX2 OEL, England

Australia and New Zealand
Harcourt Brace Jovanovich Group (Australia) Pty Limited
30–52 Smidmore Street
Marrickville, N.S.W. 2204
Australia

Japan
Igaku-Shoin Ltd.
Tokyo International P.O. Box 5063
1-28-36 Hongo, Bunkyo-ku, Tokyo 113, Japan

Asia
Info-Med Ltd.
802–3 Ruttonjee House
11 Duddell Street
Central Hong Kong

South Africa
Libriger Book Distributors
Warehouse Number 8
"Die Ou Looiery"
Tannery Road
Hamilton, Bloemfontein 9300

South America
Inter-Book Marketing Services
Rua das Palmeriras, 32
Apto. 701
222–70 Rio de Janeiro
RJ, Brazil

NOTICE

The authors and publisher have made every effort to ensure that the patient care recommended herein, including choice of drugs and drug dosages, are in accord with the accepted standards and practice at the time of publication. However, since research and regulation constantly change clinical standards, the reader is urged to check the product information sheet included in the package of each drug, which includes recommended doses, warnings, and contra-indications. This is particularly important with new or infrequently used drugs.

Current Therapy in Obstetrics

ISBN 1-55664-019-6

Library of Congress catalog card number: 88-70682

10 9 8 7 6 5 4 3 2 1

To Jean,
whose encouragement, support, and
continued confidence make everything possible

CONTRIBUTORS

EROL AMON, M.D.

Assistant Professor of Obstetrics and Gynecology, Division of Maternal-Fetal Medicine, Washington University School of Medicine; Staff, Barnes Hospital, Saint Louis, Missouri

Tocolytic Agents

MARVIN S. AMSTEY, M.D.

Professor, Department of Obstetrics and Gynecology, University of Rochester School of Medicine and Dentistry; Chief, Department of Obstetrics and Gynecology, Highland Hospital, Rochester, New York

Vaccination in Pregnancy

HUGH R. K. BARBER, M.D.

Director, Department of Obstetrics and Gynecology, Lenox Hill Hospital, New York, New York

Malignant Disease in Pregnancy

JAMES A. BARROWMAN, B.Sc., Ph.D., M.B., Ch.B., F.R.C.P.(Lond), F.R.C.P.(C), F.A.C.P.

Professor of Medicine (Gastroenterology), Memorial University of Newfoundland Faculty of Medicine, St. John's, Newfoundland, Canada

Gastrointestinal Tract Disorders

VANESSA A. BARSS, M.D.

Assistant Professor of Obstetrics and Gynecology, Harvard Medical School; Staff, Brigham and Women's Hospital, Boston, Massachusetts

Erythroblastosis Fetalis

ALAN S. BERKELEY, M.D.

Associate Professor of Obstetrics and Gynecology, Cornell University Medical College; Associate Attending Obstetrician and Gynecologist, New York Hospital, New York, New York

Prophylactic Antibiotics in Obstetrics

RICHARD L. BERNSTINE, M.D.

Professor of Obstetrics and Gynecology, Northeastern Ohio Universities College of Medicine; Director of Obstetrics and Gynecology and Education for Obstetrics and Gynecology, St. Elizabeth Hospital Medical Center, Youngstown, Ohio

Missed Abortion

MAX BORTEN, M.D., J.D.

Associate Professor of Obstetrics and Gynecology, Harvard Medical School; Director, Division of Medical Gynecology, Beth Israel Hospital and Member, Massachusetts Bar, Boston, Massachusetts

Current Medicolegal Issues

PETER C. BOYLAN, M.B., M.R.C.O.G.

Lecturer, Department of Obstetrics and Gynaecology, University College Dublin; Consultant Obstetrician Gynaecologist, National Maternity Hospital, Dublin, Ireland

Obstetric Management of the Growth-Retarded Baby

ROBERT C. CEFALO, M.D., Ph.D.

Professor, Department of Obstetrics and Gynecology, University of North Carolina School of Medicine, Chapel Hill, North Carolina

Planned Prenatal Care: Key to the Future

WELDON CHAFE, M.D., F.R.C.S.(C), F.A.C.O.G.

Assistant Professor, Division Gynecologic Oncology, Department of Obstetrics and Gynecology, University of Florida College of Medicine, Gainesville, Florida

Choriocarcinoma—Gestational Trophoblastic Neoplasia

DAVID CHARLES, M.D., F.A.C.O.G., F.R.C.O.G.

Formerly, Professor and Chairman, Department of Obstetrics and Gynecology, Marshall University School of Medicine; Chief of Obstetrics and Gynecology Service, St. Mary's Hospital, Huntington, West Virginia

Cervical Incompetence
Syphilis in Pregnancy
Yeast Vaginitis
Ectopic Pregnancy
Spontaneous Abortion
Abruptio Placentae

NeeOo W. CHIN, M.D.

Clinical Instructor and Senior Fellow, Division of Reproductive Endocrinology, Ohio State University Hospitals, Columbus, Ohio

Thyroid Disorders in Pregnancy

WAYNE R. COHEN, M.D.

Associate Professor of Obstetrics and Gynecology, Albert Einstein College of Medicine of Yeshiva University; Director of Obstetrics and Gynecology, Bronx Municipal Hospital Center, Bronx, New York

Fetal Heart Rate Monitoring

SUSAN M. COX, M.D.

Jack A. and Signe Pritchard Fellow in Maternal-Fetal Medicine, Department of Obstetrics and Gynecology, University of Texas Southwestern Medical Center, Dallas, Texas

Urinary Tract Infections

ROBERT K. CREASY, M.D.

Emma Sue Hightower Professor of Obstetrics and Gynecology and Chairman, Department of Obstetrics, Gynecology, and Reproductive Sciences, University of Texas Medical School; Attending Physician, Chief of Obstetrics and Gynecology, Hermann Hospital, Houston, Texas

Obstetric Management of the Growth-Retarded Baby

WARREN M. CROSBY, M.D.

Professor of Obstetrics and Gynecology, University of Oklahoma College of Medicine, Oklahoma City, Oklahoma

Nutrition in Pregnancy

DWIGHT P. CRUIKSHANK, M.D., F.A.C.O.G.

Professor of Obstetrics and Gynecology, University of Utah School of Medicine; Vice Chairman, Department of Obstetrics and Gynecology, University of Utah Health Sciences Center, Salt Lake City, Utah

Pregnancy-Induced Hypertension

F. GARY CUNNINGHAM, M.D.

Professor and Chairman, Department of Obstetrics and Gynecology, University of Texas Southwestern Medical Center, Dallas, Texas

Urinary Tract Infections

LAWRENCE D. DEVOE, M.D.

Associate Professor, Department of Obstetrics and Gynecology and Director, Maternal-Fetal Medicine Section, Medical College of Georgia School of Medicine, Augusta, Georgia

Antepartum Fetal Testing

RICHARD C. DICKSON, M.D.

Instructor, Division of Maternal-Fetal Medicine, Medical University of South Carolina College of Medicine, Charleston, South Carolina

Breech Presentation

JOAN V. EGGERT, R.D., M.P.H., M.D.

Faculty Lecturer, Perinatal Nutrition; Clinical Instructor, Department of Obstetrics and Gynecology, University of Nebraska Medical Center, Omaha, Nebraska

Parenteral and Enteral Nutrition in Pregnancy

DAVID A. ESCHENBACH, M.D.

Professor, Department of Obstetrics and Gynecology, University of Washington School of Medicine; Chief, Division of Gynecology, University Hospital and Harborview Medical Center, Seattle, Washington

Bacterial Vaginosis in Pregnancy

BISHARA J. FREIJ, M.D.

Assistant Professor of Pediatrics, Division of Infectious Diseases, Georgetown University School of Medicine; Attending Physician, Georgetown University Children's Medical Center, Washington, D.C.

Gestational Herpesvirus Infections

EMANUEL A. FRIEDMAN, M.D., Sc.D.

Professor, Obstetrics and Gynecology, Harvard Medical School and Health Sciences and Technology, Massachusetts Institute of Technology; Obstetrician-Gynecologist-in-Chief, Beth Israel Hospital, Boston, Massachusetts

Dysfunctional Labor

FREDRIC D. FRIGOLETTO Jr., M.D.

William Lambert Richardson Professor of Obstetrics, Harvard Medical School; Chief, Maternal-Fetal Medicine and Director of Obstetrics, Brigham and Women's Hospital, Boston, Massachusetts

Erythroblastosis Fetalis

STEVEN G. GABBE, M.D.

Professor and Chairman, Department of Obstetrics and Gynecology, Ohio State University College of Medicine, Columbus, Ohio

Diabetes in Pregnancy

RONALD S. GIBBS, M.D.

Jane and Roland Blumberg Professor, Department of Obstetrics and Gynecology, University of Texas Medical School, San Antonio, Texas

Postpartum Infection

DOUGLAS D. GLOVER, B.S. Pharm., M.D.

Professor of Obstetrics and Gynecology, West Virginia University School of Medicine and Associate Professor of Clinical Pharmacy, West Virginia University School of Pharmacy; Staff, West Virginia University Hosptial, Morgantown, West Virginia

Ectopic Pregnancy
Spontaneous Abortion
Abruptio Placentae
Lactation
Mastitis
Drug Excretion in Human Milk

HAMID A. HADI, M.D.

Associate Professor of Obstetrics and Gynecology and Director, Division of Maternal-Fetal Medicine, East Carolina University School of Medicine, Greenville, North Carolina

Renal Transplantation in Pregnancy

WILLIAM N. P. HERBERT, M.D.

Associate Professor, University of North Carolina School of Medicine; Attending Physician, North Carolina Memorial Hospital, Chapel Hill, North Carolina

Amniotic Fluid Tests of Fetal Maturity

WILLIAM M. HOLLS III, M.D.

Assistant Professor of Obstetrics and Gynecology, University of Tennessee College of Medicine; Associate Medical Director, Regional Perinatal Center, University of Tennessee Memorial Hospital, Knoxville, Tennessee

Intrauterine Fetal Demise

EDGAR O. HORGER III, M.D.

Professor of Obstetrics and Gynecology and Radiology and Director of Maternal-Fetal Medicine, Medical University of South Carolina College of Medicine, Charleston, South Carolina

Cesarean Section

JAY D. IAMS, M.D.

Associate Professor, Department of Obstetrics and Gynecology, Division of Maternal-Fetal Medicine, Ohio State University College of Medicine, Columbus, Ohio

Premature Rupture of the Membranes

LESLIE IFFY, M.D., F.R.C.S.(C)

Professor of Obstetrics and Gynecology, University of Medicine and Dentistry, New Jersey Medical School; Director, Division of Maternal-Fetal Medicine, University Hospital, Newark, New Jersey

Placenta Previa

DAVID Z. KITAY, M.D.

Staff Physician and Obstetrician Gynecologist, Halifax Hospital Medical Center, Daytona Beach, Florida

Anemia in Pregnancy
Hemoglobinopathies

MOON H. KIM, M.D.

Professor of Reproductive Endocrinology, Ohio State University College of Medicine; Director, Division of Reproductive Endocrinology, The University Hospitals, Columbus, Ohio

Thyroid Disorders in Pregnancy

JEFFREY C. KING, M.D.

Assistant Professor, Department of Obstetrics and Gynecology, Division of Maternal-Fetal Medicine, Georgetown University School of Medicine, Washington, D.C.

Oligohydramnios

MARK B. LANDON, M.D.

Assistant Professor of Obstetrics and Gynecology, Division of Maternal-Fetal Medicine, Ohio State University College of Medicine, Columbus, Ohio

Diabetes in Pregnancy

ALVIN LANGER, M.D.

Professor of Obstetrics and Gynecology, Northeastern Ohio Universities College of Medicine, Rootstown; Academic Director of Obstetrics and Gynecology, Aultman Hospital, Canton, Ohio

Intrauterine Fetal Demise

BRYAN LARSEN, Ph.D.

Associate Professor of Microbiology and Obstetrics and Gynecology, Marshall University School of Medicine, Huntington, West Virginia

Syphilis in Pregnancy
Yeast Vaginitis

J. PATRICK LAVERY, M.D.

Clinical Professor, Department of Obstetrics and Gynecology, Michigan State University College of Human Medicine, East Lansing; Perinatologist, Bronson Methodist Hospital, Kalamazoo, Michigan

Premature Labor

DESMOND J. LEDDIN, M.B., M.R.C.P.(I), F.R.C.P.(C)

Assistant Professor of Medicine (Gastroenterology), Memorial University of Newfoundland Faculty of Medicine, St. John's, Newfoundland, Canada

Gastrointestinal Tract Disorders

RICK W. MARTIN, M.D.

Assistant Professor, Division of Maternal-Fetal Medicine, Department of Obstetrics and Gynecology, University of Mississippi School of Medicine, Jackson, Mississippi

Liver Disease

PHILIP B. MEAD, M.D.

Clinical Professor of Obstetrics and Gynecology, University of Vermont College of Medicine; Hospital Epidemiologist, Medical Center Hospital of Vermont, Burlington, Vermont

Group B Streptococcal Sepsis

RICHARD K. MILLER, Ph.D.

Associate Professor of Obstetrics and Gynecology and Pharmacology and Toxicology, University of Rochester School of Medicine and Dentistry, Rochester, New York
Infectious Disease Therapy in Pregnancy

HOWARD L. MINKOFF, M.D.

Associate Professor of Obstetrics and Gynecology and Director of Maternal-Fetal Medicine, State University of New York College of Medicine, Health Sciences Center, Brooklyn, New York
Acquired Immunodeficiency Syndrome

LINDA S. MORGAN, M.D., F.A.C.O.G.

Associate Professor and Director of Gynecologic Oncology, Department of Obstetrics and Gynecology, University of Florida College of Medicine, Gainesville, Florida
Choriocarcinoma—Gestational Trophoblastic Neoplasia

JOHN C. MORRISON, M.D.

Director, Division of Maternal-Fetal Medicine, Department of Obstetrics and Gynecology, University of Mississippi School of Medicine, Jackson, Mississippi
Liver Disease

MAURICE A. MUFSON, M.D., F.A.C.P.

Professor and Chairman, Department of Medicine, Marshall University School of Medicine and Associate Chief of Staff of Research, Veterans Administration Medical Center; Attending Physician, Cabell Huntington Hospital and St. Mary's Hospital, Huntington, West Virginia
Respiratory Diseases

NANCY J. MUNN, M.D.

Associate Professor of Medicine, Marshall University School of Medicine and Chief of Pulmonary Section, Veterans Administration Medical Center; Attending Physician, Cabell Huntington Hospital and St. Mary's Hospital, Huntington, West Virginia
Respiratory Diseases

JAMES A. O'LEARY, M.D.

Professor of Obstetrics and Gynecology, University of Medicine and Dentistry, New Jersey Medical School, Newark; Chairman, Department of Obstetrics and Gynecology, Jersey City Medical Center, Jersey City, New Jersey
Postpartum Hemorrhage

MARY D. PEOPLES-SHEPS, R.N., Dr. P.H.

Assistant Professor of Maternal and Child Health, School of Public Health, University of North Carolina, Chapel Hill, North Carolina
Planned Prenatal Care: Key to the Future

ROY H. PETRIE, M.D., Sc.D.

Professor of Obstetrics and Gynecology, Washington University School of Medicine; Director, Division of Maternal-Fetal Medicine, Washington University Medical Center and Obstetrical Service, Barnes Hospital, Saint Louis, Missouri
Tocolytic Agents

W. SOYINI POWELL, M.D.

Director, Division of Gynecology, Hahnemann University Hospital, Philadelphia, Pennsylvania
Trichomoniasis During Pregnancy

WILLIAM E. M. PRYSE-PHILLIPS, M.D. F.R.C.P.(C), F.R.C.P.

Professor of Medicine (Neurology), Memorial University of Newfoundland Faculty of Medicine; Chief of Neurology, General Hospital, Health Sciences Centre, St. John's, Newfoundland, Canada
Neurologic Disorders

JAMES G. PULLANO, M.D., M.B.A.

Instructor and Fellow, Division of Maternal-Fetal Medicine, University of Medicine and Dentistry, New Jersey Medical School, Newark, New Jersey
Placenta Previa

WILLIAM F. RAYBURN, M.D.

Associate Professor, Department of Obstetrics and Gynecology and Pharmacology, University of Nebraska College of Medicine; Director, Division of Maternal-Fetal Medicine, Department of Obstetrics and Gynecology, University of Nebraska Medical Center, Omaha, Nebraska
Parenteral and Enteral Nutrition in Pregnancy

KENNETH J. REAMY, M.D., M.P.H.

Associate Professor, Department of Obstetrics and Gynecology and Behavioral Medicine and Psychiatry, West Virginia University School of Medicine, Morgantown, West Virginia
Sexuality in Pregnancy and the Puerperium

ROBERTO ROMERO, M.D.

Associate Professor of Obstetrics and Gynecology and Director, Perinatal Research, Yale University School of Medicine, New Haven, Connecticut
Coagulopathies in Obstetrics

LUIS SANCHEZ-RAMOS, M.D.

Assistant Professor, Department of Obstetrics and Gynecology, University of Florida College of Medicine, Gainesville; Director, Maternal-Fetal Medicine, University Hospital, Jacksonville, Florida
Prostaglandins

JOHN W. SEEDS, M.D.

Associate Professor, Department of Obstetrics and Gynecology, University of North Carolina School of Medicine, Chapel Hill, North Carolina

Fetal Therapy

JOHN L. SEVER, M.D., Ph.D.

Chief, Infectious Diseases Branch, National Institute of Neurological and Communicative Disorders and Stroke, National Institutes of Health, Bethesda, Maryland

Gestational Herpesvirus Infections

YOGESH G. SHAH, M.D.

Clinical Associate Professor of Obstetrics and Gynecology, University of Rochester School of Medicine and Dentistry, Rochester, New York

Infectious Disease Therapy in Pregnancy

WILLIAM N. SPELLACY, M.D.

Professor and Head, Department of Obstetrics and Gynecology, University of Illinois College of Medicine, Chicago, Illinois

Postdate Pregnancy

MICHAEL R. SPENCE, M.D., M.P.H

Professor and Chairman, Department of Obstetrics and Gynecology, Hahnemann University School of Medicine, Philadelphia, Pennsylvania

Trichomoniasis During Pregnancy

RICHARD L. SWEET, M.D.

Professor of Obstetrics, Gynecology, and Reproductive Sciences, University of California School of Medicine; Chief of Obstetrics and Gynecology, San Francisco General Hospital Medical Center, San Francisco, California

Chlamydia Trachomatis Infection

KENT UELAND, M.D.

Professor and Chairman, Department of Gynecology and Obstetrics, Stanford University School of Medicine; Chief of Obstetrics and Gynecology, Stanford University Medical Center, Stanford, California

Heart Disease

J. PETER VAN DORSTEN, M.D.

Associate Professor of Obstetrics and Gynecology and Director of Maternal-Fetal Medicine, Virginia Commonwealth University Medical College, Richmond, Virginia

Breech Presentation

HUNG N. WINN, M.D.

Assistant Professor of Obstetrics and Gynecology, Washington University School of Medicine; Attending Physician, Barnes Hospital, Saint Louis, Missouri

Coagulopathies in Obstetrics

STEVEN S. WITKIN, Ph.D.

Associate Professor of Immunology and Director, Immunology Division, Department of Obstetrics and Gynecology, Cornell University Medical College, New York, New York

Immunology of Pregnancy and Spontaneous Abortion

FRANK R. WITTER, M.D.

Assistant Professor, The Johns Hopkins University School of Medicine; Active Staff, The Johns Hopkins Hospital, Baltimore, Maryland

Drug Abuse

ROBERT A. WOLK, Pharm.D.

Clinical Assistant Professor, University of Michigan College of Pharmacy; Clinical Pharmacist, University of Michigan Medical Center, Ann Arbor, Michigan

Parenteral and Enteral Nutrition in Pregnancy

FREDERICK P. ZUSPAN, M.D.

Professor, The Richard Meiling Chair, Obstetrics and Gynecology, Ohio State University College of Medicine; Faculty, Ohio State University Hospitals, Columbus, Ohio

Chronic Hypertension in Pregnancy

CONTENTS

OBSTETRIC HEMORRHAGES

LABOR AND DELIVERY

THE FETUS

THE BREAST

MALIGNANT DISEASE

PREFACE

Modern medicine is like a tree whose branches, which divide so majestically, require the invisible roots that represent the strength of the sciences from which therapy grows. So important are the basic concepts that I would say with Democritis, ''Rather would I explain the cause of a single fact than become King of the Persians.''

With the rapid growth of new knowledge fostered by important discoveries, together with the increasing recognition that nature is of one piece, I have the pleasure of being able to explain the cause of many facts that have led to an ever-improving basis for therapy in obstetrics.

During the past several years, there has been an extensive reappraisal of the physiologic changes with pregnancy and its associated disorders, and there has been a concomitant refinement of diagnostic procedures accompanied by a sounder evaluation of therapeutic approaches, which remain of primary concern to the physician.

Clinical management is the central theme of this book, which is destined primarily for those who practice obstetrics, but it will also serve as a useful reference tool for anyone whose practice includes the gravid patient. Chapters have been written expressly for this book by a distinguished cadre, carefully selected for their clinical and investigational interest in the assigned topics, as well as their status as authorities in the field. Their views on current management have been succinctly portrayed, and the presentations are devoid of extraneous material. Thus, the book represents an authoritative distillation of current thought that is well ordered and representative of accepted obstetric practice.

A book of this type would be impossible without the wholehearted support of the contributors. The Editor wishes to thank the staff of B.C. Decker, specifically Mary Mansor for her unstinted assistance and guidance. Finally, as with any such enterprise that has many contributors, one cannot embark along the course of such a volume without a secretary who is not only capable, but has the patience of Job, and I wish therefore to express my sincere and heartfelt appreciation to Nancy Urban.

David Charles, M.D.

PRENATAL CARE

PLANNED PRENATAL CARE: KEY TO THE FUTURE

MARY D. PEOPLES-SHEPS, R.N., Dr.P.H.
ROBERT C. CEFALO, M.D., Ph.D.

Prenatal care addresses many of the medical and obstetric problems that occur during the prenatal period and that are discussed in other chapters of this book. It is the medium through which the screening, diagnosis, and therapies discussed in these chapters usually take place. In addition, prenatal care, from its earliest inception, was intended to prevent the onset of morbidity during pregnancy by identifying those at risk and reducing their risks and by promoting healthy behaviors among all pregnant women.

Specifically, prenatal care consists of a series of activities that are designed to:

1. Detect physical and psychosocial risk factors and early signs of asymptomatic diseases that may adversely affect mother and fetus.
2. Diagnose and treat maternal and fetal abnormalities as soon as they appear.
3. Provide guidance and education regarding behaviors and signs that may influence maternal and fetal well-being as well as for delivery arrangements and postpartum, family planning, and infant care arrangements.

Over time, as screening and diagnostic tests and problem-specific therapies developed, certain aspects of prenatal care, such as history-taking, selected laboratory tests, and specific schedules of visits, became "routine." In theory, routinization of these components of prenatal care allowed all women to benefit from important advances in the field relatively quickly. In practice, it also promoted a system of care in which higher priority could be assigned to objective standards of care rather than to individual patient needs.

Although adherence to standards of prenatal care has never been monitored regularly, there is evidence that some providers have deviated from what might be considered routine for many years. These deviations are due, at least in part, to variations in accepted standards across obstetric textbooks and professional societies and to the responsiveness of providers to individual patient needs.

In the latter half of the 1980s, there is a general recognition that routine prenatal care no longer exists. Still remaining are standards for certain activities, some of which are controversial. Other routines, such as the number and frequency of prenatal visits and the content of those visits, are in flux. Prenatal care is becoming a process that is planned with each individual woman based on her specific needs as derived from her history, laboratory findings, physical examination, and the progress of the current pregnancy. Prenatal care, of necessity, is mercurial and dynamic.

CONTROVERSIAL ISSUES

History—The Cornerstone of Prenatal Care

Background. A careful, systematic history is critical to identify whether there were problems in previous pregnancies that might repeat themselves in the present pregnancy and to detect known medical problems or conditions and behavioral or social circumstances that might compromise the current pregnancy. It constitutes part of the baseline information that should be available for every prenatal patient. The history, therefore, should be targeted, but at the same time it should be broad enough to detect a range of clues to potential problems. A prenatal history should include the following:

1. Medical history: diseases, conditions, and surgeries throughout the life of the individual.
2. Obstetric history: details on the course and outcome of each previous pregnancy.
3. Gynecologic history: experience with and treatment of gynecologic problems, including sexually transmitted diseases and contraceptive utilization.
4. Immunization status for communicable diseases.
5. Family medical and genetic history.
6. Nutritional problems and treatments.
7. Selected behaviors, including ingestion of cigarettes, alcohol, and drugs, and work outside the home.
8. Social history: marital status, family problems, financial status.

To complete a history, all prior medical records should be obtained and reviewed. The history should be taken as early in pregnancy as possible, preferably at the first prenatal visit, before 12-weeks gestation.

Each positive finding in a history suggests one or more activities that should be undertaken. The management of many specific medical and obstetric problems is given in other chapters of this volume. In addition to those, appropriate courses of action for behavioral, social, and nutritional problems also require attention. They are addressed below in the section on referral networks.

Controversy. What is controversial about history-taking is not whether it should be done but how it should be recorded so that the information can be put to greatest use. In the past 15 years, a number of forms for recording historical data as well as other information about the pregnancy have been developed. Some of the forms require calculation of weighted scores that determine the risk classification of the pregnancy (e.g., high, medium, low). Others do not yield scores, but relevant problems can be recorded and reviewed in a simple but systematic fashion.

The extent to which either type of instrument is used by providers of prenatal care is unknown. Moreover, the relative value of one type of form over another in improving the management of selected pregnancies has not been examined. The greatest amount of controversy is with regard to the instruments that yield weighted scores. There are several reasons for this:

1. The instruments have not been validated or modified for differences in age, race, social class, or geographic area.
2. Cut-points for high risk differ not only by population group but also by outcome.
3. The instruments are susceptible to mechanistic application, to becoming ends in themselves rather than tools for intervention, and to producing anxiety in the women labeled high-risk (whether the label is correct or not).

In addition to controversies surrounding the type of form that is most appropriate for recording a history, there is some debate about what items should be included in a history-taking instrument. Most of the forms available today request very little information on nonclinical factors, such as social, behavioral, and environmental risks. Yet, some of these factors (e.g., smoking) constitute major preventable causes of perinatal morbidity.

Recommendations. Although controversies exist, it is reasonable to conclude that: (1) a careful, systematic history should be taken on each pregnant woman, and the information should be recorded in a systematic manner. (2) A check-off history can be a helpful tool if it is used as a reminder to increase communication between humans, not as a short cut to abbreviated care. (3) One specific tool for recording historical and other relevant information during pregnancy cannot be recommended over another. All have positive and negative attributes. (4) Careful attention should be given to the nonclinical characteristics that may not be well represented in available instruments but are important determinants of pregnancy outcome, some of which (e.g., work place environment, consumption of alcohol and drugs) may require sensitive probing during the process of history-taking.

Screening Tests

Prenatal care includes a set of laboratory tests that are used to screen for selected conditions that can compromise the mother or infant or both. Recommendations for these tests have evolved over time as the capabilities to identify disorders and the technology to do screening tests have developed. For the most part, tests were absorbed into routine prenatal care before the clinical trials required to establish efficacy were conducted. As a result, there is some remaining controversy associated with several of them.

Hemoglobin/Hematocrit

Background. A blood test for hemoglobin or hematocrit levels is done at the first prenatal visit, early in the third trimester, and at other times, as needed. It is considered important to assess hemoglobin levels at the first visit in order to detect anemia early in pregnancy so that the cause may be ascertained and the condition treated. Monitoring hemoglobin levels over time allows an assessment of the amount of change in levels and provides for additional treatment, if necessary, before the blood loss associated with delivery and the postpartum period occurs.

Controversy. Since pregnancy is characterized by a dilutional anemia that is most evident at 28 to 32 weeks and is apparently normal, there is controversy about the "ideal" prenatal hemoglobin and hematocrit values. Nevertheless, values that are likely to be abnormal (e.g., <11 g per deciliter in the second and third trimesters) can be identified so that further investigation can be initiated.

Recommendations. (1) A blood sample for hemoglobin and hematocrit readings should be drawn at the first prenatal visit. The need for additional laboratory evaluation should be determined by historical factors or unusual clinical findings. Ethnic or social circumstances may dictate the need for special testing, such as sickle-cell test or hemoglobin electrophoresis or both. (2) A hemoglobin of less than 10 g per deciliter in the early part of pregnancy deserves further evaluation. (3) Early in the third trimester, repeat hemoglobin and hematocrit evaluations should be done as dilutional anemia is anticipated. If the hematocrit increases, one may become suspicious of contracted blood volume and look for evidence of intrauterine growth retardation or preeclampsia.

Cervical Cytology

Background. A cervical smear to detect invasive cancer of the cervix as well as the premalignant forms—cancer in situ and cervical dysplasia—is recommended once during pregnancy, at the first prenatal visit. The smear is recommended during pregnancy because (1) this period is the only time many women are in contact with a health care provider, (2) it can be done easily during a vaginal examination, and (3) it promotes coverage of a particularly high-risk group of women, multiparas of low socioeconomic status.

Controversy. Since all women are screened, the screening process covers a number of women who are at low risk. Studies in Great Britain have shown that the probability of developing cervical cancer—in the short term (10 years)—among women less than 25 years old is very low. In addition, women who are tested during pregnancy are more likely to have a higher rate (about six times as great) of false-positive tests than those in the general population. Such a high false-positive rate for young women during pregnancy limits the acceptability of universal screening because of the stress likely to be engendered by a false-positive finding. Also, although a few young women die each year as a result of cervical cancer, the death rate is very low when compared with that of older women. An alternative approach to screening for cervical cancer would involve using age as the primary screening test, that is, routine smears would only be done on women age 25 and older. This approach has not received widespread support, however, because the Papanicolaou smear can also yield evidence of sexually transmitted diseases, such as condylomata or herpes.

Recommendation. Because the Papanicolaou smear can detect conditions other than cancer and its premalignant manifestations, it is recommended for all women at least once during pregnancy.

Dipstick Urinalysis

Background. A simple and safe method for testing the urine for selected components is the dipstick urinalysis at each visit. The test is usually done for two reasons: (1) to detect proteinuria, which is a sign of preeclampsia and may indicate acute or chronic renal disease, and (2) to detect glycosuria, which may be a sign of gestational diabetes. Random urine testing for proteinuria is considered cost-effective, but the value of testing for glycosuria is controversial.

Controversy. Reliable estimates of the sensitivity and specificity of this test for predicting gestational diabetes have not been determined, although the random timing of the test would suggest that it would not be highly predictive. Moreover, glycosuria during pregnancy is common and frequently physiologic.

On the other hand, persistent glycosuria is associated with maternal diabetes and should signal the need for further investigation.

Recommendations. (1) A dipstick test of the urine to detect proteinuria is recommended at each prenatal visit. (2) To detect persistent glycosuria, which should signal the need for further investigation of maternal diabetes, a dipstick reading at each visit is also recommended.

Blood Tests for Glucose

Background. Currently, carbohydrate intolerance screening is not part of prenatal care unless risk factors for diabetes mellitus are present. However, detection of gestational diabetes is essential because the condition has been associated with maternal and fetal complications. When risk factors, such as family history of diabetes, previous macrosomic infant, poor obstetric history, or persistent glycosuria, are used as indicators for further screening for gestational diabetes, 30 to 40 percent of affected patients are not detected. A more sensitive screening procedure involves administration of 50 g of glucose orally, followed in 1 hour by a plasma glucose test. A definitive diagnosis of gestational diabetes should be based on a 100-g, 3-hour oral glucose tolerance procedure.

Controversy. At present, there is no clear evidence of the cost-effectiveness of universal 1-hour screening of plasma for glucose tolerance. As a result, recommendations vary. The American Diabetes Association and the Centers for Disease Control have endorsed universal screening of all pregnant women. The American College of Obstetricians and Gynecologists recommends screening of women who are 30 years of age or older. The recommendation further states that if any risk factors are present, screening should be performed regardless of age.

Recommendations. (1) All pregnant women should be screened for glucose intolerance between 24 to 28 weeks using a 50-g oral glucose load, followed by a 1-hour plasma glucose test. (2) If risk factors are present, a glucose screen should be performed early in pregnancy. If that screening test is negative, it should be repeated at 24 or 28 weeks.

Urine Culture

Background. Routine screening for asymptomatic bacteriuria is not recommended at present in the United States, although interest is growing. Women with bacteriuria of pregnancy are significantly more likely to develop pyelonephritis, which in turn is closely associated with perinatal mortality and low infant birth weight. The relationships among these factors are not clearly understood, but treatment of bacteriuria significantly lowers the risk of pyelonephritis from 28 to 3 percent and, through that route, may affect the incidence of low birth weight in a positive direction.

Controversy. The incidence of asymptomatic bacteriuria is about 2 to 10 percent; hence, a massive screening effort would involve testing a large number of unaffected people. Screening can be done relatively inexpensively, however, with a nitrite dipstick, or more expensively, by urine culture. It is estimated that routine screening could prevent 115 cases of pyelonephritis per 10,000 pregnancies.

Recommendations. (1) The urine of all pregnant women should be tested each trimester with a nitrite dipstick. (2) A urine culture and sensitivity test should be done on all pregnant women with (a) histories of urinary tract infection, preterm labor, diabetes mellitus, and sickle-cell trait or disease, or (b) a positive dipstick screen.

Maternal Serum Alpha-Fetoprotein

Background. Open neural tube defects affect 1 to 2 per 1,000 births in the United States each year. The maternal serum alpha-fetoprotein (MSAFP) screening test can detect about 80 percent of infants with open spina bifida and virtually all cases of anencephaly. Although the test has a relatively high false-positive rate because of the difficulty of firmly establishing gestational age from date of last menstrual period, subsequent diagnostic procedures (e.g., ultrasonography and amniocentesis) are widely available.

Controversy. If the diagnosis is positive, the woman or couple is faced with a choice: to terminate the pregnancy or to continue with adequate preparation for the birth of a high-risk infant. The former choice is unacceptable on moral or religious grounds for some people. Regardless of the acceptability of the choice, a well-organized network of counselors and other professionals must be in place to help deal with the emotional implications of a firm positive diagnosis as well as the anxiety associated with a positive screening test. Such networks are not available everywhere. In view of these constraints, routine screening of all pregnancies in the United States is not possible at present. However, the Department of Professional Liability of the American College of Obstetricians and Gynecologists has advised that the test and a full discussion of it should be offered to all pregnant women.

Recommendations. (1) MSAFP screening should be offered to all pregnant women. (2) All providers of prenatal care should establish and maintain linkages with comprehensive regional programs for MSAFP screening, which include expertise in ultrasonography, genetic counseling, and amniocentesis.

Ultrasound Screening

Background. The value of prenatal ultrasonography in diagnosing intrauterine growth deficits and fetal malformations is unquestionable, and the capabilities of the procedure continue to expand.

Controversy. Controversies still exist as to whether ultrasound screening of all obstetric patients is efficacious. To date, there is no conclusive evidence that routine ultrasonography improves perinatal outcome. However, future studies may indicate that with routine ultrasound screening, higher rates of detection of twins and anomalies and lower rates of post-term (by dates) inductions may be demonstrated.

Recommendations. (1) In pregnancies complicated by ill-defined last menstrual period, previous cesarean delivery, or past medical or obstetric problems, a routine scan at 18 to 20 weeks and a repeat examination 6 to 8 weeks later for dating and to rule out anomalies are indicated. (2) Additional examination should be performed as medically indicated.

Prevention of Prematurity

Background. Approximately 7 percent of infants born in the United States are of low birth weight (<2,500 g). The majority of low birth weight infants are products of preterm deliveries or premature rupture of membranes. Low birth weight is a major cause of perinatal morbidity and mortality. Over the years, many strategies have focused on improving neonatal care of the infants as well as on management of pregnancies in which preterm delivery is likely. Recently, emphasis has been placed on early recognition and prevention of signs and symptoms of preterm labor. The current approach involves several components:

1. A careful history, accompanied by a risk scoring system.
2. Intensive education of women at risk regarding the signs and symptoms of preterm labor.
3. Vaginal and cervical examinations at 24 weeks.
4. Treatment of infections detected during the examination.
5. Prompt intervention if preterm labor commences.

Controversies. Several risk scoring systems have been developed to identify women at risk for low birth weight deliveries. However, these systems have not yet been sufficiently validated to warrant inclusion as an essential component of prenatal care. The other elements of preterm birth prevention programs are currently being studied through randomized trials in several sites. As a result, empirically derived recommendations about them cannot be made at this time. Nevertheless, the main elements of preterm birth prevention, as given above, are reasonable on theoretical grounds, are unlikely to cause untoward side effects, and have been supported by some research.

Recommendations. (1) All patients should be educated regarding the signs and symptoms of preterm labor.

(2) All patients should have a vaginal and a cervical examination at 24 weeks. (3) Consideration should be given to aggressive treatment of vaginitis or cervicitis or both.

Referral Networks for Nonclinical Services

Background. There are several patient needs that can be identified during the first prenatal visit and should be addressed promptly and actively.

Smoking. Smoking is a major determinant of intrauterine growth retardation, clearly associated with lower mean birth weights from 150 to 300 g in range. The extent of the birth weight deficit is directly related to the number of cigarettes smoked. But the smoking habits of pregnant women can be modified, and improved smoking behavior has been associated with improved pregnancy outcomes, especially regarding birth weight. The earlier women quit or reduce cigarette consumption, the more their babies are likely to weigh.

Seventy-five to 80 percent of women who smoke at the onset of pregnancy (about 30 percent of pregnant women) will continue to smoke throughout. Advice to quit or modify smoking habits, in the absence of active assistance, has not been effective. However, at least three models of successful interventions are now available. The first involves home correspondence, supplemented by telephone reinforcement. The second type is a culturally appropriate self-help guide, and the third strategy involves personal home visits with telephone and mail contacts. Either of the first two approaches could be integrated into most prenatal services without major commitments of time or staff. The third approach, although highly effective in demonstration projects, is labor-intensive and likely to be more expensive. For some women, however, particularly those who lack social supports, a more personal approach may be the only effective method.

Chemical Dependency. Heavy drinking during pregnancy is the only known cause of fetal alcohol syndrome. Women who quit or reduce consumption early in pregnancy may be less likely to have infants who suffer from fetal alcohol syndrome. Some other prescription and recreational drugs have been associated with adverse effects on the mother or fetus or both. Even in cases in which a particular drug is not known to have adverse physiologic effects, maternal dependency on any chemical substance can endanger the well-being of the mother and infant in a number of social and psychological ways. Treatment of chemical dependency requires intensive intervention through organized programs established specifically for that purpose.

Nutritional Risks. Associations between maternal nutrition and pregnancy outcome have been recognized for many years. Chronic malnutrition has been associated with birth weight deficits, and wartime famine studies have shown that starvation of the mother in the third trimester can result in birth weight reductions of 300 to 400 g. The Collaborative Perinatal Project found that as maternal weight gain increased, birth weight increased and the incidences of low birth weight and neonatal mortality decreased. Despite these findings, the mechanisms through which nutrition affects pregnancy outcome are not clear. This is due, in part, to interrelationships among nutritional status, socioeconomic status, and smoking. Of particular note are findings from the 1980 National Natality Survey, which showed that women who were less likely to gain 16 or more pounds during pregnancy were those already at risk for poor outcomes by virtue of age (age 17 or younger and age 35 and older), marital status (unmarried), and educational attainment (low).

Two major approaches are used to improve nutrition in the prenatal period: (1) nutrition advice and counseling and (2) nutrition supplementation. Evidence regarding the effectiveness of nutrition advice is hard to find. The meager evidence that is available suggests that prenatal nutrition counseling is capable of improving nutrition knowledge and dietary behavior. Whether those changes are associated with improved outcomes of pregnancy is not known.

The major source of nutrition supplementation in the United States is the Special Supplemental Food Program for Women, Infants, and Children (WIC). The program provides nutrition education and vouchers for selected nutritious foods. Although details of service delivery vary across sites, WIC programs are generally linked to public prenatal care. The evaluations of those programs suggest that (1) participation in WIC is associated with improved mean birth weight, low birth weight rates, and maternal nutrition; (2) WIC may also improve the length of gestation and subsequent cognitive development of the fetus; (3) WIC appears to have a greater impact on women at increased demographic risk; and (4) longer participation in WIC is associated with improved outcomes of pregnancy.

Stress. Speculation about a relationship between maternal stress and pregnancy outcome has existed since biblical times and has appeared in medical literature for at least 200 years. Current evidence suggests that stressful circumstances (e.g., major life events or day-to-day problems) are associated with adverse outcomes of pregnancy. However, if a woman has a great deal of social and psychological support (e.g., family, friends), she is less likely to experience these effects of stress. The series of physiologic events that may link maternal psychological stress to pregnancy complications and outcomes is not fully understood. Evidence suggests that stress produces an increase in catecholamine release, increased sympathetic nervous system activity, and changes in circulating levels of adrenocortical and other hormones. These changes can affect the fetus in a variety of ways, possibly by inducing fetal hypoxia, which, in turn, may stimulate the onset of preterm labor.

There are two basic approaches to controlling stress during pregnancy: (1) reduce the amount of stress to which an individual is exposed and (2) buffer the effects of stress by providing or maximizing social support. Public social service agencies and the various types of public and private counseling services use both of these approaches. Work leave programs and home visiting services by public health nurses and other visitors have also been used to control stress.

Childbirth Education. Childbirth education (CBE) is a process that involves imparting information about the anatomy, physiology, and psychology of labor and delivery, the teaching of muscle relaxation techniques, and training in specific breathing patterns that serve as a focus of attention and distraction during labor. Generally, CBE courses involve a series of weekly classes that begin in the late second or early third trimester. They are offered by a variety of sources, including (1) independent educators often coordinated by large consumer groups (e.g., American Society of Psychoprophylaxis in Obstetrics, International Childbirth Education Association), (2) private health care providers, (3) hospitals, and (4) public health agencies. There are no national data on participation in CBE, but estimates from local areas suggest that 30 to 50 percent of pregnant women (and usually their partners) enroll in classes. Enrollees tend to be from socially advantaged circumstances: older primiparas with higher incomes and better educations. This is partly because third-party payment is usually not available for this service, and CBE is often not included in public programs of prenatal care.

Controversy. For each of the problems and needs described above, there is some disagreement regarding either (1) whether to intervene or (2) what strategy to use in the event that intervention is warranted.

Encouraging women to control smoking, heavy drinking, and drug use during pregnancy may have the unintended effect of introducing new sources of stress. There is, however, some evidence that the stress associated with changing an addictive behavior may be minimized by providing social and psychological support.

Although the relationship between heavy drinking and fetal alcohol syndrome has been well documented, any effects of consumption of moderate or small amounts of alcohol are not clear-cut. Most women who drink before pregnancy either quit or reduce consumption greatly once the pregnancy is confirmed. A conservative approach to this issue is to err on the safe side by advising those remaining occasional drinkers to abstain. But a counterargument that small amounts of alcohol might be used by some women to control stress suggests that providers avoid any involvement.

Another controversy has to do with nutritional advice: Is it worth the time and energy? Available evidence suggests that nutrition counseling can change dietary knowledge and behaviors. But whether those changes are sufficient to influence fetal health has not been demonstrated. This lack of evidence, however, is due to a shortage of studies rather than to negative findings.

A growing awareness of the potential influence of stress on maternal and fetal well-being is influencing the delivery of prenatal care in the United States. But developing interventions to combat those influences is frustrating because there are few models that have been rigorously evaluated. Despite the longstanding and intuitively logical contributions of social workers to reducing environmental stresses and to providing both psychological and tangible support, clear evidence of the effects of their work has not yet been presented. Similarly, efforts to reduce stressful barriers to care (e.g., high costs) and to remove women from stressful situations via work leave and rest at home have not been studied independently. Recent studies of the effects of home visitors, both public health nurses and others specifically trained to provide guidance and support, have yielded promising results. These studies suggest that home visiting with clear objectives and specific methods can be effective not only in providing and developing social support systems but also in changing behavior and improving infant birth weights. Teenagers seem to be particularly responsive to home visiting.

Other interventions that buffer the effects of stress are used routinely for individuals at risk for coronary and other stress-related diseases. Exercise and relaxation techniques are major elements of those interventions. They are used in some prenatal services, but their effectiveness for pregnant women has not yet been reported.

The major issues regarding CBE classes are (1) whether they have any measurable effects that go beyond their intuitive appeal, and (2) if they do, whether all women should be referred to them. With regard to the first issue, participation has been related to a variety of medical and psychological outcomes in different studies, but the most consistent finding is that women who attend classes use less medication during labor and delivery. There is some debate as to whether this indicates that those women feel less pain, whether their attendants withhold medication, or whether the women do not want or need medication. Regardless of the mechanism, however, the finding is of clinical significance, since medications used in labor can cross the placenta and affect newborn respiration, sucking, and alertness.

Since there is evidence of measurable effects of CBE on the fetus, the second issue takes on greater significance: Should all women be referred? The real issue here is whether low-income women should be referred to CBE classes. It appears that many middle- to upper-income couples find their way to classes. Some of them are referred, whereas others probably seek out the service on their own. The appeal and relevance of CBE to low-income women is less well understood because those women rarely have access to classes. Nevertheless, the data that are available suggest that low-income women do attend classes and experience benefits similar to those of their higher income counterparts if given the opportunity.

Recommendations. (1) Providers of prenatal care should have linkages established with smoking modification and chemical dependency programs that are based on supportive, nonthreatening principles of behavior change. In addition, there should be provisions for interim support and guidance for women who are not yet ready to participate in an organized program. (2) Providers of prenatal care should have established referral networks with nutrition services, social services (including those that provide home visiting), and CBE classes. (3) Providers with low-income patients should establish linkages with services that can accommodate to the financial constraints of the patient. (4) All women who smoke cigarettes, drink heavily, and use drugs at the time of the first prenatal visit should be encouraged to participate in an appropriate program. (5) Women who are at risk for dietary deficiencies, poor weight gain, and intrauterine growth retardation should receive nutrition counseling and, if available and appropriate, nutrition supplementation. (6) Women who live in stressful circumstances and have limited support in their homes and communities should receive assistance in stress management. Teenagers should receive highest priority in these referrals. (7) All women should be given the opportunity to attend childbirth education classes.

Prenatal Surveillance

Background. Prenatal care has been organized into a surveillance framework for multiphasic screening and periodic monitoring of progress. The same basic framework with few alterations has been used for prenatal care since the early part of this century. The generally accepted visit schedule for prenatal surveillance includes an initial work-up as early in the first trimester as possible, followed by monthly visits until the 28th week, visits every 2 to 3 weeks until the 36th week, and weekly visits thereafter until delivery. The early first visit is considered essential for identification of risks and appropriate planning for the pregnancy. More frequent visits in the latter weeks have been considered necessary to detect and treat serious problems, especially preeclampsia, which develop in the late second and third trimesters. The application of new technology in the prenatal period has probably contributed to an increase in the average number of visits per patient. Until recently, little consideration was given to systematically questioning, reducing, or in other ways changing the basic pattern of prenatal visits.

Controversy. A series of reports from Scotland, which started to appear in 1980, indicated that a different arrangement of prenatal visits may be more useful than the routine one. The research suggested that some of the specific conditions that should be detected promptly and managed appropriately within the prenatal surveillance framework were not identified or were mismanaged or both. In part, the investigators felt that the fact that so much of what is done in prenatal care is routine prevented the providers from focusing on the very important problems they were trying to prevent.

No study of this nature has been conducted in the United States. However, these findings, in conjunction with an insidious increase in the number of visits required to apply new technologies and the continually increasing cost of prenatal care, have encouraged critical examinations of the number, frequency, and content of prenatal visits. At present, alternative schedules have not been fully explored.

Recommendations. (1) The first prenatal visit should take place before 12-weeks gestation. (2) Assuming there are no complications, the next visits should be at 16 and 18 to 20 weeks, in order to offer MSAFP screening and to document uterine growth and fetal heart tones. A visit around 24 to 28 weeks should be included for a cervical and vaginal examination, diabetes screening, and anti-RH gamma globulin, if necessary. (3) The needs that determine the frequency of other visits should be educational, behavioral, and psychosocial as well as obstetric and medical, and each visit should have a defined purpose. (4) This open framework should not be viewed as license to decrease precipitously the total number of visits, but rather it should be seen as an opportunity to rearrange the schedule of visits to best meet the needs of individual expectant women.

CONCLUSION

The content of prenatal care has been evolving for many years, and components have shifted to emphasize new diagnostic and therapeutic developments as they have occurred. Currently, most of the components are widely available; some, as noted in the preceding review, are controversial. However, the opportunity to provide beneficial interventions for pregnancies at risk is clearly greater now than it has ever been in the past.

The existence of a variety of options, many of which were developed to address specific problems, suggests that every component is not appropriate for every woman. Therefore, the application and timing of components of care should be guided by specific circumstances, especially the comprehensive history, laboratory tests, physical examination, and the progress of the current pregnancy. A few of the components (an early first visit, the history, and baseline lab work) comprise the cornerstone for management of the entire pregnancy. With this foundation in place, each subsequent encounter should have specific goals and the timing of those encounters should be determined by the goals. In addition to encouraging appropriate care for each individual, this planned approach to the delivery of care also encourages patient participation in the management of pregnancy, which is an essential element in patient cooperation with important recommendations.

In the years ahead, the content of prenatal care will continue to evolve. New developments will lead to new components, thereby sparking new controversies. But it is unlikely in this continually developing field that a return to the days of a routine set of prenatal activities will occur. Future improvements in pregnancy outcomes will undoubtedly be linked to high quality, carefully tailored management of each pregnancy.

SUGGESTED READING

Bishop EH, Cefalo RC. Signs and symptoms of disorders in pregnancy. New York: JB Lippincott, 1983.

Hall M, MacIntyre S, Porter M. Antenatal care assessed. Aberdeen, Scotland: Aberdeen University, 1985.

Institute of Medicine. Preventing low birthweight. Washington, DC: National Academy, 1985.

Wald NJ, ed. Antenatal and neonatal screening. New York: Oxford University, 1984.

NUTRITION IN PREGNANCY

WARREN M. CROSBY, M.D.

OVERVIEW

Pregnancy nutrition cannot be approached as a simple addition of the metabolic requirements of the uterus, the placenta, and the growing fetus to those of the mother because of the fundamental changes in maternal physiology and metabolism that occur in the pregnant state. Furthermore, these changes occur much earlier in pregnancy than would be the case if they were simply responses to the demands of the fetus. Virtually all of the physiologic and metabolic alterations characteristic of pregnancy are instituted within the first trimester, long before fetal demands become large enough to have an effect upon maternal reserves. The concept of the fetus as a "parasite" is also too simple to account for the enormously successful reproductive history of the human race in the face of the extreme variability in the quality and availability of foods throughout our evolution.

Humans are omnivores, and as such can derive useful energy from a very broad variety of foods. Our history is characterized not by a constant availability of a wide variety of foods but by a less predictable cycle of periods of satiety followed by periods of near starvation. Our capacious stomachs hold large amounts of food when it is available, and our long intestine is designed to wring the last calorie from the food we eat. Our ability to store carbohydrates in the form of glycogen is limited to about a days' supply, but our ability to store energy as fat is almost unlimited.

With the exception of a few essential compounds such as vitamins or essential amino acids and some essential fatty acids, our metabolic flexibility enables us to interchange one variety of nutrient with another so that nutritional deficiencies rarely cause disease except under extreme circumstances. Ingestion of protein provides us not only with a wide variety of amino acids for cellular growth, repair, and manufacture of new proteins but also with energy if our main fuels—glucose and fat—come into short supply. We can thus "make" just about anything we need at the cellular level. It is thus not surprising that the people of sub-Sahara Africa continue to have a high birth rate in spite of an appalling famine. Although the perinatal death rate in these countries is high by our standards, much of the reproductive waste occurs among children beyond the newborn period who can no longer draw from the mother's substance for survival.

It is equally clear, however, that maternal nutrition has an effect not only on the successful completion of pregnancy but also on the optimum function of the new being. There are a plethora of animal studies relating variations in nutrition to pregnancy outcome. Most studies of alterations in animal nutrition during pregnancy bear little relationship to the human situation, however, and are usually limited to nutritional deprivation considerably beyond that seen in human starvation. Furthermore, pregnancy in most experimental animals is much shorter than it is in humans, with intensified maternal nutritional needs over a shorter period of time. The nutritional demands of pregnancy consume much more of the maternal reserve in these small laboratory animals than in human pregnancy. Some overall lessons can be learned from these animal studies. An example is that the deleterious effects of chronic malnutrition are cumulative over generations. Experimental nutritional deprivation during human pregnancy is, of course, unethical. Studies of "natural experiments" during a period of famine have shown that severe protein-calorie malnutrition imposed upon otherwise healthy and previously well-fed pregnant Dutch women during World War II reduced infant birth weight. When the period of starvation involved the third trimester of pregnancy, the effect was most pronounced. If the period of starvation involved only the first trimester with return of adequate nutrition in the third, there was no reduction in birth weight. A longer lasting and more severe period of starvation occurred during the seige of Leningrad, also during World War II. There the number of infants weighing less than 2,500 g was increased, and there was a marked increase in neonatal morbidity as well. Poor women, wherever they live, have smaller babies and higher perinatal mortality than more affluent women. Differences in race, prenatal care, chronic disease, smoking, hygiene, and drug ingestion complicate and tend to invalidate conclusions based solely on nutritional differences between any two groups.

Nutritional supplementation studies obviate some of these variables. Groups of women in undeveloped countries whose diets were inadequate have been given food supplements in controlled scientific experiments. Statistically significant increases in birth weight were observed in the group that got more to eat. Any study of human nutrition and its relationship to birth weight must take into account the effects of race, prepregnancy weight, maternal weight gain, sex of the fetus, maternal drug and smoking habits, maternal disease (including glucose intolerance), parity, age, and the length of gestation, all of which have been shown to significantly influence the baby's weight at birth. One report utilized each of these factors and added an additional number of laboratory values measured in the mother at midpregnancy to derive an equation that predicts fetal weight at every week of pregnancy. The formula was tested and found to have an 80 percent predictive value. Utilizing the formula to predict fetal size, deviations from the expected size at birth could then be used to identify babies suffering from malnutrition even when their actual birth weight was above 2,500 g. Using the formula, this report estimates that 15 to 20 percent of pregnancies in the United States result in babies who are significantly smaller than they should be. Nutritional supplementation in the form of WIC (United States Department of Agriculture, Special Supplemental Program for Women, Infants, and Children) vouchers in a controlled study resulted in a significant increase in adjusted birth weight but only in the group of babies whose mothers smoked during the pregnancy.

Many studies have shown that larger mothers have

larger babies and that there is a clear, positive, linear relationship between maternal weight gain during pregnancy and birth weight. The National Collaborative Perinatal Project reported that the lowest perinatal morbidity and mortality occurred in that group of mothers who gained between 26 and 30 pounds during pregnancy. It is clear, then, that although modern women can reproduce successfully under enormously variant nutritional conditions, there is a harmful effect of nutritional deprivation during pregnancy. This effect is most severe if the deprivation occurs throughout pregnancy, although it is most visible when deprivation involves the last trimester. The deleterious effect of nutritional deprivation on the fetus is probably increased if the deprivation has occurred over many generations, further compounding the plight of the chronically poor.

PHYSIOLOGY OF PREGNANCY

Virtually all the alterations of organ function that accompany pregnancy are already in place by the end of the first trimester, long before the fetus and placenta are large enough to cause any detectable drain on maternal reserves. Most of the changes from normal physiology seem to have both beneficial and harmful effects on the mother. Delayed gastrointestinal motility, for instance, may enable extraction of more nutrients from the same amount of food, but it also is responsible for nausea, vomiting, and constipation.

THE GASTROINTESTINAL TRACT

Morning sickness is observed in more than half of pregnant women. Its cause is unknown, and it is almost easier to explain why nausea and vomiting may occur secondary to rapid changes in the level of estrogenic hormones and the resultant decrease in gastrointestinal motility than it is to explain why the morning nausea disappears so miraculously at 12 to 14 weeks of gestation. For whatever reason, many patients obtain relief of morning sickness by eating small, frequent meals. Having a piece of toast before getting out of bed in the morning is helpful. Having part of breakfast at midmorning and part of the noon meal at midafternoon often provides complete relief.

The esophagus shares in the depression of gastrointestinal muscular tonus and motility seen throughout the gastrointestinal tract during pregnancy. Heartburn is also extremely common and can be explained at least in part by changes in the tonus of the esophagogastric sphincter. Reflux of acidic gastric juices is the principal cause of heartburn, but some studies have shown that infusion of hydrochloric acid at appropriate pH causes pain in the lower esophagus only in those women who already complain of heartburn. Those patients who had not experienced heartburn did not have any symptoms from the acid alone. It seems clear that chronic reflux and physical esophagitis are present in patients who complain of heartburn.

The reduction in motility and tonus present in the rest of the gastrointestinal tract during pregnancy was first discovered by studies of the stomach. Gastric emptying time has long been known to be delayed during pregnancy, and this delay is compounded during labor, to the extent that food in the stomach at the onset of labor is usually still there after delivery. This delayed gastric emptying during labor represents a significant problem for obstetric anesthesiologists and is a relative contraindication to using general anesthesia for delivery, particularly in the absence of an endotracheal tube with an appropriately sized cuff.

Gastric secretion is also affected by pregnancy, and studies universally show a reduction in gastric secretion and a diminution in the response to ingested meals or injected histamine. Similarly, the secretion of gastric acid is thought to be diminished during pregnancy, along with the secretion and activity of pepsin. These facts apparently explain the well-known reduction in peptic ulcer complaints during pregnancy.

Small intestinal motility and tonus are also reduced by the elevated levels of progesterone during pregnancy, but this effect is much more difficult to study than it is in the stomach and the esophagus. There is evidence of improved absorption during pregnancy, particularly in relationship to the absorption of iron, calcium, and folic acid. It is uncertain, at least with regard to the minerals, whether increase of absorption relates to fundamental changes in the lining of the small intestine or to increased demand for these nutrients, a mechanism that operates in the nonpregnant state as well. The large intestine also has been shown to have reduced tonus and motility, a feature that explains the constipation observed in many pregnancies. The slower transit time may also account for reports of increased water absorption from the large intestine during pregnancy, which may be a contributing factor in constipation.

THE LIVER AND GALLBLADDER

Liver function tests do not change during pregnancy, except for those that are related to the increased concentration of globulins in the maternal blood. Heat-stable alkaline phosphatase, derived from the placenta, contributes to the overall increase in the concentration of this enzyme during pregnancy. The liver may be more vulnerable to infection during pregnancy. A high rate of death during pregnancy reported from a few hepatitis epidemics may be accounted for by the virulence of the virus accompanied by a general state of poor nutrition in the populace rather than by the condition of pregnancy itself. There are no obvious physiologic changes in liver function during pregnancy that can clearly account for the mysterious disease known as acute yellow atrophy or its cousin, acute fatty liver of pregnancy.

Gallbladder function is apparently altered by virtue of the reduction in tonus and motility of the muscles in the wall of the gallbladder, but the content of the bile itself apparently does not change during pregnancy.

RENAL FUNCTION

The most striking feature of the anatomy of the urinary system seen during pregnancy is the physiologic dilation of the ureters and renal pelvis, known as the hydronephrosis of pregnancy. This feature is seen in nearly every pregnant woman; it is often more striking on the left than the right side and is thought to be due not only to the decrease in tonus and motility of the smooth muscles of the urinary tract but also to the hypertrophy of the condensation of connective tissues surrounding the ureter as it enters the bladder, the sheath of Waldeyer. Renal function changes dramatically during pregnancy. The principal effect responsible for all of the changes seen seems to be an increase in renal blood flow. This is not merely an effect of the increased cardiac output but represents a true increase in blood flow per gram of kidney. With more blood flowing through the glomeruli, more urine is filtered and the glomerular filtration rate can be shown to increase by as much as 50 percent in the majority of pregnant women studied. There are thus more solutes filtered. The requirement of the renal tubules for reabsorption of solutes then increases concomitantly, resulting in occasional spillage of solutes in the urine. The appearance of glucose in the urine is much more frequent during pregnancy and at one time served as a crude pregnancy test. Delayed gastrointestinal absorption and alterations in glucose metabolism also plays a role in the causation of glycosuria. Glucose reabsorption by the tubule, however, has been shown to be reduced during pregnancy. Amino acids are similarly found in the urine more frequently during pregnancy than in the nonpregnant state. Some amino acids are found in greater quantities in the urine than others. Thus there appears to be some selection by the renal tubules in their ability to reabsorb amino acids presented to them by the increased amount of filtered urine. The significance of such selection is not known at this time. Renal excretion of hydrogen and bicarbonate ions appears to be relatively unchanged during the course of pregnancy in spite of the fact that there is a relative alkalosis during pregnancy. The relative alkalosis is thought to be brought about by an increased respiratory rate and minute volume. The increased amount of air exchanged results in an increased excretion of carbon dioxide.

Water excretion is markedly altered during pregnancy, with a tendency toward increased water and sodium retention. Water retention is at least partly related to retention of sodium. During pregnancy the marked increase in glomerular filtration rate and increased progesterone production would appear to increase sodium excretion. To counter that effect, there is an elevated level of plasma aldosterone as well as other salt-retaining hormones such as estrogen and cortisol. The reduction in plasma albumin concentration decreases plasma oncotic pressure, which decreases the tendency of salt and water to remain in the vascular system. The net result of all this in normal pregnancy is to increase total salt and water in the body. Thus, with an increasing amount of salt and water retention, there is increased filling of the vascular system. This phenomenon accounts for the remarkable increase of blood volume (30 to 50 percent) and the marked tendency for pregnant women to develop dependent edema. Edema was once viewed with alarm, as it almost invariably accompanies acute preeclampsia and eclampsia. Attempts at reducing edema were thought to reduce the risk of these diseases. However, acute and chronic diuretic therapy have been shown to be ineffective in preventing preeclampsia. Furthermore, by reducing blood volume, diuretic therapy for preeclampsia or eclampsia actually contributes to an increased risk of perinatal mortality, presumably due to the reduction in uteroplacental blood flow brought about by the disease and the reduction in blood volume. It has also been reported that women who fail to expand their blood volume during pregnancy have an extraordinarily high level of fetal wastage. Indeed, this pendulum has swung so far in the other direction that one very large survey of 16,000 pregnant women reported from the National Collaborative Perinatal Project by E.W. Page indicated that women who developed edema (in the absence of hypertension) had a lower perinatal mortality rate than women who did not demonstrate edema during pregnancy. Page's conclusions were that the women who developed edema during late pregnancy had won the race to increase their blood volume to capacity and had actually exceeded that capacity. Conversely, the women who had never developed edema were those who never satisfactorily met the goal of maximum blood volume expansion and thus were never quite able to increase uteroplacental blood flow to optimum levels.

METABOLIC CHANGES

Proteins

There is a dramatic fall in the level of serum albumin during pregnancy, which begins abruptly in early pregnancy and this reduction only slows during the last trimester. The cause for the decrease in serum albumin level is unknown, but the colloid osmotic pressure drops in parallel with albumin concentration. This drop is partially accounted for by dilution, with an increase in the water content of blood. In late pregnancy the total amount of albumin found in the blood is similar to that in the nonpregnant state.

The concentration of globulins is increased during pregnancy. The carrier proteins for thyroxine, cortisol, iron and the immunoglobulins are the most studied, but virtually all serum globulins increase in concentration during pregnancy. This implies a marked increase in their production rate.

Similarly, lipids characteristically increase in concentration in the blood during pregnancy, and pregnancy can be considered a hyperlipidemic state. Cholesterol, in particular, is elevated in pregnancy in all cultures so far studied, and this occurs regardless of dietary intake of cholesterol. The metabolic significance is not known. Complex lipids do not cross the placenta but free (unesterified) fatty acids do and may play a role in fetal energy metabolism.

Amino acids generally decline in concentration during pregnancy, at least partly because of increased excretion in the urine. It is clear that retention or excretion of individual amino acids varies considerably during pregnancy and relates at least partly to the type of food eaten. The reason for variations of excretion or retention of individual amino acids and individual amino acid groups is not known. Metcoff has shown that certain patterns of blood levels of amino acids during pregnancy correlate with fetal growth. His concept is that concentrations of amino acids may constitute rate-limiting or rate-enhancing factors in biochemical reactions, particularly those that provide amino acids for placental transfer and fetal metabolism.

Vitamins

The vast majority of pregnant women in the United States receive vitamin supplements during pregnancy, presumably on the grounds that an oversupply is better than the risk of an occasional undersupply in the availability of these essential nutrients for fetal growth. There is essentially no evidence to support this concept. Indeed, some evidence exists that excessive amounts of vitamin ingestion may be harmful to fetal development. Ingestion of excessive amounts of fat-soluble vitamins, particularly vitamin A, is clearly toxic. Blood levels of the fat-soluble vitamins increase during pregnancy like the levels of the other lipids.

Water-soluble vitamins have a general tendency to decrease in concentration during pregnancy, at least partly because of the increased amount of water in the blood. Indeed, vitamin C levels fall progressively during pregnancy even if vitamin C intake is increased.

Carbohydrates

Pregnancy can be characterized as diabetogenic in that higher levels of glucose can be found in the blood of a pregnant woman following a carbohydrate meal than in the same individual in the nonpregnant state. Fasting plasma or blood glucose levels clearly diminished during pregnancy, and this reduction is usually detectable in the first trimester. Thus in early pregnancy the reduction in fasting glucose is accompanied by a diminution in the level of insulin in the fasting state. The plasma level of glucagon has been studied less frequently. Plasma glucagon apparently increases in the fasting state. Following these changes in the first trimester, the fasting level of glucose remains depressed, but the plasma glucose following ingestion of carbohydrate rises to a higher level than it did in the nonpregnant state. Furthermore, this level increases as pregnancy advances and is accompanied by an elevation in the plasma insulin level as well. The causes for these changes in carbohydrate metabolism that accompany pregnancy are not clear. Several mechanisms have been suggested. The plasma cortisol level is elevated during pregnancy, partly because of the elevation in globulin binding. If there is indeed an elevation in the circulating level of free active cortisol, it may stimulate degradation of insulin in the liver. Several reports have indicated an insulinase in the placenta that may reduce plasma levels in early pregnancy, following which there may be a compensatory increase in secretion of insulin by the pancreas. Human placental lactogen also has been described as having a diabetogenic influence by somehow diminishing the number of insulin binding sites on cell membranes.

The diabetogenic effects of pregnancy are lost within 48 hours of delivery, and indeed the immediate puerperal woman becomes much more sensitive to a given dose of insulin than she was immediately prior to delivery. Interestingly enough, the return of insulin sensitivity is not accompanied by as rapid a change in glucose tolerance in that the insulin response to ingested glucose requires more than 4 to 6 weeks to return to the normal state following delivery.

The effect of maternal hyperglycemia on fetal growth is complex, but there is a fairly straightforward relationship between the two. It has long been known that prior to the clinical diagnosis of diabetes such women have a history of delivery of large fetuses, with a progressive increase in birth weight occurring closer to the discovery of clinically evident disease. The appearance of the baby of the diabetic mother is one of both immaturity and insulin excess. The level of fetal and newborn plasma insulin is increased to compensate for the increased level of plasma glucose derived from the hyperglycemia of the mother. When the glucose supply from the mother is suddenly shut off by delivery, the excess insulin frequently brings about hypoglycemia in the newborn within the first few hours of life. For the diabetic mother, the fetal growth pattern is one of excessive fat deposition and macrosomia. The metabolic derangements produced by hyperglycemia and hyperinsulinemia are not thoroughly understood but clearly result in alterations of organ maturation such that the newborn has an excess risk of hyperbilirubinemia and respiratory distress syndrome.

Calcium Metabolism

Calcium metabolism is the result of a complex interplay between calcium absorption and excretion through the influences of vitamin D on its absorption as well as of the relationship between parathyroid hormone, calcitonin, and the plasma level of the phosphate ion on its excretion by the kidney.

In normal pregnancy, the level of total calcium and inorganic phosphate falls, at least in part due to hemodilution and the decrease in serum albumin that binds both calcium and phosphate. Calcium and phosphorus absorption are increased during pregnancy because of a rise in the secretion and plasma level of the parathyroid hormone, at least in the presence of an adequate dietary supply of vitamin D. Plasma calcitonin levels are also increased. The rise in calcium and phosphate absorption occurs well in advance of the needs of the fetal skeletal system, and there is an early increase in the amount of calcium excretion from the kidney. As fetal growth occurs, however, there is increased incorporation of calcium into both the fetal and the maternal skeletons plus an increase in the amount of turnover of calcium from maternal bone to serum and back again. Calcium balance, then, in the face of reasonably adequate supplies of calcium, phosphate, and vitamin D, does not lead to osteomalacia or osteoporosis or to loss of teeth.

Calcium deficiency even in pregnant women of developing countries is very uncommon. It is almost never seen except in conjunction with diseases of calcium absorption or excessive renal loss. More commonly, vitamin D deficiency leads to derangements in calcium metabolism.

FETAL GROWTH AND MATERNAL NUTRITION

The goal of good maternal nutrition is the delivery of a healthy baby at term. Many factors can interrupt this process, but we will discuss those nutritional factors that may relate to inadequate fetal growth.

The most rapid period of fetal growth occurs during the 20 weeks between the 14th and 34th week of gestation (menstrual age). It is during this time that the nutritional supply of the mother is most critical. The nutrient supply reaching the fetus must first pass through the placenta after being made available by the flow of maternal blood through the intervillous space. Circulatory alterations such as changes in blood pressure, toxemia of pregnancy, or thrombosis may diminish the maternal blood flow to the placenta to the point that optimal or normal fetal growth may be diminished. Indeed, blood flow may diminish so much that the flow is incapable of supporting fetal life, and fetal death occurs. Presumably there is a state of inadequate maternal blood flow through the intervillous space that is compatible with maintenance of fetal life but inadequate to continue proper growth. The condition of inadequate fetal nutrition leading to inadequate fetal growth has been termed in utero growth retardation (IUGR), small for gestational age (SGA), or fetal malnutrition (FM).

The majority of newborns found or identified as having FM cannot be shown to have clinically identifiable alterations in maternal circulation related to hypertension, hypotension, or thrombosis. The next organ in line, the placenta, is the next likely cause for inadequate transfer of nutrients to the fetus. The placenta is an actively growing, metabolizing organ. Placental transfer of nutrients to the fetus is an active process. The transplacental passage of nutrients from the mother to the fetus can be affected by the mode of transfer of a particular nutrient from maternal blood to that of the fetus. Certain nutrients such as oxygen and glucose are consumed by the placenta, and amino acids contribute to its growth during pregnancy. Following entry into the fetal blood stream, alterations in umbilical blood flow or deficiencies in uptake and utilization of nutrients by fetal cells can also affect the rate of fetal growth.

Metcoff has described three types of fetal malnutrition:

1. Type I is seen in a newborn that is uniformly small but in proportion. This type of malnutrition is exemplified in the baby that not only is low in weight but also has not gained appropriate length or head circumference. It is thought to be the result of chronic diminution of the availability of nutrients throughout pregnancy, or at least during that period associated with the most rapid growth.
2. In type II malnutrition, the infant's head size is relatively normal but he or she is remarkably underweight. It is natural to assume that during the period of malnutrition that causes this type, brain development was spared the overall inadequate amount of nutrients available to the entire fetus. This is the pattern of diminished fetal growth that was seen during the famine in the Netherlands during World War II and is probably the result of limited availability of nutrients to the fetus principally during the last trimester of pregnancy. Today this type of fetal malnutrition is also seen more commonly in cigarette smokers and in mothers with preeclampsia.
3. The type III malnourished baby is markedly underweight but has an appropriate length, and the head circumference is also normal. There is clear evidence of weight loss in these babies; skin folds are easily pulled up, and they have the clinical appearance of starvation. The operant mechanism here is a gradual but severe diminution in the availability of nutrients to the fetus during the last few weeks before birth, which requires that the fetus catabolize its own fat in order to continue energy metabolism. This must occur after the period of rapid growth has been completed. This type of malnutrition appears to have the best prognosis in that fetal cell numbers, particularly in the brain, are likely to be the greatest, since they were formed before the limitation in nutrition occurred. Such babies are often insatiable in their formula requirements following birth. Since the majority of mothers who deliver malnourished fetuses cannot be identified as having had a disease that limits either nutrition or maternal blood flow, it is likely that there is some other major explanation for fetal malnutrition. Metcoff and associates have suggested that an imbalance rather than a deficiency in nutrient concentration in the mother's blood may influence the transport of nutrients across the placenta into the fetus. In studies designed to test this hypothesis, the pattern of a large number of indicators of maternal nutrition varied between normal women and those who were destined to have malnourished fetuses when measured at midpregnancy. This group was able to predict fetal malnutrition at delivery by identifying the pattern of maternal nutrients in blood drawn at midpregnancy.

Fetal Nutrition

The fetus receives all substances required for life through the placenta. It is therefore totally dependent upon placental transfer of all substances in order to sustain life as well as growth. For that reason, any concept of fetal growth and nutrition depends on knowledge of placental transfer.

The placenta is dependent upon maternal blood flow with adequate concentration of nutrients to supply its own needs as well as those of the fetus. The concentration of nutrients in maternal blood depends on maternal nutrition. During periods of starvation, maternal concentration of amino acids and glucose may be replenished from maternal stores through gluconeogenesis at the expense of the mother. If this process goes on very long, starvation ketosis occurs.

Blood flow to the placenta is controlled by the tonus in the spiral arterioles that supply maternal blood to the intervillous space. Control upstream from the spiral arterioles is related to constriction and dilation of the branches of the uterine arteries.

TRANSFER OF NUTRIENTS

Water and electrolytes readily cross the placenta, reaching equilibrium on both sides within extremely short periods of time. There is a constant relationship between the concentration of electrolytes and water in the fetus, in the maternal blood, in the intervillous space, and in the amniotic fluid, with the exchange of such substances between the fetal and maternal circulations in the intervillous space being extremely fast and the interchange of substances between the fetus and the amniotic fluid and the amniotic fluid with the mother being considerably slower.

The fetus utilizes glucose as its principal energy supply. Most of the fat deposited by the fetus in the last few weeks of pregnancy comes from transfer of glucose, not fats. The transfer of glucose across the placenta is accomplished by facilitated diffusion, which ensures adequate flow of glucose into the fetus at all times. When there is profound hypoglycemia in the mother, it is apparent that glucose can flow from the fetus to the mother, but the blood level is always slightly lower in the fetus than in the mother. The tolerance of the fetus to hypoglycemia is not well understood, but prolonged hypoglycemia is likely to be harmful, at least to the growth and development of the fetal brain.

All proteins in the fetus, with the exception of some immunoglobulins, are made from the supply of amino acids following transfer from the mother. The transfer of amino acids across the placenta is accomplished by an active transport system in which the fetal levels of amino acids are higher than those found in the mother.

Fats

In general, nonesterified (free) fatty acids are the only lipids that are transferred intact across the placenta. The biologic importance of these substances for fetal growth is not well understood.

Vitamins

The water-soluble vitamins of the B complex are handled much in the same way as amino acids. There seems to be an active transport mechanism so that there is a higher concentration of vitamins in the fetal plasma than in that of the mother. Riboflavin, on the other hand, is broken down by the placenta and reassembled on the fetal side. Pyridoxine is similarly altered and reassembled. Vitamin B_{12}, thiamine, and pantothenic acid may be handled in this way as well, but supporting data are still lacking.

Fat-soluble vitamins are found in the fetus. Vitamin A is apparently reconstructed from placental transfer of carotene. Metcoff's group has shown that the maternal serum level of carotene correlates well with fetal growth. The mechanism for this relationship is not known, but the level of carotene in the mother's blood may in some general way reflect the efficiency of absorption of nutrients from the small bowel, clearly an important part of nutritional well-being. The mechanism of transfer of vitamin D is not well understood. It is clear, however, that vitamin D is acquired from the mother by the fetus and that fetal bone development requires its presence for proper growth. There must be more than enough vitamin D available in maternal blood, however, for the minimum daily allowance is the same for the pregnant as for the nonpregnant woman.

RECOMMENDED DAILY ALLOWANCES

Table 1 shows the total amount of energy required by the mother (in excess of her normal nonpregnant requirements) to maintain fetal and placental metabolism and the increased requirements for the uterus, breasts, and heart. The total metabolizable energy is 10 percent more than the total net energy, since it is estimated that only 90 percent of ingested protein, fat, and carbohydrates are converted to energy.

It is usually stated that the normal dietary increase required to meet the demands of pregnancy is 300 kcal per day (84, 957 kcal divided by 280 days = 303.4 kcal per day). This recommendation is divided into the four quarters of pregnancy in Table 1, showing that the largest daily need is between 20 and 30 weeks. Normal pregnant women vary considerably in their self-chosen diets during pregnancy, with some gaining more weight early and others gaining it later than the specified times according to the energy needs portrayed by this table. In general, recommended daily allowances should be taken into consideration with regard to the overall health and nutritional state of the individual patient. For instance, patients who are grossly underweight would do well to gain more than the usually recommended 26 to 30 pounds during pregnancy. Management of nutritional problems such as obesity or nutritional or gastrointestinal disease will be discussed later. The recommended daily allowances discussed here are appropriate only for the adult pregnant female in good health who is going into pregnancy.

Calories

The recommended daily allowance for nonpregnant females in the 45 to 55 kilogram weight group is 2,000 to 2,100 cal per day. It is normally stated that this should be increased by 300 cal per day during pregnancy. However, the increase in dietary needs in early pregnancy is very small compared with that of late pregnancy (See Table 1).

Protein

It is clear that both the maternal requirement for increased muscle size of the uterus and protein requirements for building the fetus and the placenta are increased considerably during pregnancy. The most appropriate amount of protein intake for any given pregnant individual is virtually impossible to ascertain. The recommended daily allowance for pregnancy is 30 g of protein above the 46 g recommended for the standard healthy woman. However, many nutritionists suggest that 100 g of protein should be the recommended daily allowance for pregnant women, with the extra 24 g being added at the expense of carbohydrate and fat in the total average caloric increase of 300 calories per day. It can be shown that pregnant women can produce healthy-appearing babies with protein and calorie intakes considerably less than these recommendations, and indeed the World Health Organization's recommendations are somewhat lower than those for the United States.

Carbohydrate and Fat

The remainder of the 2,000 and 2,100 cal of the total caloric replacement minus the calories contributed to by 75 to 100 g of protein daily should be made up by an appropriate mix of carbohydrates and fats. It is difficult to utilize a diet in which there are less than 50 g of fat without going to considerable extremes. Furthermore, reduction in essential fatty acids could conceivably cause nutritional problems if an attempt were made to totally eliminate fat from the diet during pregnancy. Some fat restrictions should occur in the calculation of diets for pregnant diabetics, in whom excessive fat metabolism may contribute excessive acidic residues that are inappropriate for fetal growth and metabolism. In the nondiabetic individual, it is difficult to show that any particular mix of carbohydrates and fat relates to poor fetal growth or nutrition.

Vitamins

Fat-soluble vitamins (A and D) are not eliminated as rapidly as the water-soluble vitamins of the B and C groups. The recommended daily allowance for vitamin A in the nonpregnant state, 4,000 U per day, is increased to 5,000 U per day during pregnancy. Again this increase is not needed until at least midpoint in pregnancy if not the third trimester. Vitamin A is important in the formation of the pigments allowing rod vision in the retina as well as being a major factor in skin metabolism. Deficiency of vitamin A is unusual in developed countries, but when it is present, night blindness and skin conditions are common.

Vitamin D requirements are unchanged by pregnancy or lactation and remain at 400 IU per day. Vitamin D is important in the regulation of calcium and phosphate metabolism, principally that related to bone growth and development. Vitamin D deficiency, or rickets, causes stunted growth and soft bones but is never seen in otherwise normal newborns.

Water-Soluble Vitamins (C and the B Group)

Vitamin C, ascorbic acid, is required in greater quantities during pregnancy. The recommended daily allowance in the nonpregnant individual is 45 mg and is increased to 60 mg per day during pregnancy. Vitamin C is important in the management of amino acid metabolism and the maintenance of ground substance. Its deficiency disease, scurvy, is accompanied by anemia, skin and collagen disorders, and poor wound healing.

The B complex vitamins (thiamine, niacin, pyridoxine [B_6] riboflavin, and B_{12}) are water-soluble and are

TABLE 1 Cumulative Energy Cost of Pregnancy Computed from the Energy Equivalents of Protein and Fat Increments and the Energy Cost of Maintaining the Fetus and Added Maternal Tissues

	Weeks of Pregnancy				
	*0–10**	*10–20*	*20–30*	*30–40*	
	Equivalent, kcal/day				*Cumulative total kcal†*
Protein	3.6	10.3	26.7	34.2	5180
Fat	55.6	235.6	207.6	31.3	36337
Oxygen consumption	19.9	62.0	110.9	186.1	26244
Total net energy	79.1	307.9	345.2	251.6	67761
Metabolizable energy (total net energy + 10%)	87	339	380	277	74537

* For the first 10 week period total increment is divided by 56 since pregnancy is dated from the last menstrual period

† Taken as 5.6 kcal/g for protein and 9.5 kcal/g for fat

From Hytten FR, Chamberlain G. Clinical physiology in obstetrics. Oxford: Blackwell, 1980:165.

excreted in the urine continuously throughout the day. Thus the recommended daily amount is almost totally excreted and must be replaced every day.

Thiamine has a recommended daily allowance of 0.9 mg per 24 hours in the nonpregnant individual, and this is increased to 1.0 mg for pregnant women. The deficiency disease associated with inadequate thiamine intake is called beriberi, and it is associated with cardiomyopathy and peripheral neuropathy. Thiamine deficiency is quite rare among pregnant women in the United States who are not alcoholics or do not have some other gastrointestinal disease.

Niacin has a recommended daily allowance of 14.5 mg for the nonpregnant individual, and this is increased to 16.8 mg per day during pregnancy. Niacin's deficiency disease, pellagra, is characterized by diarrhea, mental disorders, and skin and oral ulceration, but deficiency of niacin is quite rare during pregnancy in the United States.

Pyridoxine, vitamin B_6, has a recommended daily allowance of 2 mg in the nonpregnant individual, and this is elevated to 2.5 mg daily in the pregnant patient. Pyridoxine functions principally as a coenzyme in amino acid metabolism, and severe pyridoxine deficiency may lead to anemia and peripheral neuropathy. Pyridoxine deficiency in otherwise healthy pregnant women in the United States is very rare.

Riboflavin has a recommended daily allowance of 1.3 mg per 24 hours in the nonpregnant individual, and this is increased to 1.5 mg during pregnancy. Riboflavin is important in many metabolic reactions throughout the body. Riboflavin deficiency, uncommon in pregnant women in the United States, is characterized by glossitis and dermatitis.

In the United States, Vitamin B_{12} has a recommended daily allowance of 5 mg per day, which is increased to 8 mg during pregnancy. This vitamin has functions similar to those of folic acid in the maintenance of hemoglobin synthesis. Deficiencies of vitamin B_{12} are very rare in pregnant women in the United States.

Folic acid has a recommended daily allowance of 400 μg per day, which is increased to 800 μg per day during pregnancy because of the remarkable increase in the amount of blood cells manufactured during pregnancy for both the mother and fetus. Folic acid deficiency during pregnancy is principally manifested as a megaloblastic and macrocytic anemia accompanied by hypersegmented neutrophils. Folic acid deficiency is not uncommon during pregnancy in the United States. Folic acid is found in high concentrations in liver and green leafy and yellow vegetables, many of which are not staples of most American diets, particularly among the poor. In some categories of patients in the United States, folic acid is boiled away by excessive cooking in large quantities of water, so that even if the green vegetables contained adequate amounts of folic acid prior to cooking, the patient's folic acid intake may not be adequate. Macrocytic anemia is often the result. Folic acid deficiency anemia is often associated with iron deficiency. This combination tends to make the cells normal in size, so the diagnosis may be difficult if the blood smear or indices are the only diagnostic means used. Serum iron and folate levels should both be obtained in anemic pregnant patients.

Minerals

Iron is probably the most important mineral requiring ingestion during pregnancy, at least as far as the possibility of deficiency during pregnancy is concerned. Iron is important in the manufacture of hemoglobin and myoglobin, both of which are manufactured in large quantities by the pregnant individual. The recommended daily allowance of elemental iron in the nonpregnant woman is 18 mg per day. Various recommendations have been made to increase iron intake during pregnancy. Studies by Pritchard have indicated that normal healthy young women have poor iron reserves and consequently are subject to iron deficiency anemia in the face of increased demands for iron such as occur during pregnancy or chronic bleeding. There has been some question about the need or usefulness of iron supplementation during pregnancy, the concept being related to whether or not the decrease in hemoglobin concentration and hematocrit seen almost universally during pregnancy is physiologic or represents an iron deficiency. It is true that when iron supplementation is given during pregnancy, the fall in hemoglobin concentration and hematocrit is not as great as it is without iron supplementation. Several authors have suggested that such a nonphysiologic polycythemia may be detrimental to proper fetal development during pregnancy because of increased viscosity of blood and diminished blood flow through the placenta. At the present time this argument does not seem to be strong enough to diminish the recommendation for iron supplementation during pregnancy. However, Table 2 shows that there is no increase in the recommended allowance of iron in the United States.

Daily calcium is important in bone formation for both the mother and the fetus, and the recommended daily allowance in the nonpregnant individual is 800 mg per day; this is increased to 1,200 mg per day during pregnancy. This increase is more than managed by the average pregnant woman's diet, particularly if she drinks milk and eats other milk products such as cottage cheese or regular cheese.

Zinc is required for nucleic acid and other protein synthesis. Its concentration in maternal blood declines during normal pregnancy, probably because it is normally bound to albumin. Approximately 750 mg per day should be ingested to supply fetal needs. Many American diets are deficient in zinc, but the effects of mild zinc deficiency on the fetus are not known. Marked zinc deficiency in animals can be shown to be teratogenic.

The recommended daily allowance for iodine is 100 mg per day in the nonpregnant individual and this is increased to 125 mg per day during pregnancy. Iodine is important in the manufacture of the thyroid hormone, and the simple dietary deficiency disease of goiter with hypothyroidism is extremely rare in the United States today, thanks to the universal availability of iodized salt.

NUTRITION AS PART OF PRENATAL CARE

Basic Nutrition as Selected by Pregnant Women

Normal healthy women with standard educations and

TABLE 2 Daily Recommended Allowances of Vitamins and Calories for Nonpregnant and Pregnant Women Doing Light Work

	United Nations		*United States*		*United States*
	Nonpregnant	*Pregnant*	*Nonpregnant*	*Pregnant*	*Lactating*
Weight, kg	*55*	—	*58*	—	
Weight gain, kg	—	*10±2*	—	*11*	
Energy, kcal	2,200	2,550	2,000	2,200	2,500
Protein, g	29	38	55	65	75
Calcium, g	0.4–0.5	1.0–1.2	0.8	1.2	1.2
Iron, mg	14–28	14–28*	18	18	18
Vitamin A	750 μg	750 μg	5,000 IU	6,000 IU	6,000 IU
Vitamin D	25 μg	10 μg	none	400 IU	400 IU
Thiamine, mg	0.9	1.0	1.0	1.0	1.3
Riboflavin, mg	1.3	1.5	1.5	1.8	2.1
Niacin, mgEq	14.5	16.8	13	15	17
Vitamin B_6, mg	—	—	2.0	2.5	2.5
Folate, μg	200	400	400	800	600
Vitamin B_{12}, μg	2.0	3.0	5.0	8.0	4.0
Ascorbic acid, mg	30	30	55	60	60

* Assuming previous iron intake has been satisfactory. A lower level is the recommendation when over 25 percent of calories are from animal foods. The upper level is the recommendation when under 10 percent of calories are from animal foods.
Adapted from Hytten FA, Chamberlain G. Clinical physiology in obstetrics. Oxford: Blackwell, 1980, and Halpern SL. Quick reference to clinical nutrition. Philadelphia: JB Lippincott, 1979.

adequate incomes tend to select diets during pregnancy that they feel are best for themselves. It is not surprising, perhaps, given the educational system in the United States, that such women's diets are quite appropriate for pregnancy. Most women eat three meals a day, drink some milk, eat meat and vegetables, and have an adequate caloric intake as reflected by an appropriate weight gàin during the entire pregnancy.

Weight Gain During Pregnancy

It is quite clear that the majority of pregnant women gain weight during pregnancy. Reduction in weight during pregnancy may have a harmful effect on the developing fetus, a fact that seems known by everyone. With these general limits in mind, how can one decide what an appropriate weight gain during pregnancy is or ought to be, and how can the physician take this information and translate it into recommendations for patients?

The average weight given during pregnancy is approximately 26 lb, 20 lb of which are made up by the absolute requirements of pregnancy: the fetus (7½ lb), the placenta 1.5 lb), amniotic fluid (2 lb), plus the increase in the size of the uterus (2 lb), breasts (1 lb), and the increase in blood volume (2 lb) and total body water (4 lb). Thus at the conclusion of an average pregnancy, these 20 pounds will be lost by the nonlactating mother over the course of the 6- to 8-week period required to return to the normal nonpregnant state. Although the average weight gain during pregnancy varies enormously about this 20 lb figure, several studies have indicated that the most successful outcome of pregnancy, i.e., the lowest perinatal mortality rate, is associated with a maternal weight gain of 26 to 30 pounds. Many studies have indicated that the excess weight is largely fat, which would not necessarily be considered to have much effect on the fetus. On the other hand, the requirements of a given individual fetus cannot be estimated with any degree of accuracy, and the concept of "nutritional overshoot" on the part of the mother seems to have a beneficial effect on perinatal mortality. The relationship between maternal weight gain and well-being of the fetus, however, is much more complicated than a simple linear relationship between perinatal mortality and maternal weight gain. There is, for instance, some question as to whether overfeeding the fetus can be considered beneficial. The macrosomic baby of the diabetic mother is a clear example of this extreme. Similarly, there are the substantial effects of race, maternal height, maternal prepregnancy weight, and other relationships that are known to influence the weight of the baby at birth.

Weight loss during pregnancy produces chronic maternal starvation ketosis. Starvation ketosis has been demonstrated to be clearly harmful for fetal development in rats. Apparently glucose is the principal and preferred energy metabolite for the fetal brain. However, ketone bodies, if transferred to the fetus in large quantities, can find themselves available to the fetal brain for energy metabolism. When the fetal brain utilizes ketone bodies for energy metabolism, the hydrogen ion production may exceed the buffering capacity of the fetal brain cells and cause cell death or malfunction. Fetal rats subjected to maternal starvation failed to run the maze after they were born as well as their genetically identical siblings who were gestated in a mother without starvation ketosis.

Lactation

During lactation, the demands of the newborn for calories and protein exceed those of the developing fetus. As a result, the recommended daily allowances for the lactating mother are increased over those during pregnancy (see Table 2). The principal dietary components required for lactation in which the newborn receives all of his or her caloric intake from the breast are an increase of additional 500 kcal per day over that in the nonpregnant state, consisting of an additional 20 g of protein and the rest made up of carbohydrate and fats. The baby consumes more vitamin A, and thus the daily requirement is increased by an additional 1,000 IU. Increases are also suggested for riboflavin, niacin, and thiamine.

DIETARY HISTORY

From the scientific standpoint, diet recall is inadequate to precisely calculate the total caloric intake of an individual. However, it is quite clear that the average diet is nutritionally sound, and physicians should be able to ask their patients what they had for breakfast, lunch, and dinner in the last 24 hours and gain an idea as to whether their diet is within reasonable limits. If it is clear that the patient's dietary habits vary considerably from what the physician knows is the norm in his area, it is suggested that an expert in nutritional dietary evaluation be consulted. Most dietitians are well qualified to estimate the adequacy of any diet and make recommendations for improving its quality within the tastes and limits expressed by the patient and the increased needs of the pregnancy.

Physical examination may also give clues as to dietary deficiency. In the nonpregnant individual the presence of edema may be suggestive of hypoalbuminemia, which may reflect a profound protein deficiency. The presence of edema in the pregnant individual is so universal that this sign of protein deficiency is essentially meaningless. A variety of dermatoses are related to single or combination vitamin deficiencies. Chronic skin conditions that have no obvious explanation suggest a dermatologic consult, with the specific question of dietary insufficiency to be ruled out.

Changes in the normal appearance of the tongue and cracks at the angles of the mouth are suggestive of vitamin deficiency. Glossitis and papillary atrophy (smooth tongue) are characteristic of chronic iron deficiency and are almost invariably associated with anemia.

Serum levels of albumin below 2.5 g per deciliter may be accounted for on the basis of protein malnutrition alone, although usually they are related more significantly to excessive hydremia during pregnancy or preeclampsia or other hypertensive diseases. The normal values of lipids and cholesterol during pregnancy are all elevated, and therefore these tests cannot be used satisfactorily to identify patients with malnutrition in the absence of clear-cut gastrointestinal disease. It should be clear that there is no test of malnutrition or vitamin deficiency that can be used to screen healthy patients. The best screen for malnutrition during pregnancy is inadequate weight gain.

SPECIAL CONSIDERATIONS FOR ADOLESCENTS

Pregnant adolescents have the additional burden of growing themselves along with their babies. As a result, such patients require an increase in the availability of calories as well as of protein and calcium. Dietary counseling should be available for pregnant adolescents, since their understanding of appropriate diets for themselves and their children is likely to be inadequate. Repeated emphasis on the importance of diet in this group is essential.

DIETARY PECULIARITIES

Pregnancy is notorious for its stories of dietary cravings, particularly at odd hours of the day and night. Such cravings have never been explained satisfactorily, but there does not appear to be any straightforward connection with an identifiable dietary or nutritional deficiency in most cases.

Morning sickness or morning nausea occurs in more than 50 percent of pregnancies and can often be relieved by frequent small feedings, keeping food in the stomach and upper small bowel continuously. The physiologic basis for morning sickness is not well understood and therefore the reason for the effectiveness of this dietary intervention is likewise not understood. Frequent eating, however, may result in excessive weight gain during early pregnancy when it is least needed, and which might lead to obesity later on. The best recommendation for the patient using this dietary method of controlling morning nausea is to recommend that she set aside part of what she would normally eat for breakfast and eat it midmorning. Similarly, she should take part of what she was going to eat at the noon meal and reserve it for midafternoon. In this way the total number of calories can remain the same, but the goal of having food in the stomach at all times can be accomplished.

Cravings most often involve fruit and vegetables and occasionally pickles, ice cream, and other foods. Aversion to foods and other substances is nearly as common. Coffee, tea, and cigarette smoking lead the list of aversions. Pregnancy is thus a good time to quit smoking, not only because the cigarettes taste bad but also because of the harmful effects of smoking on the fetus. Craving for nonfoods is called pica. It is reported much less commonly than cravings for specific foods or aversions but is virtually an everyday finding when taking dietary histories in a large prenatal clinic, particularly one serving the poor. In the United States, cravings for clay, chalk, and laundry starch are frequent; sniffing various solvents has been reported, as has ingestion of library paste or other glue. The harmful effects of such substances are not thoroughly understood, but inhalation of industrial solvents has been reported to have harmful and teratogenic effects in early pregnancy. Other pathophysiologic problems produced by pica are fecal inpaction and, when the pica sufferer satisfies all her desires for food by eating starch or clay, profound anemia and poor weight gain are often seen. A nutritional history should accompany the investigation of anemia seen in pregnant women.

DISEASES AFFECTING NUTRITION DURING PREGNANCY

Alcoholism

Alcoholism is becoming a more frequent complication of pregnancy. It not only results in maternal malnutrition and possibly contributes to cirrhosis of the liver but also produces a particular combination of malnutrition and alcoholism in the fetus known as the fetal alcohol syndrome. Alcoholic women should be identified by dietary and substance abuse questions in every pregnancy, and maximum encouragement should be applied to stop or at least reduce alcoholic ingestion during pregnancy with concomitant recommendations for satisfactory nutrition.

Drug Abuse

Substance abuse of all kinds is being seen more frequently today than ever before. The effects of many drugs on pregnancy are not well understood. There is little question that substance abuse is harmful for the mother even if it cannot be identified as being harmful for the fetus. Pregnancy is a good time to identify substance abuse and, taking advantage of the parent's normal desire to have as healthy a baby as possible, to suggest detoxification and treatment as soon as this diagnosis is made.

Caffeine has been identified as a possible contributor to perinatal mortality. The scientific proof of this has not yet been established, but caffeine does readily cross the placenta and may unnaturally stimulate the fetal central nervous system. The effect of such stimulation is not fully understood but is assumed to be harmful.

Lactose Intolerance

Lactose intolerance is common, particularly in black women. It is a genetic abnormality that causes abdominal pain and severe cramps when lactose is eaten. Although not a particularly serious disease, it does force those afflicted with it to avoid milk and milk products because of their lactose constituents. In the absence of milk ingestion, the protein and B complex vitamin sources available in milk must be replaced by either supplementation or, in the case of protein, switching from milk proteins to other animal or vegetable proteins.

Malabsorption Syndromes

Malabsorption syndromes are uncommon during pregnancy and require the supervision of a gastroenterologist to control the disease while maintaining adequate food intake.

Patients who have undergone surgical procedures for weight reduction are increasing in number and many become pregnant. Pregnancy after jejunoileal bypass constitutes a larger and more serious metabolic insult than after gastric stapling or gastric bypass. Patients who continue to lose weight during pregnancy following one of these procedures may have a continuous and unavoidable ketosis, the harmful effects of which have already been discussed. Jejunoileal bypass usually results in potassium and calcium deficiencies. Patients with this problem also suffer from low levels of blood glucose and more than the usual diminution in serum albumin. It is recommended that such patients have supplementation of potasium, calcium, protein, and magnesium. Gastric bypass or stapling creates less significant nutritional abnormalities during pregnancy, and most pregnancies following these procedures have been reported to have had appropriate outcomes. The precautions against continuous ketosis have already been mentioned; additional protein and vitamin supplementation would also seem to be appropriate.

SUGGESTED READING

Arneil GC, Metcoff J. Pediatric nutrition. London: Butterworth, 1985:56.

Committee on Maternal Nutrition. Maternal nutrition and the course of pregnancy. Washington, DC: National Academy of Sciences, 1970.

Halperns L. Quick reference to clinical nutrition. Philadelphia: JB Lippincott, 1979.

Hytten FA, Chamberlain G. Clinical physiology in obstetrics. Oxford: Blackwell, 1980.

Metcoff J, et al. Effect of food supplementation (WIC) during pregnancy on birth weight. Am J Clin Nutr 1985; 41:933–947.

PARENTERAL AND ENTERAL NUTRITION IN PREGNANCY

JOAN V. EGGERT, R.D., M.P.H., M.D.
WILLIAM F. RAYBURN, M.D.
ROBERT A. WOLK, Pharm.D.

Most pregnancies are uncomplicated and require no more than a diet consisting of a sufficient caloric intake and a proper balance of nutrients. Any additional nutritional support ranges from supplementing with one or more specific nutrients to supplying the entire nutritional needs through total enteral or parenteral nutrition. Nutrients have traditionally been divided into six categories: protein, carbohydrates, fats, vitamins, minerals (electrolytes and trace minerals), and fluids. Supplemental nutritional products may contain any or all of these components.

This chapter is intended to provide an overview for the management of pregnant women who require nutritional support. These pregnancies are complicated by conditions that involve increased metabolic needs, decreased absorption, or mechanical problems with food intake. Table 1 lists specific conditions within each diagnostic category. None is unique to pregnancy, but may have detrimental effects on both the mother and the fetus.

BACKGROUND

Although the use of total enteral nutrition (TEN), including nasogastric or gastrostomy tube feeding, is a long-established mode of therapy, there are no recent reports of its long-term use during pregnancy. This may be on account of under-reporting. Since the establishment of dietetics as a specialty in the early 1900s, diet therapy manuals have contained elaborate formulas for blenderized and strained enteral feedings. Most were based on a balanced diet and contained liver, milk, potatoes, fruits, and vegetables. Since the late 1960s, more refined products, which contain lactose-free casein hydrolysate, soy proteins, corn syrup, and corn and soybean oil, have become the industry standard. We have recently used tube feedings in a pregnant schizophrenic patient who was semi-catatonic from the tenth week of gestation until delivery at term. She delivered an appropriate-for-gestational-age (AGA) term infant who is breast feeding and thriving. The mother still refuses to swallow food and inserts her own nasogastric tube three times daily in order to feed herself.

A parenteral solution, which consisted of hypertonic protein hydrolysate and glucose, was first used by Dudrick et al in 1968 to correct nutritional deficiencies in adult humans. The first report of total parenteral nutrition (TPN) during pregnancy was in 1972. A woman with anorexia nervosa at 26-weeks gestation received 3,000 kcal per day for 10 days. Forty-two reports of pregnant patients who received total parenteral nutrition have since appeared in the literature between 1972 and 1986. Most studies involved one patient, and the duration of therapy ranged from 5 to 365 (postpartum included) days. These persons usually had a gastrointestinal problem such as pancreatitis, ileus formation, malabsorption, or intestinal resection that precluded oral intake. A few patients had pregnancies that were complicated by terminal cancer, anorexia nervosa, or hyperemesis gravidarum. The majority had central venous catheters, although peripheral hyperalimentation was provided when therapy was expected to be short-term. Most infants at birth were appropriately sized. In the few cases where the infant was small, intrauterine growth retardation had been apparent before the start of hyperalimentation.

ASSESSMENT OF MALNUTRITION

A detailed nutritional assessment that is used to identify hospitalized patients at risk for nutritional depletion was developed in the late 1960s and early 1970s by Dudrick and Blackburn. This model not only identifies patients with nutritional deficiencies, but also those at risk for developing problems unless there is intervention.

This technique, which has been adapted for pregnancy, is shown in Table 2. Nutritional deprivation may be characterized as mild, moderate, or severe according to this scoring system. Physical findings may also reflect protein-calorie deficiency or specific deficiencies of various vitamins or minerals. Physical findings indicative of nutritional deficiencies are listed in Table 3.

NUTRITIONAL REQUIREMENTS DURING PREGNANCY

Proper replacement of deficient nutrients requires a knowledge of normal daily requirements. Table 4 is a version of the 1980 Recommended Daily Allowances (RDAs) published by the National Research Council, which has been modified to reflect the nutritional needs of pregnant women. The individual daily needs should reflect the RDA; additional nutritional requirements should be judged according to the type of underlying complication.

The requirements for additional nutrients in pregnancy have been calculated by two different experimental techniques. Nutritional balance studies have been performed for some, but not all, nutrients. Thus, the intake required to keep women in positive balance may easily be calculated for these nutrients. The second technique involves an animal model. Either concentrations of the nutrient are determined in maternal and fetal blood, or isotopic-labeled compounds are used to calculate fetal nutrient needs.

Several factors affect placental nutrient exchange; these include concentration differences, exchange area, thickness of the placenta, and chemical properties (lipid solubilities, degree of ionization, and molecular configuration) of the transported nutrients. Fatty acids, steroids, electrolytes, and fat soluble vitamins are transported by passive diffusion. Sugars are transported by facilitated diffusion. Amino acids, water soluble vitamins, and some

TABLE 1 Major Conditions that Require Nutritional Support

Increased Metabolic Needs	*Decreased Absorption*	*Inability to Swallow*
Trauma	Crohn's disease, ulcerative colitis	Esophageal or other stricture
Major burns	Short gut syndrome, intestinal bypass	Diabetic neuropathy
Cancer	Bowel surgery	Dental, "wired jaw"
Fever, systemic infection	Obstructive jaundice, pancreatitis	Psychiatric
	Cirrhosis, renal failure	Unconsciousness

TABLE 2 Nutritional Assessment for Degree of Severity

Factors	*Column 1**	*Column 2†*	*Column 3††*
Number of days intake <1,200 kcal	<5	5–10	>10
Number of additional days intake will be <1,200	<3	3–7	>7
Weight/height (% of standard)	>90%	60–90%	<60%
Prepregnancy weight lost	<10%	10–20%	>20%
Total lymphocyte count	>1,500	1,200–1,500	<1,200
Serum albumin	>3	2.5–3.0	<2.5
Serum transferrin	>300	200–300	<200
Anthropometrics (TSK, MUAC, MUAMC)§	>90%	60–90%	<60%
Ketonuria	Trace	Moderate	Large
Fetal body dimensions:	Within	Lagging by	
(Ultrasound compared to dates)	2 wk	2–3 wk	>3 wk

* Mild: If most values are in column 1, this patient has mild nutritional depletion. A nutritional consultation and supplemental products or improved diet are recommended.
† Moderate: If >4 risk factors are in column 2, this patient has moderate nutritional depletion and needs an immediate nutritional evaluation and decision as to whether enteral nutrition would be tolerated. Complete enteral or parenteral nutrition needs to be started promptly.
†† Severe: If >4 risk factors are in column 3, this patient has severe nutritional depletion and needs immediate nutritional evaluation and placement of an intravenous line because of the often profound mineral and electrolyte disturbances seen with this. Peripheral alimentation should be started while a decision is being made to place either a central line or enteral feeding catheter and while nutrition is being advanced via these routes to full strength.
§ TSK=Triceps skinfold
MUAC=Mid-upper arm circumference
MUAMC=Mid-upper arm muscle circumference
Adapted from Blackburn GL, et al. Nutrition and metabolic assessment of the hospitalized patient. JPEN 1977; 1:11–22.

TABLE 3 Physical Findings Associated with Malnutrition

Deficiency	*Physical Findings*
Protein-calorie	Dependent edema; hair dull, dry, color change, pluckable; weight loss; poor muscle mass; skin with blotchy pigmentation.
Essential fatty acids	Skin dry, flaky (hyperkeratosis); hair loss.
Vitamin A	Bitot's spots; dry membranes; soft, dull cornea (conjunctival and corneal xerosis and keratomalacia).
Vitamin E	Anemia unresponsive to therapy.
Vitamin K	Bruising; bleeding; abruptio placenta.
Vitamin D	Rickets; pathological fractures; epiphyseal swelling.
Thiamine (B_1)	Cardiomegaly; wrist and foot drop; encephalopathy; polyneuropathy.
Riboflavin (B_2)	Cheilosis; angular fissures of mouth or eyes; magenta color tongue.
Niacin	Pellagra (exposed skin dermatitis); red, swollen tongue.
B_6, B_{12}	Both: Peripheral neuropathy. B_{12}: megaloblastic anemia; tongue may be either red and swollen or pale and slick; skin has pallor.
Vitamin C	Bleeding gums; fragile capillaries; petechiae; rickets (interacts with copper).
Iron	Spoon-shaped, brittle nails; pale skin and mucous membranes.
Zinc	Dermatitis around mouth, perineum, elbows and knees; anorexia; dysgeusia; hair loss.
Copper	Triad of rickets, anemia, neutropenia.
Folic acid	Megaloblastic anemia; red, painful tongue; generalized skin hyperpigmentation.

TABLE 4 Recommended Daily Allowances (RDA) During Pregnancy

	*Recommended Amount**	*Additional For Pregnancy*
Energy (kcal)	2,000	+300
Protein (g)	44	+30
Vitamin A (μg)	800	+200
Vitamin D (μg)	7.5	+5
Vitamin E (mg)	8	+2
Vitamin C (mg)	60	+20
Folic acid (μg)	400	+400
Niacin (mg)	13	+2
Riboflavin (mg)	1.2	+0.3
Thiamine (mg)	1	+0.4
Vitamin B_6 (mg)	2	+0.6
Vitamin B_{12} (μg)	3	+1
Calcium (mEq)	40	+20
Iron (mg)	18	+3
Zinc (mg)	15	+5
Phosphorus (mM)	26–39	+13
Magnesium (mEq)	25	+12.5
Iodine (μg)	150	+25

* Nonpregnant women, age 19 or older
Adapted from National Research Council, 1980

minerals, such as calcium (Ca), iron (Fe), iodine (I), and phosphorus (P), are transported by active transport, and some electrolytes are transported by solvent drag. While it is not known if the human fetus handles nutrients by these exact mechanisms, these experiments serve as a beginning model for understanding the maternal-fetal nutrient requirements.

Energy

Caloric intake should be designed to achieve a total weight gain of 10 to 12 kg (22 to 27 pounds) during pregnancy. A gain of 1 to 2 kg in the first trimester and an average gain of 0.4 kg per week are desired for the second and third trimesters. The additional 300 kcal per day RDA is inadequate to achieve appropriate weight gain during periods of increased physiologic stress or trauma.

Daily caloric needs may be calculated by using the Harris-Benedict equation for women to determine the basal metabolic rate (BMR):

$$BMR = 655 + 9.563\,(W) + 1.75\,(H) - 4.676\,(A)$$
W=weight in kg, H=height in cm, A=age in years

and by multiplying this by factors listed below, which reflect the increased needs.

Bedrest	1.2	Ambulatory	1.3
Major surgery	1.2	Trauma, fracture	1.3
$>$20 percent burn	2.0	Severe infection	1.7
Fever $>38.3^{0}$ C	1.0 to 1.5		

Carbohydrate

Oral carbohydrate sources provide 4 kcal per gram. Enteral products contain glucose polymers, sucrose, corn syrup, and corn starch. They are formulated to contain from 40 to 90 percent of kcal as carbohydrate.

Dextrose at 3.4 kcal per gram is the carbohydrate source in parenteral nutrition. Up to 10 percent dextrose concentrations may be used peripherally, while a 20 to 50 percent concentration may be used only when administered centrally. The total amount of infused dextrose is usually limited by liver utilization, which is 0.4 to 1.2 g per kilogram per hour. A 70 kg pregnant woman can typically tolerate 400 to 900 g of glucose a day. Hyperglycemia may result from dextrose infusion, but this is transitory, and insulin is usually not required. Daily blood glucose monitoring and the addition of insulin if blood glucose levels are consistently above 120 mg per deciliter are recommended for the patient who receives nutritional supplementation (parenteral or enteral) during pregnancy.

Fat

There is no specific RDA for fat. The fat in enteral products provides 9 kcal per gram, and ranges from 1 to 48 percent of the total kcal. Most complete enteral formulas (except the elemental ones) contain adequate amounts of essential fatty acids. Enteral fat sources usually include corn, safflower, soybean, and medium-chain-triglyceride (MCT) oil. MCT oil is also available separately.

Essential fatty acid deficiency in the patient who is receiving TPN is usually prevented by use of a 10 or 20 percent intravenous soybean fat emulsion twice weekly. Because of their isotonicity, intravenous fat emulsions are often used to provide a significant portion of calorie needs. Fat emulsions may be used to provide up to 40 percent of kcal (no more than 3.5 g per kilogram per day) in total parenteral nutrition during pregnancy. The 10 percent fat emulsion provides 550 kcal per 500 ml, whereas the 20 percent emulsion contains 1,000 kcal per 500 ml.

The amount of tolerable fat may be evaluated by serum triglyceride levels. Elevated bilirubin and liver enzyme levels may indicate that caloric intake is too high and needs to be reduced. Either the fat emulsion (if triglycerides are elevated) or the dextrose content should be decreased if enzyme changes are not transient. Fatty infiltration of the placenta in women with endogenous hyperlipidemia has been reported, but there are no accurate reports of this occurring with intravenous fat emulsions in pregnant patients who are receiving TPN.

Protein

The RDA for protein is 0.8 g per kilogram with an additional 30 g per day for pregnancy. Hypermetabolic states, such as severe burns and trauma, may increase protein needs to as much as 2.0 g per kilogram per day. No definitive studies exist concerning the amino acid profile recommended during pregnancy. Most complete enteral formulas contain a significant amount of protein from high biologic value sources such as calcium caseinate and soy proteins. Usual protein sources for enteral products include hydrolyzed whey, meat, and egg white proteins. Protein content varies from 2.6 to 8.4 g per deciliter, providing 10 to 35 percent of total kcal.

A nitrogen:kcal ratio of 1:150 to 1:300 in parenteral formulas has resulted in the best utilization of both nitrogen and calorie sources in the nonpregnant adult. Most currently used parenteral formulas contain protein derived from synthetic free amino acids, which contain approximately 60 percent of the nitrogen contained in essential amino acids.

Minerals

No RDAs exist for sodium, potassium, and chloride because the typical diet contains adequate amounts and the person with functioning kidneys can adapt to a wide range of intake. The amounts of these electrolytes that are added to enteral and parenteral products are usually based on results of balance studies and clinical experience in nonpregnant patients. These amounts would need to be restricted in patients with renal or liver disease and increased with excessive gastrointestinal losses.

Amounts in enteral products are variable, and individual product literature should be consulted. Usual amounts of sodium, potassium, and chloride in TPN are listed in the section on guidelines for ordering total parenteral nutrition. These guidelines are general since exact ordering procedures often vary from institution to institution.

RDAs have been established during pregnancy for calcium, iron, phosphorus, magnesium, and iodine (see Table 4). Most complete enteral products (except the elemental formulas) are formulated such that about 2,000 kcal per day meets 100 percent of the RDA for calcium, iron, phosphorus, magnesium, and iodine for a nonpregnant female. Additional iron supplementation may be needed for long-term total enteral nutrition use in pregnancy. Because bioavailability of minerals is 100 percent when given intravenously and only 30 percent with oral intake, intravenous requirements are considerably less than that of the RDAs, which are based on oral intake. Guidelines for intravenous electrolyte, macro, and trace mineral administration are provided in the section on guidelines for total parenteral nutrition.

The amount of calcium in standard parenteral electrolyte additives may not be sufficient for pregnancy. An additional 4.5 mEq of calcium gluconate and phosphorus (10 to 20 mmol) per day is recommended. Iodine may be necessary, although adequate amounts seem to be provided through solution contamination and dressing changes with iodine products.

An average of 3 mg per day of intravenous elemental iron is needed for the anemic pregnant patient who is receiving TPN. Although intravenous use of iron-dextran is contraindicated by the manufacturer, several clinicians have used 20 mg per week for anemic patients. Test for allergic reaction before use by giving an intravenous test dose of 0.5 ml in 50 to 100 ml of normal saline, infused over a 1- to 2-hour period. Patients who receive iron-dextran should receive no more than 100 mg per day and should be followed closely.

Trace Minerals

Zinc and copper are the only trace minerals that have been well studied during pregnancy. Recommendations for enteral and parenteral supplementation are based on data from nonpregnant adults. Most enteral formulas do not contain adequate amounts of zinc or copper for long-term use during pregnancy. Furthermore, all parenteral formulas should have a trace mineral package added once daily. An additional 2 to 4 mg per day of zinc may also be needed. Recommended supplemental amounts are listed on the total enteral and total parenteral nutrition worksheets (see Table 5 and section on guidelines for ordering total parenteral nutrition).

Vitamins

RDAs have been established for all the essential vitamins. Most complete enteral formulas meet the daily requirements, if 2,000 kcal per day are consumed. A possible exception would be folic acid. A daily prenatal vitamin or supplemental folic acid tablet should be crushed and added to the enteral formula for patients with exceptional losses or a poor preconception diet.

Multivitamin parenteral preparations (such as MVI-12) meet the needs for pregnancy and should be added to parenteral formulas (see section on guidelines for ordering total parenteral nutrition). Vitamin K (Aquamephyton [R MSD]) may be given intravenously or subcutaneously either daily (1 mg) or weekly (5 to 10 mg). The patient needs to be monitored for any clinical signs of vitamin deficiency (see Table 2), and serum vitamin levels should be ordered if indicated clinically.

TABLE 5 Worksheet for Complete Enteral Nutrition During Pregnancy

Desired total fluids = 3,000 ml (or as calculated)
Kcal = 2,300 (or as calculated)
Select formula, and calculate ml to provide 2,300 kcal
Calculate total protein in 2,300 kcal of selected formula
Calculate total folic acid, Ca, Fe, Zn in selected formula
Add 1 crushed prenatal vitamin/day and calculate the folic acid, Ca, Fe, and Zn it provides.
Examine patient needs:
  Does this patient need a concentrated formula (>1 kcal per milliliter), or is a high nitrogen protein formula needed?
  How much additional folic acid, Ca, Fe, and Zn are needed?
Add in any modular products (such as MCT oil or glucose polymers) needed for extra fat, carbohydrate, or protein.

TABLE 5A Sample Calculation for Complete Enteral Nutrition

	Amount (ml)	*Kcal*	*Protein (g)*	*Folic Acid (μg)*	*Calcium (mg)*	*Iron (mg)*	*Zinc (mg)*
Osmolyte	2,300	2,300	85	957	1,197	21	27
Materna 1/60	1 tablet			1,000	250	60	25
Total	2,300	2,300	85	1,957	1,447	81	52

Monitoring Parameters:
  Daily weights, intake, output, and bedside clinical assessment.
  Initial and weekly anthropometrics (triceps skinfold, mid-upper arm circumference, and mid-upper arm muscle circumference).

TABLE 5B Laboratory Tests for Monitoring Complete Enteral Nutrition

	Initially	*At 1 Week*	*Monthly*
Complete blood count	x	x	x
24-hr urine, urinary nitrogen excretion (UUN)	x	x	x
Chemistries*	x	x	x
Transferrin, PT/PTT, ferritin	x		x

* Na, K, Cl, HCO_3, BUN, creatinine, Ca, PO_4, Mg, protein, albumin, SGOT, SGPT, LDH, alkaline, phosphate, bilirubin, glucose.

Guidelines

Guidelines for ordering total parenteral nutrition follow:

1. Energy requirements should be calculated using the Harris-Benedict equation, plus stress-activity factor, plus 300 kcal.
2. Calculate protein as 0.8 g per kilogram ideal body weight, plus 30 g.
3. Determine TPN formulation of amino acids and fat emulsion as follows:

   Amino acids:
   4.25% amino acids + 25% dextrose per liter = 42.5 g protein and 1,000 kcal per liter

   2.5% amino acids + 10% dextrose per liter = 25 g protein and 880 kcal per liter

   Fat emulsion:
   10% = 550 kcal per 500 ml bottle
   20% = 1,000 kcal per 500 ml bottle
4. Maintenance fluid formulation:
   100 ml per kilogram for the first 10 kg,
   plus 50 ml per kilogram for the next 10 kg (or fraction of),
   plus 20 ml per kilogram for the remaining kg of weight

   Patients may tolerate more fluid than this, and those with additional losses, such as ostomy or nasogastric, need specific fluid and electrolyte replacement. If TPN supplies less than maintenance fluids, additional fluids should be added.
5. Recommended daily requirements of electrolytes are as follows:

Calcium	10–15	mEq
Magnesium	8–24	mEq
Potassium	90–240	mEq
Sodium	60–150	mEq
Acetate	80–120	mEq
Chloride	60–150	mEq
Phosphorus	20–40	mM

   Amino acid solutions (i.e., calcium and phosphorus) contain varying amounts; thus, product information should be consulted. In addition, with potassium, chloride, and phosphorus higher amounts may precipitate.

6. Vitamin K should be added as follows: 5 to 10 mg per week or 1 mg per day subcutaneously or intravenously.
7. One unit dose of multivitamins should be added per day. A typical package contains the following:

Vitamin C	100 mg
Vitamin A	1 mg (3,300 IU)
Vitamin D	5 mg (200 IU)
Vitamin B_1	3 mg
Vitamin B_2	3.6 mg
Vitamin B_{12}	5 μg
Niacin	40 mg
Pantothenic acid	15 mg
Vitamin E (10 IU)	10 mg
Biotin	60 μg
Folic acid	400 μg

8. Trace elements should follow FDA guidelines (in parentheses); a typical package contains the following:

zinc (5.0 mg)	2.5–4.0 mg
copper (1.0 mg)	0.5–1.5 mg
manganese (0.5 mg)	0.15–0.8 mg
chromium (10.0 μg)	10.0–15.0 μg

Some packages also contain selenium, which may be required.

9. Individual elements are added as indicated below:
   Iodine (see text for guidelines)
   Iron dextran (see text for guidelines)
   Heparin 1 U per milliliter
10. Parameters that require monitoring are as follows: daily weights, intake and output, daily bedside clinical assessment. In addition, monitor the patient's initial and weekly anthropometrics (abdominal measurement is not useful in pregnancy, but triceps skinfold, mid-upper arm circumference, and mid-upper arm muscle circumference may be useful).
11. Laboratory tests are indicated in Table 6.

MODE OF SUPPLEMENTATION

A golden rule of nutrition has been, "if the gut works, use it!" A motivated patient with a functional gastrointestinal tract and who is at risk for malnutrition may avoid parenteral support by the early addition of palatable supplements. Patients with a minimum of functional bowel who cannot or will not ingest adequate nutrients may benefit from partial or complete enteral support through a nasogastric tube or percutaneous gastrostomy tube. Partial enteral support may be useful when the patient can take part, but not all, of the required calories orally. An example of this would be the burn or trauma patient who is able to eat regular meals, but who requires tube feeding at night to achieve the desired 3,000 to 6,000 kcal per day intake.

Total enteral support has the advantages of significantly less cost than parenteral support and a negligible risk of sepsis, metabolic, and technical problems. A liter of our commonly used enteral feeding product costs $2.46 at our institution and 1,000 ml of an amino acid-dextrose TPN solution (including electrolytes, vitamins, and minerals) costs $99.00. Administration and equipment costs are additional.

Most third-party payers, including Medicaid, reimburse for partial or complete nutrition supplementation if this is ordered by the physician. Diagnosis-related groups (DRG) may not cover the cost of providing total parenteral nutrition. We have also had good experience with third-party payers reimbursing costs of total enteral or parenteral nutrition in the home, and several good home hyperalimentation services are available in most communities.

There are no enteral products manufactured exclusively for use during pregnancy. In selecting an enteral product, the same guidelines should be used whether or not the patient is pregnant. We usually prescribe the lactose-free, palatable formulas (such as Ensure or Sustacal) for the patient who is able to take oral supplementation, and the isotonic, lactose-free formulas (such as Osmolyte or Isocal) for the patient who is receiving nasogastric or jejunostomy-gastrostomy feedings. Figure 1 illustrates an algorithm for product selection used at our medical center. A list of representative products and their ingredients is shown in Table 7. It should be emphasized that no product meets the needs of pregnancy without extra supplementation. Total dietary replacements with these products alone are inadequate for prolonged use,

TABLE 6 Laboratory Tests for Monitoring Total Parenteral Nutrition

	Initially	*At 1 Week*	*Weekly*	*Monthly*
Complete blood count	x	x	x 1 month	x
Chemistries*	x	x	x 1 month	x
24-hr urine, urinary nitrogen excretion (UUN)	x	x	until +	x
Transferrin	x			x
PT/PTT	x			x
Ferritin	x			x
Triglycerides	x	x	x 1 month	x

* Na, K, Cl, HCO_3, BUN, creatinine, Ca, PO_4, Mg, protein, albumin, SGOT, SGPT, LDH, alkaline, phosphatase, bilirubin, glucose

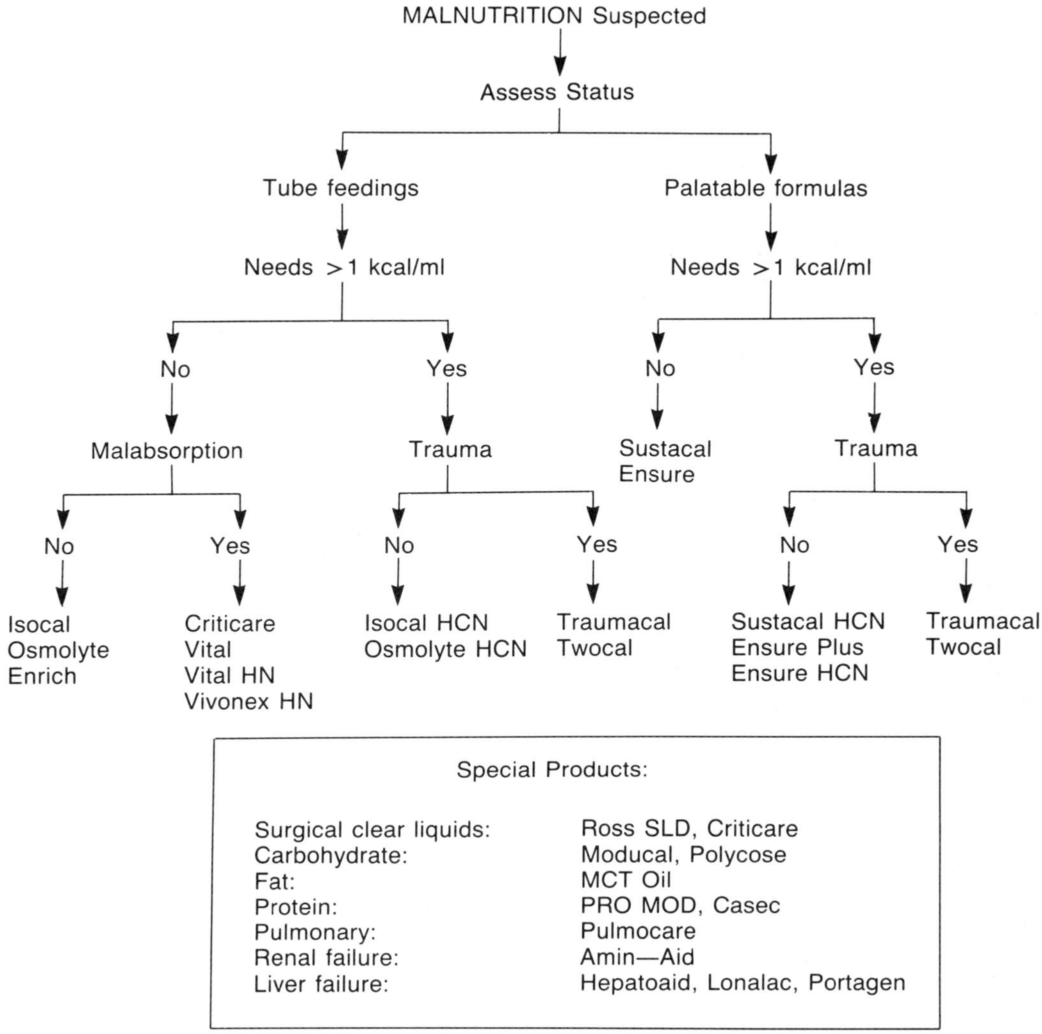

Figure 1 Choosing an enteral product.

TABLE 7 Nutritional Content of Enteral Products

Product	Kcal/ml	Protein (g/100 ml)	Carbohydrate (g/100 ml)	Fat (g/100 ml)	Folic Acid (μg)	Calcium (mg/100 ml)	Iron (mg/100 ml)	Zinc (mg/100 ml)
Criticare	1.0	3.8	22	0.3	21	53	0.9	1.0
Enrich	1.1	3.9	16	3.7	43	71	1.3	1.6
Ensure	1.0	3.7	14	3.7	21	52	0.9	1.2
Ensure HN	1.0	4.4	14	3.5	45	75	1.3	1.6
Ensure +	1.5	5.5	20	5.3	56	71	1.3	1.2
Ensure +HN	1.5	6.3	20	4.9	84	104	1.9	2.3
Isocal	1.0	3.4	13	4.4	21	63	0.9	1.0
Isocal HCN	2.0	7.5	20	10.2	42	100	1.9	3.0
Osmolite	1.0	3.7	14	3.8	42	52	0.9	1.2
Osmolite HN	1.0	4.4	14	3.7	45	75	1.3	1.6
Pulmocare	1.5	6.3	10	9.2	83	104	1.9	2.3
Ross SLD	0.7	3.7	13	0.5	50	84	1.5	1.9
Sustacal HC	1.5	6.1	19	5.8	37	101	1.7	1.4
Sustacal	1.0	6.1	14	2.3	51	85	1.5	1.3
Traumacal	1.5	8.3	14	6.8	20	75	0.9	1.5
Twocal	2.0	8.4	22	9.0	67	104	1.9	2.3
Vital HN	1.0	4.2	18	11.0	53	63	1.3	1.5
Vivonex	1.0	2.6	23	1.5	2	5	1.0	0.8
Vivonex HN	1.0	4.4	20	<0.1	<1	3	0.6	0.5

and supplementation with extra vitamins and minerals is recommended for pregnancy.

When tube feedings are used, we prefer continuous feedings, using one of the enteral feeding pumps. A 50 percent concentration is started at 75 ml per hour, increasing gradually to a 100 percent concentration at 95 ml per hour (to provide 2,300 kcal per day)(see Table 5).

Total parenteral nutrition may be the best alternative for the pregnant patient with either nonfunctioning bowel, severe malnourishment, or mechanical problems with tube feedings. For long-term use (2 weeks or more), a central subclavian or internal jugular line, rather than peripheral administration, is recommended. A baseline nutritional assessment is important to determine the patient's requirements for parenteral supplementation. Total calorie and protein needs should be calculated initially. Next, the maintenance fluid required is calculated, which may dictate the protein and carbohydrate concentrations used. Attention is then paid to the needs for electrolytes, vitamins, and trace minerals in a stepwise fashion.

The use of standardized solutions may streamline this process and should be utilized when applicable. Most clinicians start at a slow rate of 40 to 50 ml per hour of the desired solution the first day and increase by 40 to 50 ml per hour per day until the desired requirements are met. This usually takes 2 to 3 days and minimizes fluid and glucose complications. Intravenous fat emulsion may be started at 500 ml of 10 percent lipid per day and increased as tolerated, based on triglyceride levels and need, to a 20 percent solution.

Heparin is commonly added to TPN at 1 U per milliliter in order to minimize fibrin sheath formation and reduce phlebitis. Coagulopathies are rarely, if ever, seen at this low dose (see section on guidelines for ordering total parenteral nutrition).

COMPLICATIONS

Complications of total enteral or parenteral nutrition may be grouped into three broad categories: (1) metabolic, (2) infection, and (3) mechanical.

Metabolic complications are usually the result of too much or too little of a nutrient. Whereas any of these metabolic complications can be seen in the patient who is receiving total enteral nutrition, they are more likely to be seen in the patient on total parenteral nutrition. Patients on TEN are usually less critically ill, and the still-functioning gut can modulate absorption of nutrients to some extent.

Hyperglycemia is the most common metabolic complication in TPN, particularly during the first few days of therapy before endogenous insulin secretion rises. Insulin is required only if glucose levels are consistently elevated. A starting dose of 10 U of regular insulin per liter of amino acid-dextrose solution may be used and adjusted as needed. Hyperkalemia may result from tissue catabolism, decreased renal function, and sepsis. Deteriorating renal function has been reported in pregnant diabetic patients receiving TPN who have had prior renal impairment. Close monitoring of this group of patients is recommended. Both elevated and low serum levels of calcium, magnesium, and phosphorus have been reported, usually within the initial days of starting TPN.

Elevated liver enzymes occur commonly with TPN. Those enzymes usually peak about 2 weeks into therapy, remain transiently elevated for the next 2 to 3 weeks, and then resolve on their own. Liver enzymes occasionally increase, continue to rise, and remain elevated. Overfeeding is the most common cause in adults. Caloric requirements should be recalculated and adjusted downward. Elevated triglyceride levels may occur with elevated liver enzyme levels; this suggests cholestasis. Ultrasonography may be helpful in the diagnosis, and the fat emulsion should be reduced until triglyceride levels return to normal.

Increased carbon dioxide load may be a problem in women with severe pulmonary compromise. Decrease the amount of carbohydrate infused, and increase lipids to provide the equivalent calories in order to minimize the carbon dioxide load.

No infectious complications have been reported in pregnant patients who receive TEN. Bacterial gastroenteritis and diarrhea have been reported in nonpregnant patients on TEN. New closed-delivery systems and improved handling and sterilization techniques have greatly reduced the incidence of bacterial contamination of enteral solutions.

Infectious complications from TPN include catheter site infection, catheter infection, or generalized bacterial or fungal sepsis. One patient with candida sepsis and one patient with a catheter infection have been reported in the report of 44 pregnant patients who received TPN. Meticulous attention to catheter insertion, catheter care, and sterile technique, and early recognition of infection should minimize catheter infection or generalized sepsis.

Mechanical problems during total enteral nutrition include aspiration from nasogastric tubes not placed deep enough or vomiting that may be resolved by placement of the tube in the jejunum rather than in the stomach. Nasogastric tubes may also clog if not flushed regularly or if too concentrated solutions are used. Nasogastric tube placement should be verified either by radiography or by clinical assessment.

Mechanical complications in patients who receive total parenteral nutrition usually relate to catheter placement, with mediastinal hemorrhage reported in a pregnant patient on TPN. Other complications may include puncture of a nearby artery, air embolism, or pneumothorax. All central TPN catheters must be verified by radiography to ensure that they are in the correct location and have not caused a pneumothorax.

MONITORING

Daily clinical assessment for any patient who requires nutritional supplementation should include a detailed physical examination. Table 3 lists physical findings associated with malnutrition. Monitoring may also be broken down into the six basic nutrient components: fluids, energy, protein, minerals (electrolytes and trace minerals), and vitamins. Specific tests and recommended testing frequency are listed in Table 5 and in the preceding section on guidelines for ordering parenteral nutrition.

The frequency of testing varies according to the patient's clinical status and stability. Because the intestinal tract is still capable of adapting to nutritional needs by altering absorption of nutrients, patients on enteral nutrition do not need as frequent testing as those receiving total parenteral nutrition (see Table 5B).

An important component of monitoring during pregnancy is fetal growth assessment. Ultrasonography evaluations should be performed every 3 to 4 weeks to make sure the fetus is growing appropriately, but not excessively. Measurement of various body dimensions (biparietal diameter, abdominal circumference, and femur length) and estimation of fetal weight may be performed.

DISCONTINUING TOTAL NUTRITIONAL SUPPORT

Enteral feedings should be encouraged while the patient is requiring total enteral or parenteral support as long as there is not an ileus or other contraindication to using the bowel. This helps to prevent cholestasis and also facilitate gradually increasing calories as enteral feeding becomes tolerated.

When the patient is consistently taking 50 percent or more of calories by mouth, the total enteral feeding may be reduced. The nasogastric tube is discontinued so that they can eat solids more comfortably, but replaced if they are unable, over the next few days, to take in adequate calories.

Because of the hypoglycemia that results from abrupt discontinuation of concentrated intravenous dextrose solutions, withdrawal should be tapered over 2 to 3 days, and frequent blood glucose levels should be ordered. The rate is usually decreased by 40 to 50 ml per hour the first day, in a reverse of the starting stepwise titration. Capillary blood glucoses should be obtained every hour until stable, then every 6 hours. Values less than 140 mg percent and greater than 60 mg percent are desired. On the second day, the rate is decreased by another 40 to 50 ml per hour, and blood glucose levels are followed similarly. When the TPN is completely weaned, 10 percent dextrose may be infused for 4 to 8 hours at a to-keep-open rate. Some patients, who have been on TPN for only a few days, may be tapered faster.

SUGGESTED READING

Catanzarite VA, Argubright K, Mann BA, Brittain VL. Malnutrition during pregnancy? Consider parenteral feeding. Contemp Obstet Gynecol 1986:110–130.

Lee RV, Rodgers BD, Young C, Eddy E, Cardinal J. Total parenteral nutrition during pregnancy. Obstet Gynecol 1986; 68:563–571.

Pitkin RM. Assessment of nutritional status of mother, fetus, and newborn. Am J Clin Nutr 1981; 34:658–668.

Rayburn WF, Wolk R, Mercer N, Roberts J. Parenteral nutrition in obstetrics and gynecology. Obstet Gynecol Surv 1986; 41:200–214.

AMNIOTIC FLUID TESTS OF FETAL MATURITY

WILLIAM N. P. HERBERT, M.D.

Prematurity is the leading cause of neonatal morbidity and mortality. Each year in the United States, approximately 40,000 newborns develop respiratory distress syndrome (RDS) owing to surfactant deficiency. About one-quarter of these infants die, and a significant number of the survivors have long-term sequelae, particularly chronic pulmonary problems. Whenever possible, delay in delivery until the fetus is mature is certainly beneficial. A number of tests to determine fetal maturity are available, and appropriate use of these tests can help minimize the problem of RDS in newborns.

After a brief discussion of fetal pulmonary development, several of the available amniotic fluid tests of fetal maturity are discussed. Reliability of these tests, performed both singly and in combination, is reviewed. Using clinical and economic considerations, a testing strategy can be developed that provides the most clinically useful information in the shortest amount of time using laboratory personnel most effectively.

BACKGROUND

Lung Development

Development of the fetal lung begins about 3 weeks after conception and is not complete until well after birth. Mammalian pulmonary development occurs in three distinct stages. In the *glandular period*, which lasts until the 16th week of gestation, the pulmonary tree develops. Proliferating buds of endodermal cells extend into the surrounding loose mesenchymal tissue. During the *canalicular period*, which extends from 16 to 24 weeks, early bronchioles develop from endodermal tissue, epithelial cells begin to differentiate, and epithelial vascularization occurs. The *alveolar* (*or terminal sac*) *period* begins at about 24 weeks and continues into childhood. Further bronchiolar division leads to the presence of thin saccules known as alveoli. Capillaries proliferate around these terminal air spaces beginning at about 26 weeks, making effective gaseous transfer possible.

The respiratory epithelium is composed of two cell lines, simply known as type I and type II cells. Type I cells are flat and have no known function other than alveolar support. Type II cells are larger, more ovoid-shaped cells that lie between individual alveoli. Within these cells phospholipids promoting pulmonary maturity are synthesized and stored.

Background of Pulmonary Physics

Since alveoli are spherical in shape, physical laws of pressure within spheres apply. The *law of La Place* states that the pressure within a sphere is directly related to its surface tension and inversely related to the radius, i.e., at the same surface tension, the smaller the sphere, the higher the pressure within it. Applying this concept to the lung, in the absence of other factors, the pressure within smaller alveoli would be greater than that within larger ones. As a result, a net transfer of gas would occur from smaller into larger alveoli, causing collapse of the smaller alveolar sacs. Overall gaseous exchange would obviously be impaired. With a mature pulmonary system, these events do not occur because a group of compounds, collectively known as *surfactant*, line the alveoli and lower surface tension. As a result, alveoli of all sizes remain patent, allowing for adequate gaseous exchange after birth.

Surfactant

Surfactant is the name given to the group of "surface-active" or detergent compounds that lower surface tension within the alveolar spaces. Lipids, protein, and carbohydrates are present in surfactant, but lipids constitute 90 percent of its composition. In turn, 90 percent of the lipids are phospholipids, primarily phosphatidylcholine (lecithin), 70 percent of the total; phosphatidylglycerol (PG), about 10 to 15 percent; phosphatidylinositol (PI), about 5 to 10 percent; and other components, 5 to 15 percent. Often included in this list is sphingomyelin, which also has surface tension-lowering properties, but this compound is actually a sphingolipid. Its origin within the pulmonary system is not known.

Synthesis of lecithin is primarily by the choline incorporation pathway, with a second methylation pathway less prominent. The production of these surfactant compounds is low until 26 to 30 weeks, when concentrations begin to rise. Within the type II cells, synthesis of the phospholipids occurs in the endoplasmic reticulum, "packaging" of the compounds takes place in the Golgi apparatus, and storage occurs in lamellar bodies. Through a microtubular system, lamellar bodies are transported to the cell surface, where the phospholipids are discharged into the alveolus. In the alveolar spaces, the surface-active substances line the alveoli and reduce surface tension. As a result, alveoli remain patent and constant gaseous exchange is possible following delivery.

Respiratory Distress Syndrome

Respiratory distress in a neonate can occur from a variety of causes and, at times, its etiology can be difficult to determine. The RDS is characterized by deficiency of surfactant within the alveoli. The elevated surface tension promotes alveolar collapse and increases the "work" of breathing. As a result, the "classic" signs of RDS—tachypnea, grunting, retraction, and flaring—usually begin 6 to 8 hours after birth. A widespread reticulogranular pattern with air bronchograms is seen on a roentgenogram of the chest. The increased effort required to maintain adequate gaseous exchange itself adds additional work to these already compromised premature newborns. Ineffective gaseous exchange leads to a decrease in oxygen, an increase in carbon dioxide, the development of acidosis, and shunting within the lungs.

It is important to remember that RDS is not invariably seen in newborns with delivery at any viable gestational age. For example, approximately two-thirds of infants born at 29 to 30 weeks' gestation can be expected to develop RDS with a mortality rate of 35 to 40 percent. Thus, one-third of infants born at this very young gestational age will not develop RDS at all.

INDIVIDUAL AMNIOTIC FLUID TESTS OF FETAL MATURITY

Tests of fetal maturity can be classified into indirect and direct types. *Indirect tests* do not measure pulmonary function per se but rather assess the age or size of the fetus. Indirect assessment of fetal maturity includes obstetric estimate of gestational age (menstrual history, first appearance of fetal heart tones, and physical examination); ultrasound examination (measurement of the gestational sac, crown-rump length, biparietal diameter, femur length, fetal weight, and placental grading); and amniotic fluid analysis for fetal fat cells, osmolality, and creatinine concentration, among others.

Direct tests of fetal maturity are designed to measure either the concentration of particular components of lung surfactant (biochemical tests) or the surface active effects of the surfactant materials in amniotic fluid (biophysical tests). These tests depend on the principle of pulmonary surfactant accumulation in the alveolar spaces with eventual respiratory flow into the amniotic fluid.

As stated earlier, RDS does not occur invariably at any viable gestational age. Indirect assessment of gestational age or size is not a reliable predictor of RDS or mature lungs unless term pregnancy is almost assured. For this reason, direct tests have become more commonly used than indirect tests to assess fetal maturity, although indirect measures of gestational age and size are certainly important in overall management decisions.

Many amniotic fluid tests are available to evaluate fetal maturity. Several of the commonly used biochemical and biophysical tests are discussed.

BIOCHEMICAL TESTS

Lecithin-Sphingomyelin Ratio

In 1971, Louis Gluck and co-workers published a now classic article in which the change in relative amounts of two phospholipids, lecithin and sphingomyelin, was evaluated in 301 amniocentesis specimens collected across a number of gestational age weeks. Up until 32 to 33 weeks, the concentrations of these substances were quite similar, but by approximately 35 weeks, the concentration of lecithin had increased significantly, whereas the sphingomyelin concentration remained quite constant. When the size of the lecithin "spot" on thin-layer chromatography exceeded that of the sphingomyelin, the clinical interpretation was that pulmonary maturity had occurred. Data published soon thereafter by these investigators established a ratio of 2.0 as the level at or above which lung maturity had been achieved. Since sphingomyelin levels increased only slightly during the course of gestation, the use of a ratio of lecithin to sphingomyelin was a novel "internal standard" against which lecithin levels could be compared. The ratio minimized variation in concentrations due to the ever-dynamic change in amniotic fluid volume and avoided the issue of nonhomogeneous dispersal of the phospholipids through the entire amniotic fluid cavity. This study and subsequent investigations suggested that RDS was very unlikely to occur once the lecithin-sphingomyelin (L/S) ratio reached greater than or equal to 2.0. Because this direct test for fetal maturity filled an important gap in the management of a most difficult obstetric problem, the L/S ratio was enthusiastically adopted and still remains the gold standard against which all other tests are compared. Despite recommendations that laboratories establish their own "mature" L/S ratio value, few have done so, and a ratio of 2.0 or more has become widely accepted without such review.

The procedure for determination of the L/S ratio is somewhat involved. Fluid removed by amniocentesis is centrifuged, and the lipids are extracted using chloroform and methanol. The "surfactant-associated lecithin" is then precipitated from the remaining extract by cold acetone. The extracted phospholipids are separated using thin-layer chromatography, the lipid bands are stained, and the L/S ratio is calculated by densitometry or another method.

Since the introduction of this test, preanalytic and analytic concerns have been voiced. Preanalytic concerns include centrifugation speed and effects of contamination with blood and other substances. Analytic concerns include poor reproducibility of the thin-layer chromatography methods; questions regarding solvents, thin-layer chromatography plates, and quantification techniques; the need for the cold acetone precipitation step; and use of one- versus two-dimensional thin-layer chromatography systems. As a result of these concerns, myriad modifications in the procedure for L/S ratio analysis have been proposed.

Within several years of publication of the original analytic technique, a number of articles were published evaluating the use of the L/S ratio in predicting lung maturity. Although pulmonary maturity as measured by the L/S ratio of greater than or equal to 2 was associated with the development of RDS in only about 1 to 3 percent of infants, much less was known about the outcome of infants born with an "immature" L/S ratio, and it was assumed that many or almost all infants would suffer the consequences of RDS if, indeed, the L/S ratio had not reached 2.0 by the time of delivery. In 1975, Harvey, Parkinson, and Campbell summarized the outcome of infants delivered with "immature" amniotic fluid L/S ratios. In this summary of a number of studies utilizing many laboratories, 40 percent of 223 infants with a ratio of 1.5 to 2.0 developed RDS, and 4 percent died; of 162 patients with an L/S ratio less than 1.5, 73 percent experienced RDS and 14 percent died. Several years later, we reported our experience in a single hospital (and laboratory) with 69 infants born within 3 days of amniocentesis whose L/S ratio results were 1.99 or less. In comparison with the earlier multicenter review, we found that no infant developed RDS with an L/S ratio of between 1.50 and 1.99, and only 1 of 13 infants with a ratio of 1.00 to 1.49 developed RDS. At ratios below 1.0, RDS was common, as was neonatal death from pulmonary immaturity. This difference in experience probably reflects a difference in technique, since reproducibility of most thin-layer chromatography methods both within and between laboratories is difficult. Nonetheless, additional experience, while it confirmed the value of a mature L/S ratio in predicting pulmonary maturity, has continued to demonstrate the inefficiency of an immature L/S ratio in predicting subsequent development of RDS. It should be stated that all tests of fetal maturity suffer the same shortcoming, i.e., each test is ineffective in predicting the *presence* of RDS in infants delivered subsequent to the test results.

Fetal lung maturity may be accelerated in pregnancies complicated by hypertension, heroin addiction, hemoglobinopathies, twins, placental infarction, or other conditions "stressful" to the fetus.

False-positive L/S ratio results (when infants develop RDS despite a "mature" L/S) occur but are unusual in normal pregnancies. In the experience of some, false-positive results are found somewhat more often in neonates from pregnancies complicated by diabetes mellitus. The debate as to whether or not diabetes alters the pulmonary maturity sequence continues, and many laboratories establish a higher end point, say 2.5 or greater, in diabetic patients or require that two tests have results of maturity before delivery, if possible. Similar claims have been made for pregnancies complicated by isoimmunization, although the final answer is not in with either condition.

Phosphatidylglycerol

In 1976, 5 years after the original paper on the L/S ratio, Hallman, Gluck, and co-workers reported on two minor components of the surfactant system in amniotic fluid, phosphatidylinositol (PI) and phosphatidylglycerol (PG). PI, when measured as a percentage of total phospholipids in amniotic fluid, begins to increase at about 30 weeks' gestation, peaks at approximately 36 weeks, and declines thereafter. On the other hand, PG appears in significant quantities only after 36 weeks, generally after the L/S ratio exceeds two, and continues to increase steadily. This pattern of synthesis suggested that PG may act as a "final stabilizing factor" in alveolar function. Because this phospholipid appears in significant quantities only late in pregnancy, its absence does not clearly imply the subsequent development of RDS. Indeed, many healthy term infants are born in whom samples of amniotic fluid do not contain significant amounts of this phospholipid.

The procedure for determination of PG can utilize thin-layer chromatography or, more recently, a commercial slide-agglutination test. Generally, the thin-layer chromatographic method involves an additional step to the traditional L/S ratio procedure. After preparation as previously described, thin-layer chromatograms are developed twice, each time in a different dimension using different solvents. Single-dimension techniques for PG are also available. The result is expressed as a percentage of total phospholipids attributed to PG or as a phosphatidylglycerol/sphingomyelin (PG/S) ratio. Although initially a percentage PG of 3 percent was considered significant, we have found in our laboratory that PG must reach 8 percent of the total phospholipids to be clinically reliable. A PG/S ratio of greater than or equal to 0.2 indicates mature fetal lungs.

Recently, a commercially prepared slide-agglutination test has been developed called Amniostat-FLM (Hana Biologics, Inc., Berkeley, CA 94710). Using antiserum specific for PG, rapid analysis is possible. The simple procedure potentially makes this test widely available in many hospitals. Comparison between the Amniostat-FLM and PG determined by two-dimensional thin-layer chromatography has found agreement in the vast majority of cases. As also shown by others, our experience using amniotic fluid from normal and complicated pregnancies suggests that a positive Amniostat-FLM is quite predictive of a mature fetus, although the predictive value of an immature result is low.

A great advantage of the utilization of PG for fetal testing lies in the fact that it has not been found in blood, meconium, or vaginal secretions. Thus, amniotic fluid contaminated with these substances can be analyzed for PG, when other tests would be more difficult or impossible to interpret. However, we have found that such contaminated samples were suitable only for the qualitative determination of PG, as contaminants themselves may alter the concentration of other phospholipids present, thereby interfering with the practice of reporting PG as a percentage of total phospholipids.

The Lung Profile

In an effort to improve further the ability of a mature L/S ratio to predict fetal maturity and to raise the predictive value of results of immaturity to better predict infants who will develop RDS, the concept of a "long profile" has been developed by Kulovich, Hallman, and Gluck. Such a profile consists of the determination and combined interpretation of the L/S ratio, PG, PI, and percentage of saturated lecithin. Although this combination of tests has achieved some degree of popularity, it is analytically involved, time-consuming, and therefore more expensive.

BIOPHYSICAL TESTS

Shake Test, Foam Stability Index

As noted earlier, biophysical tests of pulmonary function measure the physical properties of the total surfactant substances found in the amniotic fluid. The surface tension-lowering ability, microviscosity changes detected by fluorescence polarization, optical density at 650 nm, and the Foam Stability Index (FSI) test are among such tests available.

In 1972, Clements and co-workers reported that the ability of pulmonary surfactant to generate and maintain a stable foam in the presence of ethanol could be used to predict pulmonary maturity. Ethanol was added to amniotic fluid to eliminate foam formation caused by "nonsurfactant" substances in the amniotic fluid such as proteins and biosalts. When the effect of these materials was removed, stable foam generated solely by the surfactant was visible. In a series of test tubes, varying amounts of amniotic fluid and saline were combined with a fixed volume of ethanol. The capped tubes were then shaken for 15 seconds and placed in a test tube rack for 15 minutes. The air-liquid interface in each tube was then examined for the presence of bubbles, and the test result reported as positive (at 1:2 dilution amniotic fluid to ethanol), negative (at 1:1 dilution), or intermediate (positive at 1:1 dilution, negative at 1:2 dilution). With a positive test result, RDS did not occur; with a negative test result, RDS occurred in almost all infants, and with an intermediate result, RDS developed in about one-third of the infants.

This procedure was modified by Sher and colleagues in 1978, and the test was named the Foam Stability Index Test (FSI). In this procedure, 0.5 ml of amniotic fluid was added to each of a series of test tubes containing varying amounts of 95 percent ethanol so that the final volume fraction of ethanol to amniotic fluid varied from 0.44 to 0.50 in 0.01 increments. For test interpretation, the decimal points were abandoned, so the results reported were from 44 to 50. In practice, an FSI value of 47 or greater indicates fetal lung maturity. Decreasing values suggest an increasing risk for RDS, but for practical purposes, the single end point is used.

The FSI test has been commercially prepared in a test called Lumadex-FSI (Beckman Instruments, Inc., Brea, CA 92621). The test kit is supplied as a sealed, single-use cassette that is separated into wells that provide a spectrum from immaturity to maturity, and a control. Each well contains different volumes of ethanol and a blue dye for better visibility. A constant amount of amniotic fluid is added to each well through individual ports. The cassette is then shaken and observed as above. The Lumadex-FSI test compares favorably with the manual FSI test, and its simplicity is appealing to many laboratories.

Fluorescence Polarization

Shinitzky and colleagues have described a test of fetal lung maturity involving fluorescence polarization microviscosity using the concept that increasing surface activity in the amniotic fluid would be associated with lower microviscosity. A lipid-soluble dye is incubated with a specimen of amniotic fluid for 30 minutes. The amount of dye absorbed can be determined by measuring the fluorescence of polarized light. With increasing surfactant, the fluorescence polarization declines.

This test has not become widely available because of its requirement for a microviscosimeter designed only for lung maturity testing. However, a new technique using a multipurpose analyzer may increase its usefulness.

Differences of opinion regarding the procedure of analysis, including centrifugation time and force and temperature, have been reported. Lipoproteins and cholesterol may also alter the microviscosity of the sample.

Optical Density at 650 nm

Measurement of the optical density of amniotic fluid at 650 nm is a rapid indirect biophysical test for fetal maturity. The test is based on the concept that the turbidity of amniotic fluid increases with advancing gestational age, in part due to an increasing amount of surfactant substances. An uncontaminated, fresh sample of amniotic fluid with an optical density reading of 0.15 nm or greater generally indicates pulmonary maturity. In comparison studies, this test compares favorably with the L/S ratio.

Influence of Contaminants on Test Results

Contamination of amniotic fluid with blood, meconium, mucus, and lower genital tract secretions can affect virtually all amniotic fluid test results. The L/S ratio of blood (serum) has been reported to be from 1.3 to in excess of 3.0, so L/S ratio results from bloody amniotic fluid samples must take that information into account. Meconium can interfere with fetal maturation tests even when present at levels so low that they are not visually apparent. Although reports have described consistent effects of contaminants on tests of fetal maturity, we are very skeptical of results on contaminated amniotic fluid samples. Similarly, we are wary of results of fluid samples obtained vaginally, except possibly for PG determinations, since our experience has not been as favorable as that reported by others.

Comparison of Tests

As different tests of fetal maturity have evolved over the years, it has become common practice to perform each new test in addition to those already in use rather than replacing these older testing procedures. For example, many laboratories routinely perform an L/S ratio, a PG determination, and possibly an FSI or some other combination on all specimens received.

With multiple tests available for determination of fetal maturity, selection of the "best" test to order in a given circumstance must take into account not only reliability of the test but also the time necessary to complete the procedure, availability, and expense. Using the several tests available in our laboratory, which include the L/S ratio, phosphatidylglycerol (measured as a percentage of total phospholipids or phosphatidylglycerol to sphingomyelin ratio), the FSI test, and the Amniostat-FLM, the factors listed above were evaluated in patients who delivered within 72 hours of fluid collection. The diagnostic reliability for both individual tests and combination testing was studied. Table 1 defines the terms used in this analysis. The prevalence of RDS in infants from whom amniotic fluid was obtained soon before delivery was 7.4 percent. Prevalence of the disorder, in this case RDS, must be taken into account when such statistical evaluation is undertaken.

In evaluating the diagnostic reliability for individual tests of fetal lung maturity (Table 2), we found that the sensitivity of all four tests was high, ranging from about 85 percent to almost 100 percent. That is, a high proportion of infants who developed RDS had a test result that predicted immature lungs (subsequent RDS). Specificity (the proportion of infants without RDS in whom the test predicted its absence) was high for the L/S ratio (85 percent) and the FSI (96 percent). For the tests that depend upon the presence of adequate PG, the specificity dropped to 70 percent for PG/S ratio and 47 percent for the Amnostat-FLM.

The predictive value for mature test results in all four categories was high, with the lowest being 98.6 percent

TABLE 1 Definition of Terms used to Discuss Analysis of Fetal Maturity Tests

Positive = P = respiratory distress syndrome (RDS)
Negative = N = no RDS
True-positive test = TP = immature test, RDS
True-negative test = TN = mature test, no RDS
False-positive test = FP = immature test, no RDS
False-negative test = FN = mature test, RDS

$$\text{Sensitivity} = \frac{TN}{TP + FN}$$ = proportion of infants with RDS in whom test predicted RDS

$$\text{Specificity} = \frac{TN}{TN + FP}$$ = proportion of infants without RDS in whom test predicted no RDS

$$\text{Predictive value, RDS} = \text{PV(RDS)} = \frac{TP}{TP + FP}$$ = proportion of time an immature test correctly predicted RDS

$$\text{Efficiency} = E = \frac{TP + TN}{TP + TN + FP + FN}$$ = the combined predictive values of mature and immature results

TABLE 2 Diagnostic Reliability of Individual Fetal Lung Maturity Tests

Test	*Interpretation*	*Sensitivity (%)*	*Specificity (%)*	*Predictive Value Mature Test(%)*	*Predictive Value RDS(%)*	*Efficiency*
Lecithin/sphingomyelin (L/S)	≥ 2 = mature	85	85	99	31	85
Foam Stability Index (FSI)	≥ 47 = mature	85	96	99	65	95
Phosphatidylglycerol/sphingomyelin (PG/S)	≥ 0.2 = mature	100	70	100	21	73
Amniostat-FLM	≥ positive control	100	47	100	13	51

and the highest 100 percent. In other words, with a mature or positive test using any of the available procedures in our laboratory, the absence of respiratory distress syndrome could be predicted with over 98 percent confidence. The predictive value for RDS, however, was much lower. The most useful was the FSI test, which predicted the subsequent development of RDS in 65 percent of cases. That is, the proportion of time test results of immaturity correctly predicted the development of RDS was only 65 percent. The other tests has lower predictive values, ranging from 31 percent for the L/S ratio to as low as 13 percent for the Amniostat-FLM. This finding is not surprising. *All tests of fetal lung maturity suffer from poor correlation between test results of immaturity and the development of RDS.*

The efficiency of the individual tests, which represents the combined predictive values of tests with both mature and immature findings, was 85 percent for the L/S ratio, 95 percent for the FSI, 73 percent for the PG/S ratio, and 51 percent for the Amniostat-FLM.

Completion time, availability, and the expense of individual tests were also compared. The L/S ratio technique using thin-layer chromatography requires personnel trained specifically in the procedure and takes several hours to perform. As a result, the availability of the L/S ratio is limited to week days in most facilities, including ours. Moreover, specimens must be received in the laboratory early enough in the day to allow for adequate time for the test to be completed during the standard work day. Using a detailed analysis for each test to include the expense of labor and reagent and/or supplies, we found that the single-dimensional thin-layer chromatography test cost $32. Addition of the second dimension for PG analysis increased the cost to $37.

The FSI, the Lumadex-FSI, and the Amniostat-FLM can be completed in 1 hour or less and thus should be more readily available. The cost of the FSI test in our analysis is $8. The cost of the Lumadex-FSI was $26, and the Amniostat-FLM was slightly higher at $28. However, the cost of the commercial preparations can be offset by the decreased personnel requirements. It should be remembered that the typical *charge* for any laboratory test has little bearing on the actual *cost* of the procedure! In practice, for example, it is not unusual for the charge for the L/S ratio procedure to be $125 or more.

After reviewing individual tests for diagnostic reliability, we evaluated the use of various combinations of tests. We found that performing multiple tests adds little to our clinical care but can increase the cost considerably. Since each of the tests, when mature, is predictive of a mature pulmonary function in more than 98 percent of patients in our laboratory, little is to be gained by continued testing.

Because of the widely divergent techniques used to measure fetal maturity, it is not uncommon to have inconsistent results, such as a mature L/S ratio and absent PG; therefore the requirement that multiple tests all be positive before intervention can be detrimental. For example, the proportion of infants without RDS in whom the FSI predicted no RDS (specificity) is 96 percent. If one requires that both the FSI and L/S values be positive prior to assuming lung maturity, the specificity decreases to 82 percent. Likewise, if one requires that the FSI *and* the Amniostat-FLM indicate mature fetal lungs, the specificity drops to 44.7 percent. As would be expected, the efficiency of testing for these combined tests is lower than that for individual tests.

For these reasons, the sequence with which fetal maturity tests are performed could have a significant bearing on cost as well as time. Table 3 contains several examples of the effect of sequential test procedures. It must be remembered that the prevalence of the disorder in question, in this case RDS, has an effect on such an analysis. The prevalence of RDS of 7.4 percent in our population of patients from whom amniotic fluid is obtained is representative of laboratories in general.

Reviewing Table 3, if one has the L/S ratio and the FSI as available tests, and it is accepted that *either* test, if mature, indicates fetal lung maturity, the sequence of testing has an obvious bearing on cost. If the more rapid and less expensive FSI is done first, reserving the L/S ratio for those samples in which the FSI indicates immaturity, the overall cost per specimen for the laboratory would be $11. If the more expensive and time-consuming L/S ratio is performed first and the FSI is not done unless the L/S ratio is less than 2.0, this particular strategy costs $34 per specimen. If both tests are done on all specimens, the cost would be the sum of the cost of each, or $40.

If an obstetric service requires that both the L/S ratio and the FSI indicate maturity prior to presuming adequate neonatal function, the sequence of testing has less effect than in the illustration above. However, the time factor can be important. For example, if results of maturity are required for both tests, it is logical to perform the simplest and quickest test first. Using this example, the

TABLE 3 Efficiency and Cost for Representative Combination Testing Strategies

Test Combination	*Efficiency (%)*	*Sequence*	*Cost per Specimen*
L/S ≥ 2 or FSI ≥ 47	98	FSI first; if < 47, then L/S	11
		L/S first; if < 2, then FSI	34
		Both tests on all specimens	40
L/S ≥ 2 or AMN* positive	81	LS first; if < 2.0, then AMN	38
		AMN first; if negative, then L/S	46
		Both tests on all specimens	60
L/S ≥ and FSI ≥ 47	82	FSI first; if ≥ 47, then L/S	37
		L/S first; if ≥ 2.0, then FSI	38
		Both tests on all specimens	40
L/S ≥ 2 and AMN positive	51	AMN first; if positive, then L/S	42
		L/S first; if ≥ 2.0, then AMN	54

* AMN = Amniostat FLM.

FSI could be done initially. If that test reveals fetal immaturity, further testing is not necessary because it has been established that *both* tests must indicate maturity prior to intervention.

Such analyses, which take into account the reliability of individual and combination tests, the availability of such tests, laboratory personnel requirements, and costs of reagents, are important because of the effect of such factors on fetal maturity testing patterns. As a result of our investigation, physicians and laboratory personnel have developed a strategy that maximizes the clinical use of various fetal maturity tests and promotes the best use of personnel time and resources.

At present, the first test performed on an amniotic fluid sample is the FSI test. This test is available 24 hours a day and can be completed in 1 hour or less. In addition, its cost is less than that of other tests. If the FSI results indicate lung immaturity, a second test, usually the L/S ratio, is performed. If the result is critical in clinical management, the test can be done at night or on weekends; otherwise, it is performed on the next following week day. Using this strategy, the laboratory is asked to perform considerably fewer L/S ratios, since the majority of amniotic fluid samples produce FSI results supporting lung maturity. A similar sequential testing strategy utilizing the shake test, fluorescence polarization, and the L/S ratio has been proposed by Garite and co-workers, who refer to such sequential testing as the "fetal maturity cascade." Combinations using other tests may likewise be useful.

SUGGESTED READING

Brown LM, Duck-Chong CG. Methods of evaluating fetal lung maturity. CRC Crit Rev Clin Lab Sci 1982; 16:85–159.

Chapman JF, Herbert WNP. Current methods for evaluating fetal lung maturity. Lab Med 1986; 17:597–602.

Clements JA, Platzker ACG, Tierney DF, et al. Assessment of risk of respiratory distress syndrome by a rapid test for surfactant in amniotic fluid. N Engl J Med 1972; 286:1077–1081.

Garite TJ, Freeman RK, Nageotte MP. Fetal maturity cascade: a rapid and cost-effective method for fetal lung maturity testing. Obstet Gynecol 1986; 67:619–622.

Gluck L, Kulovich MV, Borer RC, et al. Diagnosis of the respiratory distress syndrome by amniocentesis. Am J Obstet Gynecol 1971; 109:440–445.

Hallman M, Kulovich M, Kirkpatrick E, et al. Phosphatidylinositol and phosphatidylglycerol in amniotic fluid: indices of lung maturity. Am J Obstet Gynecol 1976; 125:613–617.

Halvorsen PR, Gross TL. Laboratory and clinical evaluation of a rapid slide agglutination test for phosphatidylglycerol. Am J Obstet Gynecol 1985; 151:1061–1066.

Harvey D, Parkinson CE, Campbell S. Risk of respiratory distress syndrome. Lancet 1975; 1:42.

Herbert WNP, Chapman JF. Clinical and economic considerations associated with testing for fetal lung maturity. Am J Obstet Gynecol 1986; 155:820–823.

Herbert WNP, Tyson Jimenez JM. Severity of respiratory distress syndrome with low lecithin:sphingomyelin ratio. Obstet Gynecol 1981; 57:426–430.

Kulovich MV, Gluck L. The lung profile: II. Complicated pregnancy. Am J Obstet Gynecol 1979; 135:64–70.

Kulovich MV, Hallman MB, Gluck L. The lung profile: I. Normal pregnancy. Am J Obstet Gynecol 1979; 135:57–63.

Sher G, Statland BE. Assessment of fetal pulmonary maturity by the Lumadex Foam Stability Index test. Obstet Gynecol 1983; 61:444–449.

Sher G, Statland BE, Freer DE, et al. Assessing fetal lung maturation by the Foam Stability Index test. Obstet Gynecol 1978; 52:673–677.

Shinitizky M, Goldfisher A, Bruck A. A new method for assessment of fetal lung maturity. Br J Obstet Gynecol 1976; 83:833–844.

Turner RJ, Read JA. Practical use and efficiency of amniotic fluid OD 650 as a predictor of fetal pulmonary maturity. Obstet Gynecol 1983; 61:551–555.

OBSTETRIC MANAGEMENT OF THE GROWTH-RETARDED BABY

PETER C. BOYLAN, M.B., M.R.C.O.G.
ROBERT K. CREASY, M.D.

The term intrauterine growth retardation (IUGR) implies failure of the fetus to fulfill its full growth potential. There are many reasons why a fetus fails to grow appropriately, and so infants with IUGR make up a widely heterogeneous group. The significance of IUGR in clinical practice is the associated high risk of perinatal death, increased by four to eight times, and the high rate of neonatal and long-term morbidity among those born alive. The dramatically increased perinatal mortality rate is a reflection of how notoriously difficult IUGR is to diagnose as well as of the inherent fatality of many fetal conditions causing IUGR. Management of the fetus with IUGR depends in large measure on accurate diagnosis and is directed at determining an etiology and timing delivery in a way that results in the best outcome for the fetus without placing the mother at risk from inappropriate intervention.

In this chapter we will discuss the definition and known causes of IUGR, review methods of diagnosis, and describe the management of pregnancies complicated by this condition.

DEFINITION

IUGR is variously defined as being present when birth weight is less than the 10th, 5th, or 3rd centiles, or more than two or three standard deviations below mean birth weight for gestational age. Any baby whose birth weight is less than 2,500 g is frequently labeled "low birth weight" but, depending on gestational age, the newborn may be small-, appropriate-, or large-for-gestational-age. Factors influencing centile grouping include parity, race, sex, birth order, and multiple or singleton pregnancy status. Another method of identifying less than expected body mass is to use the ponderal index, which is defined as birth weight × 100/crown-heel length. An infant may not have IUGR by centile definition but still may have an abnormal ponderal index due to in utero malnutrition. These infants tend to tolerate labor poorly and gain weight rapidly when fed adequately in the neonatal period. Although there is a wide range of definitions used in the literature the most frequently used cut-off point separating IUGR infants from normals is the 10th centile.

Normal birth weight distribution varies widely among populations. American White and British infants have almost identical birth weights, whereas other populations, Indians and American Blacks, for example, have lower birth weights for gestational age. On the other hand, there are countries, Ireland and Sweden among them, in which infants have heavier birth weights at term than either American Whites or the British. Accurate designation of centile weight therefore depends on accurate figures for the population studied and accurate dating of the pregnancy.

In the United States it is not appropriate, for example, to use the Denver birth weight centile chart derived for infants born at altitude for infants at sea level. The contrasting birth weights observed in California and at altitude in Colorado are illustrated in Figure 1. The 10th centiles diverge at approximately 32 weeks. Use of an inappropriate reference profile results in either over- or underdiagnosis of IUGR.

ETIOLOGY

Although the majority of cases of IUGR are associated with no apparent cause, a number of significant causes may have a substantial impact on management. IUGR may be divided into three broad categories (Table 1): (1) the "small normal" fetus who is genetically predetermined to be relatively small throughout life. (2) IUGR that is the result of a problem from early in pregnancy. This category includes fetuses with chromosomal abnormalities, congenital malformations, and some infections. Those in categories 1 and 2 are usually symmetrically small. There is an inherent inability to achieve normal size, which tends to affect organ systems uniformly or selectively affects different organs. (3) Late, or asymmetric IUGR; when expressed in the most extreme form, the infants exhibit the classic features of relatively normal head size and wasted body, with more specific findings

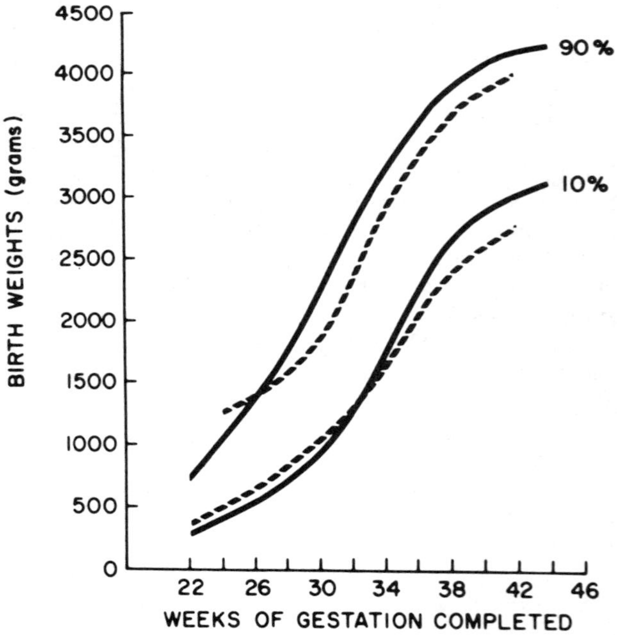

Figure 1 Birth weight percentiles for gestational age. Solid line represents California total single live births, 1970–1976; dotted line represents Colorado General Hospital live births, 1948–1960. (Modified from Williams RL, Creasy RK, Cunningham GC, et al. Fetal growth and perinatal viability in California. Obstet Gynecol 1982; 59:624.)

TABLE 1 Categories of IUGR

Symmetric	
	The constitutionally small normal fetus.
	Early pregnancy insult affecting all organ systems.
Asymmetric	
	Late-onset malnutrition with relative brain sparing.

of caved-in abdomen, meconium-stained skin, loose skin folds, and oligohydramnios, and have a characteristic "wizened old man" appearance. When presented with a suspicion of an infant with IUGR, the clinician should bear in mind the above broad categorization. Parental size, although of some influence on birth weight, is not usually helpful in discerning the etiology of the IUGR. Paternal influence on birth weight is minimal. If the Y chromosome is given to the developing fetus, it can contribute 150 to 200 g in birth weight, the difference being noted after 32 to 34 weeks. Also, the greater the antigenic dissimilarity of the parents, in general the higher the birth weight. A suspicion of very early IUGR mandates an ultrasound estimation of fetal size. If this confirms the suspicion, then an extensive level II scan should be performed to look for fetal anomalies that could explain the problem, and consideration should be given to obtaining amniotic fluid for fetal chromosomal analysis. If a fetal abnormality is found, management will depend on what the malformation is, and this is outside the scope of this chapter. Postnatally, the ponderal index is helpful in differentiating symmetric from asymmetric IUGR.

Management is directed at prolonging the pregnancy until it is apparent that the infant would do better as a neonate rather than as a fetus. The aim is to protect the fetus from deleterious effects of in utero hypoxia that may have long-term adverse affects, while at the same time not placing it at undue neonatal risk from premature delivery.

DIAGNOSIS

The major problem in the management of IUGR is diagnosis, and between 50 and 80 percent of all IUGR fetuses are undiagnosed before birth. Diagnosis is made particularly difficult when gestational age is uncertain. Certain risk factors (Table 2) predispose to IUGR, and when present, should alert the clinician. Accurate diagnosis may have a major influence in reducing perinatal mortality and morbidity associated with IUGR, and appropriate antenatal management can reduce mortality and morbidity to levels comparable with those for the normally grown fetus.

It is essential that gestational age be accurately known early in pregnancy if IUGR is to be reliably diagnosed in later pregnancy. Gestational age can be reliably calculated from menstrual history if the first day of the last menstrual period is accurately recorded, the mother is seen early in pregnancy, and there is no history of irregular menses or use of oral contraceptives immediately prior to conception. Uterine size should correspond with gestational age, at least until 22 to 24 weeks, as IUGR is rarely diagnosed clinically before this. Early ultrasound measurement has become the most accepted and widely used method of estimating gestational age when there is some discrepancy between dates and size.

Between 6 and 12 weeks crown-rump length (CRL) is the most accurate method of assessing gestational age. After 12 weeks, flexion of the fetal spine makes this method unreliable. A single CRL measurement is accurate within 5 days and within 3 days if three CRLs are averaged. After 12 weeks, biparietal diameter (BPD) and femur length measurements are standard methods of estimating gestational age. BPD is best measured in the middle of the second trimester at 16 to 20 weeks. This is the time when there is the best correlation between gestational age and BPD. With increasing gestational age, biologic variability in BPD increases, and so the measurement is a less reliable method of estimating gestational age. It is important to understand that BPD measurement has an accuracy of no better than 10 days on either side of the actual dates. Therefore, if the BPD is within 10 days of the expected value for gestational age calculated by dates, the dates may be considered accurate and the expected date of delivery should not be altered. If there is a 4-week difference, it is highly likely that the dates are wrong. Femur length measurement is at least as accurate as BPD in estimating gestational age. Repeated measurement during the same scan improves dating accuracy.

Fundal Height Measurement

Regular fundal height measurement appears to be a useful screening method to clinically detect retarded growth. Graphic representation of fundal height growth at each antenatal visit from 20 weeks onward may give an early warning of less than optimal growth. Some have reported a greater than 80 percent positive predictive value using this method, although this is not a universal experience. Fundal height measurement is useful as a screening method when dates are known accurately and when attendance at antenatal care visits is regular. If fundal height lags more than 4 weeks behind gestational age, further investigation should be undertaken.

TABLE 2 Risk Factors Associated with IUGR

Chronic Maternal Conditions	
	Chronic hypertension
	Diabetes with microvascular disease
	Renal disease
	Prepregnancy weight <50 kg
	Cyanotic heart disease
Pregnancy-Associated Conditions	
	Previous infants with intrauterine growth retardation
	Pregnancy-induced hypertension
	Poor weight gain (<0.9 kg per month)
	Anemia, HCT <30 mg per deciliter
	Fundal height 4 cm less than expected
	Multiple gestation
	Decreased amniotic fluid volume

Ultrasonography

A wide variety of ultrasonic screening tests have been used in efforts to improve diagnostic accuracy. BPD measurement alone is a poor method of diagnosing IUGR and therefore is not useful as a screening method. Brain sparing can occur, due to redistribution of blood flow to essential organs such as the brain, in chronic placental insufficiency. Head growth may therefore continue normally for a considerable period of time despite wasting of the rest of the body. Serial BPD measurements, if started early in pregnancy, may be useful in differentiating "early" from "late" growth retardation. The early pattern is associated with symmetric IUGR, whereas the late pattern is more characteristic of asymmetric IUGR.

Hobbins and co-workers have been advocates of the use of total intrauterine volume in screening for IUGR. Total intrauterine volume takes into account fetal mass, placental volume, and amniotic fluid volume (AFV) but requires a static scan. Fundal height measurement is the clinical correlate of ultrasonic total intrauterine volume measurement.

Fetal weight estimation by ultrasonography is accurate in experienced hands, although errors may occur in oligohydramnios, and the range of error increases with increasing fetal weight. At 1,000 g, for example, 95 percent of weights fall within 160 g, whereas at 3,000 g the corresponding figure is 450 g. A single measurement of abdominal circumference, where the umbilical vein branches into the portal sinus, is an accurate way of estimating fetal weight, provided amniotic fluid volume is normal, whereas the combination of BPD and abdominal circumference may predict fetal weight with an accuracy of plus or minus 106 g per kilogram; again, however, the range of error increases with increasing fetal weight. If gestational age is known accurately, a scan at 32 to 34 weeks may be a satisfactory method of screening for IUGR, particularly in a high-risk population. The combined measurement of abdominal and head circumference, expressed as head:abdominal circumference ratio (H:A ratio), is a useful method of helping to differentiate asymmetric from symmetric IUGR. Abdominal circumference reflects fetal liver size, which is determined in large part by hepatic glycogen stores in late pregnancy. Normally head and abdominal circumference are approximately equal at 34 to 36 weeks; after 34 to 36 weeks, abdominal circumference increases more than head circumference, and the H:A ratio should be less than 1. In asymmetric IUGR the H:A ratio may remain greater than 1 after 36 weeks, whereas in symmetric IUGR the ratio may remain close to normal.

Recently the ponderal index has been calculated antenatally by estimating fetal weight and length. Vintzileos and colleagues utilized estimated fetal weight and calculated fetal length to measure in utero ponderal index in 113 patients. They were able to confidently exclude IUGR in 96 percent of cases, although only 36 percent of those with an abnormally low fetal ponderal index also had a low neonatal ponderal index (36 percent positive predictive value). Yagel and associates used a modified in utero ponderal index, estimated fetal weight/$(FL)^3$, in 51 cases of suspected IUGR. They had a similarly high negative predictive value, 97 percent, but a more impressive positive predictive value, 52 percent than Vintzileos and co-workers.

The unexpected finding of reduced AFV immediately places the pregnancy in a high-risk category and should prompt the initiation of further antenatal testing procedures (as will be discussed).

ANTENATAL MANAGEMENT

In general, management is strongly influenced by whether the IUGR is symmetric or asymmetric. Diagnosis of symmetric IUGR warrants a detailed search to exclude structural malformation. Exclusion of chromosomal abnormality may be considered, either by amniocentesis or cordocentesis (to be discussed). Exclusion of recent maternal infection by serial TORCH (toxoplasmosis, rubella, cytomegalovirus, and herpes simplex) titers estimation may be considered, although in practice it is rarely diagnostic. It is unusual to have to intervene and deliver prematurely with symmetric IUGR. Asymmetric, or late-onset, IUGR infants are generally without structural abnormalities and are capable of achieving normal postnatal growth and intellectual attainment. Asymmetric IUGR is associated with pregnancy-induced hypertension, particularly when proteinuria is present, and in many cases may be the end result of impaired uteroplacental perfusion. Asymmetric IUGR fetuses benefit most from intensive antenatal monitoring.

Underlying maternal disease should be controlled and bed rest should be encouraged, since it may increase uterine blood flow and have a positive effect on fetal growth. Smoking should be discontinued, anemia corrected, and dietary advice to increase protein consumption should be given.

Until recently biochemical tests of fetoplacental function were the mainstay of antenatal management of suspected IUGR, or placental insufficiency. Biophysical testing, ultrasound, and fetal heart rate monitoring have largely supplanted biochemical testing.

BIOCHEMICAL TESTING

Estriol. Estriol synthesis involves the fetal adrenal gland and liver and the placenta. Decreased levels of estriol in either maternal plasma or urine are associated with IUGR. However, there is a wide range of normal values and many infants (up to 30 percent) with IUGR have normal values. In an individual patient there may be some merit in following serial values and intervening on the basis of a downward trend. Isolated values are rarely helpful in management and may indeed precipitate unwarranted intervention. Estriol measurement for the management of IUGR has largely been abandoned in contemporary practice.

Human Placental Lactogen. Human placental lactogen (hPL) is produced solely by the placenta. Because of the association of a small placenta with a small fetus, there is reasonable correlation between low hPL levels and IUGR. Again there is considerable overlap between IUGR and normal hPL values, probably reflecting the wide variation in causes of IUGR. In late pregnancy a level below 4 μg per milliliter places the patient in a high-risk category for IUGR. Like estriol measurement, hPL is no longer widely used in practice.

BIOPHYSICAL MONITORING

Fetal Heart Rate Monitoring. Antenatal fetal heart rate monitoring is performed either as an isolated timed observation such as the nonstress test or accompanied by induced contractions that are aimed at producing transient episodes of relative hypoxia similar to labor: the contraction stress test or oxytocin challenge test. Institutional preferences vary and are likely to be carried into practice when residents complete their training. In general, there is more experience with the nonstress test.

Nonstress Test. For a nonstress test to be classified as normal, fetal heart rate should be normal (120 to 160 beats per minute), variability should be normal ($\geq$5 beats per minute), and there should be at least two fetal heart rate accelerations of not less than 15 beats per minute and lasting not less than 15 seconds in association with fetal movements, over a 20- to 30-minute period of observation. This definition is somewhat complicated by the knowledge that the fetus may spend considerable periods of time, up to 80 to 90 minutes, asleep, with reduced variability and little or no movement. To overcome this problem, some have stimulated the fetus with sound or vibration to produce an in utero Moro response.

Predictive Value of a Normal, Reactive, Nonstress Test. A reactive nonstress test, if repeated weekly, is rarely associated with perinatal mortality. Sudden unexpected deaths have been reported, however, within 1 week of a normal nonstress test. Some do not place complete reliance on the test in the management of a fetus with suspected IUGR but do include it as part of the biophysical profile (as will be discussed).

Oxytocin Challenge Test. Uterine contractions for an oxytocin challenge test may be generated either by nipple stimulation or by intravenous infusion of oxytocin until three contractions occur in a 10-minute period. Of necessity an external contraction monitor is used, and this gives an indication of duration but not of the strength of contractions. Oxytocin is begun at 1 mU per minute and increased every 15 minutes until there are three contractions, lasting at least 1 minute each, in a 10-minute window, when the test is completed. Many women may find nipple stimulation more acceptable than intravenous infusion of oxytocin but because of the uncontrolled and uncontrollable nature of the uterine stimulation, we personally currently do not encourage its use in clinical practice for evaluation of IUGR.

Oxytocin Challenge Test Interpretation

Negative:	Normal rate and no late decelerations.
Positive:	Persistent late decelerations.
Suspicious:	Intermittent late decelerations, or variable decelerations, or abnormal baseline rate.
Unsatisfactory:	Poor quality or inability to achieve three contractions lasting 1 minute in a 10-minute window.

A positive oxytocin challenge test usually mandates delivery, or further fetal evaluation, since there is poor fetal outcome in up to 50 percent of cases. A positive test indicates the possibility of poor fetal reserve and inability to tolerate labor. If the cervix is favorable and it is likely that fetal scalp pH and blood gas estimation will be feasible early in labor, then a trial of labor is indicated. The clinical circumstances usually dictate the course of management. For example, a multiparous patient at 42 weeks, suspected fetal IUGR, a positive oxytocin challenge test, and a favorable Bishop's score should be given the opportunity to labor, whereas a primigravida at 34 weeks with an unfavorable cervix, oligohydramnios, and suspected fetal IUGR with a positive oxytocin challenge test should be delivered by cesarean section. A negative oxytocin challenge test is associated with better than 99 percent fetal survival for 1 week. It is worth pointing out that even with a 1 percent mortality rate, equivalent to a perinatal mortality rate of 10 per 1,000, we should strive to reduce the incidence further.

Biophysical Profile Testing in IUGR. The Biophysical Profile (BPP), developed by Manning and colleagues, is a mainstay of many in the contemporary management of the fetus with IUGR and has supplanted biochemical testing in most institutions. The component parts of the BPP are listed in Table 3. The nonstress test has been discussed. Amniotic fluid volume is perhaps the single most important component of the BPP. Fetal breathing movements may be absent in the normal fetus for periods up to 100 minutes and prolonging a BPP to this length to ensure absence of fetal breathing movements is unrealistic outside a research setting. Fetal tone is open to subjective interpretation and may therefore be difficult to assess. Visualization of fetal body movements may require a prolonged observation period. Amniotic fluid volume assessment, on the other hand, is a semiobjective measure. Oligohydramnios has been defined as present when there is either no detectable amniotic fluid on ultrasonography or the largest pool is less than 1 cm in two perpendicular planes. Amniotic fluid volume has been defined as marginal when the largest pool is less than 2 cm in two perpendicular planes. Although some may find a 2-cm pool too small and prefer to use a 3-cm pocket, the results from Manning's group would appear to justify a 2-cm pool as the lower limit of normal. Interestingly, perinatal mortality shows a sharp increase at less than 3 cm, and this is the level we work with (Fig. 2). More important than the actual figure chosen is an appreciation that reduced amniotic fluid volume may be an ominous sign.

Frequency of Testing. How often should a BPP be repeated? There is no standard response to this question, as it depends on a variety of circumstances, such as gestational age, degree of reduced fetal growth, and results of

TABLE 3 Criteria for Fetal Biophysical Profile Scoring*

Variable	*Score Assigned* 2	0
Fetal breathing movements (FBM)	The presence of at least 30 sec of sustained FBM in 30 min of observation.	Less than 30 sec of FBM in 30 min of observation.
Fetal body movements	Three or more gross body movements in 30 min of observation. Simultaneous limb and trunk movements are counted as a single movement.	Two or less gross body movements in 30 min of observation.
Fetal tone	At least one episode of motion of a limb from a position of flexion to extension and a rapid return to flexion.	Fetus in a position of semi- or full-limb extension with no return to flexion with movement. Absence of fetal movement is counted as absent tone.
Fetal reactivity	The presence of two or more fetal heart rate accelerations of at least 15 bpm, lasting at least 15 sec, and associated with fetal movement in 40 min.	No acceleration or less than two accelerations of the fetal heart rate in 40 min of observation.
Qualitative amniotic fluid volume	A pocket of amniotic fluid that measures at least 1 cm in two perpendicular planes	Largest pocket of amniotic fluid measures <1 in two perpendicular planes.
Maximal score	10	—
Minimal score	—	0

* From Manning FA, Baskett TF, Mossison I, Lange I. Fetal biophysical profile scoring: a prospective study in 1,184 high-risk patients. Am J Obstet Gynecol 1981; 140:289. Reprinted by permission.

previous BPP. As a rule of thumb, when amniotic fluid volume is 4 cm or less, we recommend that a BPP should be performed in X−1 day's time, where X = amniotic fluid volume; so, if amniotic fluid volume is 4 cm, the test should be repeated in 3 days. This is to emphasize the importance attached to amniotic fluid volume as a measure of fetal reserve. Most authors recommend that the test be repeated on a weekly basis. If the nonstress test component is nonreactive but amniotic fluid volume is normal, the nonstress test should be repeated within 48 hours.

TIMING OF DELIVERY

When a diagnosis of IUGR has been made, the most critical decision is when to deliver, and by what method. There is no simple answer to the question of when a fetus with IUGR should be delivered, as it depends on the certainty of diagnosis, exclusion of lethal anomalies, gestational age, and results of antenatal testing. The aim is to prolong in utero development for as long as there are no signs of fetal compromise, or until maturity is reached, and then effect delivery without causing avoidable maternal morbidity. The most useful method of following a fetus is by repeated amniotic fluid volume assessment by ultrasound examination. It is most unlikely that a fetus with IUGR will be compromised if the largest vertical pocket of amniotic fluid is greater than or equal to 3 cm. The addition of the nonstress test provides further reassurance.

Development of oligohydramnios, to less than 3 cm, at a gestational age at which fetal lung maturity is unlikely, e.g., at 32 weeks, warrants amniocentesis to check a lecithin-sphingomyelin ratio, although this may be a difficult procedure in the presence of oligohydramnios. Bed rest for 24 to 48 hours may result in reaccumulation of amniotic fluid in some cases of IUGR, sufficient to permit amniocentesis or continuation of the pregnancy. The combination of persistent oligohydramnios, an abnormal nonstress test, and documented IUGR warrants intervention to effect delivery. Late in the third trimester, after 37

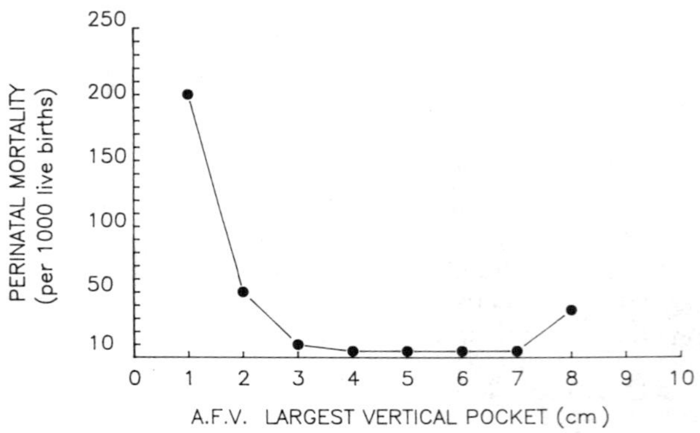

Figure 2 Increase in perinatal mortality at both extremes of amniotic fluid depth measurement using ultrasonography. (Data courtesy of Dr. F. Manning.)

weeks' gestation, the decision regarding timing of delivery is less difficult, since pulmonary maturity is almost assured. Indications for delivery may therefore be slightly relaxed, although the effect of intervention on maternal outcome is an important consideration. Induction of labor with an unfavorable cervix, for example, may not be successful, and cesarean section may be necessary. With an unfavorable cervix it may not be wise to undertake induction unless the benefits from delivery clearly outweigh the risks from remaining in utero. We would regard oligohydramnios, less than 3 cm of amniotic fluid per vertical pocket, with documented IUGR, as sufficient to justify attempted delivery, even if cesarean section for failed induction of labor eventually became necessary. In the presence of a favorable cervix, however, one may safely intervene with less stringent criteria in the knowledge that vaginal delivery is a more likely outcome.

In the final analysis, the decision to deliver a fetus with IUGR must be individualized, taking into account gestational age, severity of IUGR, amniotic fluid volume, nonstress test results, and from the maternal point of view, favorableness of the cervix for induction of labor and likelihood of achieving vaginal delivery. The latter may be influenced by parity, with successful induction more likely to occur in the multiparous woman.

MANAGEMENT OF DELIVERY

During labor, whether induced or spontaneous, electronic fetal monitoring is advisable. The likelihood of developing fetal distress de novo in labor may be influenced by the color and volume of amniotic fluid. A normal volume of clear amniotic fluid, for example, makes the development of fetal distress unlikely, whereas thick meconium, often a reflection of preexisting oligohydramnios, substantially increases the chances of an adverse outcome.

At the time of delivery it is important to have pediatric help readily available and, depending on the circumstances, it may be advisable to have a neonatologist present.

RECENT DEVELOPMENTS IN ANTENATAL MANAGEMENT

Blood Flow Measurement. Recent developments in ultrasound and application of the Doppler shift principle have enabled measurement of uteroplacental and fetal blood flow velocity waveforms. There are a variety of indices measured, but the aim is to estimate both blood flow and resistance to flow and to use these measurements in the management of particular problems.

When confronted by hypoxia, the fetus responds by redistributing blood flow toward vital areas such as the brain, coronary arteries, and adrenal gland, and away from less vital areas such as the skin, muscle, lungs, and kidney. Reduced blood flow to the kidney causes reduced fetal urinary output and accounts, in part, for the oligohydramnios seen with IUGR.

IUGR is associated with increased resistance to flow in the uteroplacental and fetal circulations. Resistance is more likely to occur in asymmetric IUGR, whereas symmetric IUGR is commonly associated with normal flow, emphasizing the "small normal" nature of these fetuses in many instances. In normal pregnancy end-diastolic blood flow velocity increases progressively as pregnancy advances, reflecting progressive reduction in resistance to flow. If end-diastolic velocity is substantially reduced, or blood flow ceases, increased risk of fetal death, low 5-minute Apgar scores, or neonatal death occurs. It is likely blood flow velocity measurement will become a standard method of following pregnancies complicated by IUGR and will increasingly determine the timing of delivery.

Cordocentesis. Fetal blood sampling for metabolic and hematologic measurements and karyotyping is now a practical reality prior to the onset of labor. Cordocentesis, or percutaneous umbilical blood sampling, involves aspiration of a fetal blood sample from an umbilical cord vessel by passage of a needle transcutaneously under ultrasonographic guidance, similar to amniocentesis. Hemorrhage from the punctured vessel has not been a significant problem, nor has transplacental passage of the needle, but problems can occur. When IUGR has been diagnosed, cordocentesis may be employed to measure fetal pH and blood gas composition, blood glucose and lactic acid levels, and a sample may be sent for rapid karyotyping to exclude a lethal chromosomal anomaly. Several groups have documented fetal acidosis and other metabolic derangements prior to the onset of labor in cases with documented IUGR. The true place of cordocentesis in the management of IUGR and its usefulness compared with currently used methods of investigation and management have yet to be established. It is likely that cordocentesis will have a role to play in selected cases of severe IUGR, particularly when diagnosed early in the third trimester when premature delivery is to be avoided if possible.

SUGGESTED READING

Campbell S, Thomas A. Ultrasound measurement of the fetal head to abdomen circumference ratio in the assessment of growth retardation. Br J Obstet Gynaecol 1977; 84:165–174.

Hogan G, Boylan P. The diagnosis of intrauterine growth retardation and its influence on perinatal outcome. Ir Med J 1987; 80:63.

Manning FA, Baskett TF, Morrison I, Lange I. Fetal biophysical profile scoring: a prospective study in 1,184 high risk patients. Am J Obstet Gynecol 1981; 140:289–294.

Pearce JM, Campbell S. Intrauterine growth retardation. Birth Defects 1985; 21:109–130.

Trudinger BJ. The umbilical circulation. Semin Perinatol 1987; 11(4):311–321.

PREGNANCY-INDUCED HYPERTENSION

DWIGHT P. CRUIKSHANK, M.D., F.A.C.O.G.

The hypertensive disorders resulting from vasospasm induced by pregnancy have been grouped together under the somewhat archaic term "toxemia." In an effort at more specificity, the Committee on Terminology of the American College of Obstetricians and Gynecologists defines *hypertension* in pregnancy as a rise in the systolic pressure of 30 mm Hg or in the diastolic pressure of 15 mm Hg above nonpregnant or first trimester levels. If such levels are not known, an absolute systolic pressure of 140 mm Hg or a diastolic pressure of 90 mm Hg defines hypertension in pregnancy. *Preeclampsia* is the development of such hypertension with proteinuria (> 0.3 g per 24 hours), edema, or both after the 20th week of gestation; *eclampsia* is the occurrence of grand mal seizures or coma, not caused by any coincidental neurologic disease, in a patient with preeclampsia. There are varying degrees of severity of preeclampsia, the definition of *severe preeclampsia* being rather standard (Table 1). Since less serious forms of preeclampsia are difficult to categorize as mild or moderate, those terms are avoided in this chapter. Instead, the term *nonsevere preeclampsia* is used. Included in this group are patients whose disease would have previously been termed gestational hypertension—patients with significant pregnancy-induced blood pressure elevation but without proteinuria or significant edema. In the development of preeclampsia, hypertension usually precedes the onset of proteinuria and marked edema and may do so by days or weeks. Therefore, patients with pregnancy-induced hypertension without the other stigmata of preeclampsia are probably at the beginning of the spectrum of the disease.

Preeclampsia and eclampsia are leading causes of perinatal mortality, both because of the vasospasm-induced placental insufficiency and because of the association of abruptio placentae with these hypertensive diseases. Although the 1 to 2 percent incidence of abruption among patients with nonsevere preeclampsia is not much higher than that of the general obstetric population, the incidence is 10 percent in patients with severe preeclampsia and eclampsia and 15 percent among patients with preeclampsia superimposed on underlying chronic vascular disease. A recent survey from the southeastern United States identified maternal hypertension, both chronic and pregnancy-induced, as the leading cause of preventable term stillbirth, being responsible for nearly 50 percent of such fetal deaths.

Preeclampsia and eclampsia also continue to be significant causes of maternal death. In 1987, as for the past 100 years, those disorders rank in the top two or three direct obstetric causes of death of pregnant women.

TREATMENT OF NONSEVERE PREECLAMPSIA

Patients whose blood pressure has risen 30 mm Hg systolic or 15 mm Hg diastolic over nonpregnant or first trimester levels, or who have a blood pressure of 140/90 with unknown earlier blood pressures but no proteinuria or symptoms of preeclampsia, should be prescribed bed rest at home. It is important that a definite and specific amount of bed rest be prescribed by the physician. I have found that patients seldom take seriously a general admonition to "get more bed rest." Rather, the patient should be specifically counseled to be at bed rest in the lateral recumbent position 6 to 8 hours per day in addition to her nightly sleep. It is often helpful to be specific, i.e., to recommend bed rest from 9 AM to noon and 2 PM to 6 PM. While the patient is at home bed rest, frequent blood pressure determinations are essential. The ideal is for a qualified family member or visiting nurse to check blood pressures twice each day, with daily reporting to the physician. If that is not feasible, the patient should be seen at least twice weekly in the physician's office for blood pressure determinations. These patients should also be advised to report immediately symptoms such as persistent severe or throbbing headaches, visual changes, epigastric or right upper quadrant abdominal pain, and reduced fetal activity. It is also useful to instruct the patient in the use of urine dipsticks and to have her check for proteinuria once or twice each day, especially with the first voiding each morning.

Hospitalization

The patient whose hypertension remains unchanged or worsens with home bed rest should be admitted to the

TABLE 1 Criteria Defining Severe Preeclampsia*

1. Blood pressure ≥ 160 mm Hg systolic or 110 mm Hg diastolic on two occasions at least 6 hours apart with patient at bed rest.
2. Proteinuria ≥ 5 g in 24 hours.
3. Oliguria with urine output ≤ 400 ml in 24 hours.
4. Cerebral or visual disturbances such as headache, altered consciousness, scotomata.
5. Pulmonary edema or cyanosis.
6. Epigastric or right upper quadrant pain.
7. Thrombocytopenia, elevated liver enzyme levels, hemolysis.

* Any one criterion is sufficient for the diagnosis.

hospital. Furthermore, any patient with pregnancy-induced hypertension whose blood pressure is higher than 140/90 or who has significant proteinuria (1+ or more by dipstick, > 300 mg in a 24-hour collection) should be hospitalized without a trial of home bed rest. The three cornerstones of hospital management are reduced activity, maternal monitoring, and fetal surveillance. I believe, as do most investigators, that activity for these patients should be limited to bed rest with bathroom privileges. It should be pointed out, however, that the group at Parkland Hospital in Dallas has reported excellent results from hospitalizing such patients in a unit where they can be somewhat more ambulatory (spending part of the day sitting up, watching television, or reading). The Parkland group hastens to add that the activity and life stress levels for such patients are far below what they would be at home or in an outpatient setting and, in fact, condemns outpatient attempts at management.

With bed rest in the hospital, up to 80 percent of nonsevere preeclamptic patients become normotensive. This must not be interpreted as a cure of their disease, however. Studies using placental dehydroepiandrosterone sulfate to estradiol clearance rates have shown that bed rest does not necessarily improve uterine blood flow, nor does it improve these patients' abnormal vascular responsiveness to infused angiotensin. Further evidence that bed rest is not curative is that at least 50 percent of such patients have a recurrence of hypertension prior to delivery, even though they remain at bed rest. Therefore, it is a management error to discharge the nonsevere preeclamptic patient if she becomes normotensive in the hospital. Rather, once the patient's disease is severe enough to warrant hospitalization, she should remain hospitalized until delivery.

Maternal monitoring in the hospital (Table 2) is directed toward ascertaining whether the mother's disease is stable, improving, or worsening. The patient should be weighed daily. The preeclamptic patient who is improving with bed rest will diurese and lose weight. Rapid weight gain during bed rest is a sign that the disease is worsening. The patient's blood pressure should be measured every 4 to 6 hours, although it may not be necessary to awaken the patient in the middle of the night for blood pressure checks if she is otherwise stable. The patient or nurse should determine qualitatively (by dipstick) the degree of proteinuria each time the patient voids, and

TABLE 2 Maternal Monitoring of Hospitalized Preeclamptic Patients

Daily weight checks.
Blood pressure monitoring every 4 to 6 hours.
Qualitative proteinuria reading, each voiding.
Quantitative proteinuria and creatinine clearance determinations twice per week.
Blood studies once or twice per week.
- Hematocrit
- Platelet count
- BUN, creatinine, uric acid
- Liver enzymes (aspartate aminotransferase, alanine aminotransferase)

Elicit symptoms from patient twice daily.

24-hour urine collections should be obtained twice weekly to quantify protein excretion and creatinine clearance. Blood studies to detect hemoconcentration (hematocrit), worsening renal function (blood urea nitrogen (BUN), creatinine, uric acid), or the insidious onset of thrombocytopenia (platelet count) and hepatocellular damage (liver enzymes) should be done once or twice per week. At least twice daily the patient should be questioned about symptoms of headaches, visual disturbances, and upper abdominal pain.

Fetal surveillance is important in order to attempt to identify those patients at risk of intrauterine fetal death. The patient should be questioned about fetal activity at least twice daily, or she can be asked to do formal fetal movement counts for 30 minutes after each meal. There are no absolute standards for how often a fetus should move in 30 minutes, but a persistent downward trend may be an indication of fetal compromise. Fetal heart rate testing in the form of nonstress tests should be done at least weekly; in more severe degrees of maternal disease, twice weekly is preferable. Nonreactive tests should be followed immediately by contraction stress tests (oxytocin challenge test, nipple stimulation tests) or biophysical profiles. An ultrasound examination should be performed weekly, both for measurement of fetal growth and of amniotic fluid volume. Although accurate determinations of fetal growth require a 2- to 3-week interval between ultrasound examinations, oligohydramnios can develop within 1 week and is an ominous sign that the fetal condition is deteriorating.

There is no drug therapy appropriate or necessary for the nonsevere preeclamptic patient hospitalized at bed rest. Many have used phenobarbital in oral doses of 30 to 60 mg every 6 to 8 hours in such patients. This therapy may make the patient more inclined to stay at bed rest because she is sleepy, but it has no effect on the underlying disease and really is unnecessary. Diuretic therapy should be scrupulously avoided. By further reducing the already contracted maternal intravascular volume, these agents reduce renal perfusion as measured by creatinine clearance, and more importantly, reduce uteroplacental perfusion. They can also cause significant maternal electrolyte depletion. The thiazide diuretics, when used to treat preeclampsia, have occasionally been associated with maternal hemorrhagic pancreatitis and neonatal thrombocytopenia as well.

As with diuretics, antihypertensives are not indicated in the management of nonsevere preeclampsia. There is no evidence that reduction in maternal blood pressure with drugs alters the course of the underlying disease, and such treatment may worsen the prognosis for the fetus by reducing uteroplacental perfusion. In addition, such therapy may mask one of the symptoms of worsening maternal disease and lead the physician into a false sense of security. Some of the newer antihypertensives such as the calcium-channel blockers and the angiotensin–converting enzyme inhibitors (e.g., captopril) are appealing on theoretical grounds when one considers what is known about the pathophysiology of preeclampsia. However, both these classes of drugs have been associated with disastrous fetal consequences when administered to pregnant animals and should be avoided until much more data are available. Magnesium sulfate therapy is not indicated in the management of nonsevere preeclampsia until the time of labor and delivery (as will be discussed).

Delivery

The curative treatment of nonsevere preeclampsia is delivery. The critical decision is the timing of that delivery. In three circumstances the decision to deliver is a relatively easy one. First, if the mother's condition deteriorates to the point that she satisfies the criteria for severe preeclampsia, delivery is indicated regardless of the duration of gestation (to be discussed). Amniocentesis for determination of fetal lung maturity is not indicated in such circumstances. Second, if fetal surveillance indicates a likelihood of death in utero at any time after the age of viability, delivery is indicated, and again amniocentesis is not appropriate. Examples of ominous fetal surveillance findings include positive contraction stress tests or cessation of fetal growth coupled with oligohydramnios on ultrasound examination. Third, if the pregnancy has reached term, delivery is indicated, and again, amniocentesis is superfluous. However, the definition of term requires some discussion. Because of the increased risk of fetal death from abruptio placentae among preeclamptic women and because this risk increases the further one progresses in pregnancy, I believe any patient with nonsevere preeclampsia who has a favorable cervix at 38 weeks' gestation should have labor induced. If the cervix is unfavorable but the mother and fetus are stable, it is acceptable to wait another week, but all patients with nonsevere preeclampsia should be delivered by 39 completed weeks of gestation. Some authorities permit waiting for the cervix until 40 weeks, but it is never acceptable to allow a patient with preeclampsia of any degree to go beyond her estimated date of confinement undelivered.

In circumstances other than the three previously outlined, the decision about when to deliver becomes more complex. For instances, if the mother's disease is gradually worsening but is not yet severe, if the fetus is growing but at a slower than normal rate, if there is reduced amniotic fluid but not true oligohydramnios, or if the fetal heart rate testing is suspicious but not clearly abnormal and the patient is not at term, when should one deliver? In such circumstances, all indices of maternal surveillance, fetal well-being, and fetal maturity must be factored into an equation and the course selected which, in the clinician's judgment, seems most compatible with intact neonatal survival. In these circumstances amniocentesis for fetal lung maturity studies may be helpful. In these complex cases a mature lecithin-sphingomyelin ratio should make one favor delivery, whereas an immature ratio might tilt one toward continued observation.

The same sorts of deliberations that determine the timing of delivery are necessary to select the route. Individualized judgment is necessary in all cases, but for the most part, patients with preeclampsia who need to be delivered at or beyond 34 weeks' gestation deserve a trial of induction of labor. This is true even in the face of a relatively unfavorable cervix. Even many fetuses with abnormal nonstress or contraction stress tests tolerate labor without developing fetal distress. Patients who need to be delivered prior to 34 weeks' gestation have, almost by definition, some degree of fetal compromise. In such cases, if the cervix is unfavorable, one could not be faulted for electing cesarean delivery without a trial of induction of labor.

Magnesium Sulfate

Patients with nonsevere preeclampsia should be treated with parenteral magnesium sulfate ($MgSO_4$) during labor, delivery, and the early puerperium. The drug is given solely to prevent maternal seizures (eclampsia), the risk for which is greatest during the peripartum period. The drug is not given to lower blood pressure or promote diuresis and seldom does either to any significant degree. The anticonvulsant effects of $MgSO_4$ are thought to be due to the antagonism of calcium by magnesium at the myoneural junction; a central mechanism has been postulated by some, but if it exists, it is probably of lesser significance. Magnesium sulfate also greatly increases the renal excretion of calcium. A 400 percent increase in urinary calcium concentration has been observed, even in oliguric patients with severe preeclampsia. This increased excretion leads to a 10 to 15 percent fall in the maternal serum ionized calcium concentration, further depression being prevented by a 25 percent rise in maternal parathyroid hormone output. Although this degree of maternal hypocalcemia is well tolerated, an occasional patient treated with parenteral magnesium sulfate for many days may become seriously hypocalcemic. This possibility should be remembered, especially in the patient who becomes progressively more obtunded after delivery. Before entertaining the diagnosis of a cerebral bleed or other neurologic disaster in such patients, investigate the possibility of hypocalcemia.

Although the intramuscular route of administration of $MgSO_4$ is time-honored and efficacious, I prefer the intravenous regimen. It is equally effective and safe and is associated with less patient discomfort. The usual regimen is 4.0 g of $MgSO_4$ in 100 ml of 5 percent dextrose in water, given as a loading dose over a 15-minute period. This is followed by an intravenous maintenance dose of 1.0 to 3.0 g per hour. It is an error to omit the 4.0 g loading dose, for without it the patient will not achieve therapeutic serum magnesium levels for 4 to 6 hours. With it, she will reach such levels in 30 minutes. The loading dose of 4.0 g may even be given to an anuric patient without danger of magnesium toxicity. However, such a patient should not receive a subsequent maintenance dose until urine output is established or serum magnesium levels are measured. Many patients need only a 1.0 g per hour $MgSO_4$ intravenous maintenance dose, and almost all will be controlled on 2.0 g per hour. I have seen an occasional patient who required a maintenance dose of 3.0 g per hour to control hyperreflexia, however. The deep tendon reflexes are used to determine the maintenance dose. The goal is to use whatever dose is necessary to keep the reflexes just barely detectable. In such circumstances monitoring serum magnesium levels is unnecessary; the patient will not develop respiratory or cardiac arrest due to magnesium toxicity if she still has detectable deep tendon reflexes. This is different from the situation in which $MgSO_4$ is being used as a tocolytic agent, when it is frequently necessary to use a dosage that abolishes reflexes in order to stop uterine contractions and when serum magnesium level monitoring is important. It should be emphasized that the reflexes are not used to determine when to start $MgSO_4$ therapy. All preeclamptic patients in labor, not only those with hyperreflexia, need $MgSO_4$ treatment. Rather, the reflexes are used to determine when to *stop* $MgSO_4$ therapy or to reduce the dosage. Reflexes should be checked hourly during $MgSO_4$ infusion, and if they are absent, the infusion should be stopped until they return. Reflexes are usually lost at serum magnesium levels of 8 to 10 mEq per liter, and respiratory depression or arrest occurs at about 12 mEq per liter. If respiratory depression or arrest occurs, the treatment is 1.0 g calcium gluconate given by intravenous push over 30 to 60 seconds. One-gram ampules of this drug should be kept near the bedside when $MgSO_4$ is being infused. The maternal urine output should also be monitored during $MgSO_4$ infusion, and the infusion usually should be discontinued if urine output is less than 30 ml per hour. In this circumstance serum magnesium levels may be helpful. In the past some have advocated placement of an in-dwelling Foley catheter in all patients receiving $MgSO_4$. I believe such a practice is not necessary as long as the patient is able to void and have her urine output measured every 1 to 2 hours.

All patients with preeclampsia should be maintained on parenteral $MgSO_4$ therapy throughout labor and delivery and for the first 24 hours of the puerperium. Thereafter when the signs and symptoms of the disease, especially hypertension and proteinuria, begin to abate, the infusion may be stopped. Diuresis is a useful sign of improvement—once the typical postpartum diuresis begins the infusion may be discontinued, especially since it is then probably impossible to maintain therapeutic serum magnesium levels with ordinary doses of $MgSO_4$. Some severely ill patients may require 3 to 4 days of therapy post partum before they begin to improve and diurese. These patients need careful monitoring of serum calcium levels.

Two coexisting maternal diseases warrant special mention with regard to the magnesium sulfate therapy of preeclampsia. Magnesium sulfate may precipitate a myasthenic crisis in patients with myasthenia gravis, because it diminishes the action and amount of acetylcholine at the motor end plate. Such crises do not respond to calcium therapy but do respond to edrophonium (Tensilon). Thus, myasthenia gravis represents the one circumstance in which $MgSO_4$ should be avoided in the treatment of preeclampsia. Patients with myasthenia gravis who develop preeclampsia should be treated with another anticonvulsant such as parenteral phenytoin (Dilantin).

Patients with primary hyperparathyroidism have elevated serum calcium levels and may not respond to ordinary doses of $MgSO_4$. I cared for a preeclamptic patient with unrecognized hyperparathyroidism who developed eclampsia despite treatment with 4.0 g of $MgSO_4$ per hour. Patients with this disorder who develop preeclampsia may also be candidates for parenteral phenytoin therapy.

If, in these two conditions, parenteral phenytoin therapy is elected, the dose is 10 to 15 mg per kilogram, or between 700 to 1,200 mg for the typical pregnant woman. This should be given in intermittent boluses of 50 mg each minute for 15 to 20 minutes. Each bolus should be flushed with copious amounts of intravenous fluid, as parenteral phenytoin is quite alkaline. Continuous infusions rapidly lead to sclerosis of vessels. Continuous maternal cardiac monitoring is essential during intravenous phenytoin administration, as the drug can induce cardiac arrhythmias.

TREATMENT OF SEVERE PREECLAMPSIA

Women with any of the criteria for severe preeclampsia (see Table 1) need to be delivered promptly, regardless of the duration of gestation. This decision is easy after the patient is beyond the gestational age of fetal viability and in the rare patient who develops severe preeclampsia before 24 weeks' gestation. However, in the patient who develops severe preeclampsia at 24 to 25 weeks, it is tempting to try to temporize, to gain some time in an effort to improve the chances for neonatal survival. Such temptation should be resisted, however. Recent studies from the University of Tennessee have shown that such temporizing rarely gains any significant improvement in fetal or neonatal outcome and is associated with unacceptable risks to maternal health. In the patient who develops severe preeclampsia prior to 32 weeks' gestation, consideration is sometimes given to maternal betamethasone therapy to accelerate fetal pulmonary maturation. However, no studies have demonstrated improved neonatal outcome with betamethasone therapy in the face of severe preeclampsia. Early studies actually showed a worse perinatal mortality in such circumstances, undoubtedly due to the 48-hour delay of delivery while awaiting the desired effect on the fetus of the betamethasone. When the mother has severe preeclampsia, the intrauterine environment is seriously compromised, and both mother and fetus are better served by prompt delivery than by a 48-hour delay. Therefore, betamethasone therapy should be avoided in these patients.

When the diagnosis of severe preeclampsia is made, certain baseline maternal laboratory studies should be obtained, if they have not been previously done as part of the process of making the diagnosis. These include a complete blood count, platelet count, coagulation indices (fibrinogen, prothrombin time, partial thromboplastin time) blood urea nitrogen, serum creatinine and uric acid, and hepatic enzymes (alanine aminotransferase and aspartate aminotransferase, formerly called serum glutamic-pyruvic transaminase and serum glutamic-oxaloacetic transaminase). Once these are obtained, the patient should be started on intravenous $MgSO_4$ therapy. The details of $MgSO_4$ therapy for these patients are the same as those described for patients with nonsevere preeclampsia and are not repeated here.

Once the patient has achieved therapeutic magnesium levels (30 to 60 minutes after the loading dose of 4.0 g

$MgSO_4$), efforts should be begun to effect delivery. The route of delivery is determined exactly as described for nonsevere preeclampsia. Many of these patients can be successfully induced and delivered vaginally. However, with fetal compromise and a very unfavorable cervix, especially at gestational ages of less than 34 weeks, cesarean delivery is an acceptable alternative.

The anesthetic management of patients with severe preeclampsia is controversial. Although all agree that epidural analgesia and anesthesia are appropriate in patients with nonsevere preeclampsia, there are those who argue it is contraindicated in the severe form of the disease. Maternal hypotension invariably complicates 20 to 30 percent of epidural anesthetics, and such hypotension leads to dramatic reduction in uterine perfusion and may cause fetal distress. One is then in the rather bizarre situation of giving pressors such as ephedrine to patients whose basic problem is vasospasm and hypertension. Furthermore, the 500 to 1,000 ml intravenous preload given to prevent such complications of epidural anesthesia may lead to pulmonary edema in some severe preeclamptic patients. Thus, the patient with preeclampsia that is severe by criteria numbers 1, 3, 4, or 5 in Table 1 should have an arterial line and a Swan-Ganz catheter placed prior to instituting epidural anesthesia, and the epidural should be performed by an anesthesiologist experienced in the use of this technique in preeclamptic women. This physician should remain with the patient throughout the duration of the anesthetic. If these criteria cannot be met, the severe preeclamptic patient undergoing cesarean delivery is better served by general anesthesia, and those undergoing induction of labor by intravenous narcotic analgesia and pudendal-local anesthesia. All would agree that epidurals are contraindicated in patients with thrombocytopenia or other forms of coagulopathy.

Some have stated that all patients with severe preeclampsia or eclampsia need a Swan-Ganz catheter and arterial line for proper management. Several studies have shown that patients with severe preeclampsia may have any of three cardiovascular dynamic states: high cardiac output-high peripheral resistance, high output-normal resistance, or low output-high resistance. The Swan-Ganz monitoring technique may help one determine which category a patient falls into, but the experience of decades clearly shows that this invasive form of monitoring is unnecessary for the successful management of the majority of patients with severe preeclampsia or eclampsia. I believe it is only necessary in selected patients, for example, those undergoing epidural anesthesia, those with anuria that is unresponsive to a fluid bolus, those with pulmonary edema, and those in whom intravenous antihypertensives other than hydralazine (e.g., sodium nitroprusside) are deemed necessary.

Unlike the situation with nonsevere preeclampsia, patients with severe preeclampsia may need antihypertensive therapy. If the diastolic pressure is persistently 110 mm Hg or greater, there is a risk of maternal intracranial hemorrhage, and efforts should be made to lower the blood pressure. The goal, however, is not to lower it to normal levels, for this may well result in reduced uteroplacental perfusion and fetal distress. Rather, the maternal blood pressure should be lowered to the range of 140/90 to 150/95, a level that protects the maternal central nervous system without causing fetal compromise. An excellent drug for controlling severe maternal hypertension is hydralazine, given intravenously. It does not reduce maternal cardiac output and works promptly. Either the intermittent or continuous infusion regimens may be used. The intermittent regimen consists of 5.0 mg intravenous push every 15 minutes until the blood pressure begins to fall. Once a response is seen, it is prudent to increase the injection interval to every 20 to 30 minutes until pressures of 140/90 mm Hg are achieved. Then 5.0-mg doses every 30 to 60 minutes usually maintain the blood pressure in the desired range.

The continuous infusion method involves diluting 150 mg of hydralazine in 150 ml of 5 percent dextrose in water. This is then piggy-backed into another intravenous line, and the infusion is started at 0.05 mg per minute, or 0.05 ml per minute. The infusion rate is doubled every 5 minutes until the desired effect is achieved. The rate can then be titrated to keep the blood pressure at 140/90 to 150/95.

Other intravenous antihypertensives should be used with caution, if at all. Diazoxide has been associated with profound and prolonged maternal hypotension when used in patients with severe preeclampsia and should be avoided. In the undelivered patient who does not respond to hydralazine, sodium nitroprusside may be useful for short-term therapy. However, because long-term therapy with this drug is associated with the accumulation of cyanide radicals in the fetus, it should be reserved for those patients who are still dangerously hypertensive after delivery.

Many patients with severe preeclampsia (or eclampsia) do not become normotensive again for 4 to 6 weeks after delivery. Unless the diastolic blood pressure is still 105 mm Hg or higher, it is unnecessary to send these patients home on oral antihypertensive therapy. If such therapy is elected, a reasonable drug of choice is clonidine. This drug can be safely used by the lactating woman. These patients should be seen at least weekly for blood pressure determinations, however. When the pregnancy-induced hypertension abates, as it eventually will, treated women can become seriously hypotensive. It should be emphasized that the need for such oral antihypertensive therapy should be rare. Once the preeclamptic patient is delivered, her disease is on the route to being cured, and patience on the part of the physician is usually the best course.

Two other drugs that theoretically could be useful in treating severe preeclampsia are mentioned here only to warn against their use. Aspirin and heparin may be useful as prophylactic measures in women with certain antiphospholipid antibodies (lupus anticoagulant and anticardiolipin) who are prone to develop early severe preeclampsia, but neither of these drugs has any place in the management of severe preeclampsia once it has developed.

The syndrome of hemolysis, elevated liver enzyme levels, and thrombocytopenia is a variant of severe preeclampsia. Like preeclampsia itself, the syndrome has a spectrum of severity—most patients with it present with thrombocytopenia and evidence of hepatocellular injury but without hemolysis, while a few present with the full syndrome. In the past there has been some controversy about whether such patients need prompt delivery. However, the incidence of placental abruption in untreated patients with the syndrome is 20 percent, and maternal morbidity and mortality are significant. I believe this variant should be managed like all other cases of severe preeclampsia, with prompt delivery. Platelet transfusions are usually not necessary. Excessive blood loss at surgery is observed only in patients with platelet counts below 50,000 per cubic millimeter. Therefore, patients with platelet counts less than 50,000 who require cesarean delivery should receive prophylactic platelet transfusions just prior to incision and interoperatively. Patients with counts above 50,000 do not need such prophylaxis, but may need platelet transfusions if the count falls and excessive bleeding occurs during surgery. Patients in whom a vaginal delivery is contemplated should not receive prophylactic platelet transfusions regardless of their platelet count. Such patients with severe thrombocytopenia may need platelet transfusions if significant episiotomy bleeding occurs, however.

TREATMENT OF ECLAMPSIA

The management of eclampsia is similar to that of severe preeclampsia in that prompt delivery is indicated regardless of the duration of gestation. The route of delivery is selected using the same considerations described for preeclamptic patients, and the anesthetic considerations and the necessity for invasive cardiovascular monitoring (Swan-Ganz catheter) are as outlined above for severe preeclampsia. The principles of magnesium sulfate and antihypertensive therapy are the same as those outlined for preeclamptic patients and need not be repeated.

The immediate management of the eclamptic seizure involves protecting the patient from injury. A padded tongue blade or similar device should be placed in the mouth to prevent serious tongue injury, and the patient should be prevented from striking her head against objects and from falling out of bed. Forceful restraint of the extremities should be avoided, however. The usual eclamptic seizure lasts 60 to 75 seconds. During this time the patient is not breathing, and attempts at oxygen therapy are superfluous. Once the seizure has ceased and the patient is postictal, mask oxygen should be started at 5 L per minute. Intravenous access should be obtained and magnesium sulfate therapy instituted. As in the case of preeclampsia, the patient should receive a 4.0-g intravenous bolus of $MgSO_4$ in 100 ml of 5 percent dextrose in water over 10 to 15 minutes followed by an initial maintenance dose of 2.0 g per hour. If the patient has another seizure after the 4.0-g bolus, an additional 2.0 g should be infused over 15 minutes. As soon as seizures are controlled, the maintenance dose should be adjusted based on the status of the deep tendon reflexes. Because these patients cannot be expected to void voluntarily every 1 to 2 hours, a Foley catheter should be placed to monitor urine output.

In the unusual circumstance of the patient who continues to convulse after administration of 6.0 g of $MgSO_4$, one dose of intravenous sodium amobarbital (Amytal), 250 mg, may be given over 2 to 3 minutes.

Fetal bradycardia usually follows an eclamptic seizure, and it can be quite remarkable. Its onset is anywhere from immediately to 5 minutes after the seizure. The heart rate may drop as low as 80 beats per minute and may remain there for anywhere from 30 seconds to 10 minutes. However, the fetus recovers when the maternal-fetal oxygenation and acid-base status return to normal. Such bradycardia is usually *not* an indication for cesarean delivery. Uterine hyperactivity may be seen after a seizure and may persist for 1 to 15 minutes. Placental abruptions can also occur shortly after an eclamptic seizure. This diagnosis can be difficult to make, since, bradycardia and uterine hypertonus, the usual signs of abruption, may be present as a result of the seizure alone. If there is vaginal bleeding, or if the fetal bradycardia and uterine hypertonus persist for more than 15 minutes, abruption should be seriously considered. Obviously, close monitoring by the physician at the bedside and excellent clinical judgment are required.

One should avoid rushing to cesarean delivery immediately after a maternal seizure if possible. Both mother and fetus are hypoxic and acidotic and will not tolerate a major anesthetic and surgery well. Knowledge of this fact has given rise to the concept of the stabilization interval, a period of time after the development of eclampsia before which one should attempt to effect delivery. In previous times this interval was stated to be anywhere from 12 to 24 hours, but very few would advocate such a lengthy delay in this era. However, a period of 1 to 3 hours after the cessation of maternal seizures is reasonable before cesarean delivery or induction of labor is undertaken. This time is used to achieve therapeutic maternal serum magnesium levels and correct maternal hypoxia and acidosis. Mask oxygen at 5.0 L per minute should be administered, and maternal arterial blood gas determinations obtained. If the maternal arterial pH is less than 7.10, intravenous sodium bicarbonate should be administered because such a serious degree of maternal acidosis leads to marked declines in uterine blood flow. Also during the stabilization interval, serum electrolytes, platelet count, prothrombin and partial thromboplastin times, and plasma fibrinogen levels should be measured. These should all be corrected toward normal before induction of labor or cesarean delivery is undertaken.

MANAGEMENT OF SUPERIMPOSED PREECLAMPSIA AND ECLAMPSIA

Patients who develop severe preeclampsia or eclampsia superimposed on preexisting chronic hypertension are managed exactly as those who develop those diseases de novo, and such management is not reiterated here.

Patients with chronic hypertension who develop superimposed, nonsevere preeclampsia should be managed in a fashion similar to that described for those who develop the disease de novo, and only the differences in management are discussed here. Many of these women are taking antihypertensive drugs, and such therapy should be continued. The best drugs for the management of chronic hypertension in pregnancy are alpha-methyldopa (Aldomet) or the beta-blocker metoprolol (Lopressor). If the blood pressure begins to worsen in pregnant women taking these drugs, the dosage can be increased until maximal dosages are being administered. For alpha-methyldopa, the maximal dose is 2.0 g per day, usually given in divided doses of 1.0 g every 12 hours. For metroprolol the daily maximal dose is 200 mg, again given in divided doses of 100 mg every 12 hours. As is true for other preeclamptic patients, diuretic therapy should not be instituted in these patients. If maximal dosages of alpha-methyldopa and/or metoprolol do not control blood pressure in these patients, further attempts at pharmacologic therapy are probably not warranted. Consideration should be given to delivery.

The timing of delivery should be earlier in patients with superimposed nonsevere preeclampsia, in part because the incidence of placental abruption is reported to be as high as 15 percent in this group of patients, the risk increasing as term approaches. The stable patient with superimposed nonsevere preeclampsia and a favorable cervix should have labor induced at 37 weeks' gestation. All other patients with superimposed nonsevere preeclampsia should be delivered by the end of the 38th completed week. Induction of labor usually should be undertaken in such circumstances, regardless of the condition of the cervix.

SUGGESTED READING

Abdella TN, Sibai BM, Hays JM, Anderson GD. Relationship of hypertensive disease to abruptio placentae. Obstet Gynecol 1984; 63:365–370.

Clark SL, Greespoon JS, Aldahl D, Phelan JP. Severe preeclampsia with persistent oliguria: management of hemodynamic subsets. Am J Obstet Gynecol 1986; 154:490–494.

Cruikshank DP, Linyear AS. Term stillbirth: causes and potential for prevention in Virginia. Obstet Gynecol 1987; 69:841–844.

Cruikshank DP, Pitkin RM, Donnelly E, Reynolds WA. Urinary magnesium, calcium and phosphate excretion during magnesium sulfate infusion. Obstet Gynecol 1981; 58:430–434.

Paul RH, Koh KS, Bernstein SG. Changes in fetal heart rate—uterine contraction patterns associated with eclampsia. Am J Obstet Gynecol 1978; 130:165–169.

Pritchard JA, Cunningham FG, Pritchard SA. The Parkland Memorial Hospital protocol for treatment of eclampsia: evaluation of 245 cases. Am J Obstet Gynecol 1984; 148:951–963.

Sibai BM, Taslimi M, Abdella TN, Brooks TF, et al. Maternal and perinatal outcome of conservative management of severe preeclampsia in midtrimester. Am J Obstet Gynecol 1985; 152:32–37.

Watson KV, Moldow CF, Ogburn PL, Jacob HS. Magnesium sulfate: rationale for its use in preeclampsia. Proc Natl Acad Sci USA 1986; 83:1075–1078.

OLIGOHYDRAMNIOS

JEFFREY C. KING, M.D.

The fetus lives and develops surrounded by amniotic fluid. The source, function, and significance of this fluid have stimulated significant research efforts in an attempt to understand fetal pulmonary, renal, and somatic growth. In addition, analysis of various substances in amniotic fluid provides valuable clinical information regarding fetal hemolysis, lung maturity, and chromosomal complement. However, in spite of our current knowledge, we must admit incomplete understanding of amniotic fluid and its significance.

In spite of previous suggestions that the amniotic fluid represents a stagnant pond, it is in reality a dynamic fetal compartment. However, studies designed to evaluate the mechanisms of amniotic fluid production and clearance are hampered for several reasons, including: (1) species differences, (2) compositional changes with advancing gestational age, (3) volume changes in the amniotic fluid compartment during pregnancy, (4) variations of normal, (5) invasive nature of investigative techniques, and (6) ethical and legal problems related to human study.

In this chapter, the physiology of amniotic fluid production and removal is briefly reviewed. This is followed by an introduction to the multiple clinical problem situations that place the fetus at risk from oligohydramnios. Last, conclusions and recommendations regarding the management of reduced or absent amniotic fluid volume are presented.

AMNIOTIC FLUID PHYSIOLOGY

The volume of total uterine contents (fetus, placenta, and amniotic fluid) increases almost linearly during the second and third trimesters. However, the percentage that each component contributes differs significantly during this same period. Amniotic fluid volume at various gestational ages has been studied using direct volumetric methods and dye dilution techniques. It has been shown that there is a progressive increase in amniotic fluid volume from approximately 250 ml at 16 weeks to a mean of 980 ml at 34 to 35 weeks. After this, there is a gradual decrease in amniotic fluid until 40 weeks, at which point the fluid volume begins to fall sharply. During the first half of pregnancy, amniotic fluid volume has been shown to increase proportional to fetal weight, but during the second half of pregnancy, these variables are not found to be directly related.

In early pregnancy amniotic fluid has been shown to closely resemble both maternal and fetal sera. At 20 weeks' gestation, the osmolality is 276 mOsm per kilogram, sodium is 136 mmol per liter, and urea is 3.0 mmol per liter, which represent 98 percent, 99 percent, and 100 percent of maternal serum concentration, respectively. During the second half of gestation the osmolality and sodium gradually decrease to 92 percent of the maternal serum value, whereas the urea and creatinine concentrations in amniotic fluid increase by 70 to 250 percent. Although urea and creatinine concentrations are higher in amniotic fluid than in maternal serum, the concentration of most other solutes is lower. Since the concentrations of maternal and fetal sera are almost identical during pregnancy, a similar relationship exists between amniotic fluid and fetal serum levels.

The amniotic cavity is a fetal compartment filled with fluid surrounded by other fetal structures. Although amniotic fluid is originally derived from the mother, its components are modified as it passes through such fetal structures as the chorioamnion and the fetal-placental unit on its way into the amniotic cavity. This passage provides the possibility for fetal control over the composition of this compartment, either passively via its membrane characteristics or actively via various homeostatic control mechanisms. The fetal urinary tract and the respiratory tract are known to be the major contributors to amniotic fluid production. Whereas fetal swallowing and transport across the chorioamnion represent major sites of amniotic fluid disappearance, other sites, such as fetal skin and the umbilical cord, provide for quantitatively less important flux.

Fetal urinary tract output represents the major source of amniotic fluid production. This factor becomes progressively more important as gestational age increases. Urine can be seen within the fetal bladder as early as 10 weeks' gestation. Various studies have demonstrated that fetal urine production increases linearly from 3.6 ml per hour at 25 weeks' gestation to 26 ml per hour at 39 weeks' gestation. Fetal urine production is known to decrease sharply at this point. There is also a linear relationship between fetal weight and gestational age between 25 to 39 weeks, resulting in the calculated urine production, increasing from 110 ml per kilogram per 24 hours at 25 weeks to 190 ml per kilogram per 24 hours at 39 weeks' gestation. Studies in chronically catheterized sheep have shown that the fetus excretes 200 to 1,000 ml per day of urine. The normal term human fetus has been shown to have a similar daily urinary output.

Since fetal urinary volume increases progressively during pregnancy, the quantity of oncotically active substances added to amniotic fluid must also increase. However, although amniotic fluid volume at 38 weeks is almost identical to that at 20 weeks, the osmolality at term is less. Therefore, an increasing amount of water, electrolytes, and solutes must be removed from the amniotic fluid compartment with advancing gestation. There is no doubt that fetal urine production is the result of fetal renal function. The glomerular filtration rate at term has been shown to average 34 ml per 1.73 m^2, which is about 25 percent of the normal adult value. Tubular reabsorption has been shown to average 90 percent of adult values. These data confirm that the fetal kidneys are actively functioning. Other studies show that expansion and contraction of fetal blood volume directly affect the volume of fetal urine production, indicating intrinsic control mechanisms.

The fetal lung also represents a significant site for amniotic fluid production. In sheep the amount of fetal pulmonary fluid increases linearly from 30 ml per kilogram per 24 hours to 50 ml per kilogram per 24 hours during the final 30 days of gestation. Vasopressin administration to the fetus has been shown to reduce tracheal fluid production without changing the osmolality or electrolyte concentration, indicating that fetal pulmonary fluid is at least partially under fetal control. The contribution of tracheal fluid to amniotic fluid dynamics in the human is unknown; however, the findings of surface-active substances (lecithin, sphingomyelin, and phosphatidylglycerol) in the amniotic fluid demonstrates that some of the pulmonary-tracheal fluid reaches the amniotic cavity. At present it remains unclear what fraction of tracheal fluid is swallowed even prior to entering the amniotic fluid compartment. The lungs have also been suggested as a site for amniotic fluid reabsorption; however, no significant absorption has ever been demonstrated in the normal human fetus.

Fetal swallowing is an extremely important mechanism for amniotic fluid clearance and is the only accepted route of entry for amniotic fluid entry into the fetus. Using radioactively labeled red blood cells, it has been found that human fetal swallowing of amniotic fluid increases from 7 ml per 24 hours at 16 weeks to approximately 500 ml per 24 hours at term. If these values are corrected for estimated fetal weight, fetal swallowing increases from 50 ml per kilogram per 24 hours to 150 ml per kilogram per 24 hours at term. Near term, the volume of amniotic fluid swallowed per day almost equals the total amniotic fluid volume. Studies in chronically instrumented sheep suggest swallowing values of 375 ml per kilogram per 24 hours, but it is unknown whether this is an artifact or a true species difference. One possible explanation for this difference is the fact that the techniques used for measuring volume removed cannot take into account the tracheal fluid that is swallowed prior to mixing with the amniotic fluid. Therefore, human values may be as much as 30 percent higher than previously noted.

Although the fetus has been shown to swallow large quantities of amniotic fluid each day, gastrointestinal atresia or experimental esophageal ligation does not result in significant disturbance in amniotic fluid volume or composition. This fact suggests that the reduced intake of fluid is compensated for by a reduced production of urine and/or tracheal fluid rather than that fetal swallowing is not a major factor in amniotic fluid homeostasis.

Fetal swallowing is episodic, and the periods are variable during the day. Each episode of swallowing lasts between 1 and 8 minutes. To determine if taste affected the rate and volume of fetal swallowing, amniotic fluid was sweetened, and it was found that this had no effect on the volume swallowed per day. It has been speculated that decreased fetal blood volume or increased fetal osmolality may stimulate fetal swallowing with its secondary effects on amniotic fluid volume control. All studies suggest a close relationship between fetal swallowing and urine production. However, with intermittent swallowing but rather continuous urine production, many hours may be necessary to demonstrate equality of flows.

In early pregnancy the fetal skin consists of only a few cell layers interposed between a basal and a superficial cell layer. The superficial layer, or periderm, gradually disappears by 17 to 20 weeks. However, until then these cells have been shown to contain intracellular structures suggestive of functional activity. Various in vitro and in vivo experiments have shown permeability to water and sodium plus transportation of urea. Therefore, transudation of fluid across the fetal skin provides a significant percentage of fluid until keratinization is completed, which occurs at 25 weeks' gestation; subsequently, the skin must be considered impermeable. The umbilical cord allows bidirectional water flux, but it is an ineffective site for solute exchange.

CLINICAL INTRODUCTION

Oligohydramnios is defined as absent or little amniotic fluid. The estimate of amniotic fluid volume using physical examination is difficult and often inaccurate. Since the relationship between fetus, amniotic fluid, and umbilical cord can be easily determined by ultrasound examination, this technique is the most appropriate evaluation modality. The ultrasonographic criterion for oligohydramnios is the finding of a pocket of amniotic fluid that measures less than 1 cm in vertical dimension. The incidence of this complication of pregnancy varies from 0.7 percent to 5.5 percent. Multiple etiologies for oligohydramnios have been proposed, including dysplastic or absent urinary tract, obstructed urinary tract, premature rupture of membranes, postdate pregnancy, and intrauterine growth retardation. Oligohydramnios has been recognized for a long time as an associated finding in cases of severe perinatal compromise. Other complications of oligohydramnios include (1) decreased fetal growth, (2) pulmonary hypoplasia, (3) deformation syndrome, (4) fetal distress, (5) maternal or neonatal infections, and (6) stillbirth or neonatal death.

SECOND TRIMESTER OLIGOHYDRAMNIOS

The gestational age when oligohydramnios is discovered may have great significance with regard to pregnancy outcome. The greatest fear is that second trimester oligohydramnios indicates that fetal pulmonary development will be adversely affected. Additionally, the adequacy of fetal renal function is often questioned. In 1984 Barrs reported on the outcome of 12 pregnancies complicated by oligohydramnios discovered during the second trimester. Termination of pregnancy was elected in four cases based on ultrasonographic findings of anomalies incompatible with life that were confirmed at delivery. Premature labor following premature rupture of membranes occurred at 22 weeks' gestation in one patient, which resulted in a neonatal death deemed secondary to pulmonary hypoplasia. Seven pregnancies continued to a viable gestational age, but five neonates died from severe renal anomalies (Potter's syndrome and hypoplastic lungs). Of the two remaining pregnancies, one fetus had severe symmetric intrauterine growth retardation and died shortly following birth at 34 weeks, and the other was stillborn at 34 weeks, further complicated by a triploid chromosomal complement and severe growth retardation. This report suggested a dismal prognosis for pregnancies complicated by oligohydramnios in the second trimester.

However, in 1986 Mercer reported on 34 pregnancies fulfilling the criteria for second trimester oligohydramnios without occurrence of rupture of the membranes. Nine fetuses were found to have congenital anomalies. Of the 25 remaining pregnancies, intrauterine deaths complicated 10 and one stillbirth resulted from abruptio placentae. Although eight pregnancies terminated in live births, all infants had an adverse perinatal outcome secondary to either premature labor (seven) or abruptio placentae (one). It is noteworthy that two of these eight fetuses survived. Six pregnancies continued in the face of persistent oligohydramnios and eventually the women delivered normal term infants unaffected by intrauterine growth retardation.

There is no question that second trimester oligohydramnios is associated with a higher incidence of perinatal morbidity and mortality, but it should not be considered uniformly hopeless. In summary, eight of 34 pregnancies (24 percent) safely progressed through gestation, resulting in healthy neonates. Therefore, when oligohydramnios is discovered during the second trimester, careful ultrasonographic evaluation for malformations is essential. Genetic amniocentesis, if possible, is recommended, since triploidy and X-isochromosome abnormality may be discovered.

Deformation Syndrome

The oligohydramnios-induced deformation syndrome was originally described by Thomas and Smith in 1974. The classic features of this syndrome occur whether the oligohydramnios is caused by renal agenesis or rupture of membranes. The components of the syndrome include flattened craniofacial features, aberrant position of the limbs, dislocated hips, redundant skin, displaced ears, and a small thoracic cavity often resulting in hypoplastic lungs.

In 1984 Nimrod reported on the effect of prolonged membrane rupture and noted that 12 percent of infants had craniofacial or skeletal deformities that required orthopaedic evaluation, most notably talipes equinovarus. These problems were most often associated with ruptured membranes between 16 and 26 weeks' gestation with a latency interval of 5 to 12 weeks. In 1986 King reported that induced oligohydramnios in an animal model (rabbit) resulted in a 14 percent incidence of deformation syndrome, with facial asymmetry and positional abnormalities of the limbs being most frequently observed.

Disturbance of Fetal Growth

The adequacy of fetal growth following rupture of the membranes has been seriously questioned. In 1977 Cefalo described four cases of ruptured membranes and noted that fetal biparietal diameter growth was unaffected. This is not totally unexpected, since the fetal skull bones develop some structural integrity with advancing gestation. Nimrod reported on 100 cases of prolonged membrane rupture and found that birth weight was unchanged compared with that of controls. After studying 97 cases of premature rupture of the membranes, in 1984 Tamura showed that the biparietal diameter, abdominal circumference, and birth weight were adversely affected. It is possible that alterations in biparietal diameter might occur subsequent to severe oligohydramnios and/or labor onset, resulting in compression of the head and abdomen. No study has determined if there is an alteration of head circumference following membrane rupture. Nakayama in 1983 and King in 1986 separately studied the effects of induced oligohydramnios on body weight, lung weight, and organ-to-body ratios. Both investigators showed that there was a significant reduction in fetal body and lung weight subsequent to amniotic fluid loss. Analysis of lung to body weight ratios showed no significance, but studies of liver to body weight proved significant. It has been postulated that oligohydramnios from any source results in alterations of umbilical blood flow with their subsequent impact on liver weight and ultimately on lung and body weight. This alteration in blood flow may disrupt nutrition delivery to the fetus and may help explain the increased incidence of stillbirth associated with oligohydramnios.

Pulmonary Hypoplasia

The fetus has the ability to survive many complications of pregnancy; however, if pulmonary hypoplasia develops, neonatal death is a certain result. Kitzmiller suggested that 16.7 percent of pregnancies complicated by oligohydramnios resulted in pulmonary hypoplasia. In his study of 100 patients with prolonged membrane rupture, Nimrod noted a 9 percent incidence of fatal pulmonary hypoplasia; in addition, 8 percent of the neonates required chest tube placement for pneumothorax. It was suggested that the need for chest tube drainage indicated the need for higher peak inspiratory and mean airway pressures associated with nonfatal pulmonary hypoplasia. Nimrod proposed that the risk of developing pulmonary hypoplasia was low (1.4 percent) when rupture of the membranes occurred after 26 weeks' gestation. This is probably explained by the fact that significant numbers of terminal air sacs have already developed by 26 weeks' gestation.

When examining lung development and pulmonary hypoplasia, it is important to review the various stages. In humans, the glandular stage is completed by 112 days, with the canalicular stage taking place between 112 and 168 days. The final stage, saccular, occurs between 168 days and term (280 days). If there is an early enough adverse impact on lung growth and development in utero due either to a vascular accident or to oligohydramnios, the result will be pulmonary hypoplasia. In 1983 Moessinger reported decreased lung DNA content as an indicator of decreased cell numbers in cases of fetal pulmonary hypoplasia. DNA content analysis eliminates the variables of edema fluid, hemorrhage, or inhaled amniotic fluid, which may alter lung weight. Progressively later insults during pregnancy may result in reduced alveolar sac development but not in neonatal death from absolute hypoplasia. No test definitely predicts pulmonary hypoplasia, although Callan (1985) and Johnson (1987) have reported that the thoracic-to-abdominal-circumference ratio is helpful.

In an attempt to examine the effect of oligohydramnios on lung function, King performed pressure-volume studies on in situ fetal rabbit lungs after timed amniotomy. He found that there was a relatively high rate of air leakage, making interpretation of those pressure-volume studies impossible. However, in those fetuses that underwent successful pressure-volume analysis, the following results were noted compared with controls. The maximum lung volume was unchanged, but as the duration of oligohydramnios increased, the lung volume became smaller and approached statistical significance. The lung volumes expressed as percentages of maximum lung volume at a transpulmonary pressure of 35 cm of water during inflation revealed essentially identical curves. However, during the deflation limb, increasing duration of oligohydramnios resulted in the lungs becoming more stable and resisting collapse. Additionally, there was a tendency for a larger residual lung volume at 0 cm of water. These results suggested that when rupture of the membranes occurs in mid- to late pregnancy, the effect is on the collagen and supporting substance in the fetal lung along with increased surfactant release rather than on suppression of the growth and development of functional alveoli.

The physiologic importance of fetal breathing movements was suggested as critical to normal lung development. Therefore, the presence of normal rates of fetal breathing was believed to be indicative of normal lung function. However, in 1987 Moessinger reported on the predictability of fetal breathing movement in pregnancies complicated by oligohydramnios. He found that all fetuses with renal anomalies (agenesis) and oligohydramnios and those that ultimately died from pulmonary hypoplasia spent more time breathing, as observed by ultrasonography, than did controls.

THIRD TRIMESTER OLIGOHYDRAMNIOS

When oligohydramnios is discovered in the third trimester, numerous potential implications must be considered. Most important, the fetus must be evaluated morphologically. Bastide in 1986 reported that there were 15 perinatal deaths in 113 patients with oligohydramnios, resulting in a gross perinatal mortality rate of 132.7 per 1,000. Of the 15 deaths, 13 (86.6 percent) were associated with a major fetal anomaly, including seven with multiple malformations, five with renal agenesis, and one with a neural tube defect. In 1984 Chamberlain found that 12 perinatal deaths occurred in 64 patients with decreased qualitative amniotic fluid volume, resulting in a gross perinatal mortality rate of 187.5 per 1,000. Seven deaths occurred in structurally normal fetuses, and five were discovered to have renal agenesis. Combining these studies, 10 of 177 (6 percent) pregnancies complicated by third trimester oligohydramnios had lethal renal anomalies.

Urinary Tract—Physiology

The fetal urinary system develops from the intermediate mesoderm and the cloaca. At about 3 weeks, transverse folding allows ventral migration of the intermediate mesoderm, resulting in bilateral nephrogenic cords. These cords give rise to the renal tubules and produce the urogenital ridges. The evaluation of the definitive kidney follows the development of the three sets of excretory organs: the pronephros, mesonephros, and metanephros.

The pronephros is of no significance as an excretory organ, but the pronephric duct is important in the development of the mesonephros. There is no proof of mesonephric function in the human embryo, although mesonephric nephrons develop during the fourth week and represent the first true glomerulonephron unit. The metanephros begins to develop in the human fetus in the fifth week, and function is present within 3 weeks.

The growth of a collecting system begins with the ureteric bud, a branch from the mesonephric duct near the cloaca. The ureteric bud then grows into mesoderm (metanephric blastema), which begins to develop into actual nephrons by 8 weeks. Nephrons continue to form in a centrifugal pattern until 34 weeks' gestation, at which time there are approximately 800,000 in each kidney.

During the sixth week, the primitive urinary tract separates from the gut. The ureters become functional by 9 weeks. Functional renal development is continuous with attainment of "adult" renal function at 2 years of age.

Urinary Tract—Malformations

Unilateral renal absence is relatively common, but bilateral renal agenesis is a rare and lethal malformation. Renal agenesis may result from failure of the ureteric bud to develop or to grow into the metanephric mesoderm and to induce nephron development.

Renal hypoplasia is a result of a reduced number and/or size of nephrons, which leads to small kidneys that appear normal. Renal dysplasia results from alteration in structural differentiation of metanephric components leading to incompletely or abnormally developed ducts. The development of renal hypoplasia or dysplasia may result in deficient amniotic fluid volume and may be associated with the adverse perinatal outcomes seen with renal agenesis.

Renal hypoplasia is generally sporadic but may be familial or in association with 13q-syndrome. Therefore, it is recommended that the parents and siblings of affected fetuses be carefully evaluated for "silent" renal dysfunction by ultrasonographic and renal clearance studies.

Dysplastic kidneys may be solid or cystic, large or small, and normal or misshapen. Associated abnormalities of the ureters, bladder, and/or urethra frequently coexist. It is believed that these abnormalities are important to the pathophysiology of renal dysplasia. The multicystic fetal kidney represents a particular type of dysplasia and consists of a severely malformed kidney without normal pyelocalyceal structures. This results in cysts of various sizes separated by thick fibrous septa. Since urethral or ureteropelvic junction obstruction is usually seen with multicystic kidneys, an abnormal development of the ureteral bud is suggested. The multicystic kidney is easily diagnosed in utero using ultrasonography, which allows visualization of the characteristically distorted fetal anatomy and calculation of renal-to-abdominal-circumference ratio.

Polycystic renal disease can result from two major forms: infantile (autosomal recessive) and adult (autosomal dominant). Infantile polycystic disease is often associated with hepatic involvement and generally has a poor outcome. Adult polycystic disease is associated with depressed renal function and hypertension, with some of these abnormalities presenting during the newborn period.

As previously suggested, urinary tract obstruction is almost certainly related to the pathogenesis of renal dysplasia. In addition, it is extremely important to distinguish between dysplasia and simple hydronephrosis, since fetal renal damage secondary to hydronephrosis may be reversible by diversion of the obstructed urine flow.

Ureteropelvic junction obstruction is the most common obstructive uropathy and is bilateral in 20 to 30 percent of cases. The obstruction may be caused by adhesions, aberrant vessels, or valve-like folds in the mucosa, but most often it is intrinsic. The obstructed kidney may fill the entire abdomen and result in dystocia or pulmonary hypoplasia.

Posterior urethral valves are a common cause of urinary tract obstruction and may result in massive renal damage. Early urethral obstruction may lead to the typical deformation syndrome or to multiple extrarenal defects, primarily involving the lungs (hypoplasia) and anterior abdominal muscles (prune-belly syndrome).

The evaluation of alterations of amniotic fluid volume resulting from renal abnormalities is difficult. Eventual outcome cannot be predicted with certainty except in cases of bilateral renal agenesis. The proposed management of the abnormal renal tract includes an initial evaluation of function based on amniotic fluid volume and bladder size. If function is good, management is dependent on serial sonography. If function remains good, term delivery is suggested. In the face of deteriorating function, the possibility of early delivery versus decompression in utero must be considered, using either a percutaneous shunt or surgical nephrostomy. If poor function is initially found, pregnancy termination should be considered. The function of the fetal kidney can often be stimulated by the furosemide (Lasix) stimulation test. However, the absence of urine flow response to a Lasix challenge is not confirmatory of renal dysfunction.

Ultrasound examination allows assessment of kidney size and structure plus evaluation of echogenicity. As predictors of renal dysplasia, sonographically determined renal cortical cysts (100 percent) and increased echogenicity (89 percent) were the most specific. Aspiration of fetal urine from the bladder is also helpful to predict renal function. Those fetuses whose renal function was later proved to be good, compared with those in whom renal function was proved to be poor, had lower urinary sodium and chloride levels and osmolarity.

PREMATURE RUPTURE OF THE MEMBRANES

Premature rupture of the membranes complicates 10 percent of pregnancies at term and 0.7 to 2 percent of pregnancies before 37 weeks' gestation. Although the management of premature rupture of membranes at term usually includes induction of labor, a conservative approach to the management of preterm premature rupture of the membranes has been advised in an attempt to reduce the incidence and severity of respiratory distress syndrome. Almost 80 to 90 percent of patients with premature rupture of the membranes at term can be expected to be in labor within 24 hours. However, when premature rupture of the membranes occurs at a time remote from term, a longer latency period prior to labor can be expected. Mead showed that 20 to 25 percent of such fetuses remained undelivered after 7 days. Taylor and Garite in 1984 reported that when premature rupture of the membranes occurred prior to fetal viability, 25 percent were undelivered at 1 month following the rupture.

The management of pregnancies complicated by premature prolonged rupture of the membranes is difficult. Although avoiding pulmonary hypoplasia and the deformation syndrome is important, the timing of delivery following rupture of the membranes prior to fetal infection or sepsis is critical to neonatal survival.

Garite in 1982 showed that there was a significant increase in the incidence of neonatal death, respiratory distress syndrome, and serious neonatal infection in infants delivered from mothers with chorioamnionitis and fever. Therefore, it is reasonable to attempt to predict the development of chorioamnionitis prior to the development of maternal fever. Numerous studies have shown that amniocentesis following rupture of the membranes was helpful in predicting chorioamnionitis. A Gram's stain positive for bacteria correlated highly with a subsequent positive amniotic fluid culture and chorioamnionitis, whereas leukocytes on Gram's stain were not indicative of an increased risk of infection. It has been suggested that if the Gram's stain for bacteria is positive, patients should be treated with antibiotics for incipient chorioamnionitis and delivered.

However, multiple studies have confirmed that only 50 percent of patients have an accessible pocket of amniotic fluid for amniocentesis following premature rupture of the membranes. Therefore, it became essential for other testing criteria to predict early infection. Numerous studies have been published advocating various therapeutic approaches to the management of premature rupture of the membranes.

Vintzileos in 1985 showed that the degree of oligohydramnios was positively correlated with an unfavorable outcome of pregnancy. His study showed that when there was no amniotic fluid remaining in the uterus, the latency period decreased while infection and fetal distress increased. Later he showed that a modified biophysical profile was a useful tool for evaluating patients with ruptured membranes. The biophysical score was found to be unaffected by rupture of the membranes in a healthy fetus, but a low score was a good predictor of impending fetal infection.

Further attempts to identify the infected fetus centered on fetal breathing. He showed that the presence of fetal breathing was a good predictor of a noninfected fetus (negative predictive value 95.3 percent), although its absence does not necessarily indicate impending infection (positive predictive value 50 percent). In 1987 Vintzileos reported on 73 patients managed with the biophysical profile. Its daily use resulted in a lower incidence of overall infectious outcome. The percentage of patients who developed infection in the study group (10.9 percent) was significantly less than in the control group (30.1 percent). However, there was no difference in the perinatal death rate.

There is no standard approach to the management of premature rupture of the membranes. In patients with membrane rupture prior to viability, a short hospitalization is indicated to evaluate for subclinical or incubating chorioamnionitis. Following this observation period, the patient may be managed as an outpatient after being instructed on the signs and symptoms of infection. Between 25 and 30 weeks, the pregnancy should be managed expectantly, since prematurity is the principal risk. Increased surveillance is indicated between 30 and 34 weeks. Between 25 and 34 weeks, continued hospitalization is most often advised. Many recommend amniocentesis if possible, whereas others prefer serial nonstress tests or biophysical profiles. If amniocentesis reveals a mature lecithin–sphingomyelin ratio or the vaginal amniotic pool fluid is positive for phosphatidylglycerol, delivery should be carefully considered. Currently, prophylactic antibiotics or tocolytics have not been proved of benefit in the management of premature membrane rupture.

INTRAUTERINE GROWTH RETARDATION

Intrauterine growth retardation is not a common problem but may complicate 3 to 7 percent of pregnancies. Fetal birth weight is less than the tenth percentile by definition. Decreased perfusion of the fetal kidneys and reduced fetal urine production may explain the decreased amniotic fluid volume so commonly seen. In 1981 Manning showed that when fluid pockets were less than 1 cm^2, 96 percent of fetuses were growth-retarded, whereas only 6 percent of cases with normal amniotic fluid exhibited fetal growth retardation.

When growth retardation is suspected, the furosemide (Lasix) stimulation test may not result in increased urine flow because of contracted fetal blood volume. The obstetric patient should be encouraged to increase rest in the lateral decubitus position and stop any tobacco or alcohol ingestion. Twice weekly nonstress tests are indicated. Sonographic assessment of fetal head growth is critical to the management plan. If no head growth is seen over 2 to 4 weeks or an ominous fetal heart rate tracing develops, delivery should be accomplished promptly.

PROLONGED PREGNANCY

As mentioned earlier, the postdate or prolonged pregnancy is at risk for oligohydramnios and its complications. After 280 days, the volume of amniotic fluid progressively decreases. In 1986 Leveno showed that when oligohydramnios complicated prolonged pregnancy, the incidence of cesarean section for fetal distress increased threefold. Similarly, the occurrence of thick meconium was doubled in the presence of oligohydramnios. Last, neonatal outcome was adversely affected when decreased amniotic fluid was present, since meconium aspiration and stillbirth occurred more frequently.

Phelan in 1985 studied postdate pregnancy and showed that when reduced amniotic fluid volume is found, a trial of labor using direct fetal monitoring should be carefully considered. Direct fetal monitoring is essential, since the incidence of variable deceleration is almost 75 percent. Cesarean delivery for fetal distress was noted in 43 percent of patients with oligohydramnios but in only 16 percent of patients with "adequate but decreased" fluid.

AMNIOINFUSION

Any pregnancy complicated by oligohydramnios has an increased frequency of fetal heart rate alterations, particularly variable decelerations associated with cord entrapment. Although alterations of maternal position may alleviate the abnormal fetal heart rate pattern in some patients, cesarean section for fetal distress is a common outcome. Miyazaki in 1985 reported on a prospective randomized study on intrauterine saline infusion for the relief of repetitive variable decelerations. Since the saline infusion corrects the oligohydramnios and makes the cord less vulnerable to compression, improved outcome was expected. Variable decelerations were relieved in 51 percent of patients, and the rate of cesarean delivery of nulliparous patients was reduced from 47 to 14 percent. Subsequent studies by Nageotte in 1985 confirmed the benefits of amnioinfusion. Specifically, umbilical vein and artery pH was significantly higher at delivery in patients treated with amnioinfusion. Amnioinfusion studies suggest that this technique reduces the incidence and severity of fetal distress and improves the metabolic status of the newborn infant in most patients with oligohydramnios from any cause.

CONCLUSIONS

The finding of oligohydramnios at any time during gestation should signal the physician to begin increased surveillance of the fetus. Its discovery during the second trimester necessitates detailed sonographic scanning to discover congenital malformations, particularly lethal renal agenesis. Even if fetal kidneys are visualized, the prognosis for a healthy fetus must remain guarded, and serial evaluation of fetal growth and development becomes essential.

When oligohydramnios results from premature rupture of the membranes, the fetus is at increased risk for pulmonary hypoplasia, infection, and stillbirth from a cord accident. Serial ultrasound examination to evaluate chest circumference may be predictive of pulmonary hypoplasia, whereas the presence of normal fetal breathing is not always reassuring. The combined modalities of antepartum fetal heart rate monitoring and biophysical testing appear to be the current technique for discovery of the fetus who remains in an increasingly hostile intrauterine environment and requires delivery.

Abnormal development of the fetal urinary tract often results in decreased amniotic fluid volume. Detailed ultrasound evaluation of fetal kidneys, ureters, and bladder has proved to be helpful in predicting the need for and/or benefit of invasive fetal therapy. In the face of normal amniotic fluid volume, unilateral obstructive uropathies should not be subjected to evaluation by invasive methods. The inclusion of pediatric urologists in the assessment of severity of urinary tract obstruction may be invaluable in planning for delivery and neonatal evaluation.

Postdate pregnancy and intrauterine growth retardation are both associated with decreased amniotic fluid volume. In addition, meconium staining of the remaining fluid places the fetus at risk for aspiration and subsequent pulmonary insufficiency. The mere finding of oligohydramnios in these clinical situations should prompt the physician to consider induction of labor using direct fetal monitoring.

Cord compression resulting in variable fetal heart rate decelerations is often seen during labor in patients with oligohydramnios. Amnioinfusion techniques have proved beneficial in reducing the incidence and severity of these heart rate abnormalities. In addition, the fetal metabolic status is often improved. However, correction of variable decelerations is not helpful in improving neonatal outcome in the face of lethal renal malformation.

Oligohydramnios should be recognized as an important warning signal. The ultimate perinatal outcome is dependent on the underlying cause of decreased amniotic fluid, the gestational age, and the metabolic well-being of the fetus at delivery. Management of this complication of pregnancy requires that the physician institute increased fetal surveillance, including serial ultrasonography, appropriate testing for chromosomal abnormalities, and intensive intrapartum monitoring. The patient must be made aware of the serious nature of oligohydramnios and brought into the decision-making process regarding subsequent management decisions.

SUGGESTED READING

Crenshaw C, ed. Premature rupture of membranes. Clin Obstet Gynecol 1986; 29(4):735–1004.

Garite TJ. Premature rupture of the membranes: the enigma of the obstetrician. Am J Obstet Gynecol 1985; 151:1001–1005.

Miyazaki FS, Nevarez F. Saline amnioinfusion for relief of repetitive variable decelerations: a prospective randomized study. Am J Obstet Gynecol 1985; 153:301–306.

Resnick R. Amniotic fluid. In: Creasy RK, Resnick R, eds. Maternal-fetal medicine. Principles and practice. Philadelphia: WB Saunders, 1984:135.

Romero R, Pilu G, Jeanty P. The urinary tract and adrenal glands. In: Prenatal diagnosis of congenital anomalies. Norwalk, CT: Appleton and Lange, 1988:255.

Rosenfeld CR, ed. Dynamics of amniotic fluid in health and disease. Semin Perinatol 1986; 10:93–162.

Vintzileos AM, Gaffney SE, Salinger LM, et al. The relationships among the fetal biophysical profile, umbilical cord pH, and Apgar scores. Am J Obstet Gynecol 1987; 157:627–632.

SEXUALITY IN PREGNANCY AND THE PUERPERIUM

KENNETH J. REAMY, M.D., M.P.H.

SEXUALITY IN PREGNANCY

Historically, the pregnant woman in our culture has been regarded as being without sexual desires or as having to deny herself sexual activity during gestation and for weeks after delivery. Maternal sexuality either was ignored in dialogues between the gravida and her physician or an arbitrary abstention period (presumably to help ensure the successful outcome of the pregnancy) was recommended to every prospective mother. The resulting confusion or anxiety caused women to limit sexual contact with their husbands or to feel guilty about sexual participation.

In recent years, researchers have expressed concern that coitus and orgasm may have adverse perinatal consequences, including premature labor and premature amniorrhexis. In the majority of subprimate species, the pregnant female is not sexually receptive and coitus does not occur. Traditionally, various religious groups have prohibited coitus in pregnancy according to references in the Talmud, the Koran, and Hindu scripture.

Recently, the opposite approach has been advanced: that unnecessary sexual restrictions could create stress that might be detrimental to successful gestation. Highly aroused pregnant women who do not experience the physical and emotional release of orgasm may be more likely to deliver prematurely than orgasmic gravidas. Potentially serious consequences for the marriage also may result from sexual frustrations. Of 71 men married to pregnant women for whom coitus was prohibited from 4 weeks to 3 months before their babies were due, 18 were involved in extramarital sexual liaisons either before or after delivery.

Sexual Patterns

Although there are individual variations, the first trimester of pregnancy is characterized by a decrease in sexual interest and activity. During the second trimester, there is either an increase in sexual feelings and behaviors to prepregnant levels or a continued decline in libido and sexual activity. Lack of sexual activity in the third trimester appears to be the predictable pattern for most pregnant women. Most researchers have reported a decreased frequency of orgasm as pregnancy progresses. Perkins has indicated that pregnancy itself may be the most important or overriding variable influencing sexuality in pregnancy.

A pregnant woman's interest in sexual activity also may be affected by her changing physical appearance. In a society that prizes a youthful, slender body, she may not feel attractive and desirable. Some women, of course, feel more attractive when pregnant and are very happy with their bodies. Women often report enjoying their enlarged and more sensitive breasts. Some experience pregnancy as such a fulfilling period in their lives that they are described as "radiant," "beautiful," or "never lovelier."

The complex psychological and physiologic demands of pregnancy may promote insecurities, anxieties, and somatic complaints such as fatigue or nausea in the expectant mother. She may seek to diminish these discomforts and add to a sense of security and closeness with her spouse through physical contact such as cuddling or being held.

A pregnant woman's view of her sexuality is influenced by her partner. A man who experiences decreased sexual desire during his spouse's pregnancy may be influenced by one or more of the following feelings: fear of harming the pregnant woman or fetus; finding his wife "asexual"; being "turned off" by the pregnant body; believing that sex with a pregnant woman is immoral; feeling inadequate to satisfy his wife as she experiences heightened sexual or emotional needs; fearing that somehow the fetus would be an observer to sexual activity or could hurt the male's penis; or needing to withdraw from his wife while dealing with the stresses of pregnancy himself. Many men experience no change in their sexual desires from prepregnancy levels, whereas others feel increased desire, reporting feeling "turned on" by their pregnant wives and the increased emotional closeness, intimacy, and happiness.

Dyspareunia

Research by Reamy and White revealed that by the third trimester, 18 percent of the women were experiencing coital discomfort more than half the time and 40 percent were apareunic. Coital discomfort during pregnancy can be caused by numerous factors. Vaginal congestion occurs because of increased vascularity and venous stasis. Vulvar varicosities, hemorrhoids, and varicosities of the broad ligament may be precipitated and aggravated by pregnancy. Progressive pelvic congestion of pregnancy and its associated pressure can be aggravated by coitus; although congestion may cause increased desire in the second trimester, by the third trimester it can become increasingly exaggerated, prolonged, and less responsive to orgasm. As the pregnant uterus enlarges, the usual uterine elevation does not occur as plateau levels of sexual arousal are approached. Deep-thrust dyspareunia can occur as the phallus prods the exposed cervix rather than the posterior fornix. Infection with *Candida vaginalis* or *Trichomonas vaginalis* and herpes genitalis and condyloma acuminatum can cause painful coitus.

Avoidance of coitus (apareunia) may occur because of decreased interest or anticipation of pain. The physiologic concomitants of inhibited sexual excitement are decreased vaginal lubrication and decreased vaginal accomodation of the penis. Vaginismus may result from guilt or fear or may be secondary to dyspareunia from a physical source.

Maternal and Perinatal Health

For many years myths, fears, taboos, and various religious and social teachings surrounding coitus during pregnancy have perpetuated an atmosphere of mystery and ignorance concerning the effects of maternal sexual behavior on the physical health of the mother-to-be and her infant. The vast majority of spontaneous abortions of 12 weeks or less are related to severe and lethal chromosomal defects resulting in early embryonic death. Miscarriage occurs in 10 to 25 percent of all pregnancies, but miscarriage due to trauma, injury, or physical activity is rare. The deep intrapelvic location of the uterus and the cushioning effect of the amniotic fluid appear to protect the fetus effectively from external trauma. During the late first and second trimesters abortions may be caused by cervical incompetence, submucous myomata, and müllerian fusion defects.

Coitus can indirectly result in maternal, fetal, and neonatal morbidity and mortality through the spread of sexually transmitted diseases. Maternal syphilis has been associated, although rarely, with abortion after 16 weeks. Abortion can also be precipitated by the venereal transmission of herpes simplex, *Listeria monocytogenes, Mycoplasma,* human immunodeficiency virus, and acute hepatitis B, the prevalence of which has been related to increasingly frequent sexual tramission. Pregnancy can stimulate growth of venereally transmitted condylomata acuminata, and treatment with podophyllin has resulted in abortion.

In addition to abortion, syphilis can result in stillbirths and congenital syphilis. Congenital cytomegalovirus infection has been described as the most prevalent intrauterine infection and has surpassed rubella as a cause of fetal injury. Congenital listeriosis can be associated with disseminated fetal infection, intrauterine death, and premature labor. Newborns can contract potentially lethal infections through maternal birth canals that have been venereally infected by *Neissina gonorrhoeae,* herpes virus, group B *Streptococcus, Listeria monocytogenes,* hepatitis B, and *Chlamydia.* Mycoplasmas are thought to be sexually transmitted pathogens associated with puerperal infection. Occasional reports of neonatal *Trichomonas* vaginitis have been reported with apparent transmission during passage through the infected birth canal of the mother. *Gardnerella vaginalis* has been isolated from the blood of women with puerperal infections and septic newborns and may be of clinical significance. Untreated *Candida* (monilia) vaginitis can result in characteristic neonatal thrush. Candidal chorioamnionitis and puerperal endometritis, although unusual, have been reported.

Maternal deaths from air embolism following the forceful blowing of air into the vagina associated with cunnilingus or sex play have been reported during the second and third trimesters of pregnancy.

Premature Labor

It has been theorized that prostaglandins in the seminal ejaculate may incite premature labor in susceptible gravidas. In vitro evaluation of human chorioamnionic membranes revealed that seminal fluid did not adversely affect their tensile strength. In a study of 500 women, Pugh and Fernandez reported no significant association between coitus and premature rupture of the membranes or puerperal infection. More than 20 years later, Wagner and colleagues concluded that coitus during pregnancy per se was not related to prematurity. Perkins, on evaluating 25 premature deliveries among a pregnancy study group of 155 women, found no association between coitus, premature labor, premature rupture of membranes, and low birth weight infants.

Naeye published a collaborative study of 26,886 pregnancies and determined that women who reported sexual intercourse once or more per week during the month prior to delivery had a higher incidence of amniotic fluid infections as well as a higher incidence in the neonates of low Apgar scores, respiratory distress, hyperbilirubinemia, and mortality compared with women who reported no history of coitus. Both his methodology and his criteria for the diagnosis of amnionitis, however, have undergone considerable criticism.

Mills and co-workers, in a collaborative study of 10,981 Israeli puerperas, found no association between coitus and premature labor, premature rupture of membranes, low birth weight, or perinatal mortality, irrespective of gestational age. Studies by Rayburn and Wilson and Zlatnik and Burmeister found no statistical association between coitus and premature labor and delivery. A recent retrospective study of third trimester coitus in more than 39,000 pregnant women from the Collaborative Perinatal Project showed no relation between coitus in pregnancy and adverse effects.

Masters and Johnson's research on pregnant women demonstrated orgasmic uterine contraction patterns suggestive of labor. Goodlin reported a significantly higher incidence of orgasm after 32 weeks' gestation in 50 women who delivered prematurely. Methodological bias, however, was evident in that the orgasmic group had an incidence of prior premature deliveries three times that of the anorgasmic or control group. Naeye and Ross reported orgasm as an important cofactor with chorioamnionitis in premature amniorrhexis among sexually active gravidas.

Perkins, on the other hand, found that pregnant women who were orgasmic had a lower incidence of premature deliveries than did anorgasmic women. He suggests that "those women oppressed by unrequited sexual frustration" experienced emotional distress that might have precipitated early delivery. Other recent investigators have found no relationship between orgasm and prematurity.

When pregnancy occurs a couple may be facing life reorganizational demands or crises that can affect their sexual bonds. Social and psychological factors, folklore, religious beliefs, sexual value systems, physical health, and hormonal milieus also help determine sexual attitudes and behaviors during pregnancy. A gravid woman's changing body image, her needs for nurturance and physical closeness, and her husband's sexual desires may affect her sexual needs and expression as well.

Physiologic and behavioral studies of sexual variables during gestation have shown, in general, decreases in sexual desire, coitus, and orgasm as pregnancy progresses.

There is no conclusive evidence that normal sexual activity in an uncomplicated pregnancy jeopardizes fetal or neonatal health, and blanket proscriptions concerning coitus are inappropriate. It seems likely that a subset of pregnant women—those who have multiple sexual partners (or those whose partners do not have an exclusive sexual relationship with them) and those who are young and single—are at risk of acquiring sexually transmitted infection of the endocervix, leading to premature amniorrhexis and on occasion to amnionitis and perinatal death. Since many hours of uterine contractions are well tolerated by the normal fetus during parturition, it appears unlikely that fetal distress is produced by the uterine contractions or orgasm.

SEXUALITY IN THE PUERPERIUM

The psychosocial transition to parenthood has been described as a developmental crisis. The demands of the new parental roles and responsibilities and the need to integrate these into activities of daily living can create stress in new parents. Hence, adjustments to birth of a child may entail marital discord and sexual dissatisfaction. Many women who seek sex therapy relate the onset of their sexual problems to the period following the birth of a child.

In addition to the psychological and interpersonal demands of the postpartum period, the woman experiences profound hormonal alterations. The delivery of the infant and placenta (the fetoplacental unit), eliminating the primary source of estrogen and progesterone provided during the second and third trimesters of pregnancy, results in a state of "steroid starvation" approximating the postmenopausal state. This causes vaginal atrophy, decreased vaginal lubrication, and decreased expansion of the vagina on sexual stimulation. Prolactin, responsible for the lactation maintained by breast-feeding, depresses pituitary gonadotropin secretion. This, in turn, depresses ovarian estrogen production. Additionally, there is a precipitous drop in placental chorionic gonadotropin, which has been associated with postpartum blues (although causation has not been established).

Jennings and Edmundson emphasized the profound biopsychosocial adjustments of the puerperium and suggested that an important priority for pregnancy care is facilitation of successful passage through the "fourth trimester of pregnancy."

Anatomic and Physiologic Changes of the Vagina and Breasts

The vagina in the early puerperium is a lax, capacious, swollen, smoothwalled cavity. By 3 weeks' post partum, normal rugal folds reappear, and congestion and edema lessen markedly. Consequent to parturition, there are generally multiple tiny superficial vaginal lacerations, too small to require suturing. These tend to heal by the sixth week after delivery.

During gestation, estrogen and progesterone act synergistically to evoke a rapid increase in breast size with growth of glandular and vascular elements. Puerperal changes in the breast are dramatic with further engorgement, enlargement, and increased pigmentation of the areolae between the second and fourth postpartum days. The effects of pregnancy and lactation on subsequent breast configuration, size, and consistency are variable. Since the breast is identified with feminine attractiveness, many women are concerned that lactation will cause diminution in size and loss of desired contour. The increased weight during nursing can produce stretching of the ligamentous support and eventuate in sagging or ptosis. A good nursing brassiere can help maintain support of the increasingly full mammary glands. A study by Oski revealed that 40 percent of lactating women who have suckled for more than 2 weeks had a subsequent decrease in breast size; 14 percent had an increase in breast size; and 46 percent experienced no change. Isolated reports of mammary atrophy and hyperinvolution following pregnancy and lactation have appeared sporadically in the literature. Dushoff has written that "the incidence of women seeking augmentation (mammaplasty) after progressive breast loss with each pregnancy is striking."

Exogenous androgenic hormones may have an adverse effect on breast structure. Ryan and Pernoll, in a letter to the editor of a medical journal, asked: "Is postpartum atrophy of the breast at least partially an iatrogenic disease?" They reported that of 20 women seeking augmentation mammaplasty, 16 gave a history of having received hormone injections to prevent milk production and breast engorgement. Deladumone OB contains 360 mg of testosterone enanthate in addition to 16 mg of estradiol valerate. Although defeminizing or virilizing complications have not been established, the advisability of administering high doses of androgens for lactation suppression has been questioned. The 360 mg of testosterone enanthate cited, the most frequently used amount, is "equivalent to several years of testosterone production by the normal female."

Postpartum Sexual Patterns

American obstetrics texts have traditionally prohibited coitus from 6 weeks prior to delivery to 6 weeks afterward. Coital restrictions often reflect societal taboos more than scientific findings. Influenced by primitive magical beliefs and superstitions concerning the uncleanliness of the postpartum woman and of lochia as well as menstrum, Hindu, ancient Persian, Talmudic, Old Testament, and Islamic scripture incorporated many taboos and regulations, concerning sexual activity. Although many American obstetricians still advise against coitus for 6 weeks post partum, more and more physicians have recently shortened and individualized coital prohibitions in the puerperium.

Masters and Johnson studied the sexual responses of six pregnant women during pregnancy and post partum under laboratory conditions. At 6 to 8 weeks post partum, genital vasocongestion was slower to develop following stimulation as reflected in slower vulvar swelling, vaginal lubrication, and vaginal distention. Rugal patterns were flattened or absent. Orgasmic contractions were reduced in intensity and duration. At 12 weeks, sexual response patterns returned to the prepregnancy state, and normal rugal patterns were reestablished. Masters and Johnson additionally described subjective responses of 101 postpartum women early in the third postpartum month. Forty-seven women reported low or absent sexual tension. The remaining 54 women expressed varying levels of sexual desire. In spite of the minimal desire in the substantial proportion of the women, all except those with coital prohibitions had resumed sexual intercourse by 6 to 8 weeks after delivery.

Tolor and DeGrazia reported data on 55 women seen at 6 weeks post partum. Over 80 percent of the women had resumed coitus. More than one-third of the group reported coitus four or more times each week. One-third of the total, interestingly, indicated that they would prefer more frequent sexual intercourse. Baker interviewed 54 British primiparas between 11 and 15 weeks post partum. Women reporting increased, decreased, and unchanged sexual interest and orgasmic capability constituted approximately equal groups, i.e., each comprised one-third of the total. Robson and Kumar studied a group of 119 British primiparas. Nearly all women had resumed sexual intercourse by 12 weeks post partum; 57 percent described their sexual desire as below prepregnancy levels, 33 percent reported no change, and only 10 percent reported an increase in sexual desire. By 1 year after delivery, a majority of women reported a decrease in coital frequency compared with before pregnancy, with only 11 percent reporting an increase. Lumley prospectively studied a group of 30 married primigravidas during pregnancy and after childbirth. Interviews during the third postpartum month recorded percentage changes in sexual desire and coital frequency. Libido was increased in 23 percent, remained the same in 61 percent, and decreased in 15 percent of the women compared with prior to pregnancy. The corresponding figures for coital frequency were 11 percent increase, 43 percent unchanged, and 46 percent decrease.

Postpartum Dyspareunia and Episiotomy

The judiciously performed episiotomy does help prevent lacerations, which are often difficult to repair and may result in poor wound healing. The purported benefits of preventing fetal brain damage and pelvic relaxation (weakening of fascial support of the uterus, vagina, rectum, and urinary bladder) have not been adequately substantiated.

Although episiotomy has been cited as one of the causes of dyspareunia, this complication has received remarkably little attention in the obstetric literature until recently. The midline or median episiotomy has been clearly contrasted with the mediolateral episiotomy. Wabrek and Wabrek report the incidence of dyspareunia following midline episiotomy to be less than 1 percent. In a British article, 60 of 68 respondents complained of dyspareunia at 3 months post partum, 80 percent attributing this to the mediolateral episiotomy. Another British study noted complaints of soreness and dyspareunia relating to episiotomy; the incidence at 3, 6, and 12 months was 40 percent, 18 percent, and 8 percent respectively. Secondary vaginismus may be produced subsequent to dyspareunia from surgical procedures on the vagina such as a mediolateral episiotomy. Reviews and editorials on the risk and benefits of episiotomy question the need for its routine use.

Lactation and Sexuality

Weichert sees lactation as part of a "psychosexual continuum." She has championed the breast-feeding of babies, criticized lactation suppression, and castigated apathetic obstetricians who do not promote breast-feeding. She has argued that a "functional castration of women has occurred [and that] forces...have eventuated in the use of the breast as a primary sex symbol and yardstick of feminine desirability, divorced from its nurturing role." She has asked, "Would anybody suggest, seriously, that males abstain from intercourse, bind themselves, take drugs to relieve congestion, or be mechanically relieved routinely, and that it would be as good?"

Newton has written that "the survival of the human race, long before the concept of duty evolved, depended upon the satisfaction gained from the two voluntary acts of reproduction—coitus and breast-feeding." Contemporary research by Robinson and Short has indicated a dramatic increase in breast sensitivity within 24 hours of parturition that lasts several days. They see this as a "key event" for activating suckling-induced oxytocin and prolactin release and suppressing ovulation during lactation. Physiologic responses common to both coitus and lactation include nipple erection, mammary venous dilation and breast warmth, and uterine contractions. Milk ejection can be triggered by sexual excitement as well as breast-feeding. Nipple stimulation, used clinically in antepartum fetal monitoring, predictably produces strong uterine contractions. Neurohumoral reflexes involving oxytocin secretion may be similar in coitus, lactation, and parturition.

Masters and Johnson reported that postpartum vaginal atrophy due to "steroid starvation" was especially true in the nursing mothers evaluated in the laboratory. Further laboratory assessment revealed that the enlarged lactating breast was found not to (further) increase in size consistently during sexual arousal from general stimulation. Lactating mothers reported sexual arousal, often to plateau levels of response, during nursing. Orgasm was reported on three occasions.

Various research studies have demonstrated a positive as well as a negative association between breast-feeding and sexual desire and responsiveness. A positive attitude toward breast-feeding has been related to comfort with sexuality. Likewise, aversive feelings toward lactation have been associated with a dislike of nudity and sexuality. On the other hand, some women's affectional and sensual needs may be met through nursing and caretaking of their infants.

Although sexual pleasure manifested during lactation—and incompatible with the concept of asexual motherhood—is believed to be uncommon by some, it may be more frequent than is realized in uninhibited, unrestricted breast-feeding. Twenty-five percent of lactating mothers in a small sample experienced sexual arousal during nursing. There are women who openly enjoy the sexual stimulation that breast-feeding may afford. Others find it uncomfortable, distasteful, guilt-producing, and intolerable to the extent that they wean their infants early. Riordan has written that if the sensual feelings the mother experiences during breast-feeding "are accepted as a natural, gratifying maternal experience [they can] strengthen the feeling of tenderness and commitment to her baby."

Psychosocial Factors

Profound psychological, interpersonal, social, and biological changes occur during pregnancy and the puerperium. The resolution of conflict, adjustment of roles, and the incorporation of changing relationships within and outside the family make this psychosocial transition period a developmental crisis. Physical, financial, social, and emotional challenges to the couple demand a stable marital relationship. Without this, the pregnancy and the arrival of a child may act as a wedge to drive the couple irreparably apart. The idea that a child will bring harmony and intimacy into a dysfunctional marriage is erroneous if not ludicrous. The husband traditionally has been relegated to a supportive if not tangential role during pregnancy and childbirth. "The obstetrician assumes many of the directive and nurturant roles, often usurping those of the husband." If this replacement is aggravated by coital prohibitions, the expectant father is likely to feel more displaced. Ambivalence, if not resentment, toward the infant is predictable if infant demands and maternal fatigue diminish the wife's sexual interest.

As is true with sexuality in pregancy, postpartum sexuality (including interest, coital resumption, and enjoyment) is influenced and complicated by many variables. In the past, the cultural desexualization of the pregnant, puerperal, and lactating woman was accomplished through widespread taboos. Successful maternal adaptation has been shown to be more dependent on the motivations for pregnancy than on whether or not the pregnancy was planned. Maternal needs for nurturance may be expressed sexually or as a desire to be held. Many of these affectional needs are fulfilled in the puerperium by touching and holding the infant and putting him or her to the breast. The most frequently given reasons for poor postpartum sexual adjustment in the women include episiotomy discomfort, fatigue, vaginal bleeding or discharge, dyspareunia, insufficient lubrication, fears of awakening the infant or not hearing him or her, fear of injury, and decreased sense of attractiveness.

SEXUAL COUNSELING

Sexual expression is crucial for marital communication and affirmation of love, trust, and commitment within marriage. Marital success and happiness depend to a large extent on a sound and satisfying sexual relationship.

Sexual attitudes, behaviors, and expectations have been influenced not only by the sex researchers but by the sexual (r) evolution, the women's liberation movement, the holistic health cause, and media promotion. In spite of hedonistic distortions, excesses, and license (freedom without responsibility) and the epidemic of sexually transmitted diseases and teenage pregnancies, an increase in openness, enlightenment, and human potential has been realized. Optimal wellness demands an emphasis on preventive medicine and health maintenance, including psychological and sexual health. There is an emphasis on self-responsibility, but, additionally, there is the expectation that the primary care physician will be concerned with the patient as a person and with her emotional as well as her physical needs. Renewed physician interest in psychosomatic and behavioral medicine has been one corollary of social and sociosexual change. The progressive, responsive physician looks at the psyche and the soma in a sociocultural-ecologic context. Sexual concerns are seen as genuine, health-related issues rather than simply "recreational handicaps."

In 1973 at a House of Delegates meeting of the American Medical Association, it was stated that patients currently identify the physician "as a primary source of sexual information and counseling...but the physicians often are not prepared to meet this responsibility." Harold Lief, a Philadelphia psychiatrist, was one member of the medical profession to recognize and publish this deficit, thus providing an important impetus for change. In 1960, human sexuality was a formal part of the curriculum of three medical schools. In 1968, about 30 medical schools had such courses, and by 1983, almost all medical schools were providing some formal instruction in human sexuality.

Counseling Techniques

To be an effective counselor, a physician must develop a sense of sexual self-awareness and sexual comfort in addition to knowledge of sexual physiology, psychology, sociocultural norms, and the effects of drugs, illness, pregnancy, and aging. Sexual comfort can be enhanced by exercises, which include role modeling of the counselor and patient/client situation (optimally with video or audio feedback), attending interactional and experiential sexuality seminars, and participating in the implosive sexual attitude reassessment workshops characterized by the viewing of explicit movies and small group process.

The invaluable tool of interviewing as a diagnostic and therapeutic skill has been ignored or deemphasized by many schools of medicine. Comfort as well as skill can be enhanced by the practice of regularly and systematically taking a sexual history from all patients. A list of counseling axioms, which constitute the style and substance of the sexual interview, with subsequent explanations, follows:

I. Primum non nocere (first do no harm)
II. Create the climate (ambience)
   Privacy without interruption
   Definite time limits
   Avoid indignities

III. Effective physician attitude and posture
   Warm permissiveness
   Active listening
   Observation—affect and body language
   Use of silence
IV. Effective verbal skills
   Level
   Sexual words
   Myths
   Normalcy queries
   Ubiquity and open-ended questions
   From more to less sensitive issues
   Avoid "why" questions.

Primum non nocere—first do no harm. Embarassed silence, misinformation, imposing one's personal values on the patient, a surprised or shocked expression, apparent boredom or preoccupation, personal discounting or belittling—these are to be avoided. It is crucial to attempt to create a relaxed, nonthreatening environment and form a therapeutic alliance with the patient.

An initial few minutes of small talk and shared commonalities (e.g., birthplace, pastimes, children, weather) may mitigate anxiety. Privacy without interruption, a quiet, soundproof office, a stated time period, and assurance of confidentiality are important considerations. Recording the interview, although it is good practice for the novice, distracts and inhibits discussion. Endearments, presumptuous familiarity (e.g., the use of first names), and patronizing or infantilizing the patient should be assiduously avoided.

The physician must balance his or her authoritative status with a gentle, caring, and attending manner, communicating acceptance of the patient as a unique individual with personal worth. Active listening requires the avoidance of distraction, awareness of intonation, and attention to feelings as well as content. It is necessary to listen until the patient completes her "train of thought" before formulating a response. Periodic nods, encouraging sounds, and appropriate paraphrases indicate active listening and hearing. The observation of the patient's facial expressions, movements, and posture can supply important information. Constant dialogue is unnecessary; occasional silence may be comforting and useful for assimilation or processing to occur.

Medical or psychological jargon may confuse rather than clarify. The patient's intelligence, education, and degree of sophistication will help to determine the level of communication. One must not accept a patient's labels, such as "He is oversexed" or "I am frigid." It is important to ask, "What do you mean by that?" Most sexual words are either euphemisms or "street" language. I explain to the patient that I use medical or scientific terms because I am more comfortable with them and because they have exact or precise meanings. On the other hand, I make it clear that I have no expectation that she will use the same terms unless she wishes to. It is essential that myths be tactfully and sensitively corrected at the risk of interruption. If this is not done at the time, you have, in effect, tacitly or implicitly validated the misconception.

A knowledge base permits you to inform and educate, a primary component of counseling. Patients frequently wish to know whether their behavior or their husband's requests are "normal" and seek informed support or reassurance.

A good technique for introducing the sexual history as part of the medical history is to begin by a universal or ubiquitous statement such as "Most people experience sexual concerns or problems at times during their lives." This is followed by a question such as "What problems, if any, have you experienced?" or "What concerns would you like to share with me?" Thus, sexual concerns are legitimized and normalized and sexual health is acknowledged as a vital part of total health. Sexual dialogue is often forthcoming and direct questions can follow.

Another approach is to ascertain the patient's expectations of a sexual situation, e.g., the marital sexual relationship as compared with her actual experiences or behavior. Information about the quality of the overall relationship, including ongoing conflicts or unresolved issues, is as important as specific sexual information. Questions about sexual desire, arousal, gratification, coital frequency, pain on intercourse, and sexual assault are useful. One should ask one question at a time and allow time for an answer. It is advisable to avoid "why" questions, which are typically heard as blaming and critical. One can ask a similar question using "how" or "what," e.g., "How do you think the problem came to be?"

The PLISSIT Paradigm

Annon devised a conceptual scheme for the rapid treatment of sexual concerns, which he has labeled the PLISSIT mode. PLISSIT (or P-LI-SS-IT) stands for four increasingly deep levels of therapeutic intervention—permission, limited information, specific suggestions, and intensive therapy. It is a concept that can be used by therapist and nontherapist alike. The first three levels are considered brief therapy (or counseling), and the fourth level is intensive therapy as stated. The PLISSIT approach can be used in a variety of settings and is suitable when there is little time available. The model can be tailored to the degree of competence (knowledge, comfort, counseling skills) of the physician, because each level requires increasing amounts of training and experience.

The first level is permission, described as giving permission to the patient to experience certain attitudes, feelings, or behaviors. (I like to think of it as enabling the patient to give herself permission. In this context I facilitate or enpower the patient's/client's coping abilities rather than problem-solving or "rescuing.") Often patients want to know if they are "normal."

"Limited information" provides the patient with specific factual information that is directly relevant to her concerns. Concerns about breasts and genital size or shape, the normality of coital positions other than the "missionary position," and orogenital sex are typical. Patients often want to know whether certain behavior is "wrong" or "bad." Appropriate, informative reassurance can be remarkably helpful.

The "specific suggestion" level, according to Annon, necessitates administering a sexual problem history. It is essential that premature, inappropriate suggestions not be given upon hearing a patient's presenting "labels." The specific, unique circumstances must be heard and unwoven first. Special suggestions might include coital proscription, sensate focus (nondemand caressing sessions), self-awareness tasks, or the admonition to the male partner "Don't use your penis sexually if you are anxious or not aroused."

Marital discord accounts for a substantial proportion of sexual problems. If a patient is married or has an ongoing sexual relationship, it is useful to see her with her husband or sexual partner at some point in order to observe their communication. Seeing the sexual partner individually is helpful in obtaining a different viewpoint. It is mandatory that information obtained at individual sessions not be shared with the other partner without expressed consent.

Intensive therapy is indicated when brief therapy (or sexual counseling) incorporating the first three levels of the PLISSIT model has been unsuccessful after a few sessions. For most physicians without formal training, referral to a sex therapist or a psychologist with special skills in this area is indicated. Intensive therapy or sex therapy, as distinguished from sex counseling, involves the capacity to deal explicitly in a more sophisticated fashion with problems of interaction between the partners and of individual psychopathology. There are times in the course of sexual counseling when it becomes obvious that significant psychopathology exists or that marital disharmony is extreme or primary. Inhibited sexual desire may be secondary to depression. Decompensated psychotic patients may present with sexual problems and should be referred to a psychiatrist. Patients whose primary problem appears to be marital dysfunction should usually be referred to a marriage counselor.

Sexual Counseling and Treatment Implications for Pregnancy and the Puerperium

The physician can be invaluable in supplying guidance concerning psychosexual aspects of pregnancy and the puerperium. Conjoint counseling, i.e., counseling the pregnant patient and her husband, is ideal. When practical, the husband can accompany his wife during her antepartum visits, childbirth education and parenting classes, and parturition.

A brief sexual history can be taken as part of the reproductive history or can follow the physical examination when other psychophysiologic aspects such as nutrition, drugs, sleep, rest and relaxation, exercise, and lactation are discussed. A ubiquitous statement such as "Most women experience noticeable sexual as well as emotional changes during pregnancy," followed by the open-ended question, "What changes if any have you experienced?", enables a patient to share her attitudes, experiences, and concerns. Physiologic leukorrhea of pregnancy should be discussed so that increased vaginal discharge is not perceived as infection and does not become a deterrent to sexual relations. On the other hand, leukorrhea with associated pruritus vulvae, vulvodynia, dysuria, or dyspareunia deserves careful assessment. Nurturant and affectional needs that are not explicitly sexual can be met by touching, caressing, massaging, and holding. Manual partner stimulation and masturbation are noncoital options for sexual pleasure, intimate communication, and sexual release. In advanced gestation, coital positions including the female superior and rear entry ("spoon") are suitable. Pillows can enhance comfort.

Coital and orgasmic prohibitions are appropriate for threatened abortion, habitual abortions of unknown cause, an incompetent cervix, müllerian fusion defects, placenta previa, threatened premature labor, premature cervical dilation, premature amniorrhexis, multifetal gestation, and dyspareunia. Patients with an incompetent cervix or threatened premature labor should be made aware that nipple stimulation may be associated with uterine contractions. The risk of air embolism from the forceful blowing of air into the vagina during sex play and the possibility of maternal and perinatal infection, premature rupture of membranes, and prematurity from sexually transmitted diseases should be mentioned. Gentleness and fastidious genital hygiene have been recommended precautions. Women with new or multiple sexual partners should consider the prophylactic benefit of condoms.

The touching and holding of the infant shortly after birth may enhance bonding with the new family addition and aid marital harmony and intimacy. Contraceptive needs must be met prior to hospital discharge.

Fatigue caused by the demands of pregnancy and childbirth, an erratic demanding feeding schedule, and interrupted sleep can compromise the coping ability of the new mother and damage the marital and sexual relationship. Sufficient sleep and rest and the husband's emotional and physical support are crucial issues. Nursing the baby just prior to sexual relations and the wearing of a bra with absorbent pads can help. Sensual and possibly sexual feelings evoked by lactation can be mentioned and their normalcy articulated.

The mediolateral episiotomy should be avoided, with rare exceptions, because of frequent and prolonged pain, tenderness, and dyspareunia. The midline episiotomy should be individualized rather than routinized for childbirth; if it is performed, the skin edges should be carefully approximated with fine suture material. Like the mediolateral episiotomy, the vertical skin incision for the cesarean section is rarely indicated. The Pfannenstiel incision is not subject to wound separation (dehiscence), as is the vertical incision, and it is cosmetically superior to the often unsightly vertical incision. Additionally, some women complain of painful spasm of a vertical scar at the time of orgasm. There are generally no medical contraindications to resuming coitus by 3 weeks post partum. It has been said that resumption of coitus after delivery, however, should be based on the couple's sexual feelings, the healing of the episiotomy, and the absence of uterine bleeding. (The last proviso is probably an extension of the menstrual taboo.) Masters and Johnson have recommended that physicians individualize rather than arbitrarily assign postpartum periods of continence.

Prior to attempted intromission, the woman can inspect the episiotomy incision with a hand mirror and can insert a clean finger or tampon to test for healing and residual soreness. The use of copious amounts of water-soluble lubricant, especially in lactating mothers in whom vaginal atrophy is maximal, is helpful. Kegel exercises should be started prior to hospital discharge and are beneficial in increasing cognitive awareness of vaginal tension, promoting healing, and strengthening the pubococcygeal muscles and improving vaginal tone. Partial intromission can precede full intromission if episiotomy tenderness or vaginospasm is inhibitory. Passive vaginal containment prior to active thrusting minimizes coital discomfort. Coital positions such as side-to-side and female superior minimize episiotomy soreness. Pressure on the episiotomy site can also be avoided by placing pillows under the woman's buttocks to direct penile pressure anteriorly.

Body image is an important factor in postpartum sexuality. Muscle toning exercises can usually be started prior to hospital discharge. Present-day obstetricians are permissive concerning allowable weight gain in pregnancy in order to avoid "starving the baby." Consequently many gravidas who are not restricted to the traditional 20 lb allowance find postpartum obesity a problem. Although early conservative dieting is prudent, it is realistic for the puerpera to set her goal of attaining her pregnancy weight at 3 to 6 months rather than 6 weeks. Protein, iron, and vitamins are essential for postpartum tissue repair and organ involution. A nutritious diet, exercise, rest and relaxation, and physical and emotional support are necessary for the release of libidinal energy that is frequently diminished in the puerperium.

SUGGESTED READING

Annon JS. The behavioral treatment of sexual problems: brief therapy. New York: Harper & Row, 1976.

Perkins RP. Sexuality during pregnancy. Clin Obstet Gynecol 1984; 27:706–716.

Reamy KJ, White SE. Sexuality in pregnancy and the puerperium: a review. Obstet Gynecol Surv 1985; 40:1–13.

Reamy KJ, White SE. Sexuality in the puerperium: a review. Arch Sex Behav 1987; 16:165–186.

Reamy KJ, White SE, Daniell WC, LeVine ES. Sexuality and pregnancy: a prospective study. J Reprod Med 1982; 27:321–327.

Swanson J. The marital sexual relationshp during pregnancy. JOGN 1980; 9: 267–270.

ANTEPARTUM FETAL TESTING

LAWRENCE D. DEVOE, M.D.

The modern history of antepartum fetal testing is now entering its third decade. During its development, a wide variety of assessment techniques has been used in the management of high-risk pregnancy. From the late 1960s to the mid 1970s, indirect evaluation of fetal-placental condition relied on determinations of pregnancy-associated hormones in maternal blood and urine, including progesterone, estrogens, and human placental lactogen. Management of pregnancy was effected by following trends in the levels of these hormones, was reliant on relatively complex laboratory assays, and was hampered by delays in obtaining results and the need for serial samples to account for normal biologic fluctuations. Approximately 15 years ago, clinical studies of maternal perception of fetal movements showed that such data could provide a useful means of antepartum evaluation that was not dependent on the availability of a sophisticated clinical chemistry laboratory. Even more recently, technologic advances in medical instrumentation resulted in the availability of obstetric ultrasound imaging and electronic fetal heart rate (FHR) monitoring in the antepartum period. These advances have led to a gradual shift away from biochemical testing methods and toward biophysical evaluation of the high-risk fetus. Several biophysical screening tests now exist to determine the level of fetal well-being at the actual time of observation. Because fetal compromise may have different etiologies and may evolve either gradually or acutely, the role of modern fetal testing has been continually reevaluated. The present chapter provides the physiologic basis, description, interpretative guidelines, and clinical applications of contraction stress testing, nonstress testing, the biophysical profile, and Doppler-directed fetal-placental blood flow studies. Its aim is to enable clinical practitioners to understand the relative importance of each of these testing methods as well as their inherent limitations in the management of complicated pregnancies.

GENERAL GUIDELINES FOR ANTEPARTUM TESTING

Biophysical testing of high-risk fetuses requires that each method be initiated not only at the first suspicion of high-risk status, but at a point in gestation where the following conditions obtain: (1) expected physiologic and/or pathologic responses are well established; (2) fetal age and/or state of maturity would result in a viable infant should delivery occur; (3) sufficient expertise and equipment for test performance and interpretation are available; and (4) contingent plans for subsequent perinatal management have been developed so that test results may be useful to the clinician.

In practical terms, this generally translates into the initiation of antepartum testing after the completion of 30-weeks gestation. While pathologic patterns observed in antepartum testing may be equally valid before 30 weeks, normative data for extremely premature fetuses is scanty. Therefore, errors in classification of normal early third trimester fetuses are possible, thereby increasing the risks of unnecessary early intervention and prematurity if such testing were used as a sole determinant for management.

The interval for test repetition may be variable. Initial recommendations that normal test outcomes require only weekly follow-up have given way to a variety of management algorithms, ranging from biweekly to daily testing in special circumstances. It is generally agreed that any test begins to lose predictive power as the time interval from its performance to delivery increases. Consequently, repeated testing at intervals of less than 1 week is strongly recommended for any of the methods described that follow.

Conditions for antepartum testing have not been standardized with respect to maternal variables such as preceding activity levels, diet, time of day, or, in some instances, length of observation. Therefore it becomes quite difficult to compare data of previous studies and nearly impossible to make valid sequential comparisons of tests performed in the same fetus. It is suggested that uniform conditions be established within any testing center so that reproducibility and sequential follow-up may be consistent. This is most important for performing biophysical profile testing as fetal breathing can be strongly affected by the maternal-fed state and the length of observation.

Equipment used in antepartum testing should be of sufficient quality so that signal loss is minimized and imaging is reliable. Individuals using test equipment should be experienced in observing fetal biophysical activity and familiar with potential artifacts seen when factitious Doppler-induced fetal heart rate variability, cardiac arrhythmias, or passive maternal movements may be present.

Interpretative criteria for fetal biophysical testing are diverse and numerous rating systems have been published. As no consensus on testing standards has been achieved, clinicians should be extremely careful when applying arbitrary criteria for nonstress test (NST) reactivity or biophysical profile scoring until adequate experience has been obtained in a population similar to their own.

Clinical management of test results should not be performed in a vacuum, but should consider all available features of the pregnancy at risk before intervention is selected. The limitations of these antepartum testing approaches raise significant concerns as to the practice of relying on any one test as a single factor in obstetric decision making.

ANTEPARTUM TESTING METHODS

Electronic Fetal Heart Rate Testing

Contraction Stress Test

Background. The contraction stress test (CST, oxytocin challenge test, nipple stimulation test) arose from intrapartum observations of fetal heart rate responses to uterine activity in both normal and pathologic pregnancies. Under conditions of relative intrauterine hypoxia, when contraction intensity exceeded 35 mm Hg, a healthy fetal-placental unit would provide sufficient reserve and maintain adequate blood gas hemostasis; therefore, little or no cardiovascular alteration was required to maintain adequate tissue oxygenation. Fetal heart rate responses, as a marker for fetal condition, during the period of stress imposed by moderate to strong uterine contractions would show no changes in normal, well-oxygenated fetuses, but would exhibit intermittent or persistent late decelerations when arterial oxygen pressures fell below 18 mm Hg. The frequency, duration, and amplitude of late fetal heart rate decelerations were related to the baseline level of fetal oxygenation prior to uterine contractions, the intensity and duration of each contraction, and the inherent responsiveness of the fetal myocardium. As fetal condition deteriorated, the ability to recover a normal baseline rate after each contraction diminished, the lag in onset of late decelerations relative to the peak of uterine contractions decreased, and, in terminal or agonal states, late decelerations might become increasingly subtle (i.e., of low amplitude) or disappear as fetal bradycardia ensued prior to death.

Under certain circumstances, especially when the fetus is either growth retarded or postmature and where oligohydramnios is present, the CST has become useful in eliciting potentially dangerous umbilical cord compression events. Sporadic or recurrent variable heart rate decelerations may reflect the intensity of cord compression or occlusion and the integrity of reflex mechanisms for recovery. Such observations have been particularly useful in predicting fetuses at risk for cord problems during labor and may be beneficial in planning the optimal mode of delivery.

Technique. In the original description of the CST, uterine activity, if not spontaneous, was induced by an infusion of intravenous oxytocin, delivered by a controlled-pump system. The patient was placed in either semi-Fowler's or lateral recumbent position in order to avoid supine hypotension. An initial baseline fetal heart rate record was begun, ranging from 10 to 30 minutes in length, to assure that a pathologic pattern was not already present, and oxytocin was infused at a rate beginning at 0.5 to 1.0 milliunits per minute, with doubling of the infusion rate every 20 to 30 minutes, until a pattern of moderate to strong uterine contractions occurring at a frequency of three in 10 minutes was achieved. Testing was concluded when a diagnostic window was achieved, when it became apparent that uterine hyporesponsiveness to oxytocin was present or, on rare occasions, when uterine hyperstimulation occurred.

A newer alternative to infused oxytocin induction of uterine activity has been provided by maternal nipple massage, i.e., the nipple stimulation CST. Palmar massage of the nipple is performed by the patient for 2 to 5 minutes and the subsequent contraction response recorded. A similar pattern of uterine activity can be achieved by this method, and it avoids the need for an intravenous line and pump controller. Moreover, nipple stimulation usually results in a more rapid onset of satisfactory uterine activity, often within 15 to 20 minutes, as opposed to 90 minutes for oxytocin infusion techniques. The actual mechanisms for producing contractions by this method are not known. Its reported rates of hyperstimulation and failure are higher than for oxytocin, and it has not been established that the uterine activity generated is comparable to that of exogenous oxytocin infusions.

Test Indications and Contraindications. The CST is indicated in any circumstance where placental insufficiency is suspected, such as postdatism, intrauterine growth retardation, or maternal vascular disease. CSTs have been successfully performed in multifetal gestations, although it may be technically more difficult to maintain satisfactory simultaneous tracings of each fetus.

Contraindications to performing the CST exist. These include the following high-risk conditions: (1) third trimester bleeding; (2) preterm rupture of membranes; (3) prior preterm labor or advanced cervical ripening when fetal maturity has not been established; and (4) documented previous classic cesarean section. While the incidence of inadvertent premature rupture of membranes or stimulation of labor is low prior to term, the potential for these results suggests that such testing be performed near or in a labor and delivery area.

Interpretation of the CST. In general, there are five classifications of test outcomes (Table 1): (1) positive—late heart rate decelerations occur after most contractions, occurring within a diagnostic window of 10 to 30 minutes; (2) negative—no late or variable heart rate decelerations are present; (3) suspicious or equivocal—occasional late or variable heart rate decelerations are present; (4) unsatisfactory—an adequate contraction pattern could not be established or fetal heart rate signal quality is insufficient for interpretation; and (5) hyperstimulation—uterine tetany or tachysystole occurs during the test. While the actual frequency of late decelerations required for a positive reading may vary among institutions, it has been suggested that a minimum of 30 percent of contractions accompanied by late decelerations is sufficient to predict fetal distress during labor.

The addition of reactivity criteria to test interpretation has refined the predictive accuracy of the CST. A reactive test, characterized by the presence of movement-associated accelerations, connotes a lower level of fetal risk than when such accelerations are absent. The majority of reactive fetuses with positive CSTs can be delivered vaginally in good condition. Conversely, a nonreactive positive CST has the highest positive predictive value and is most commonly seen in instances where fetal hypoxemia is present and/or perinatal asphyxia is imminent.

Clinical Follow-Up of the CST. A negative test confers a high probability of fetal health, but should be followed up in less than 1 week, as numerous reports of fetal demise have followed negative tests performed at intervals of greater than 6 days. A nonreactive positive CST is highly suggestive of fetal compromise and mandates acute intervention, generally by cesarean delivery, unless the cervix is favorable and early amniotomy and internal electronic fetal monitoring with scalp blood sampling can be instituted. A reactive positive CST, in the presence of a favorable cervix, and/or established fetal maturity, and/or intrauterine growth retardation (IUGR), should also result in obstetric intervention. Otherwise, it would be appropriate to consider performing an adjunctive test, such as a comprehensive biophysical profile, and include the results of that test in clinical management. Suspicious or equivocal tests should be repeated within 24 hours until a clearly negative or positive result occurs. Persistently equivocal tests should be managed on an individual basis and may be backed up with the biophysical profile if the uterine cervix is unfavorable or fetal maturity has not been established. When uterine hyperstimulation occurs, the patient

TABLE 1 Contraction Stress Test: Clinical Summary

Test Outcome	*Interpretative Criteria*	*Clinical Response*
Negative	No late or variable FHR decelerations	Repeat <7 days
Positive	Repetitive late FHR decelerations associated with at least 30 to 50% of uterine contractions in a 30-minute window of 3 contractions per 10 minutes	Mature fetus or absent reactivity→delivery Immature fetus or reactivity present→confirm with biophysical profile Consider delivery if IUGR is present
Equivocal	Occasional late or variable FHR decelerations present	Repeat test within 24 hours If positive or negative, manage as listed above; if persistently equivocal, consider delivery if fetus is mature; otherwise, back up with biophysical profile
Unsatisfactory	Inadequate pattern of uterine activity or excessive FHR signal loss	Repeat test or perform biophysical profile
Hyperstimulation	Uterine tetany or tachysystole occurs	Rest patient for 2-6 hours and repeat test

should be allowed a rest period of several hours before resuming testing.

Nonstress Test

Background. The nonstress test was introduced into clinical obstetrics approximately 10 years ago. It is based on the observations that healthy fetuses exhibited frequent movements that were associated with FHR accelerations. The linkage of fetal movement with heart rate acceleration is influenced by the state of cardiovascular maturity and becomes a common finding in fetuses beyond 30-weeks gestation.

The rationale for using FHR accelerations as an indicator of fetal well-being is based on the following observations: (1) the sympathetic reflexes involved require adequate adrenal medullary reserve, providing a reservoir of cardioactive catecholamines; (2) fetal activity needed to stimulate accelerations depends on adequate energy stores in fetal liver and heart; (3) chronically stressed or acutely hypoxemic fetuses decrease their frequency of movements so that either a low incidence of accelerations is present or myocardial response is blunted; and (4) extremely compromised fetuses generate little or no spontaneous body movements. Acceleration amplitude is inversely related to baseline FHR, which in turn declines gradually with advancing gestational age. Immature fetuses or those with tachycardia produced by exogenous drugs or stress factors may exhibit low amplitude accelerations that may fail to meet most commonly accepted reactivity criteria. There are also instances where a false impression of fetal compromise may be created when baseline reactivity is reduced by maternal sedation or beta-blockade or when fetal supraventricular arrhythmias occur.

Technique. The nonstress test is easy to perform and requires an electronic fetal heart rate monitor with a second channel for documentation of baseline uterine activity and fetal movement. As with the CST, the patient should be positioned to avoid maternal hypotension. It is extremely helpful to prepare the mother to be a cooperative observer so that fetal movements can be tracked accurately. This allows subsequent interpreters to be more assured that the accelerations produced during testing are most likely the consequence of endogenous fetal stimulation.

Numerous manipulations have been used to provoke fetal reactivity: (1) external physical stimulation; (2) glucose or glucose-containing substance administration; and (3) acoustic stimulation. Controlled studies of physical manipulation of the fetus have failed to demonstrate that this results in "enhanced" fetal responsiveness; it is more probable that the increased frequency of reactive tests following this maneuver is a function of extended observation time. Glucose administration has not been shown to elicit a significant increase in fetal movement incidence and may only be indicated when there has been documentation of maternal hypoglycemia. Acoustic stimulation, using an artificial larynx or sound generator, has been shown to provoke fetal accelerations, analogous to "startle" responses after 25-weeks gestation. Preliminary studies suggest that such information is highly predictive of fetal well-being and correlates well with subsequently normal or reactive NSTs.

Indications and Contraindications. The clinical conditions indicating nonstress testing are the same as those for the CST. There are no known contraindications to performing this test.

Interpretation of the NST. At present, more than two dozen interpretative schemes have been reported. Most share a common requirement for a minimal frequency of FHR accelerations (e.g., two per 20 minutes, three per 30 minutes; and of a minimum amplitude, e.g., 10 or 15 beats per minute, and duration, e.g., 15 seconds) associated with active fetal movements. Whereas other parameters, such as baseline FHR, long-term variability of FHR, and the presence or absence of spontaneous heart rate decelerations, have been suggested as additions to improve the diagnostic accuracy of nonstress testing, no comprehensive universally acceptable multiple parameter scheme has been developed. In addition, the designations "reactive" and "nonreactive" are somewhat misleading and arbitrary as there may be gradations in fetal decompensation, which would be overlooked by the application of absolute minimal criteria for test normalcy. NSTs may be classified as unsatisfactory if signal loss precludes interpretability or if FHR baseline is indeterminate because of an intrinsic cardiac arrhythmia. A final classification, sinusoidal pattern, has been identified in association with fetal compromise secondary to severe Rh-isoimmunization wherein profound fetal anemia or hydrops is present. This pattern, characterized by regular, recurrent baseline oscillations of five to ten beats per minute, with a frequency of three to five cycles per minute has also been reported in cases of significant fetal-maternal transfusion and twin-to-twin transfusion when fetal anemia is present. Its etiology is unknown, but the persistence of a true sinusoidal pattern, even in the face of periodic normal baseline events, should be considered an ominous finding.

Clinical Follow-Up of the NST. Several management options exist for the follow-up of NSTs (Table 2). A reactive or normal test, as in the case of a negative CST, should be followed up with a repeat examination as indicated by the severity of the clinical condition; biweekly testing is recommended as a minimum "safe" interval. A nonreactive or abnormal test may be followed up using one of the following schemes: (1) extension of the original observation period for as long as 90 minutes, unless a reactive window is achieved earlier; (2) repetition of the test later in the day if nonreactivity is ascribed to maternal hypoglycemia or drug ingestion; (3) subsequent performance of a CST, using its outcome as previously described for clinical management; and (4) performance of a biophysical profile, using its outcome to plan management.

Under the following selected circumstances, a persistently nonreactive NST mandates acute obstetric intervention: (1) the fetus is mature and the test is nonreactive for 90 minutes in the absence of fetal anomalies, drug influences, or maternal metabolic imbalance; (2) spontaneous, late, or severe variable decelerations are consistently

TABLE 2 Nonstress Test: Clinical Summary

Test Outcome	*Interpretative Criteria*	*Clinical Response*
Reactive	FHR accelerations of adequate frequency, amplitude, and duration accompany fetal movement	Repeat test within 3–4 days
Nonreactive	Inadequate or absent FHR accelerations; fetal movement reduced or absent	Extend test up to 90 minutes If reactivity appears, manage as above; if test remains nonreactive, perform CST or biophysical profile
Spontaneous	FHR decelerations occur with fetal movement	Consider possibility of cord entanglement or oligohydramnios Perform ultrasound for amniotic fluid volume, anomalies
Sinusoidal	Repetitive, uniform FHR oscillations, 5–10 beats per minute, 3–5 cycles per minute Reactivity usually absent	Consider delivery if fetus is mature or Rh-isoimmunization is present Perform Kleihauer-Betke test to rule out fetal-maternal bleed
Unsatisfactory	Excessive signal loss or indeterminate baseline	Repeat test Consider M-mode echocardiogram or abdominal ECG if fetal arrhythmia is suspected

present; (3) there is documented oligohydramnios; and (4) a sinusoidal pattern is present.

The Biophysical Profile

Background. Multiple parameter biophysical testing, or the "biophysical profile," has evolved over the past 7 years as an attempt to refine fetal evaluation. This approach uses additional parameters that examine both dynamic and static data generated by the fetus and placenta. In principle, biophysical profile testing includes dynamic or acute observations (fetal heart rate patterns, fetal breathing movements (FBMs), fetal body movements (FMs), fetal reflex activity, or neurologic tonus) and static or chronic information (semiquantitative or qualitative amniotic fluid volume, placental grading).

The rationale for this test is based on both acute and long-term studies of activity in normal and compromised animal and human fetuses, coupled with the notions that oligohydramnios is a marker for intrauterine hypoxemia and accelerated placental senescence indicates an increased risk for intrauteria hypoxia and acidemia. Since a variety of parameters are examined, biophysical profile testing gives a more comprehensive view of intrauterine fetal status, and aids in the detection of fetal anomalies and conditions associated with increased risk for intrapartum fetal distress, such as oligohydramnios. The components of a biophysical profile can be regarded as providing two complementary types of information about intrauterine well-being. The dynamic or acute parameters of FHR, breathing and body movements, and neurologic tonus may reflect states of oxygenation, acid-base balance, and caloric reserves, as all of these activities require an adequate level of fetal homeostasis for their normal appearance and frequency. The static or chronic parameters of amniotic fluid volume and placental grade reflect longer-term conditions such as chronic uteroplacental insufficiency. Amniotic fluid volume (AFV) may be reduced as a consequence of fetal circulatory shunting. Placental senescence may be accelerated when intervillous perfusion is suboptimal. Whether the dynamic parameters of the biophysical profile are equally reflective of neuromuscular maturation remains to be determined as they may be normal in cases of central motoneuron aberrations (e.g., anencephaly) and may be abnormal when decreased amniotic fluid volume restricts fetal movements and promotes flexion contractures and pulmonary hypoplasia.

Technique. The original description of this test utilized a nonstress test, followed by ultrasonographic visualization of the other dynamic and static parameters. An alternate approach is to perform the electronic fetal heart rate monitoring and ultrasonographic observation simultaneously, thus eliminating artifacts attributable to changes in fetal state that may occur during the testing session. Recent developments in technology have enabled computerization of data acquisition and analysis, allowing greater precision in their measurements.

Although test length has not been standardized, at least 30 to 45 minutes is generally needed to complete a biophysical profile, with an ideal minimum period accounting for activity fluctuations due to physiologic cycles being closer to 60 to 90 minutes. Maternal state conditions during testing have not been standardized, although it is recognized that prolonged fasting or hypoglycemia may result in unusually decreased frequency of fetal breathing movements. Circadian rhythms governing fetal activity cycles mandate that each fetus should be tested at approximately the same time of day if serial testing is anticipated.

Indications. The indications for biophysical profile testing are similar to those for nonstress testing, although most centers have used the biophysical profile as a selective primary test in cases where amniotic fluid volume is likely to be decreased, e.g., intrauterine growth retardation or postdatism. The biophysical profile is also recommended as a back-up test for abnormal or nonreactive NSTs or persistently equivocal CSTs. Although there are no known contraindications for this test, its relatively greater cost, time requirements, and equipment needs make it a less desirable primary test than FHR testing alone.

Interpretation. Initial studies of biophysical profile testing used an arbitrary scoring system related to each of the parameters, which was compiled as a "planning" or management score (Table 3). A normal parameter was assigned a score of 2; an abnormal parameter, 0. Subsequent investigators have attempted a further refinement of this system by either adding an intermediate score of 1 for borderline or equivocal parameters or by considering placental grading. Consequently, the assignment of a normal score depends on the system used and may range from 0 to 10 in a five-parameter system, with the normal cutoff greater than 6, or 0 to 12 in a six-parameter system, with a normal cutoff greater than 7. Such approaches have been criticized for the following reasons: (1) the scoring system is not only arbitrary but unweighted, assuming independence and equal importance of all parameters; (2) comparative studies against nonstress testing alone have not shown that diagnostic accuracy has been significantly improved except for the detection of anomalies and oligohydramnios; (3) the threshold values chosen for each dynamic biophysical parameter bear little relationship to established physiologic norms; and (4) quantitation of amniotic fluid volume is controversial and no "gold standard," short of dye-dilution studies, exists. Recently, normal reference values for dynamic parameters have been determined for a normal obstetric population. Application of a rating scale for these values has shown that the predictive power of biophysical testing may be enhanced by such an approach and is maximal once any two test parameters fall more than two standard deviations from the norm.

Clinical Follow-Up of Biophysical Profile Outcomes. A normal test result, regardless of interpretative criteria, is highly predictive of an intact, well-oxygenated fetus. In most cases, this observation retains its validity for up to 7 days. An abnormal test should be viewed in the following two ways: (1) the nature of the factors contributing to the test abnormality, e.g., reduced amniotic fluid or nonreactivity; and (2) the gestational age and maturity of the fetus. As most abnormal tests contain two or more abnormal parameters, a weighting system would be most useful in realizing the maximum potential of this modality and should be developed in the near future. As most biophysical profile schemes have relatively high positive predictive values, a test that is abnormal in all of its parameters should lead to obstetric intervention, whereas one that has only one or two abnormal parameters should be backed up with a CST.

Doppler Flow Velocity Studies of Fetal Umbilical Vessels

Background. For the past decade, technologic adaptation of Doppler signal devices, in either a pulsed or continuous wave mode, has allowed investigators to perform noninvasive assessments of fetal and placental vessels. The rationale for using these observations for fetal well-being determination is derived from the theory that when uteroplacental compromise exists, there is a gradual perturbation of blood flow characteristics in umbilical arterial circulation, leading to a loss of compliance of vessels in the placenta and a higher, rather than lower, resistance to umbilical blood flow.

TABLE 3 Biophysical Profile: Clinical Summary

Test Outcome	*Interpretative Criteria*	*Clinical Response*
Normal	NST: Reactive AFV: Maximum pocket $>1 \times 1$ cm FBM: Present for at least 30 seconds per 30 minutes FM: >3 per 30 minutes Tone: Flexion-extension present; normal fetal attitude present Placenta grade <3	All parameters normal →Repeat in <7 days One parameter abnormal →Repeat in 24 hours
Abnormal	At least two of the above fail to meet minimum standards	Consider delivery if fetus is mature Back-up with CST if fetus is immature or drug effects are present

Technique. Although most of the fetal great vessels are accessible to Doppler scanning probes operating at frequencies from 2 to 10 MHz, the concerns for emitted ultrasonographic energy output of these instruments have limited diagnostic studies primarily to the use of continuous wave probes that have a limited resolution. Therefore, the study of isolated vessels, such as those in the umbilical cord, becomes their most practical application.

The study technique is relatively simple, involving the location of umbilical arteries by imaging their characteristic Doppler waveforms produced during systole and diastole. An indirect estimate of blood flow velocity can be determined by measuring the difference between systolic and diastolic peaks of the umbilical artery waveform and by dividing it by the mean flow velocity over one cardiac cycle, thus yielding the "pulsatility index." The advantage of using this approach for evaluating vascular flow is that it is relatively independent of angle of insonation and, therefore, alterations in the position of the umbilical arteries caused by fetal movement are less critical. Use of the pulsatility index or systolic:diastolic ratio also obviates the need for continuous visualization of these vessels. Most Doppler flow studies reflect averages of several cardiac cycles obtained within a time frame of 10 to 30 minutes.

Indications. Most reports have focused on fetuses at risk for uteroplacental insufficiency; therefore, the logical groups for Doppler assessment are (1) suspected cases of intrauterine growth retardation; (2) twin gestations; and (3) maternal diabetes or hypertension with vascular complications. No known contraindications exist.

Interpretation of Doppler Flow Studies. At present, a relatively small population of normal patients have been reported, thus limiting the availability of normative data on longitudinal or cross-sectional variation in umbilical flow parameters during pregnancy. While most authors have calculated either systolic:diastolic peak ratios or pulsatility indices, study techniques, methodologic approaches for data analysis, and length of data collection have varied considerably. Thus, the normal values for these parameters must be related to the specific scheme reported, with subsequent testing methods conforming to those described therein. In general, nomograms for flow-related parameters can be determined successfully from midgestation to term and show a gradual decline in their values. When intrauterine growth retarded fetuses have been studied, sequential flow studies produce measurements that exceed the laboratory means by more than two standard deviations.

Clinical Follow-Up of Doppler Flow Studies. This modality should be considered as investigational and not be relied upon for primary fetal management. Until more data become available, the place of these studies may be regarded as an adjunct to the previously described biophysical testing methods.

As the discussion in this chapter points out, antepartum fetal testing now relies primarily on biophysical testing techniques. The most widely used approaches are the NST and CST, both of which have been studied for more than one decade in large obstetric populations. While reported clinical experience with antepartum fetal heart rate testing includes more than 50,000 cases, numerous interpretative standards and management algorithms available have produced confusion for practitioners. Both heart rate tests are characterized as accurate predictors of fetal health, but are considerably poorer indicators of fetal compromise. The matter of selecting the best primary testing approach is still unresolved, although there are circumstances in which the CST is contraindicated or when uterine insensitivity to exogenous oxytocin or nipple stimulation makes this test impractical. Conversely, the NST is regarded as a less "rigorous" test of uteroplacental competence, unless its evaluation includes baseline features other than acceleration frequency alone. Both tests lose predictive accuracy as the interval between testing and delivery increases and, thus, it is recommended that such intervals should not exceed 3 to 4 days.

The development of multiple parameter biophysical testing or biophysical profile, using a combination of ultrasonographic visualization of fetal breathing and body movements, placental morphology, amniotic fluid volume, and external electronic recording of fetal heart rate, has proven useful in identifying fetal anomalies, oligohydramnios, and potential disturbances of fetal oxygenation and acid-base balance. It is a more complex, time-consuming approach, which has been hampered by a lack of consensus on interpretative standards. The biophysical profile has not been shown conclusively to be a more accurate test than the NST, one of its components, and at present must be considered a first-line test for a limited number of fetal disorders or as a potential back-up test when the CST is contraindicated.

Doppler flow studies of the fetal-placental vasculature are still an investigative technique that warrants further study before clinical usefulness can be determined.

A final consideration in this overview of antepartum testing is that all approaches used in medical decision making should require at least three stages of evaluation before being accepted into practice and assigned a definitive role in high-risk pregnancy management. These stages encompass the development of test methodology, assessment of data reproducibility, ability to detect both well-being and compromise accurately, and, as a bottom line, the reduction of perinatal mortality and morbidity when viewed prospectively. It should be noted that none of the testing methods described in this chapter has successfully satisfied all of these demands in a proper randomized, controlled trial. Ultimately, the results of any antepartum test should be weighed within the context of the specific pregnancy under investigation. The fact that antepartum testing has been associated with contemporary reductions in the incidence of poor fetal outcomes cannot be solely ascribed to the tests themselves. Rather, the testing environment has compelled clinicians to spend more time with patients and to consider their antepartum problems and management in greater detail.

SUGGESTED READING

Devoe LD, Castillo RA, Sherline DM. The nonstress test as a diagnostic test: a critical reappraisal. Am J Obstet Gynecol 1985; 152:1047–1053.

Freeman RK. The use of the oxytocin challenge test for antepartum clinical evaluation of utero placental respiratory function. Am J Obstet Gynecol 1975; 121:481–489.

Manning FA, Platt LD, Sipos L. Antepartum fetal evaluation: development of a fetal biophysical profile. Am J Obstet Gynecol 1980; 136: 787–795.

Shulman H, Fleischer A, Stern W, et al. Umbilical artery velocity waveforms in human pregnancy. Am J Obstet Gynecol 1984; 148:985–990.

CERVICAL INCOMPETENCE

DAVID CHARLES, M.D., F.A.C.O.G., F.R.C.O.G.

A functional weakness of the cervix, referred to as cervical incompetence, was first reported in 1865; albeit, at that time, no studies had been conducted on the histopathology of the cervix. Today it is accepted that the cervix is predominantly composed of connective tissue in which collagen provides the mechanical strength that is required to retain the conceptus in the uterus. Various studies have shown that the connective tissue component of the uterine cervix changes during pregnancy and parturition. Effacement and dilation of the cervix probably involve partial breakdown of the collagen, which requires the action of a specific collagenase. Recent studies indicate that elastin also plays a role in the mechanism of cervical dilation. Decreased elastin content in incompetent cervices has been observed, and this may be of significance in cervical insufficiency.

At the beginning of this century, it was suggested that cervical lacerations resulted in abortion in subsequent pregnancies, and as a result, repairs of such lacerations were considered to be a means of circumventing these losses. Various forms of trauma have been blamed for structural defects in the cervix and the resulting cervical insufficiency. However, there is no unanimity as to whether cervical conization is associated with an increased incidence of abortion or incompetence of the internal cervical os. It is agreed the more extensive the conization procedure, the greater the risk of cervical incompetence and midtrimester abortion in a subsequent pregnancy. There is no available evidence to indicate that treatment of cervical dysplasia by laser or cryosurgery predisposes patients to cervical incompetence.

Various reports have indicated that there is an increased incidence of cervical incompetence that follows the termination of pregnancy at the end of the first trimester. There is some evidence that cervical dilation attained by the use of Hegar's dilators carries a greater risk of subsequent cervical incompetence as compared with dilation of the cervix by the use of Laminaria tents (which are the dried stems of *Laminaria digitata*). Laminaria tents have the advantage of being the only method available that acts directly on the cervix without necessarily stimulating uterine contractions. These tents probably act mechanically by swelling and slowly dilating the cervix, but it is of interest to note that they do contain a considerable amount of arachidonic acid, which is a prostaglandin precursor. During cervical dilation, arachidonic acid or its metabolites may stimulate collagen breakdown. Therefore, it is possible that Laminaria tents produce a softening of the cervix by changing the ground substances, which means that this effect is not purely mechanical as previously presumed. Follow-up of cases in which Laminaria tents have been used has shown a low incidence of cervical incompetence in subsequent pregnancies. It has been estimated that termination of pregnancy in the first trimester results in subsequent cervical incompetence in at least 4 percent of patients.

Although approximately 20 percent of second trimester abortions have been ascribed to cervical incompetence, it is frequently difficult to define the etiology. Cervical incompetence is encountered in both primigravidas and multigravidas, and frequently no apparent etiology is discernible.

Approximately 2 percent of such patients are considered to have congenital cervical incompetence. Intrauterine exposure to diethylstilbestrol (DES) is considered to be a congenital cause of cervical incompetence. Much controversy has evolved as to the role of this nonsteroidal agent in the entity, but there is no doubt that DES exposure does cause some structural defects in the uterus. It is now generally accepted that there is a higher prematurity rate for infants of individuals who were exposed to DES in utero.

When patients with a poor reproductive history initially attend for prenatal care, it is often difficult to investigate all the possible etiologies. Likewise, patients who have had a successful outcome to a pregnancy subsequent to a cerclage procedure may have an identical operative procedure performed in future pregnancies without physicians necessarily determining the presence of cervical incompetence. Consequently, in many reports, a significant proportion of patients do not have cervical incompetence recorded as the etiology of previous second trimester abortion.

In most instances, the diagnosis of cervical insufficiency or incompetence has been made predominantly on clinical grounds. A patient history of recurrent second trimester abortion in the absence of painful uterine contractions and the demonstration that a No. 8 Hegar's dilator can readily pass through the internal cervical os are major factors in formulating a diagnosis. After conception, this clinical entity should be suspected if repeat examinations by speculum during the second trimester document progressive cervical dilation. Of late, ultrasonography has proven useful in establishing a diagnosis of cervical incompetence. Ultrasonography can also help to determine when a cerclage procedure should be utilized as well as to evaluate the success of a cerclage procedure. Today, identification and measurement of the internal cervical os plays an extremely important role in the diagnosis of cervical incompetence, and such studies should be considered in any individual who furnishes a prior history consistent with incompetent cervix. Studies should be conducted in individuals who have had a first trimester termination, because at least 4 percent of such individuals develop incompetence of the cervix in a subsequent pregnancy.

In the nongravid patient, hysterosalpingography should be performed because this radiologic study also provides information that pertains to the status of the internal cervical os. Hysterosalpingographic studies should be performed in all patients who have had in utero exposure to DES, prior to commencement of a reproductive career. This can furnish information concerning the configuration of the endometrial cavity and the endocervical canal. When such patients become pregnant, they should undergo frequent examinations by speculum in order to establish any clinical evidence of cervical incompetence, thereby ensuring that an appropriate operative procedure can be instituted at the opportune moment.

Counseling patients with repeated pregnancy loss is difficult because few empiric data are available, and the role of certain specific risk factors frequently remains unclarified in the couple's history. In many instances, the wife undergoes a cerclage procedure for putative cervical incompetence. Consequently, this surgical procedure has become commonplace in many obstetric units, although frequently the rationale for the performance of the operation is inadequate. The incidence of incompetent cervix varies greatly among hospitals and is reported to occur in anywhere from 0.1 to 1.0 percent of all deliveries. This occurrence may be as much a reflection of the diagnostic criteria and populations studied as it is a reflection of the true incidence of the condition. When any institution reports an incidence of 1 percent of all deliveries, there is no doubt that physicians at that center resort to cerclage procedures in an arbitrary and haphazard fashion. In many instances, the classic features of cervical incompetence, which include painless dilation of the cervix with or without effacement, rupture of the fetal membranes in the absence of significant contractions, or passage of the gestational sac in toto, cannot be enunciated from the patient's history.

Controlled prospective studies on therapy of cervical incompetence are not available. Unfortunately, prospective trials to assess the efficacy of cerclage procedures cannot be undertaken because of ethical issues posed by control groups of patients. However, during the past few years, randomized trials of cerclage procedures have been reported, and they give rise to doubt about the established practices of many physicians, particularly those obstetricians who perform a prophylactic cerclage without properly establishing the diagnosis of cervical incompetence. A history of repeated fetal loss in the second trimester may raise suspicion of the presence of cervical incompetence, but this information is usually subjective and often incomplete.

Most physicians now advocate treating cervical incompetence by surgical procedure, which involves encirclement of the cervix in order to reduce the diameter of the internal cervical os. However, some still advocate medical therapy, and this remains controversial because it consists of bed rest, progestational agents, tocolytic agents, and antibiotics. The majority of clinicians agree that bed rest, which is included in all perioperative procedures, has a role in therapy. However, there are criticisms of bed rest as therapy, specifically because of the increased incidence of phlebitis and phlebothrombosis. Complete bed rest for any length of time is virtually impossible for a woman who has other children who need her care or who works outside the home. Consequently, the majority of patients are treated by a modified Shirodkar or McDonald procedure. Although many modalities of treatment have been suggested for cervical incompetence, cerclage procedures have received the greatest acclaim. The basic principle of the surgical procedure for this condition is the insertion of a nonabsorbable suture material at the level of the internal os, which rectifies any defective tissue resistance. Although in former years cerclage procedure in the nongravid patient was widely performed, such operations have now fallen out of favor because, in many instances, the surgical procedure resulted in damage to the cervix and produced such troublesome symptoms as dyspareunia, vaginal discharge, and, on occasion, infertility.

Contraindications to an operative procedure in patients with an incompetent cervix must be noted. These include a history of active bleeding, rupture of the fetal membranes, excessive uterine irritability, a gestational age of less than 12 weeks, intrauterine fetal demise, fetal abnormalities, and herpesvirus infection or pathogenic organisms in the vagina, which could result in bacteremia. One should also remember that a patient with evidence of preeclampsia or hydramnios is not a suitable candidate for a cerclage procedure. Cervical dilatation greater than 4 cm is a relative contraindication. Careful selection of cases for surgical treatment is essential, as is meticulous attention to detail during the operative procedure. As instruments on the surgical border may accidentally perforate the membranes, use of a tenaculum should be avoided. Plasma alpha-fetoprotein estimations should be conducted before the procedure in order to exclude, as far as possible, neural tube defects of the fetus. The use of ultrasonography, not only to diagnose the potential cervical incompetence but also to rule out hydatidiform mole or fetal death in utero, is mandatory.

Shirodkar was first to demonstrate that encirclement of the cervix at the level of the internal os during pregnancy can drastically reduce the patulous internal os. The Shirodkar method involved incising the cervicovaginal junction in a transverse manner and elevating the bladder in order to insert a suitable suture material for occlusion of the cervix. Likewise, a small vertical incision was made posteriorly so that the material could be inserted by means of an aneurysm needle and then sutured in place. Shirodkar originally used three strands of chromic catgut, but subsequently employed fascia lata. Various modifications of this technique have been used since, and satisfactory results have been obtained by the majority of individuals who have adopted this operative approach to the incompetent cervix. In the Shirodkar procedure today, a 5-mm width mersilene tape is used instead of fascia lata. This is available on swedged atraumatic needles and can be readily ligated in order to reduce the endocervical canal to less than 5 mm. This band is placed deeply in order to avoid the descending cervical artery on either side, thereby averting serious intraoperative or postoperative hemorrhage. Due care and attention must be taken in the insertion of the band in order to avoid rupture of the fetal membranes or too superficial placement of the band, which can lead to slipping, thereby defeating the purpose of the procedure.

The McDonald procedure is probably preferable because of its simplicity and because it does not involve the dissection of the bladder and is not associated with risk of hemorrhage or urinary tract problems. There are few cases in which a cervix is so damaged or foreshortened that this procedure cannot be undertaken.

Mersilene suture, used on an atraumatic needle, is inserted at four points circumferentially around the cervix and then tied with sufficient tension to reduce the width of the internal os. The ends of the knot are left long enough to facilitate division of the suture at a later date. This purse-string suture is adequate as a primary measure in the majority of instances and produces less trauma than the Shirodkar method.

On occasion a vaginal approach is not feasible; this is particularly true after failed cerclage procedures, when the cervix has been attenuated, or when there has been high amputation of the cervix such as occurs in the Manchester operation. In such instances, a transabdominal approach is necessary. When the transabdominal approach is used, the ligature is permanent, and subsequent deliveries must be performed by cesarean section.

It cannot be stressed too strongly that careful patient selection and meticulous attention to detail are essential if cerclage procedures are to be successful. Such procedures may initiate myometrial activity, and this is more likely to occur if the operation is delayed until there is evidence of cervical dilatation. Ideally, the operative procedure should be performed prior to 18-weeks gestation. Naturally, there is an increased incidence of sepsis if amniorrhexis occurs during the procedure.

Again, it must be emphasized that it is preferable not to perform any operation on the gravid patient until the gestation is of 14-weeks duration. As the risk of abortion associated with chromosomal abnormalities is markedly decreased after the 14th week, any patient with a proven diagnosis of cervical incompetence should ideally undergo a cerclage procedure between the 14th and 16th week. In the case of multiple pregnancy, there is no evidence to indicate that a cerclage improves the prognosis.

Postoperatively, the patient should remain in hospital for 24 to 48 hours, but should be mobilized early and given routine analgesia for any discomfort. There is no evidence that the use of uterine relaxants or tocolytic agents improves the outcome for the patient. Likewise, there is no evidence to demonstrate that progestational agents are wholly effective in preventing uterine contractions.

The patient is encouraged to lead a reasonably normal life after leaving hospital, but is kept under constant surveillance as regards any cervical dilation and should be seen and examined by speculum every 2 weeks. Since seminal fluid contains large amounts of prostaglandins, the subject of sexual intercourse after cerclage must be discussed with the patient. Although there is no indication for total abstinence, it is preferable that the male partner use a condom to circumvent any prostaglandin-mediated stimulation of the uterus.

Sepsis is an important complication of cerclage, and careful surgical technique and microbiologic control should always be adopted in order to minimize the risk. The incidence of amnionitis increases greatly if the membranes have been exposed prior to the cerclage procedure, and consequently, this author prefers to do the procedure prior to the 18th week of gestation.

Evaluation of fetal maturity is of importance; when the gestation is in the 38th week, the McDonald-type suture can be removed and spontaneous labor allowed to ensue. There is rarely a need for induction of labor. In the case of the Shirodkar procedure, in which the cerclage has been buried in the cervix, cesarean section is preferable to attempting to divide the mersilene band under general anesthesia.

When the vaginal approach is being used, cervical dystocia in labor subsequent to the removal of the suture may necessitate cesarean section. However, even those patients who have had a McDonald suture removed must be carefully followed in labor because during vaginal delivery further lacerations of the cervix may be sustained.

Unless prospective trials produce evidence to the contrary, cervical cerclage must continue to play an important role in the care of patients who have proven cervical incompetence. If the operative procedure is not performed unless cervical incompetence is proven, many unnecessary ligatures will not be applied, and the operation will not fall into disrepute. The major cerclage procedures have been discussed, and the patient who has undergone such a procedure can expect a good prognosis for the pregnancy, with a live birth rate of at least 85 percent. However, in conclusion, it must be stated that cervical incompetence is a relatively rare cause of abortion and is misdiagnosed far too frequently.

SUGGESTED READING

Charles D, Glover DD. Incompetent cervical os. In: Cibils L, ed. Surgical diseases in pregnancy. New York: Springer-Verlag, in press.

Charles D, Edwards WR. Infectious complications of cervical cerclage. Am J Obstet Gynecol 1981; 141:1064–1071.

Harger JH. Cervical cerclage: patient selection, morbidity and success rates. Clin Perinatol 1983; 10:321–341.

Leppert PC, Cerreta J, Mandl I. Orientation of elastic fibers in the human cervix. Am J Obstet Gynecol 1986; 155:219–224.

McDonald IA. Cervical cerclage. Clin Obstet Gynaecol 1980; 7:461–479.

Toaff R, Toaff ME, Ballas S, et al. Cervical incompetence: diagnostic and therapeutic aspects. Isr J Med Sci 1977; 13:39–49.

DRUG ABUSE

FRANK R. WITTER, M.D.

Drug abuse in pregnancy is a serious problem requiring high-risk management. The pregnant drug abuser is a complex patient with obstetric, medical, social, and psychological problems, which must be met with a team effort in order to optimize the pregnancy outcome. They are best managed in the setting of a special drug abuse prenatal care center where obstetric expertise, physicians versed in the medical and psychological aspects of addiction therapy, social workers, and social services are available.

This chapter discusses the therapy for maternal narcotic abuse, cocaine abuse, phencyclidine (PCP) abuse, barbiturate abuse, and polydrug abuse, in addition to the general therapy for drug overdose.

NARCOTIC DRUG ABUSE

Therapeutic Alternatives

In the narcotic-addicted mother there are two therapeutic alternatives, methadone maintenance and withdrawal in the second trimester. Methadone maintenance coupled with psychosocial support can decrease the incidence of fetal wastage and perinatal mortality while probably increasing the duration and intensity of neonatal withdrawal. Narcotic withdrawal during pregnancy can result in pregnancy wastage, stillbirth, premature labor, and neonatal death from meconium aspiration and should only be undertaken between 16- and 32-weeks gestation. Withdrawal requires first methadone maintenance and then slow decreases in methadone dosage (not to exceed 5 mg every 2 weeks) with careful fetal surveillance. The preferred treatment course is methadone maintenance.

Methadone Maintenance

Oral methadone maintenance in narcotic-addicted mothers should be instituted as soon as the patient registers for her pregnancy. The earlier in pregnancy it is instituted, the more likely a favorable pregnancy outcome can be achieved. The initial replacement dose should be sufficient to prevent maternal withdrawal symptoms and to suppress craving for narcotics. An initial oral dose of 50 mg per day is frequently sufficient, although, on occasion, higher doses may be needed. Once the initial dose has been established, the dose should be gradually decreased by 5 mg every 2 weeks until the minimal dose that prevents maternal withdrawal and narcotic craving is achieved. A good goal, if it can be reached, is a dose of less than 20 mg per day as this minimizes neonatal withdrawal.

During the stabilization and dose reduction phases of this therapy, careful observation of the fetus for withdrawal should be carried out by the use of daily fetal kick counts and weekly biophysical profiles. Additionally, monitoring should include serial sonography in order to monitor fetal growth on a monthly basis.

Signs and symptoms of narcotic withdrawal include drug seeking behavior, lacrimation, rhinorrhea, yawning, sweating, restlessness, nausea, vomiting, intestinal spasm, diarrhea, weakness, depression, tachycardia, elevated blood pressure, and pains in bones and muscles. Withdrawal should be treated by upward titration of the methadone dose.

Signs and symptoms of narcotic overdose include stupor, coma, pinpoint pupils (dilated with anoxia), gastrointestinal and biliary spasm, irregular, slow, shallow respirations, cyanosis, respiratory arrest, weak pulse, hypotension, spasticity and twitching of the musculature, and hypothermia. Therapy for overdose is discussed under General Treatment of Drug Overdose.

Methadone maintenance alone is ineffective in improving perinatal outcome and must be accompanied by psychosocial support. Intensive social and psychological support may be provided by a professional-paraprofessional team and should be at the same site as the prenatal care to improve patient compliance. It should include individual and marital counseling, prenatal classes, frequent collaboration between team members on management problems and prejudicial attitudes, and maternal aid information on financial aid and transport to and from the special drug abuse prenatal care center, the hospital, and the antepartum testing center.

An important component of prenatal care for narcotic dependent mothers is to screen for noncompliance and the use of other elicit drugs. This can be achieved by a drug screen of blood and urine at each prenatal visit. Those individuals abusing additional drugs should be treated as listed under the specific drugs. Alcohol and tobacco use, which are more prevalent in addicts, should be discouraged.

Screening should be performed for significant associated disease that might adversely affect the fetus. Syphilis, gonorrhea, hepatitis, and human immune virus (HIV) screening are necessary.

Pros and Cons of Therapy for Narcotic Abuse

Obstetric complications associated with untreated narcotic abuse include abortion, abruptio placentae, amnionitis, breech presentation, previous cesarean section, preeclampsia and eclampsia, placental insufficiency, intrauterine growth retardation (IUGR), fetal death in utero, premature labor, premature rupture of membranes, and septic thrombophlebitis. Withdrawal and overdose are associated with stillbirth. Medical complications of narcotic abuse that complicate pregnancy include anemia, cardiac disease secondary to subacute bacterial endocarditis, cellulitis, poor dental hygiene, diabetes, sexually transmitted disease, hepatitis, AIDS, and HIV infection.

Methadone maintenance alone is inadequate. Methadone maintenance with intensive psychosocial support can clearly improve pregnancy outcome and aid in early detection of medical complications of drug abuse. Psychosocial support is therefore indicated. Although neonatal withdrawal can be more prolonged and intense with methadone, the ultimate outcome for the neonate is normal development in infancy. Monitoring for neonatal withdrawal should, however, occur over the first week of life.

The one outcome variable not improved by methadone maintenance is birth weight. Use of narcotics appears intrinsically to decrease birth weight. Additionally, the increased risk of sudden infant death syndrome (SIDS) seen with maternal narcotic addiction also occurs with methadone-treated patients. The infant should therefore have SIDS monitoring for at least the first 3 months of life when the risk is maximal.

NON-NARCOTIC DRUG ABUSE

Therapy

The treatment for all forms of drug abuse other than narcotic abuse is withdrawal with intensive psychosocial support. As polydrug use is quite prevalent, it is important to screen substance-abusing mothers for multiple drug use by drug screens of blood and urine at each prenatal visit. This also enables monitoring for noncompliance. The withdrawal should be conducted under controlled conditions. Fetal monitoring should be used, consisting of daily kick counts and weekly biophysical profiles.

As with narcotic abuse, intensive social and psychological support is essential to obtaining continued abstinence. It may be provided by a professional-paraprofessional team and should be at the same site as the prenatal care to improve patient compliance. Included in the support should be individual and marital counseling, prenatal classes, frequent collaboration between team members on management problems and prejudicial attitudes, and maternal aid information on financial aid and transport to and from the special drug abuse prenatal care center, the hospital, and the antepartum testing center.

As substance-abusing mothers are likely to be heavy alcohol and tobacco users, the use of these substances should be actively discouraged because of their known adverse effect on pregnancy. Screening should be performed for significant associated disease, which might adversely affect the fetus—syphilis, gonorrhea, hepatitis, and HIV screening being necessary.

All substance abusing mothers are at risk for giving birth to infants with IUGR, neonatal withdrawal, and SIDS. Monitoring for adequacy of growth should be conducted with monthly sonography. After birth the infant should be monitored for withdrawal for the first week of life and for SIDS, at least, for the first 3 months of life when the risk is greatest.

Cocaine Abuse

Cocaine is the most addictive drug known. Intensive psychosocial support and screening for recidivism are essential. Because of cocaine's ability to suppress appetite, careful observation for poor weight gain is needed, and nutritional intervention may be required. Infant outcome is worse when cocaine and opiates are abused together; therefore, special efforts should be extended to treat mothers who abuse both substances with methadone maintenance and cocaine abstinence. Cocaine, especially when given intravenously, may be associated with abruptio placentae. Mothers who present with cocaine intoxication should be carefully evaluated for the possibility of placental abruption with sonography, fetal heart rate testing, and observation in a labor- and delivery-type intensive care setting.

Signs and symptoms of cocaine withdrawal include craving for the drug, prolonged sleep, generalized fatigue, lassitude, hyperphagia, and depression. Psychological support in a structured setting should be offered to patients experiencing withdrawal.

Symptoms and signs of cocaine overdose include restlessness, excitability, sensory aberrations, hallucinations, tachycardia, dilated pupils, chills and fever, abdominal pain, vomiting, numbness and muscle spasms, irregular or Cheyne-Stokes respirations, circulatory failure, convulsions, and coma. Withdrawal from cocaine should be treated as listed under General Treatment of Drug Overdose.

Phencyclidine (PCP) Abuse

PCP is the most common drug found on drug screens. It is often abused in conjunction with other drugs and obtaining abstinence during pregnancy is difficult. Intensive screening for drug use and psychosocial support are imperative in mothers abusing PCP. Near term, special effort should be extended to achieve abstinence because of the prolonged adverse affect of prenatal PCP on neonatal adaptive behavior.

Signs and symptoms of PCP withdrawal include craving for PCP and difficulties in recent memory, speech, and thinking. Psychological support should be offered for this withdrawal syndrome.

Signs and symptoms of PCP overdose include hyperactivity, rigidity, peripheral anesthesia, nystagmus, incoordination, wild movements, salivation, sweating, muscle rigidity, stupor, coma, hyperthermia, hypertension, laryngeal stridor, decreased or absent reflexes, respiratory depression, convulsions, and acute rhabdomyolysis. The treatment is symptomatic as listed under General Treatment of Drug Overdose. The psychotic state produced by PCP overdosage may take up to 2 weeks to resolve.

Barbiturate Abuse

Barbiturate abuse requires a slower withdrawal because of the danger of convulsions and should be undertaken only on an inpatient basis in the setting of a special detoxification center. Seizures are a potential complication of withdrawal and should be treated acutely with diazepam, 2 to 10 ml intravenously. Seizures are best treated by prevention through adequate treatment of barbiturate withdrawal symptoms, which consist of tremulousness, anxiety, weakness, insomnia, and delirium. Treatment should be with paraldehyde, 0.2 mg per kilogram body weight rectally or intramuscularly in oil. Paraldehyde has a duration of action of 12 hours and has the advantage of causing little respiratory depression. Therapy should be titrated to symptomatology and the individual doses should be tapered gradually to nothing.

Infant outcome is worse when barbiturate and opiates are abused together; therefore, special effort should be extended to treat mothers who abuse both substances by means of methadone maintenance and barbiturate abstinence. Fetal growth retardation is less likely to occur in mothers who abuse only barbiturates when compared to other substance-abusing mothers.

Pros and Cons of Therapy for Non-Narcotic Drug Abuse

Obstetric and medical complications of non-narcotic drug abuse are similar to those seen with narcotic abuse. They reflect the complications inherent to the drugs themselves, the complications of nonsterile injection techniques, and the complications brought about by the unfavorable social setting associated with drug abuse. Intervention through withdrawal and psychosocial support offers the only hope for improvement in the perinatal outcome.

GENERAL TREATMENT OF DRUG OVERDOSE

The general treatment for drug overdose consists of maintaining vital functions, removal of drug, and delay of drug absorption. The first priorities of vital function maintenance in drug overdose are to secure the airway, support the circulation, and control seizures.

In the mother presenting with a drug overdose, every effort should be made to identify the drug or drugs involved. If available, history or a sample of the drug would be useful, but, in most instances, one must rely on drug screens in blood, urine, and vomitus. Additionally, baseline studies should be obtained consisting of arterial blood gases, central venous pressure monitoring, chest roentgenogram, electrolytes, creatinine, blood urea nitrogen, liver function tests, and electrocardiogram. Results of these studies enable monitoring of the course of potential pulmonary, renal, liver, and cardiac complications. The fetal heart rate should be monitored during the treatment, but no intervention for fetal distress should be considered until the maternal status is stabilized. As with stabilization of the mother's physiology, fetal stress will be relieved and the infant resuscitated in utero.

During therapy, the maternal arterial pO_2 should be kept above 60 torr and the maternal arterial pCO_2 should be kept below 40 torr. The maternal central venous pressure should not exceed 15 cm of water and the maternal systolic blood pressure should be kept above 90 torr. The patient should be treated on her left side to avoid supine hypotension and to improve uterine blood flow.

If the drug was recently injected, absorption may be delayed by application of a tourniquet and cold packs to the extremity where the injection occurred. If the drug was ingested, it is possible to decrease absorption by inducing emesis. Emesis is contraindicated in the patient who is obtundent, in the presence of convulsions, or when drugs that may produce convulsions have been ingested. Syrup of ipecac in a maximum dose of 30 to 60 ml should be used to induce emesis. The initial dose should be 10 to 30 ml followed by several large glasses of water. The dose may be repeated once in 20 to 30 minutes, if no vomitus has occurred.

If the drug was orally ingested and emesis is contraindicated or if ipecac fails, proceed to gastric gavage. The mother should be in the head-down, left-lateral decubitus position and, if unconscious, should have the airway protected by a cuffed endotracheal tube. Gavage should be through a large bore tube (30 to 36 F) with 0.5 normal sodium chloride in 100 to 200 ml aliquots until clear. The quantity of fluid given at any one time should not exceed 50 ml per 10 kilogram body weight. After emesis or gavage, activated charcoal should be given as a slurry with water in a dose of 1.0 g per kilogram body weight. This will delay drug absorption.

Specific Treatment

Coma

Coma should be treated with endotracheal intubation with a cuffed endotracheal tube to prevent aspiration. Maternal arterial pO_2 and pCO_2 should be followed with an arterial line. The pCO_2 should be kept below 40 torr and the pO_2 between 70 to 100 torr. Mechanical ventilation may be required to maintain gas exchange at this level. Although naloxone hydrochloride in a dose of 0.01 ml per kilogram body weight reverses coma due to narcotics, it also precipitates withdrawal, thereby causing possible adverse effects to the fetus. For this reason mechanical ventilation is preferred.

Hyperexcitability

Hyperexcitability may be treated with phenobarbital, 30 to 90 mg every 6 hours. In the presence of barbiturate abuse, paraldehyde in a dose of 0.2 mg per kilogram body weight rectally or intramuscularly in oil every 12 hours is preferred.

Convulsions

If delivery is not anticipated, convulsions should be treated with diazepam, 2 to 10 mg, given at a rate of 1 mg per minute intravenously. If delivery is anticipated, convulsions should be treated with intravenous magnesium sulfate utilizing a 4-g loading dose followed by a maintenance dose of 1 to 2 g per hour by continuous infusion. Occasionally higher or lower doses of magnesium sulfate may be needed, depending on clinical response and the patient's renal status. Therapy may be followed by serum magnesium levels; a level between 4 and 6 mEq per liter should be sought.

Hypertension

Hypertension should be treated if the diastolic is greater than 110 torr. The treatment of choice is intravenous hydralazine given as an initial test dose of 5 mg as an intravenous bolus. This initial dose may be repeated twice in 20 to 30 minutes. If hypertension recurs after this initial therapy, treat with a continuous intravenous infusion beginning at 2 to 4 mg per hour. The dose may be increased 2 mg every 30 minutes until blood pressure control is achieved. The diastolic should not be lowered below 90 torr.

Hypotension

The systolic blood pressure should be maintained above 90 torr. Place the patient on her left side to optimize uterine perfusion and to rule out supine hypotension. Restoration and maintenance of blood pressure in drug overdose situations is best achieved by fluid expansion with Ringer's lactate or normal saline, while carefully monitoring central venous pressure, which should not exceed 15 cm of water. If fluid expansion fails, ephedrine (10 to 15 mg) may be given intravenously to carefully titrate the patient's blood pressure.

Hyperthermia and Hypothermia

These conditions are treated with a cooling blanket and with warm blankets respectively.

Symptomatic Treatment of Drug Withdrawal Symptoms

The symptomatic treatment of drug withdrawal symptoms is the same as listed for specific symptoms under General Treatment of Drug Overdose. Narcotic withdrawal is treated as indicated under Methadone Maintenance.

SUGGESTED READING

Chasnoff IJ, Burns WJ, Schnoll SH, Burns KA. Cocaine use in pregnancy. N Engl J Med 1985; 113:666–669.

Davis RC, Chappel JN, Mejia-Zelaya A, Madden J. Clinical observations on methadone-maintained pregnancies. Addict Dis 1975; 2:101–112.

Witter FR, Niebyl JR. Drug intoxications and anaphylactic shock in the obstetric patient. In: Berkowitz RL, ed. Critical care in the obstetrical patient. New York: Churchill Livingstone, 1983:527.

MEDICAL DISORDERS

GASTROINTESTINAL TRACT DISORDERS

DESMOND J. LEDDIN, M.B., M.R.C.P.(I), F.R.C.P.(C)
JAMES A. BARROWMAN, B.Sc., Ph.D., M.B., Ch.B., F.R.C.P.(Lond), F.R.C.P.(C), F.A.C.P.

Two principles guide the choice of therapy of gastrointestinal disorders in pregnancy. First, pharmacologic treatment should be avoided in the management of conditions that may respond to nonpharmacologic therapy. Second, if drugs must be used, the therapeutic agent chosen should act locally and have minimal systemic distribution.

Many gastrointestinal disorders are caused or exacerbated by dietary factors and may respond to nonpharmacologic therapy. Constipation, for example, is common in pregnancy and may be treated simply by increasing dietary fiber. Another characteristic of the gastrointestinal tract is that many therapeutic agents for dysfunction or disease of this system are active topically in the gut and are poorly absorbed.

As regards systemically absorbed agents, there is always a risk of adverse effects on the mother or fetus, and their use must be reserved for situations in which the therapeutic benefit clearly outweighs the risk associated with therapy.

This chapter first describes the physiologic changes in pregnancy that affect gastrointestinal function and motility. Thereafter the treatment of gastrointestinal disease as it presents, continues, or relapses during pregnancy is discussed. Lastly, the use of medical therapy in the postpartum period and during lactation is described, with particular attention to the transfer of drugs from mother to child. Concentration is primarily on medical gastroenterologic conditions, although consideration is given to the need for emergency surgical procedures when these are indicated.

Adequate data on the teratogenicity of many drugs used in the treatment of gastrointestinal disease are lacking. Furthermore, the adverse effects of drugs on the fetus may be subtle. Detection of such abnormalities would require large-scale follow-up trials extending over many years. It is unlikely that such trials will be performed on all therapeutic agents. Therefore caution should be exercised before proceeding with drug treatment of gastrointestinal disease in the pregnant woman.

Although major unwanted effects and interactions are described, the list is not intended to be comprehensive and the drug package insert should also be consulted.

PHYSIOLOGIC ALTERATIONS IN THE GASTROINTESTINAL TRACT DURING PREGNANCY

A striking increase in appetite is a feature of pregnancy, and accompanying this are qualitative changes in food habits. These include cravings for certain foods, such as fruit and highly flavored materials, and aversion to other dietary items, such as fried foods, eggs, tea, and coffee.

Reflux of gastric juice into the distal esophagus is considered to be responsible for heartburn, which is a frequent complaint in pregnancy. This effect may be related to increased abdominal pressure, but there is also good evidence that there is reduced tone in the lower esophageal sphincter in pregnancy and that the response of this sphincter to hormonal, pharmacologic, and physiologic stimuli is reduced.

Although satisfactory studies of gastric secretion in pregnancy are lacking, there is little evidence that pregnancy markedly affects gastric acid secretion. Unlike small intestinal motility, gastric motility is probably not markedly reduced, although some decrease does occur. Peptic ulcer is relatively rare in pregnancy, and it has been suggested that this may reflect a protective effect of estrogen on the gastric mucosa.

Pregnancy produces marked alterations in small bowel function. Small bowel transit time is increased, and this reduction in smooth muscle activity is usually attributed to high circulating levels of progesterone. The mucosal villi hypertrophy, and there is an increase in mucosal enzyme content with a corresponding increase in the absorption of many nutrients.

The general depression of smooth muscle contractility seen in pregnancy is partly responsible for the common complaint of constipation. Enhanced water absorption from the colon, possibly due to increased amounts of circulating angiotensin and aldosterone, also contributes in that stool bulk is reduced and consistency increased.

ORAL DISEASE

Pregnancy is associated with an increase in dental caries, gingivitis, and epulis. The cause of the increase in caries is not clear, but estrogen has been shown experimentally to cause gingival hyperplasia. Epulis, an inflammatory lesion resembling a tumor, is generally found in patients with preexisting poor dental hygiene.

NAUSEA AND VOMITING

As early as the first missed menstrual period, nausea and vomiting, chiefly in the morning, are experienced by a very large number of pregnant women. Two-thirds of those with these symptoms are primigravid. The condition is benign and usually limited to the first trimester of pregnancy. No clear precipitating factors have been identified.

This condition is distressing but not usually associated with metabolic deterioration. Since the symptoms are most prominent at the time when the fetus is extremely vulnerable to adverse drug effects, pharmacologic intervention should be avoided.

Supportive measures and, occasionally, psychological counseling may be useful. Some help has been obtained from the use of a combination of vitamins K and C together with pyridoxine.

Hyperemesis gravidarum, an extreme form of the problem, is rare but carries a high risk for both mother and fetus. Severe metabolic effects occur, which include dehydration, acidosis, and hepatic and renal failure. This condition is associated with hydatidiform mole.

The major therapeutic efforts are directed toward parenteral correction of fluid and electrolyte abnormalities and nutritional deficiencies. Enteral or parenteral hyperalimentation is often required, together with vitamin supplements. The hazards of total parenteral nutrition are discussed in the section dealing with inflammatory bowel disease. In this condition, in which the risk–benefit ratio is entirely different from the mild condition of nausea and vomiting described above, cautious drug therapy has been advocated by some authors. Nevertheless, the teratogenic and other risks for the pregnancy from drug therapy do not generally warrant this.

ESOPHAGITIS AND GASTROESOPHAGEAL REFLUX

A majority of pregnant women experience at least occasional symptoms of retrosternal burning or reflux. Many patients quite adequately treat themselves with milk or proprietary antacids, and the symptoms are never severe enough to warrant more aggressive therapy. Alterations in gastric emptying, increasing abdominal pressure, and a progesterone-mediated fall in sphincter pressure are probably the causes. In patients with frequent vomiting, the vomitus itself may cause esophageal inflammation.

Diagnosis

The diagnosis is based on a history of retrosternal burning and regurgitation. Specific diagnostic procedures, such as endoscopy and esophageal biopsy, are not necessary unless complications such as bleeding or dysphagia occur.

Therapy

Diet. A diet low in fat and high in protein may be beneficial. Elevation of the head of the bed on 8-inch blocks is useful but not always tolerated. Avoidance of injurious agents or agents known to decrease the lower esophageal pressure, such as alcohol, chocolate, excessive tea or coffee, colas, and nonsteroidal anti-inflammatory agents (NSAIDs), is to be encouraged.

Antacids. Many patients require doses of antacids in liquid or tablet form only as needed. For patients with severe symptoms or those with complications of esophagitis such as bleeding, the therapeutic regime as described under Peptic Ulceration is necessary.

Side Effects and Interactions. These are discussed under Peptic Ulceration.

Sodium Alginate Compound. The acid-buffering capacity of these compounds is minimal. The primary effect is to form a viscous foam on the surface of the gastric contents and thus reduce the number of reflux events. This compound is probably safe for use in the pregnant patient. Aluminum and magnesium absorption does occur, but the significance of this is unknown and probably inconsequential.

Dosage is 10 or 20 ml of liquid or two to four tablets from one to four times daily.

Unwanted Effects and Interactions

The cations of magnesium and aluminum may interfere with phosphate and iron absorption. The significance of this in normal pregnancy is not likely to be great. Absorption of magnesium and aluminum is not likely to be of concern except in patients with renal failure in whom hypermagnesemia can cause neurologic symptoms.

The liquid contains 6 mg of sodium in each milliliter and the tablets 22 mg of sodium. This may be a problem in patients on sodium-restricted diets. Nausea, vomiting, and flatulence have been reported.

DISEASES OF THE STOMACH

Gastritis

This disorder is most commonly manifested by burning epigastric discomfort that may be associated with nausea, anorexia, and vomiting. The etiology is diverse, but whatever the precipitating factor, it is likely that bile, pepsin, and acid contribute to the mucosal injury. As discussed above, pregnancy does not markedly inhibit gastric motility, and bile stasis per se is not usually responsible for the development of symptoms. Alcohol intake and ingestion of NSAIDs may cause gastric inflammation, as may excessive ingestion of coffee, tea, or colas.

Diagnosis

It is rarely necessary to make a specific diagnosis. The symptoms, though not specific, clearly point to a gastric source and a trial of therapy usually resolves the question. Endoscopy is accurate in diagnosing this condition, especially if histologic evidence is obtained.

Therapy

Avoidance of known exacerbating agents such as alcohol, NSAIDs, and caffeine, with the addition of antacids on an as needed basis, may be the only therapy required. If symptoms persist, treatment as for peptic ulcer disease may be effective.

Peptic Ulceration

Both gastric and duodenal ulceration are uncommon in the pregnant patient. Estrogen may actually protect against the development of duodenal ulcers.

The presenting symptoms of peptic ulcer disease are similar to those in the nonpregnant patient except that confusion with obstetric causes of abdominal pain may occur. Nausea, epigastric pain (characteristically relieved by antacids), and vomiting are common. Differentiation from gastritis on clinical grounds may be difficult. Although duodenal ulcers are rarely, if ever, malignant, this is always a possibility with gastric ulcers, and biopsy is required.

Diagnosis

If a specific diagnosis is felt to be necessary, endoscopy can be performed with minimal risk to the fetus.

Therapy

Agents known to be injurious to the gastroduodenal mucosa such as alcohol, caffeine, and NSAIDs should be eliminated. The primary pharmacologic agents used should be antacids. There is extensive experience with these drugs, absorption is minimal, and they are effective in healing peptic ulceration.

If an additional or alternative drug is required, the drug of choice is probably sucralfate, although experience to date with this medication is limited and its use in pregnancy has not been approved. Other commonly used drugs will be briefly reviewed.

Drugs Used in the Management of Acid/Peptic Disease

Oral antacids act by decreasing gastric acidity, by binding bile salts, and by decreasing pepsin activation. More recently, it has been recognized that these agents may increase mucosal prostaglandin production and stimulate bicarbonate secretion. Both of these effects are beneficial.

Dosage regimen of magnesium hydroxide and aluminum hydroxide liquid is 10 to 30 ml at 1 and 3 hours after meals and at bedtime. The preparations of antacid available vary widely in potency. An antacid containing 400 mg of each hydroxide should be used.

Antacid tablets are also useful. These have the advantage of being easily transported and more palatable. The tablet preparations are generally less potent, but high-dose tablets are available.

Unwanted Effects and Interactions.

Antacids containing only aluminum hydroxide should usually be avoided because they tend to decrease gastric emptying and may cause constipation. Aluminum is absorbed to a minor degree, but the significance of this is not known. There is some epidemiologic evidence, in patients with renal disease, linking chronic aluminum absorption to neurologic deterioration.

Magnesium-containing antacids, in contrast, tend to cause diarrhea, and this effect may be beneficial in the constipated patient. Systemic absorption of magnesium also occurs and may cause seizures and other neurologic symptoms in patients with renal disease.

If constipation becomes a problem, the antacid containing only magnesium should be used. If diarrhea is troublesome, the magnesium-containing antacid may be alternated with one containing aluminum. Impaired absorption of iron, calcium, and phosphorus may result. Note that some patients cannot tolerate these preparations because of nausea.

Antacids interfere with the absorption of tetracyclines, but these antibiotics should not be used in the pregnant patient.

Sucralfate. Sucralfate is a minimally absorbed medication that inhibits the action of pepsin and bile, blocks the back diffusion of acid, and forms a chemical barrier at sites of ulceration. This drug may also increase mucosal prostaglandin synthesis. Although sucralfate is most likely safe for use during pregnancy, experience with this drug is limited, and it should not be used unless the risk–benefit ratio is favorable.

Dosage regimen is 1 g by mouth four times a day, 1 hour before meals.

Side Effects and Interactions. The only common side effect of sucralfate is constipation. This may make pregnancy-induced constipation worse. Nausea, epigastric discomfort, skin rash, dizziness, and vertigo also have been reported.

The major interaction is with antacids in that simultaneous administration of antacids may decrease mucosal binding of sucralfate. If antacids are also being administered, at least 30 minutes should be allowed before ingestion of sucralfate. Sucralfate binds to many ingested drugs and may decrease the bioavailability of these agents.

Histamine Receptor Blockers. Drugs in this class include cimetidine and ranitidine. In the nonpregnant patient, these are widely used and are highly efficacious. Unfortunately, these drugs are known to have antiandrogenic effects. They cannot be recommended for use in pregnancy at present.

Acetylcholine Receptor Blockers. Pirenzepine is an anticholinergic agent relatively selective for the gastric cholinergic receptors. Experience with this drug in pregnancy is very limited, and although animal studies have not shown any adverse fetal effects, its use should be avoided until further data are available.

Prostaglandins. Misoprostol is a synthetic prostaglandin that decreases acid production and increases mucus and bicarbonate secretion. Until much more experience has been gained with this drug, it should be avoided because of possible adverse effects on the fetus and the possibility of its precipitating labor.

Gastroparesis

A decrease in gastric motility may occur in pregnancy but is not as marked as the decrease seen in small intestinal and colonic motility. Gastric stasis may, however, be seen in diabetic patients with autonomic neuropathy and in patients on medications with anticholinergic effects. The presenting symptoms are those of nausea associated with vomiting of undigested or old food. The volume of vomitus may be large. There may be associated epigastric discomfort.

Diagnosis

The history may be very suggestive. A specific diagnosis without using radioisotopes or radiology is difficult to make. Nonradioisotopic breath tests are dependent on small bowel transit as well as gastric emptying, and pregnancy is known to increase intestinal transit time. Endoscopy is useful; food may be found in the stomach after an overnight fast.

Therapy

Dietary fat decreases gastric emptying, and alteration of the diet to one relatively higher in protein may help. Smaller, more frequent meals with plenty of fluids are advantageous. Medications that have anticholinergic side effects should be discontinued or reduced in dosage.

In the nonpregnant patient both metoclopramide and domperidone are effective therapy. These medications appear to act by antagonizing dopamine.

Dosage regimen is as follows: metoclopramide 5 mg or 10 mg by mouth four times a day; domperidone 10 mg by mouth four times a day, 30 minutes before meals.

Unwanted Effects and Interactions

Both metoclopramide and domperidone increase plasma prolactin levels and should not be used in pregnancy unless there is a very clear indication and the risks of fetal toxicity are appreciated.

Metoclopramide not uncommonly causes drowsiness, fatigue, and lethargy. Parkinsonism and extrapyramidal signs may occur. This drug should not be used concomitantly with anticholinergic medications, since the therapeutic effect of metoclopramide is antagonized. Potentiation of the unwanted effects of metoclopramide may occur if this drug is used in conjunction with sedatives or monoamine oxidase inhibitors.

Domperidone has less central nervous system toxicity than metoclopramide, probably because it does not readily cross the blood-brain barrier. Headache, insomnia, and irritability occur, and dry mouth, dizziness, and lethargy have been reported. Skin rashes occur but are uncommon.

The therapeutic efficacy of domperidone may be markedly decreased by simultaneous administration of high-dose antacids or H_2 blockers. This appears to be due to the requirement of this drug for an acidic gastric pH for absorption.

Contraindications

Use of either of these medications is contraindicated if an obstructive lesion of the gastrointestinal tract is present. They should not be used if there is a prior history of allergic reactions to the medication.

PANCREATIC DISEASE

Debate exists as to whether a specific acute pancreatitis of pregnancy exists. Plasma triglycerides are known to rise during pregnancy, and hypertriglyceridemia is associated with an increased risk of pancreatitis. The presenting symptoms are those of epigastric pain (which may radiate to the back), nausea, and vomiting. In severe cases, hypotension may occur.

Pregnant patients are no less at risk of developing pancreatitis from the more common precipitants such as gallstones, drugs, and alcohol. Hypertriglyceridemia, which may have been present prior to the pregnancy, and hypercalcemia may be occult causes.

Diagnosis

This is based on the clinical presentation and on the finding of an elevated serum or urinary amylase level. Liver function tests may be abnormal and biliary obstruction, usually transient, may occur. Ultrasonography is useful mainly in helping to exclude gallstone-induced pancreatitis but may show pancreatic edema.

Therapy

With the exception of intravenous fluids, there is no known effective therapy. Third space fluid losses may be enormous. Blood pressure, pulse, and urine output should be monitored closely and hydration adjusted accordingly. In hemorrhagic pancreatitis, the hematocrit may fall as blood is lost into the retroperitoneal space, and blood transfusion may be needed.

Analgesia is usually required. Meperidine is said to be the drug of choice because it is thought to produce less spasm of the sphincter of Oddi.

Nasogastric suctioning is useful if vomiting is a problem and is used routinely by some. It is certainly indicated if ileus is present. A second rationale for the use of nasogastric suction is that by decreasing gastric secretion, reflex pancreatic secretion is abolished. H_2 blockers are frequently used on the same basis. Neither of these treatments, however, has been shown to be of benefit.

Serum electrolytes, glucose, and calcium concentrations should be monitored and abnormalities treated.

Occasionally pulmonary involvement with an adult respiratory distress syndrome occurs, and oxygen is needed.

Drugs known to precipitate pancreatitis, such as thiazides and furosemide, should be discontinued.

Gallstone Pancreatitis

If gallstones are present on ultrasound examination, then the likelihood that the stones have precipitated the pancreatitis must be considered. If the stones are not removed, the risk of a recurrence of the pancreatitis may be as high as 40 percent in the next 3 months. In patients in whom the gallbladder is in place, the optimal therapy is cholecystectomy with exploration of the common bile duct. In those patients who have had a cholecystectomy in the past, the choice of therapy is between surgical removal and endoscopic sphincterotomy. The risks of general anesthesia and laparotomy must be weighed against those of sphincterotomy. The major disadvantage of sphincterotomy is the need for fluoroscopy. The choice of approach depends to a large extent on the level of expertise available at a particular center.

Timing of intervention is difficult. If possible, any major procedures should be delayed until later in the pregnancy.

SMALL BOWEL DISEASE

The only commonly encountered small bowel diseases in the pregnant patient are Crohn's disease and gluten-sensitive enteropathy. Crohn's disease is discussed under the treatment of Inflammatory Bowel Disease.

Gluten-Sensitive Enteropathy

This disorder is due to sensitivity to a fraction of gluten. It is characterized by total or subtotal atrophy of the intestinal villi with subsequent malabsorption. The presentation may vary from isolated deficencies of iron and other nutrients to florid malabsorption with life-threatening diarrhea. Since iron and folate deficiencies are common in the pregnant patient it may be very difficult to recognize the disease if it appears for the first time during pregnancy. There is evidence to suggest that the height of the intestinal villi may increase during the normal pregnancy, as may intestinal enzyme content. Some patients with gluten-sensitive enteropathy actually improve during pregnancy.

Diagnosis

This is based on the clinical and biochemical picture of malabsorption but must be confirmed by biopsy evidence of villous atrophy. Following the demonstration of abnormal villous architecture, the response of the mucosa to a gluten-free diet should be documented, and ideally the patient should then be rechallenged with gluten. The reason for this rather lengthy process is that the pathology is not specific and furthermore there are many causes, some transient, of villous atrophy.

Therapy

This is based on strict avoidance of dietary gluten. Gluten is found in many staple foods and is also used as an additive in many preparations. A highly motivated, well-informed, and suspicious patient is necessary to ensure dietary adherence.

Lactose intolerance may complicate the picture, and avoidance of milk products until the mucosa improves may be useful in controlling diarrhea.

Vitamin and iron supplementation may be required. In severely ill patients, hospitalization and hyperalimentation may be necessary until the disease is under control.

Rarely, corticosteroids may be required for the management of refractory sprue, but prior to initiating therapy consideration should be given to alternative diagnostic possibilities such as lymphoma, pancreatic insufficiency, or bacterial overgrowth.

COLONIC DISEASE

Constipation

A majority of women experience alterations in bowel habit during pregnancy. Stool consistency may increase and stool frequency may decrease. This may, in part, relate to dietary alterations, but may also be due to the effects of progesterone on colonic motility and water absorption. Oral iron supplementation may also contribute.

Therapy

Treatment consists of increasing nonabsorbable fiber in the diet. One or two tablespoons of psyllium hydrophilic mucilloid twice a day or four to six tablets of bran and fruit fiber daily are generally sufficient.

Unwanted Effects and Interactions

There are no serious side effects associated with these medications. Some preparations of psyllium contain over 200 mg of sodium per dose, and this may be a problem in patients on salt restriction.

Stool softeners such as docusate sodium are frequently used, but specific data on safety are lacking. Nonabsorbable laxatives such as magnesium hydroxide or lactulose are not usually required. Lactulose has the advantage of being minimally absorbed. The dose can be titrated until the desired effect is reached.

Hemorrhoids

Rectal bleeding from internal or prolapsed hemorrhoids is a common, though rarely serious, problem. Constipation with straining at stool, the increased plasma volume, and the effects of hormones on rectal tone may all contribute.

Therapy

Treatment consists of relief of the constipation, maintenance of a soft stool, and local treatment such as Sitz baths. Constipation may be effectively treated with psyllium (see above).

Application of nonabsorbable or minimally absorbed ointments such as zinc sulfate may provide relief. Ointments used in the treatment of hemorrhoids frequently contain hydrocortisone. Although absorption of topical steroids is small, compounds containing steroids should be avoided if possible.

If pain is a major symptom, then creams containing the combination of a topical analgesic agent such as pramoxine or lidocaine with the emollient are indicated.

Unwanted Effects and Interactions

The only common side effect is that of local hypersensitivity. Systemic absorption of steroids may occur.

INFLAMMATORY BOWEL DISEASE

Crohn's Disease

This is a disease of unknown etiology characterized by transmural granulomatous inflammation of the bowel. Any part of the gastrointestinal tract from mouth to anus may be involved. A majority of patients have ileal involvement in combination with colonic disease.

Diagnosis

This can be very difficult, especially in pregnancy, because radiologic evaluation of the ileum or colon is often required to demonstrate the lesions. The presenting symptoms are very variable, but most commonly diarrhea and abdominal pain are prominent complaints. Clinically, the findings of fever, weight loss, and extraintestinal manifestations of the disease may suggest the diagnosis. There are no specific diagnostic tests, but sigmoidoscopic or colonoscopic evidence of ulceration in a discontinuous pattern is highly suggestive. Stool cultures for the common enteric pathogens and for *Yersinia enterocolitica* should be performed.

Ulcerative Colitis

This is an inflammatory disease of the colon of unknown etiology. The inflammation is primarily of the colonic mucosa, but in severe disease the inflammation may extend more deeply.

Diagnosis

Fortunately this is easier than for Crohn's disease and is based on the clinical history of diarrhea, often bloody, and sigmoidoscopic evidence of mucosal disease. Enteric pathogens should be excluded.

Indications for Therapy of Inflammatory Bowel Disease

The major indication for therapy in both Crohn's disease and ulcerative colitis is the presence of symptoms of inflammation such as rectal bleeding and diarrhea.

Therapy of Inflammatory Bowel Disease

There is no evidence that dietary alteration changes the course of inflammatory bowel disease. A low residue diet may be useful in patients with active disease and in patients with bowel narrowing. Maintenance of good nutrition is extremely important.

Two agents, sulfasalazine and corticosteroids, are the mainstay of treatment of these disorders. As discussed below, they are effective in inducing remission of active disease.

In patients with ulcerative colitis, prophylactic treatment with sulfasalazine may decrease the risk of relapse. There is no indication for prophylactic therapy in patients with Crohn's disease.

Sulfasalazine. Sulfasalazine is a combination of 5-aminosalicylic acid (5-ASA) and sulfapyridine linked by a diazo bond. Given orally, the diazo bond of the drug is split by colonic bacteria, releasing the constituent agents. It is now reasonably clear that the active moiety is the 5-ASA and that most of the side effects are related to the sulfapyridine fraction.

Sulfasalazine is useful in the induction of remission of active disease in both patients with Crohn's disease and those with ulcerative colitis. As might be expected from its mode of activation, sulfasalazine is less effective in Crohn's disease patients with disease confined to the small bowel.

In patients with Crohn's disease, the efficacy of this drug in maintaining remission is doubtful. In contrast, sulfasalazine significantly reduces the frequency of relapse in patients with ulcerative colitis.

For the dosage regimen, a reasonable starting dose is 1 g by mouth once daily. At this level both efficacy and side effects are minimal. Dosage may be gradually increased to a maximum of 1 g by mouth four times daily provided that careful monitoring to detect unwanted effects is carried out.

Increasing the dose above this level results in a high incidence of unwanted effects without a corresponding increase in therapeutic efficacy. Many of the unwanted effects associated with use of this drug are dose-related, and individual titration of the dose is necessary.

Unwanted Effects and Interactions

Systemic absorption of both 5-ASA and sulfapyridine occurs. Side effects may be either dose-related or idiosyncratic.

Dose-related side effects include nausea, anorexia, epigastric distress, fatigue, and a toxic hemolysis that may be associated with Heinz's bodies. These side effects often improve with reduction in drug dosage, are more common in slow acetylators, and correlate with the serum level of sulfapyridine.

Idiosyncratic side effects are more serious, and discontinuation of the drug is required. These include agranulocytosis, aplastic anemia, autoimmune hemolytic anemia, exfoliative dermatitis, and hepatic or pulmonary toxicity.

Skin rash is not uncommon. If the rash occurs in isolation, an attempt may be made to desensitize the patient by using very small doses of sulfasalazine. If the rash is associated with involvement of other systems, it may actually be part of a more generalized serum sickness reaction, and reintroduction of the drug is unwise.

Almost any system may be adversely affected by sulfasalazine. Proteinuria, hematuria, nephrotic syndrome, vertigo, tinnitus, peripheral neuropathy, pulmonary eosinophilia, fibrosing alveolitis, dyspnea, and hepatitis have been reported. In addition, there are occasional reports of bone marrow depression, urticaria, Stevens-Johnson syndrome, exfoliative dermatitis, and epidermal necrolysis. This list is not complete. Many of these reactions may be associated with the disease process itself, and it is sometimes difficult to know if the drug is responsible.

Contraindications

Patients known to be allergic to sulfonamides or salicylates should not receive this drug. Patients with hepatic, renal, hematologic or allergic conditions (including asthma) may be at increased risk of adverse effects.

Corticosteroids. Corticosteroids are useful in the induction of remission in both Crohn's disease and ulcerative colitis but not in the maintenance of remission in either disease. Once remission has been achieved, these drugs should be slowly withdrawn. In some patients, however, it is not possible to withdraw the drug without exacerbation of the disease.

The mechanism of action is not fully understood but probably relates to the anti-inflammatory and immune-modulating effect of these drugs.

The decision as to whether to initiate treatment with sulfasalazine alone or to add corticosteroids from the start can be difficult. In general, patients with mild symptoms may respond to sulfasalazine alone, whereas those with more severe symptoms also need steroids. In patients with Crohn's disease involving the small bowel, many physicians routinely use steroids as part of the initial management.

Dosage should be initiated at 40 to 60 mg of prednisone by mouth daily. When the desired therapeutic response is achieved and the disease is firmly in remission (generally after 1 to 3 weeks), the dose may be tapered by 5 mg every 3 to 5 days with careful monitoring of disease activity.

Most relapses of disease occur as the dose is reduced below 15 mg, and reduction by 2.5 mg every 5 days may be required.

Unwanted Effects and Interactions

Side effects are common, but fortunately many are dose-related and disappear as the dosage is reduced. The most commonly observed unwanted effects are those related to the sodium-retaining and metabolic effects of these drugs. Moon facies, weight gain with increased body fat and decreased muscle bulk, edema, and hypertension are common. Abdominal striae and easy bruising may be seen. Musculoskeletal effects include steroid myopathy, osteoporosis, aseptic necrosis of the hip, and vertebral collapse. Peptic ulceration may be more frequent, and there is an association with pancreatitis. Diabetes and hypokalemia with alkalosis may occur. Glaucoma may be precipitated in susceptible patients. Headache is not uncommon, but pseudotumor cerebri is rare.

The possibility of adrenal insufficiency must be considered in patients receiving steroids. If the patient is unable to continue oral medication and is severely stressed or requires anesthesia, parenteral steroids should be given. Babies born to mothers on steroids are also at risk for adrenal insufficiency.

Corticosteroid enemas are useful in the management of patients with distal colonic disease. They have the advantage of delivering topical therapy with less systemic side effects. Systemic absorption does occur, and all of the side effects listed above are possible though much less common.

Betamethasone enemas containing 5 mg of the active ingredient in 100 ml of buffered solution should be administered once or twice daily. It is preferable to administer these agents in the morning and on retiring at night. The longer the retention of the enema, the greater the efficacy. Hydrocortisone enemas are also available, generally containing 100 mg of hydrocortisone. There is probably little difference in efficacy between the preparations.

Therapeutic response may be assessed by monitoring the frequency of bowel movements, amount of bleeding, and general well-being. More objective assessment may be made by estimating one of the Crohn's disease activity indices or by using Truelove's criteria for ulcerative colitis.

Other Therapeutic Agents

In addition to the medications discussed above, other agents are being introduced for the management of inflammatory bowel disease.

In enteric-coated 5-aminosalicylic acid, the 5-ASA is contained in an acrylic resin. Release of the drug is pH-dependent and occurs in the proximal colon. The major advantage of this dosage form is that the unwanted effects of the sulfapyridine moiety of sulfasalazine are avoided.

5-Aminosalicylic acid has also been suspended in a wax matrix. The 5-ASA is released as the medication passes through the small bowel. The advantage is that the drug is delivered at the site of inflammation in patients with Crohn's disease affecting the small bowel. Colonic activation is not required.

5-Aminosalicylic acid enemas have been used with success in the management of distal colonic disease including proctosigmoiditis and proctitis. High concentrations of the active moiety of sulfasalazine are delivered directly to the mucosa. These enemas may be useful in patients who do not respond to corticosteroids.

The Management of Unresponsive Disease

Occasionally a patient does not respond to treatment with sulfasalazine and corticosteroids. In such cases treatment with bed rest, intravenous steroids, oral sulfasalazine, and steroid enemas may be effective.

If no response is obtained, then consideration should be given to bowel rest and total parenteral nutrition (TPN). Apart from the usual hazards of TPN such as pneumothorax and sepsis, there may be an added risk in pregnancy if lipid emulsions are used. Pregnancy tends to produce hypertriglyceridemia, and lipid emulsions may augment this tendency with subsequent ketosis to the detriment of the fetus. There is also concern that TPN may lead to placental insufficiency. Such risks have to be balanced against the possibility of fetal loss in patients with severe disease or patients who become malnourished.

Effect of Pregnancy on the Activity of Inflammatory Bowel Disease

The fertility rate of patients with inactive inflammatory bowel disease is comparable to that of the general population. Pregnancy exerts little effect on the Crohn's disease activity, but there may be an increased risk of relapse in the postpartum period. It is likely that patients with severe disease at the onset of pregnancy experience an increased risk of fetal loss.

As is the case with Crohn's disease, women with ulcerative colitis whose disease is inactive at the time of conception are unlikely to encounter major problems. If the disease is active at conception, the subsequent course may be difficult to predict. There is some evidence to suggest that women with severe disease during the pregnancy are at increased risk of fetal loss.

Effect of Inflammatory Bowel Disease on the Fetus

It does not appear that the disease per se predisposes to fetal abnormalities. As discussed above, there may be an increased risk of fetal loss in women with active disease.

Sulfasalazine does not appear to cause fetal abnormalities. The sulfapyridine moiety may displace bilirubin from albumin and therefore may predispose to kernicterus. Clinically this does not seem to be a major problem, since the bilirubin-displacing capacity of sulfapyridine is small.

Corticosteroids, in animals, are associated with fetal abnormalities. The data in humans suggest that they are not associated with a higher risk of fetal abnormalities. Certainly, given the risk–benefit of using these drugs, it would appear that they should be used in the treatment of inflammatory bowel disease in the pregnant patient.

Management of Stomas in Inflammatory Bowel Disease

The presence of a stoma is not a contraindication to pregnancy. Pregnancy may make management of the stoma more difficult, especially in the second and third trimesters, as the uterus enlarges and intra-abdominal pressure rises. The available evidence suggests that the majority of women with stomas have an uncomplicated course and a vaginal delivery.

GASTROINTESTINAL INFECTIONS

These illnesses are a common cause of morbidity and occur as frequently in pregnancy as in the nonpregnant state. The major threat to the pregnancy is the risk of fetal loss as a result of severe maternal dehydration.

The infectious diarrheas include those due to organisms that invade the intestinal mucosa, resulting in a febrile illness with bloody or mucoid diarrhea and lower abdominal cramps. Organisms causing diarrhea by tissue invasion include *Shigella* species, *Salmonella* species, *Campylobacter jejuni, Entamoeba histolytica, Yersinia enterocolitica, Vibrio parahaemolyticus,* and some strains of *Escherichia coli.*

Alternatively, diarrhea may be due to toxin production by microorganisms, and this is usually of high volume, without blood or mucus in the stool (except for *Clostridium difficile* enterocolitis); there is usually no fever. Cramps are usually felt in the lower abdomen. Organisms producing toxin-induced gastroenteritis are *Bacillus cereus, Clostridium difficile, Vibrio cholerae, Escherichia coli, Clostridium perfringens,* and *Staphylococcus aureus.*

Two other important microorganisms causing infectious diarrheas are *Giardia lamblia* and viruses of the reovirus and parvovirus types. These organisms tend to produce diarrhea that is large volume and foul-smelling and may be associated with periumbilical cramps. Mucus and blood are not usually found in the stools.

Diagnosis

The pattern of diarrhea (i.e., volume, presence of mucus or blood, site of the cramps) is a useful indicator of whether it is of small bowel or colonic origin. Small bowel diarrhea is usually of viral origin, whereas colonic diarrheas are usually bacterial. Three stool cultures and examinations for ova and parasites detect most treatable enteric pathogens. Viruses cannot be detected on routine culture, and the stool may be negative for *Giardia* even if the organism is causing symptoms. Small bowel aspiration may be necessary to detect *Giardia*. Sigmoidoscopic examination is not usually required but is important if amebiasis is being considered.

Therapy

The principles of treatment of infectious diarrheas in the pregnant patient are essentially similar to those for the nonpregnant patient. Attention to fluid and electrolyte balance is essential in view of the threat of maternal dehydration to the viability of the fetus, and intravenous rehydration should be considered early in the management. Agents that reduce motility should not be used because they delay the elimination of the causative organism.

Drug therapy is generally to be avoided but may be necessary in very severe cases or when there is systemic infection (i.e., positive blood cultures in *Salmonella* infections). The reader is referred to the July 1987 issue of the *Medical Letter* for a current assessment of the safety of antimicrobial agents in pregnancy.

Ampicillin appears to be safe in the treatment of severe *Salmonella* or *Shigella* infections, although bacterial resistance is common.

Chloramphenicol has been proposed as an alternative to ampicillin, although its use is somewhat controversial and maternal blood level monitoring is strongly advised.

Ceftriaxone is very effective against *Salmonella* species, but its teratogenic potential has not been fully established.

For *Yersinia* and *Vibrio parahaemolyticus* infections, drug therapy is seldom required, though chloramphenicol may be considered in severe cases. *Campylobacter* infections, similarly, should be treated conservatively.

Erythromycin appears to lack teratogenic effects, is useful in the treatment of *Campylobacter* infections, and has been shown to shorten the duration of excretion of the organism.

Paromomycin, which is poorly absorbed, is effective in the treatment of amebic colitis and is probably safe during pregnancy.

Chloroquine is a powerful amebicide and is probably safe in pregnancy, although fetal mice concentrate the drug in the retina.

Metronidazole is useful for treating patients with amebic liver abscess, but its potential teratogenicity, especially in the first trimester, is a very serious drawback.

For all the forms of toxin-induced gastroenteritis, conservative treatment with parenteral rehydration is the best approach. Pseudomembranous enterocolitis is the exception, for which the drug of choice is oral vancomycin.

Viral gastroenteritides should be treated conservatively with supportive rehydration.

Giardia lamblia infection poses a problem, since metronidazole has carcinogenic and mutagenic effects in rodents and one human study showed an increase in congenital defects when the drug was used in the first trimester. It may be safe to use this drug in later pregnancy. Quinacrine is mutagenic in microorganisms and is contraindicated in pregnancy.

Pharmacologic Treatment of Gastrointestinal Disease During Lactation

A very limited number of medications have been provisionally recommended for the treatment of gastrointestinal disease in pregnancy. With the exception of the drugs listed below, these medications are active primarily by a topical effect, and absorption (with subsequent excretion in milk) is minimal. This section deals with the medications that are absorbed and thus may have an effect on lactation and be excreted in breast milk. The antibiotics have not been discussed simply because of the number of drugs available. The package insert should be consulted before administering any drug to the lactating mother.

Metoclopramide and domperidone should not be used in the lactating mother until more data are available on possible effects on the neonate. Both of these drugs affect prolactin secretion.

The question as to whether it is safe to continue sulfasalazine during breast feeding remains somewhat controversial. It is clear that little of the intact drug is excreted in milk. However, sulfapyridine concentrations of 40 percent of those found in maternal serum may be found in breast milk. The major concern in the past has been that sulfapyridine might predispose to kernicterus because of the ability of sulfa drugs to displace bilirubin from protein in the serum. It appears that the bilirubin-displacing ability of sulfapyridine is small and the risk of kernicterus minimal. However, it is prudent to discontinue use of this drug if the neonate is jaundiced. The neonate theoretically should be at risk from idiosyncratic side effects of sulfapyridine. We are not aware of any such reports.

The serum level of 5-ASA in women receiving sulfasalazine is low. It is not known whether 5-ASA in breast milk reaches the neonatal blood in appreciable concentrations. Whether 5-ASA in neonatal serum would predispose the child to Reye's syndrome, as has been reported with ASA, is not known, but this possibility appears extremely unlikely.

In contrast to many drugs, the excretion of prednisolone in breast milk has been well studied. Prednisolone at doses of 80 mg per day is excreted in breast milk at concentrations of 20 percent of those found in plasma. Peak concentrations may reach 300 ng per milliliter of milk. Six hours after the dose, breast milk concentrations were minimal. If high-dose prednisone therapy is being employed, it is preferable to wait at least 8 hours after ingestion of the drug before feeding. A practical approach would be to express the breast milk prior to ingesting the prednisone. If refrigerated, the milk may then be used during the time when plasma concentrations of the drug are at their peak.

SUGGESTED READING

Burrow GN, Ferris TF, eds. Medical complications during pregnancy. 3rd ed. Philadelphia: WB Saunders, 1988.

Cherry SH, Berkowitz RL, Kase NG, eds. Medical, surgical, and gynecologic complications of pregnancy. 3rd ed. Baltimore: Williams & Wilkins, 1985.

Farmer RG, ed. Inflammatory bowel disease. Clin Gastroenterol 1980; 9(2).

Lawrence R, ed. Breast feeding. Clin Perinatol 1987; 14(1).

Rustei VK, Cooper JN, eds. Gastrointestinal and hepatic complications in pregnancy. New York: John Wiley & Sons, 1986.

ANEMIA IN PREGNANCY

DAVID Z. KITAY, M.D.

Anemia is always a symptom. The principal concern in pregnancy is therapy of the underlying problem causing the anemia, and whether or not anemia is actually present. Indirect screening tests are used (packed cell volume, hemoglobin) rather than direct measurements of equilibrium between erythrocyte production and destruction. The hematocrit* may reflect normal hydremia (no therapy), a nutritional anemia (the specific nutrient or nutrients), or other problems such as a hemoglobinopathy (occasionally vigorous therapy). In all cases, therapy of the problem causing the anemia, and not the anemia itself, influences reproductive outcome. Table 1 includes the more common causes of anemia in pregnancy. Hemorrhage and the hemoglobinopathies are discussed in the chapter entitled *Hemoglobinopathies.*

IRON DEFICIENCY

The goal of therapy of iron deficiency and iron-deficiency anemia is to reestablish adequate erythrocyte proliferation by providing the absent or deficient nutrient. In the final analysis, response to iron with reticulocytosis and elevation of hematocrit is both diagnostic and therapeutic.

Oral Therapy

There are no therapeutic alternatives to provision of oral or parenteral iron. The patient should be encouraged to ingest a diet containing a wide variety of nutrients from the various food groups. Nevertheless, it is practically impossible to treat iron-deficiency anemia with dietary therapy alone because no single food contains sufficient iron to be therapeutically effective, and costs would be prohibitive. For example, an average serving of steak contains approximately 3 mg of iron; in order to provide enough iron from this source to fully recover from iron-deficiency anemia, a woman would have to eat roughly 10 lbs per day.

TABLE 1 More Common Causes of Anemia in Pregnancy

Hypoproliferative (decreased production)
Iron deficient erythropoiesis
Relative (hemorrhage)
Iron deficiency
Erythropoietin lack
Renal disease
Stem cell dysfunction
Erythrocyte aplasia or hypoplasia
Ineffective
Folic acid deficiency
Thalassemia
Hemolytic (increased destruction)
Hemolytic hemoglobinopathies
Hereditary spherocytosis
Microangiopathic

Oral iron salts are the therapy of choice. There are certain principles to follow in selecting the most efficacious preparation. The American Druggist Red Book lists at least 100 pharmaceuticals promoted for therapy of iron deficiency.

Each tablet or capsule should contain roughly 60 mg of elemental iron. At this dosage level, side effects are minimal or absent, and smaller doses may result in delayed or incomplete recovery. This amount is contained in the popular prenatal multivitamin preparations used for prophylaxis in pregnancy.

The iron-containing, prophylactic, prenatal multivitamin must be formulated and ingested in a manner that promotes iron release and absorption in gastric and duodenal juice. Enteric-coated or delayed release iron preparations may present iron to a portion of the gastrointestinal tract where absorption is inefficient or virtually nonexistent. The amount of calcium and magnesium administered simultaneously should be less than one-fifth the recommended daily dietary allowance in pregnancy, since both interfere with iron absorption.

It has been common practice to administer either therapeutic or prophylactic iron with meals in an attempt to minimize side effects. A host of food substances, such as tea, have been shown to inhibit iron absorption, while others, such as citrus juices, have the opposite effect. Iron should be given between meals or prophylactically at bedtime with a small glass of citrus juice.

Iron is absorbed in the ferrous form. Only ferrous salts should be used in prophylaxis or therapy, and the cost to the patient should be small.

The three commonly used iron preparations are ferrous sulfate, ferrous gluconate, and ferrous fumarate. The sulfate and fumarate contain 60 mg per tablet; the gluconate contains half this amount and, therefore, is about 1.5 times more expensive per treatment regimen. Dosage is one tablet (two for the gluconate) between meals and at bedtime (total 180 mg iron) or alternatively, ferrous sulfate 320 mg (60 mg iron) three times per day, 1 hour before meals.

There is no evidence that any one of these salts is superior with regard to side effects; indeed, patient complaints assure proper compliance. Roughly 10 to 20 percent of patients complain of diarrhea, constipation, or a metallic taste. Stools will blacken. In some cases side effects may be psychological in origin, and occasionally side effects may be dosage-related. This can be helped by reduction in the number of tablets per day and switching to another preparation that has a different external appearance. A pregnant woman may prefer ferrous sulfate solution, concentrated, which has 25 mg iron per cubic centi-

* Packed cell volume is the correct term since the word "hematocrit" actually refers to a machine. However, since physicians and automated counters use the terms interchangeably, "hematocrit" is retained in this text.

meter. Dosage would be 2.5 to 3 cc three times per day.

The only important complication of oral iron therapy is acute iron poisoning, which occurs in children and is almost always accidental.

Parenteral Therapy

The few indications in pregnancy for the use of parenteral iron are as follows: (1) iron malabsorption, (2) noncompliance, (3) oral iron intolerance, and (4) iron need greater than can be provided orally. Iron dextran is the only parenteral compound available in the United States and is currently manufactured by at least 17 generic pharmaceutical firms. The minimum required dose in an adult is at least 1,000 mg or 20 ml.

Parenteral iron in pregnancy is justified when one or more of the above indications exists, and there is laboratory evidence of iron deficiency using any of the following parameters:

1. Serum iron below 63 μg per deciliter
2. Mean corpuscular volume 79 or less in the absence of beta-thalassemia minor or a hemolytic hemoglobinopathy
3. Elevated red cell distribution width (above 15)
4. Serum ferritin 10 μg per liter (or lower)
5. Microcytosis, hypochromia on peripheral smear.

The presence of pica (ingestion of "normal" or "abnormal" substances with possible caloric but definite deficient nutritive value, with simultaneous exclusion or limitation of nutritionally beneficial foodstuffs) in pregnancy can also be regarded as presumptive evidence of iron deficiency.

Iron-dextran is supplied as 50 mg per milliliter in 2- and 10-ml vials. It can be administered intramuscularly or intravenously. A dose of 0.5 cc is given intravenously to test for the possibility of anaphylaxis, which occurs in less than 1 percent of patients. If no reaction occurs after an hour, the remainder of the dose may be given.

Table 2 shows total dose requirement in milliliters of iron-dextran to correct iron deficiency anemia. One of the problems in therapy is the manufacturer's recommendation that no more than 2.0 ml be given at one time and that it not be used in pregnancy.†

Iron-dextran is given either by deep intramuscular injection or by intravenous infusion at a rate no faster than 1.0 ml per minute. Intramuscular administration is painful and is associated with skin staining. To avoid leakage or injection into the skin, the "Z track" technique (displacement of the skin laterally prior to the injection) is used. Total dose intravenous infusion has been used extensively and successfully by a number of physicians, but is currently not approved in the United States.

The frequency of systemic side effects varies markedly depending on the series reported. By far the most important problem is anaphylaxis, although this occurs in less than 1 percent of patients and is independent of the route of administration. It is advisable to have at hand 0.5 ml of a 1:1,000 aqueous epinephrine solution when initiating therapy. Other side effects, which may appear as delayed reactions (after hours to days), include chills, fever, myalgias, dizziness, headache, nausea, and malaise.

The expected responses to either oral or parenteral iron preparations in the treatment of iron deficiency are, for all practical purposes, identical in timing and magnitude. Reticulocytosis begins after 5 to 7 days, reaches a maximum after 7 to 12 days, and then decreases. In pregnancy, especially if therapy is begun in midtrimester, normal hydremia may mask the expected rise in hematocrit. In addition, the extent of plasma volume rise differs among women and is higher in multiple pregnancy where iron loss to the products of conception is greater. If the hematocrit remains at a reasonable level (30 percent) or rises as pregnancy proceeds, it can be assumed that therapy is adequate. If there is no excessive delivery blood loss, therapy with prophylactic iron dosage (60 mg per day) should be continued for at least 12 weeks post partum.

If the hematocrit falls in the face of adequate therapy and good compliance, the diagnosis should be suspect or some other reason for either iron deficiency or anemia (inflammation, hepatic or renal disease, neoplasia) should be sought. If the patient obtained oral iron by prescription, she should be asked to display the tablets to negate the possibility that an enteric-coated product had not been dispensed.

The serum ferritin is of some value in pregnancy. Normally, serum ferritin falls because of pregnancy hydremia. In an iron-supplemented patient, when prophylaxis is begun before or at 20 weeks, the serum ferritin should not fall below 10 μg per liter. An adequately treated patient should have a puerperal ferritin level a number of times this amount.

TABLE 2 Milliliters of Iron-Dextran Required to Obtain a Desired Hemoglobin Response

		Pretreatment Hgb			
lbs	*kg*	*4.0 (g/dl)*	*6.0 (g/dl)*	*8.0 (g/dl)*	*10.0 (g/dl)*
80	36.3	35	28	22	16
90	40.8	39	32	25	18
100	45.4	44	35	28	20
110	49.9	48	39	30	21
120	54.4	53	42	33	23
130	59.0	57	46	36	25
140	63.5	61	50	39	27
150	68.1	66	53	41	29
160	72.6	70	57	44	31
170	77.1	74	60	47	33
180	81.7	79	64	50	35

Reprinted with permission from Physicians' desk reference. 38th ed. Oradell, NJ: Medical Economics, 1984:1337.

† The recommendation that only 2.0 ml be given in a single dose came from the experience of one hospital in Florida with a single lot number of the drug. A number of pregnant women developed fever, hematuria, and arthralgias in temporal relation to intramuscular administration. The recommendation about use in pregnancy is based on animal studies and a stillbirth some weeks after a reaction to iron-dextran.

FOLIC ACID DEFICIENCY

The development of megaloblastic anemia secondary to folic acid deficiency in late pregnancy (or earlier if hemolysis from any associated condition is present) was not uncommon in the United States prior to 1970. In 1966, the Physicians' Desk Reference listed 48 preparations for use as prenatal multivitamin supplements although only five contained folic acid in varying dosage. In 1968, the Food and Nutrition Board of the National Research Council noted that the daily requirement of folate in pregnancy might be ten times that of the nonpregnant state. The requirement in lactation is even higher since the breast preferentially extracts folate from serum. In 1987, the vast majority, if not all, of the popular prenatal supplements contain folic acid in a dosage of 400 μg to 1 mg. One milligram covers all pregnancy requirements and all pregnancy-associated medical or surgical problems causing an increase in folic acid need.

Since prophylaxis with 1 mg of folate daily has been so effective in reducing the incidence of florid megaloblastic anemia in pregnancy, the patients who may develop this problem are as follows:

1. Those with minimal to absent prenatal care
2. Those noncompliant in taking the vitamin supplement
3. Those with malabsorption of folic acid
4. Those ingesting drugs that are known folate antagonists (e.g. phenytoin in epilepsy).

Megaloblastic anemia appearing in pregnancy is presumptive evidence of folic acid deficiency. The only other nutritional etiology, vitamin B_{12} deficiency, is exceedingly rare. When megaloblastic anemia appears, the hematocrit is usually quite low (10 to 16 percent), glossitis is common, and the patient is pale.

Therapy is begun with 1.0 mg folic acid tablets daily. The patient should be hospitalized for the first several days of recovery. The patient is usually close to term and may begin labor. Folic acid deficiency may cause profound thrombocytopenia, which is associated with a significant incidence of hemorrhage at delivery.

There are no significant side effects associated with either oral or parenteral folic acid therapy.

Recovery begins with a rapid-onset, occasionally profound, reticulocytosis, which starts at approximately 72 hours. The hematocrit has been observed to double in 2 weeks and, with continued puerperal therapy, will be normal 6 weeks post partum.

Indications for parenteral folic acid are the same as for parenteral iron. The patient may be too ill from an associated medical or surgical problem to ingest the oral form. One of the drawbacks of the prenatal folate and iron-containing multivitamin preparation is noncompliance because of iron side effects.

In patients with sickle cell disease-complicating pregnancy, the normal gestational demand for folic acid is greatly increased because of hemolysis. Antepartum folate administration is critical. Since these patients do not require iron (and a modicum of iron deficiency induced by pregnancy may actually be beneficial), the prenatal vitamin is withheld and only oral or parenteral folate is given. Parenteral folic acid comes as vials containing 15 mg per cubic centimeter. One cc intravenously, subcutaneously, or intramuscularly every week should be sufficient.

Combined iron and folate deficiency in pregnancy is not uncommon because dietary sources of both nutrients overlap. In the course of treatment of folic acid deficiency, iron availability may become the limiting factor in obtaining a complete hematologic response.

VITAMIN B_{12} DEFICIENCY

It would be inappropriate to discuss vitamin B_{12} therapy of megaloblastic anemia in pregnancy. Patients with true addisonian pernicious anemia are generally older than child-bearing years, infertile, and cannot be treated with oral medication. Case reports of pernicious anemia in pregnancy are so rare (I am aware of one) as to be a curiosity.

SUGGESTED READING

Horan C, Kitay DZ. Folic acid deficiency. In: Kitay DZ, ed. Hematologic problems in pregnancy. Oradell, NJ: Medical Economics, 1987:49.

Meeks GR, Gookin K, Morrison JC. Iron deficiency. In: Kitay DZ, ed. Hematologic problems in pregnancy. Oradell, NJ: Medical Economics, 1987:27.

HEMOGLOBINOPATHIES

DAVID Z. KITAY, M.D.

Four principles govern therapy of the hemolytic hemoglobinopathies in pregnancy:

1. If the patient has survived to the childbearing years, she must have milder disease that is potentially but not necessarily life-threatening.
2. The location of care is important—sickle cell disease patients are usually found in medium to large cities in the South and Northeast; in a recently conducted survey of 20 medical centers, half the patients were treated with "conservative" management and the others with routine or indicated transfusion therapy; the term "indicated" refers to the patient's clinical condition and reticulocyte count—it should not

refer to her packed cell volume or amount of hemoglobin S, A, or other.
3. Review of the literature and experience in anesthesiology reveal that in such patients, any anesthetic agent for any procedure, including parturition, may be safely employed in the presence of adequate oxygenation. The level of hemoglobin A should not be arbitrarily raised prior to surgery or delivery, especially if the patient's history and course have been benign. Raising the level of hemoglobin A (by straight or exchange transfusion) increases blood viscosity which may be detrimental.
4. Almost all pregnant women with a hemolytic hemoglobinopathy should have a good outcome at delivery; the fetus may be compromised, but that is a problem in antepartum testing and care.

DEFINITIONS

Hemoglobinopathies are molecular disorders in which the structure and possibly the function of normal hemoglobin are altered, and the hereditable pattern of these disorders is well defined. The thalassemias are problems in hemoglobin production rate and are not addressed in this chapter unless they interact with an abnormal hemoglobin. Table 1 lists the most common hemoglobinopathies encountered in the United States Black population; it does not include the recent influx of Southeast Asians from Vietnam, Thailand, and Cambodia, who have a relatively high incidence of hemoglobin E as trait, in combination with beta-thalassemia minor, or as homozygous hemoglobin E disease.

The hemoglobinopathy must be properly defined by hemoglobin electrophoresis and properly named. Therapy in this chapter refers only to the following disorders: sickle cell disease (SS); sickle cell–hemoglobin C disease (SC); sickle cell beta-thalassemia (S-thal); and other hemolytic hemoglobinopathies, such as homozygous hemoglobin C or E disease. Trait problems (hemoglobin AC, AS, AE) are not addressed because the pregnancy course and outcome in such women (with the exception of a high incidence of urinary tract infections in those with sickle cell trait), are virtually identical to those of the general population. In documenting the disorder, electrophoresis with quantitated A_2 hemoglobin should always be employed; screening tests for sickle hemoglobin may be inadequate and misleading. Hematologic conventions name hemoglobinopathies by the amino acid changes in alpha or beta chains; for obstetricians, this is cumbersome. The easiest way to document the disease is to name it (e.g., sickle cell–hemoglobin C disease) and to abbreviate the hemoglobins with the majority hemoglobin named first:

sickle cell trait AS (60% A, 40% S)
sickle cell disease SS (90+% S, remainder F)

In Grady Memorial Hospital, Atlanta, Georgia, most crises of SS, SC, and S-thal disease in pregnancy have been managed expectantly with analgesics and hydration. In the University of South Alabama, Mobile, Alabama, half are expectantly treated and half require exchange transfusions for one or another maternal or fetal complication. In the University of Mississippi, Jackson, Mississippi, all pregnant patients with sickle cell disease are routinely transfused or exchange transfused on intake, and perinatal mortality has been greatly reduced.

Regardless of the location, certain factors seem evident.

1. The city in which patients live (and receive therapy) determines disease severity because the phenotype of sickle cell disease is determined by the genetic makeup of ancestors who entered the country via a specific slave port. For example, in the eastern province of Saudi Arabia, there are many asymptomatic patients with sickle cell disease and similarly in Atlanta, where many slaves entered via Charleston, thus carrying a phenotype that caused their descendents to suffer only mild disease.
2. The only specific therapy at present is to reduce sickling in pregnancy with transfusion of AA erythrocytes; no therapy is yet available that consistently reduces or prevents crises.
3. Following reticulocytosis during prenatal care appears a better method of determining hematologic status than packed cell volume; the patient with SS disease, adequately provided with folate supplementation, has a reticulocyte count of approximately 7 to 25 percent; similarly, the patient with SC disease has a value of 5 to 10 percent. The reticulocytosis demonstrates that bone marrow erythrocyte production is at least adequately compensating for hemolysis.

TABLE 1 Most Common Hemoglobinopathies in U.S. Black Population

Hemoglobinopathy	*Designation*	*Incidence*
Sickle-cell trait	HbA/S	1:12
Hemoglobin C trait	HbA/C	1:33
Sickle-cell anemia	HbS/S	1:500
Sickle cell–hemoglobin C disease	HbS/C	1:600
Sickle cell–B thalassemia	HbS/Thal	1:650
Hemoglobin C disease	HbC/C	1:4400

From Horger EO. Hemoglobinopathies. In: Kitay DZ, ed. Hematologic problems in pregnancy. Oradell, NJ: Medical Economics, 1987:118.

SPECIFIC THERAPY

The patient's past medical and obstetric history should to a large degree determine her course in the present pregnancy; if her past history has been relatively benign, with few pain crises and successful completion of a previous pregnancy, one would tend to withhold transfusion therapy.

The patient is seen every 2 weeks after intake until the 32nd to 34th week, then every week until delivery. Virgorous genetic counseling should be provided. Although most women with sickle cell disease (SS) know of their problem, it is not at all unusual to have a patient with SC disease enter pregnancy totally unaware of her hemoglobinopathy. Amniocentesis may be performed, if desired, in early pregnancy to determine fetal hemoglobin type by DNA analysis.

Oral folic acid, 1.0 mg per day, must be given either by itself or as that contained in most popular prenatal vitamin preparations. This dosage is adequate to cover both the demands of pregnancy and the hemolysis of the disease. Parenteral folic acid (supplied as 15 mg per milliliter) is indicated if the patient will not take oral medication and in the presence of a malabsorption syndrome. SS disease patients who are not supplemented with folate therapy risk cardiac failure in midtrimester.

After the initial routine laboratory studies, including a hemoglobin electrophoresis with quantitated A_2 hemoglobin to define the disease, a reticulocyte count is obtained every other visit until term.

A urine culture is obtained at the first visit, in the presence of any real or remote complaints, and in each trimester. Asymptomatic bacteriuria or obvious clinical infection should be treated acutely with sulfa drugs or ampicillin, depending on sensitivities. If infection persists or recurs, after acute therapy is provided, the patient may be placed on chronic sulfa or nitrofurantoin prophylaxis until delivery. Pregnant women with the sickling disorders have at least a three times greater incidence of urinary infection.

Serial ultrasonic fetal growth measurement and stress testing (or other biophysical measurements) should be routine—the most important fetal complication is growth retardation.

Hospitalization is indicated in the presence of pyelonephritis, pneumonia, absence of reticulocytosis (possible aplastic crisis), and any pain crisis. A pain crisis near term may be associated with onset of premature labor.

Exchange transfusion with AA red cells is done routinely in some centers. It should be considered (and perhaps repeated) in the presence of fetal growth retardation, in the pain crisis that is not relieved by opiates, and in the presence of severe maternal infection. The goal is to achieve a hemoglobin A level (as measured by electrophoresis) of approximately 40 to 50 percent. In general, this requires about four units of packed cells in the exchange. The protocol for exchange transfusion is detailed in Table 2.

THE PUERPERIUM

Cord blood samples for hemoglobin electrophoresis should be obtained at delivery. Although these show hemoglobin F as predominant, the presence of any other hemoglobin or the absence of hemoglobin A indicates a hemoglobinopathy, and the pediatrician should be notified. (Although rare, homozygous persistence of fetal hemoglobin—FF—has been reported).

All patients with sickling disorders should be given pneumococcal vaccine (Pneumovax); current recommendations include repetition of the vaccine every 3 years.

Puerperal bilateral partial salpingectomy for sterilization is preferred when indicated. Although patients with mild disease may use oral contraceptives (sickling is a mechanical, not thrombotic phenomenon), many obstetricians prefer to avoid this method.

Medroxyprogesterone (Depo-Provera) in a dosage of 150 mg intramuscularly every 3 months is extremely effective as reversible contraception. The Federal Drug Administration has not approved Depo-Provera for contraception, although a number of centers are routinely using it as such along with informed consent. Clinical experience has shown it to be safe and effective in sickle cell disease patients.

FUTURE THERAPEUTIC MODALITIES

Clinical and experimental evidence suggests that stimulation of fetal hemoglobin production benefits patients with sickle cell disease by inhibiting sickling. In adults, fetal hemoglobin appears to be restricted to a subpopulation of erythrocytes, the F cells. Stimulation of F-cell formation has been achieved with 5-azacitidine, a drug that induces gamma-globin gene demethylation. Other drugs, such as hydroxyurea, cytarabine, and vinblastine have been found to stimulate F-cell formation in primates and

TABLE 2 Partial Exchange Transfusion Protocol

Packed cell volume, hemoglobin A and A_2, and type and cross-match at 28 weeks' gestation
1,000 ml 1:6 molar lactate; infuse 200–400 ml (1 hour)
Phlebotomize 500 ml blood into Vacutainer (30 minutes)
Give two units (150–300 ml/unit) buffy coat–poor washed red cells (warmed, under pressure; 1–2 hours)
Repeat procedure in afternoon and allow overnight equilibration
Obtain packed cell volume and hemoglobin A next morning
If over 35 and 40%, respectively, discharge patient, if not, repeat procedure until desired levels are obtained
Repeat entire procedure: (1) at 36–38 weeks; (2) when packed cell volume is less than 25% and hemoglobin A less than 20%; and (3) if crisis occurs

After Morrison JC, Schneider JM, Whybrew WD, et al. Prophylactic transfusion in pregnant patients with sickle hemoglobinopathies: benefit versus risk. Obstet Gynecol 1980; 56:274.

patients, and most recently pulses of erythropoietin have stimulated tremendous increases in F-reticulocyte levels.

SUGGESTED READING

Adil Al-Khatti, et al. Stimulation of fetal hemoglobin synthesis by erythropoietin in baboons. N Engl J Med 1987; 317:415–420.
Horger EO. Hemoglobinopathies. In: Kitay DZ, ed. Hematologic problems in pregnancy. Oradell, NJ: Medical Economics, 1987:116.

RESPIRATORY DISEASES

MAURICE A. MUFSON, M.D., F.A.C.P.
NANCY J. MUNN, M.D.

Particularly during pregnancy, the exacerbation of a chronic respiratory disease (mainly asthma in this age group) or the onset of an acute respiratory tract infection requires astute diagnosis and judicious treatment, taking into account the health of both the mother and the fetus (Table 1). Exacerbations of asthma and chronic obstructive pulmonary disease complicate the course of the pregnancy, and the treatment of these respiratory diseases requires prompt attention. Pregnant women who smoke increase their risk of pulmonary complications—mainly aspiration pneumonia and pulmonary embolism—especially when they require a cesarean section delivery.

The acute respiratory infections likely to complicate the pregnancy of normal women (women whose immune system mechanisms are intact and who may not be otherwise considered "high risk" for acute respiratory infections because of underlying diseases or habits) include acute viral infections of the upper respiratory tract, such as undifferentiated upper respiratory tract illness, influenza, pharyngitis, and laryngitis; viral and mycoplasmal pneumonia; and bacterial pneumonia. Very infrequently, pulmonary tuberculosis and lung abscess and, rarely, acute fungal infection occur in the pregnant woman.

PHYSIOLOGIC CHANGES IN PULMONARY SYSTEM DURING PREGNANCY

The stress placed on the maternal pulmonary system by the demands of the fetus complicates the management of acute and chronic respiratory disease in the pregnant woman. During pregnancy, a mild degree of hyperventilation occurs that may be the result of respiratory stimulation by progesterone. This produces an increase in the minute ventilation caused primarily by an increase in tidal volume; the increase in minute ventilation varies in individual women from 20 to 50 percent, and oxygen consumption also increases by 20 to 35 percent. The respiratory rate remains unchanged. The hyperventilation also results in a persistent decrease in the pCO_2, which plateaus at about 27 to 30 mm Hg. However, blood pH remains normal because of a compensatory increase in the renal excretion of bicarbonate. The pO_2 usually increases during pregnancy, but the alveolar-arterial oxygen gradient does not change until term, when it may increase slightly, perhaps reflecting the decreased functional residual capacity and airway closure at that time.

TABLE 1 Respiratory Diseases of Concern During Pregnancy

Category	*Disease*	*Occurrence*
Noninfectious	Asthma	Common
	Chronic obstructive disease	Uncommon
Infectious	Viral upper respiratory tract	Very common
	Influenza	Very common
	Viral pneumonia	Uncommon
	Mycoplasmal pneumonia	Uncommon
	Bacterial pneumonia	Uncommon
	Tuberculosis	Rare

During pregnancy, the diaphragm becomes elevated, although its movement remains unimpaired, and the configuration of the thorax changes. Lung volumes show only mild reductions. Vital capacity does not decrease. Expiratory reserve volume, residual volume, and functional residual capacity decrease 15 to 25 percent in pregnancy. Total lung capacity decreases slightly, from 4 to 6 percent. Forced expiratory volume in 1 second (FEV_1) remains unchanged.

Although hyperventilation is a normal physiologic alteration in pregnancy, many pregnant women experience symptoms of dyspnea as a consequence. In the first trimester, 15 to 30 percent of women may experience dyspnea. The proportion of women with dyspnea increases to 70 percent in the second and third trimesters.

Considering the character of these physiologic changes in the pulmonary system, the pregnant woman faces increased risks from exacerbation of existing chronic respiratory disease and the onset of acute respiratory tract infections. The prevention of acute respiratory infections and the control of chronic respiratory disease assume the highest priority during pregnancy. Treatment of respiratory disease in the pregnant woman must be prompt and aggressive, employing drugs that do not pass the placental barrier or, if they do, that do not affect the fetus (Table 2).

ASTHMA

Asthma is a common respiratory disease that occurs in about 0.4 to 1.3 percent of pregnant women. Except for status asthmaticus, asthma in pregnant women represents a slightly more serious respiratory condition than in nonpregnant women. Pregnancy in women with

TABLE 2 Recommended Drugs in the Treatment of Respiratory Disease During Pregnancy

Disease	*Recommended Classes of Drugs*
Asthma	Theophylline; $beta_2$-agonists (ephedrine, epinephrine, isoproterenol hydrochloride); steroids; cromolyn sodium
Chronic obstructive disease	Same as recommended for asthma
Viral upper respiratory tract	Acetaminophen; non-narcotic cough syrups; antihistamines
Influenza	Amantadine
Viral pneumonia	Acetaminophen; non-narcotic cough syrups; antihistamines
Mycoplasmal pneumonia	Erythromycin
Bacterial pneumonia	Penicillins; erythromycin; cephalosporins
Tuberculosis	INH; ethambutol; rifampin

asthma generally has a favorable outcome, but some increased risk of fetal and perinatal mortality and of spontaneous abortions exists. Status asthmaticus must be avoided because the hypoxemia and alkalosis that accompany it adversely affect the fetus. Fetal oxygenation may be depressed more by the alkalosis than by the hypoxemia; prompt and effective reversal of airway obstruction represents the most urgent goal of therapy during acute bronchospasm. The pregnant woman with asthma needs careful regulation of therapeutic modalities and thoughtful selection of antiasthmatic drugs.

Among the group of women who have asthma, about one-third experience no change in their disease, one-third become worse, and one-third improve during pregnancy. Pregnant women who have previously experienced severe asthmatic episodes seem more likely to worsen. Among asthmatic women, pregnancy may mildly increase their risk of morbidity and mortality, but the risk is lessened by satisfactory control of their disease.

Asthma in the pregnant woman can be effectively treated with several classes of drugs. Theophylline and $beta_2$-agonists are the drugs of first choice, and several studies suggest that these are safe for use during pregnancy. Cromolyn sodium and steroids can be used if necessary, but they are not routinely recommended. Few treatment studies have been reported of cromolyn sodium and of high-dose steroids; apparently, these drugs appear to be safe for use in pregnancy.

The most commonly used drugs, theophylline and the $beta_2$-agents, do not cause serious side effects in the fetus. For good control, maintain the theophylline blood levels between 10 to 20 μg per milliliter. Among the $beta_2$-adrenergic agonists, ephedrine, isoproterenol hydrochloride, and epinephrine are preferred for use in pregnant women; these can be used in inhaled form or orally. For the newer drugs of this class, such as terbutaline and metaproterenol, the question of safety remains unanswered. Although cromolyn sodium apparently does not have teratogenic effects, its use should be limited to those persons in whom good control and relief of bronchospasm cannot be achieved with theophylline and the $beta_2$-drugs. Steroids should be used as necessary when other classes of drugs do not provide satisfactory control; for example, a dose of 6 to 10 mg of prednisone daily may be adequate. Steroids in modest doses do not appear to be harmful to the human fetus; nonetheless, in animals experimental doses of steroids have been shown to cause congenital defects and an increased rate of stillbirths. Inhalation steroids, such as beclomethasone dipropionate, appear safe for use in pregnancy and their use three or four times daily can serve to decrease the dose of oral steroids required. When used with caution, immunotherapy has been found to be safe in pregnancy and offers one other approach to the treatment of asthma in pregnant women.

Status asthmaticus requires immediate and aggressive therapy. Therapeutic levels of theophylline can be achieved rapidly by intravenous infusion of aminophylline at 5 to 6 mg per kilogram over 30 minutes' time; therapy should then be continued with a maintenance infusion of 0.5 mg per kilogram per hour. Theophylline levels at the middle to high end of therapeutic levels need to be maintained by regular monitoring.

Nondrug therapeutic measures also help the course of asthma in pregnant women. These include deep breathing and coughing exercises to prevent mucus plugging and atelectasis. Bacterial infections should be treated promptly (see below). Iodine and iodine-containing preparations should be avoided.

CHRONIC OBSTRUCTIVE LUNG DISEASE AND SMOKING

Few pregnant women suffer from chronic obstructive pulmonary disease because it is mainly a disease of longstanding insult to the pulmonary system. Those who do need careful monitoring during pregnancy. The increase in minute ventilation does not appear to be a pulmonary burden to women with underlying chronic respiratory disease. Acute viral and bacterial infections cause significant impairment of respiratory function, and they need to be treated promptly and appropriately. Women with chronic pulmonary disease must avoid smoking, as it compromises their pulmonary reserve and it has been associated with an increase in pregnancy complications.

Smoking has been implicated on a consistent basis with high incidence of low birth weight infants. Infants born to mothers who smoke are on the average about 200 g lighter than infants born to women who do not smoke. Smoking during pregnancy has been associated with a greater risk of intrauterine growth retardation, and a weak association between smoking and spontaneous abortions has been identified. Congenital malformations apparently do not occur any more often in pregnant women who smoke than among those who do not smoke, although there is lack of consensus in this regard.

VIRAL INFECTIONS OF THE UPPER RESPIRATORY TRACT: MINOR ACUTE UPPER RESPIRATORY TRACT ILLNESS, INFLUENZA, PHARYNGITIS, AND LARYNGITIS

Viral infections of the respiratory tract represent the most commonly occurring acute respiratory disease in pregnant women. These infections occur throughout the year, although most of them develop during the winter months in temperate climates. As a group, influenza, parainfluenza, and respiratory syncytial viruses, adenoviruses, coronaviruses, and rhinoviruses cause most of the respiratory illnesses experienced by young adult women. Influenza virus infections most commonly cause serious acute respiratory tract disease in pregnant women, usually febrile undifferentiated upper respiratory tract illness, pharyngitis and laryngitis, and primary influenza pneumonia. The other common virus infections produce only mild respiratory tract disease; these infections cause pneumonia infrequently in pregnant women. They begin abruptly, last only a few days, and usually pose no threat to the life of the mother, except for influenza A virus infection in the high-risk woman or the fetus. No evidence exists that placental transmission occurs or that the fetus is at risk from any of the common virus infections of the respiratory tract.

Respiratory syncytial virus and the parainfluenza viruses, rhinoviruses, adenoviruses, and coronaviruses cause minor upper respiratory tract illness almost exclusively, usually without fever and only modest or no systemic symptoms. Pharyngitis, sometimes associated with exudate, can accompany adenovirus infection. In respiratory syncytial virus infection, ribavirin (1-beta-D-ribofuranosyl-1,2,4-triazole-3-carboxamide) hastens recovery and shortens the duration of virus shedding when administered by aerosol to infants and children with serious illness; however, ribavirin is contraindicated for treatment of the mild respiratory illness associated with respiratory syncytial virus infection of pregnant women, as the drug crosses the placental barrier and is toxic to the fetus. No specific antiviral drug therapy is available for the other common virus infections of the respiratory tract.

In pregnant women, the therapeutic approach to viral respiratory disease involves treatment of the symptoms and signs of disease. Drugs to lessen fever, cough, and rhinorrhea should be used in virus infections of the respiratory tract; however, prescribe only the minimum number of medications for minor illness. Use acetaminophen, a non-narcotic cough syrup containing as its active ingredient either dextromethorphan or guaifenesin or both, and a nasal decongestant, such as oxymetazoline. Infrequently, drowsiness or slight nausea and dizziness may ensue from the use of non-narcotic cough syrups. Narcotic-containing cough syrups should not be used during pregnancy, especially in the first trimester. Adequate fluids and frequent use of a room humidifier add to the comfort of the pregnant woman who is ill with a viral upper respiratory infection.

Influenza virus infection characteristically presents with high fever, nonproductive cough, diffuse muscle aches, and malaise, unlike the other respiratory viruses. Pharyngitis, laryngitis, and bronchitis can be features of influenza virus infection. In women with underlying chronic disease such as heart disease and pulmonary disease, influenza virus infection can cause life-threatening pneumonia. During the winter months, influenza virus infections reach epidemic levels; pregnant women should avoid contact with persons suffering from influenza.

Recognition of women in the group at high risk for serious influenza virus infection, especially influenza A virus, should be accomplished before they become pregnant and appropriate prophylactic measures taken at that time; however, often this is not the case, and it may become necessary to treat the influenza A virus infections with amantadine. Women who are judged to be at high risk for serious influenza virus infection should be immunized with the available inactivated trivalent influenza virus vaccine, preferably before they become pregnant. The recommended dose is 0.5 ml of the split products vaccine (ether-Tween treated to lessen local reactivity), administered once intramuscularly. The vaccine is contraindicated in women who are allergic to eggs or egg products.

Influenza A virus infection can be treated by the oral administration of amantadine (1-adamantanamine hydrochloride), 200 mg daily. Amantadine is absorbed promptly, and it is excreted unchanged by the kidneys. It is not effective in influenza B virus infection, and it should not be used in these cases. Amantadine should be used for prophylaxis and therapy only in the high-risk pregnant woman. Although controlled studies of the use of amantadine in pregnant women are lacking, the drug should be used cautiously and only when the necessity for its use overrides any potential risk to the fetus. For the treatment of influenza A virus infection, administer amantadine 200 mg daily in a single dose; it reduces the severity of symptoms and may shorten the duration of illness. For prophylaxis of influenza A virus infections, amantadine should be begun in high-risk women before the virus begins to spread in the community and before the woman becomes infected, and it should be continued until after the epidemic subsides. Adverse reactions include mild nausea, drowsiness, and insomnia.

Avoid antibiotic treatment of respiratory disease associated with any of the respiratory viruses, unless secondary bacterial infection occurs. Usually, secondary bacterial infection complicates only influenza virus infection. Then the diagnosis of the bacterial pathogen must be confirmed and appropriate treatment initiated promptly and continued for the required time period.

The respiratory disease associated with *Chlamydia* and human immunodeficiency virus (HIV or AIDS virus) infections are discussed in the chapters on *Chlamydia Trachomatis Infections* and *Acquired Immunodeficiency Syndrome*.

VIRAL AND MYCOPLASMAL PNEUMONIA

Viral and mycoplasmal pneumonia occur infrequently among pregnant women and no more often than among normal adults younger than 40 years of age. Influenza virus is the predominant virus pathogen of pneumonia; the other viruses that infect the respiratory tract rarely cause pneumonia in pregnant women. *Mycoplasma pneumoniae* is the only human mycoplasmal species that is pathogenic for the respiratory tract.

Influenza virus causes pneumonia mainly in high-risk persons, including pregnant women, who have underlying heart disease and lung disease. Amantadine is used for the treatment of influenza A virus pneumonia; the regimen is the same as described for the treatment of influenza A virus infection of the upper respiratory tract. Use 200 mg daily in a single dose; all measures to improve symptoms and signs of the illness should be taken, including administering acetaminophen (to reduce fever) and non-narcotic cough medications.

Mycoplasma pneumoniae infection of the respiratory tract can be associated with afebrile or febrile upper respiratory tract disease, bronchitis, and "atypical" pneumonia. These infections most often develop in young adults, including pregnant women, in their second or third decades of life. Pneumonia develops in 3 to 10 percent of persons infected with *M. pneumoniae*. Deaths from *M. pneumoniae* infection are very rare. No data exist confirming that other *Mycoplasma* species possess pathogenic potential for the respiratory tract of the pregnant woman.

M. pneumoniae pneumonia occurs mainly in young adults, including women of child-bearing age. Its occurrence in pregnancy is infrequent. The insidious onset of symptoms and signs of pneumonia, characterized by nonproductive cough, slight fever, and minimal auscultatory findings on examination of the lungs, suggests the diagnosis of mycoplasmal pneumonia. *M. pneumoniae* pneumonia can be effectively treated with erythromycin. Erythromycin crosses the placental barrier and appears in breast milk. It is not known to be toxic to the fetus. The dosage of erythromycin—base, stearate, and estolate—is 500 mg orally every 6 hours, on an empty stomach; the estolate form absorbs best. The dosage of erythromycin ethyl succinate is 400 to 600 mg orally every 6 hours. Parenteral administration of erythromycin is rarely necessary for the treatment of *M. pneumoniae* pneumonia in pregnant women. The adverse reactions associated with the oral administration of erythromycin include abdominal cramping and, infrequently, nausea, vomiting, and diarrhea. Although *M. pneumoniae* pneumonia can be successfully treated with tetracycline or one of the tetracycline analogs, the use of this group of antibiotics in pregnancy is contraindicated because these drugs cross the placenta and bind to calcium in bones, causing deformity, discoloration, or enamel dysplasia.

BACTERIAL PNEUMONIA

When bacterial pneumonia occurs in pregnant women, the pathogens are most often *Streptococcus pneumoniae* (pneumococcus) and *Haemophilus influenzae*. These infections occur predominantly in the winter months because *S. pneumoniae* is the main and *H. influenzae* is a common secondary bacterial complication of influenza virus infection. The risk of death from nonbacteremic pneumococcal pneumonia in normal gravid women is nil, as it is in nonpregnant women. Bacteremic pneumonia in normal gravid women younger than 40 years of age carries a very low case fatality rate, estimated at less than 5 percent, not unlike the rate expected in the nonpregnant young adult woman.

Bacterial pneumonia occurs uncommonly during pregnancy, especially in healthy women. It may complicate influenza A virus infection in women with underlying chronic heart or lung disease or develop in women at high risk for bacterial infection because of immune disorders. Women with sickle cell anemia or nonfunctioning spleens because of underlying disease or women who have had a splenectomy are at especially high risk for developing life-threatening pneumococcal infections.

The leading bacterial pathogens involved include the pneumococcus and *H. influenzae*. Penicillin is the drug of choice in pneumococcal pneumonia; a first-generation cephalosporin, such as cefazolin, is effective also. Neither of these antibiotics adversely affects the fetus. More aggressive antibiotic therapy is necessary when bacteremia occurs in pneumonia. In the penicillin-allergic (and cephalosporin-allergic) pregnant woman, use erythromycin. Do not use tetracycline, not only because of its destructive effects on the teeth of the fetus but also because 5 to 15 percent of pneumococci are resistant to it.

The recommended treatment regimens are aqueous penicillin G, 600,000 U every 12 hours, increasing to 1.2 million U every 6 to 12 hours intravenously, depending on the severity of the illness; or, cefazolin, 500 mg to 1 g every 6 hours intravenously; or in penicillin-allergic women, erythromycin, 1 g every 6 hours. Treatment should be continued for 10 days or 3 days after fever subsides (with a minimum treatment duration of 5 days).

The adverse reactions associated with penicillin therapy include rash and drug fever. Cefazolin administration is associated occasionally with fever, rash, leukopenia, positive Coombs' test results, and increased transaminase activity, which subside after stopping the antibiotic.

In *H. influenzae* pneumonia, the recommended treatment regimen includes either a second- or third-generation cephalosporin, for example, cefotaxime, ceftazidime, or cefuroxime. Chloramphenicol, although it is effective in the treatment of *H. influenzae* infections, should not be administered to pregnant women because transplacental passage is almost complete and it is toxic to the fetus.

The dosage of cefotaxime is 1 g every 8 hours and for ceftazidime the dosage is 1 to 2 g every 8 hours, intramuscularly or intravenously. Adverse effects of these antibiotics include pain at the site of intramuscular injection, phlebitis, and rash. These antibiotics do not affect the fetus.

PULMONARY TUBERCULOSIS

Pulmonary tuberculosis occurs uncommonly in pregnant women; its prevalence is estimated at less than 1 percent, although the rate is higher in certain high-risk groups, such as women who reside in the inner city or in rural areas. Pregnant women are not at higher risk for acquiring pulmonary tuberculosis than comparable groups of nonpregnant women. Positive tuberculin skin test reactivity in pregnant women varies from 1 to 10 percent, depending on the group of women tested. Tuberculosis in the pregnant woman rarely represents a threat to the fetus, and its transmission to the fetus occurs in very few cases; therapeutic abortion is not indicated. When treated appropriately, tuberculosis in pregnant women appears to respond as well as it does in nonpregnant women.

The recommended treatment of active pulmonary tuberculosis in the pregnant woman consists of administration of isoniazid (INH), 300 mg daily in a single dose, and ethambutol, 15 mg per kilogram daily for at least 18 months. Respiratory isolation precautions should be followed with all patient contacts. Within a few weeks after the start of therapy, the mycobacteria will be cleared from the sputum and the respiratory isolation procedures can be stopped. INH crosses the placenta, but neither INH nor ethambutol apparently causes fetal abnormalities. Hepatitis is the major adverse effect of INH therapy; when it occurs, the drug must be stopped. Pregnant women treated with INH should be given oral pyridoxine supplements, 10 mg daily.

Rifampin, an alternative choice in the treatment of tuberculosis in the pregnant woman, traverses the placenta and, since it inhibits DNA-dependent RNA polymerase, it potentially can affect the fetus. Thus far, however, rifampin has not been linked to fetal abnormalities. Rifampin in combination with INH should be given for 9 months. The dose of rifampin is 10 mg per kilogram daily, not to exceed 600 mg daily.

When INH resistance is suspected, three drugs should be used in the treatment of tuberculosis: INH, ethambutol, and rifampin. Resistance to INH is likely to occur when tuberculosis develops in those previously treated with the drug, or in those exposed to a patient infected with drug-resistant organisms, or when the disease was acquired in endemic areas, usually outside of the United States.

Pregnant women in their teens and twenties with a positive tuberculin skin test should be given INH alone as prophylaxis. The dose is 300 mg daily for 12 months.

SUGGESTED READING

Greenberger PA, Patterson R. Management of asthma during pregnancy. N Engl J Med 1985; 312:897–902.

Mufson MA. Diagnosis and treatment of pneumonia. In: Marr JJ, ed. Infectious diseases in general medical practice. Menlo Park, CA: Addison Wesley, 1982:229.

Snider D. Pregnancy and tuberculosis. Chest 1984; 86 (Suppl 3):10S–13S.

LIVER DISEASE

RICK W. MARTIN, M.D.
JOHN C. MORRISON, M.D.

Liver disease in pregnancy represents a broad spectrum of disorders, which vary from mild biochemical changes to hepatic failure and maternal death. New developments in the diagnostic and prophylactic measures for infectious hepatitis have increased the practitioner's overall interest in liver disease. This chapter deals with the various disorders that occur during coexistent pregnancy and those which present only during pregnancy.

Physiology

An understanding of the normal physiology is important to the management of liver problems. In pregnancy, liver morphology is essentially unchanged, and hepatic blood flow remains unaltered. However, the usual laboratory tests of liver function can vary during pregnancy. Although the serum transaminases and bilirubin are unchanged, alkaline phosphatase is elevated from the contribution of placental alkaline phosphatase. Total serum protein and serum albumin are decreased because of dilution by an expanding plasma volume. Fibrinogen and clotting factors VII, IX, and X are elevated, but prothrombin time (PT) and partial thromboplastin time (PTT) are unchanged. The normal liver is not palpable nor is there tenderness during pregnancy. Palmar erythema and spider angiomata, which are frequently found in liver disease in the nonpregnant woman, are normally present during gestation in 60 percent of patients.

INFECTIOUS HEPATITIS

At least five types of viral hepatitis have been identified: hepatitis A, B, D, and two types of non-A/non-B. The clinical presentation of all forms is similar. After an incubation period, the patient becomes symptomatic. Jaundice is rarely an initial symptom. A prodromal period of malaise, anorexia, nausea, and vomiting follows. Headache, myalgia, and fever may also be present, and the condition may initially be diagnosed as a flu-like illness. Urticaria, arthralgias, and arthritis can mimic an immune-complex disease. A history of abdominal discomfort may be given. In the next phase, jaundice appears, and the patient's symptoms usually improve. Dark-colored urine and light stools may accompany the jaundice. In rare cases, fulminant hepatitis and coma occur.

Bilirubin rises slowly, comes sharply to a peak, then declines. Jaundice appears when the total bilirubin reaches 2 to 3 mg per 100 milliliters. Serum transaminase levels rise before the bilirubin does and remain elevated for 1 to 3 months. The usual range for alanine aminotransferase (ALT), formerly SGPT, and aspartate aminotransferase (AST), formerly SGOT, is 500 to 1,000 IU per liter with the ALT being greater than the AST. Mild disease is associated with lower transaminase levels, albeit even patients with mild disturbances should be investigated for hepatitis.

Pregnant women with viral hepatitis are encouraged to rest and to avoid unnecessary drugs that may cause hepatotoxicity. A nutritionally adequate diet without protein restriction or excessive carbohydrates is preferred. Corticosteroids are no longer given for chronic viral hepatitis as the drug may actually cause more severe disease. In one series of patients with chronic hepatitis B, aminotransferase levels were improved during therapy, but after treatment, rebounded to levels higher than before, and the disease was prolonged as compared to controls. However, corticosteroids and other immunosuppressants, such as azathioprine, may be used for autoimmune hepatitis. Various antiviral agents may be of benefit for the non-pregnant patient with chronic active hepatitis, but it is unlikely that these drugs are investigated during pregnancy.

Hepatitis A (HAV) is a ribonucleic acid (RNA) virus that is usually transmitted by the fecal-oral route. It accounts for about 25 percent of hospitalized cases of hepatitis. The incubation period is 15 to 50 days. Most patients have subclinical disease, but icteric hepatitis A can appear abruptly; the symptoms resolve within 2 to 3 weeks. Maternal infection with HAV has been associated with a higher incidence of preterm delivery. Immunoglobulin M (IgM) anti-HAV antibody is present from the onset of disease, persists for several months, and then declines, albeit, in a few cases, a persistent anti-IgM antibody has been seen for as long as 1 year. Its presence in serum confirms the diagnosis. Immunoglobulin G (IgG) anti-HAV antibody is only indicative of previous infection. There is no chronic form of HAV. The period of maximum viral excretion is the 2 weeks before the onset of symptoms and the early prodromal period. No special isolation procedures are recommended for hospitalized patients with HAV, but each hospital may have different infection control guidelines. Postexposure prophylaxis is recommended for household contacts and sexual contacts, but not for school contacts or hospital employees. Immune globulin 0.2 mg per kilogram IM should be given within 2 weeks of exposure in order to prevent infection and can be given to pregnant women. No cases of acquired immunodeficiency syndrome have been transmitted from immune globulin to date. Perinatal transmission is uncertain, but congenital abnormalities are not found with HAV in early pregnancy, and pregnancy termination is not recommended. Although HAV causes only acute hepatitis and no chronic form exists, prophylaxis with immune globulin is appropriate for the neonate when active maternal disease is present.

Hepatitis B virus (HBV) is a DNA virus that is basically bloodborne or sexually transmitted. Approximately 50 percent of cases of viral hepatitis are caused by HBV. The incubation period is from 45 to 160 days, but longer intervals have been reported in patients treated with hepatitis B immune globulin. Clinically, the onset of HBV is more insidious than HAV. Certain high-risk groups should be screened for carrier status. These include Asian, Pacific island, Eskimo, Haitian, and sub-Saharan African women, prostitutes, IV drug abusers, and household contacts of hemodialysis patients or hepatitis B carriers. Workers in hemodialysis units and institutions for the mentally retarded should also be screened.

The presence of hepatitis B surface antigen (HBsAg) indicates infectivity and is usually the first specific marker present for the disease. Antibody to hepatitis B surface antigen (anti-HBs) indicates previous infection and immunity to HBV. The presence of antibody to hepatitis B core antigen (anti-HBc) indicates infection sometime in the past. This test may be helpful during the so-called "window" period when HBsAg has become negative and anti-HBs is not yet present. If HBsAg is positive, a test for hepatitis B e-antigen (HBeAg) is useful because, if positive, there is a greater likelihood of infectivity. Those patients who are HBsAg positive and who have antibody to HBeAg are less likely to be infected. Five to 10 percent of cases of HBV remain HBsAg positive for longer than 6 months and become chronic carriers. Those with chronic persistent hepatitis have mild elevations of liver enzymes, and chances for recovery are good although remission may take years. Diagnosis is made by characteristic changes on biopsy. Those with chronic active hepatitis (30 percent) on biopsy have a poor prognosis because of eventual progression to cirrhosis. A strong association exists between chronic active hepatitis and primary hepatocellular carcinoma. Strict isolation of HBsAg carriers with masking, gloving, or gowning is unnecessary, but blood, lochia, and surgical dressings should be handled with gloves, and personnel should take care to avoid accidental needle puncture.

Two products provide prophylaxis for HBV. Hepa titis B immune globulin (HBIG) is prepared from plasma with a high titer of anti-HBs and provides passive immunity. Hepatitis B vaccine is a suspension of inactivated, alum-absorbed 22-nanometer surface antigen particles that have been purified from human plasma. A three-step treatment process has been shown to inactivate all classes of viruses found in human blood. Postexposure prophylaxis is recommended for percutaneous or permucosal exposure to HBsAg-positive blood and for the sexual contacts of HBsAg-positive persons. A regimen of two doses of HBIG (0.06 ml per kilogram IM within 24 hours - repeat in 1 month) after percutaneous exposure and one dose (0.06 ml per kilogram IM within 14 days) after sexual exposure is about 75 percent effective in preventing hepatitis B. For high-risk medical personnel, a single dose of

HBIG, combined with hepatitis vaccine, provides protection and is more cost-effective. These employees are likely to be working in high-risk areas, and a risk for further exposure remains present. Preexposure prophylaxis for HBV is provided with hepatitis B vaccine. A 20 μg injection is given IM with a repeat dose at 1 and 6 months. In adults, it is important that the vaccine be given in the deltoid muscle as greater success is achieved there than at other sites. High-risk groups that should be vaccinated include medical workers, patients and staff of mental institutions, abusers of injectable drugs, household contacts and sexual partners of HBV carriers, recipients of certain blood products such as those with clotting abnormalities, and travelers to areas where hepatitis B is endemic.

Perinatal transmission occurs during the birth process in 70 to 90 percent of infants if the mother is both HBsAg- and HBeAg-positive. If the mother is HBsAg-positive and HBeAg-negative, transmission occurs less frequently. A hepatitis B carrier state can occur in the infant or, worse, fulminant hepatitis may result. Therefore, prophylaxis for newborns is indicated when the mother is HBsAg-positive. HBIG, 0.5 ml IM, should be given within 12 hours of birth. Hepatitis B vaccine, 10 μg IM, should be given concurrently at an alternate injection site. Two subsequent doses of vaccine are administered at 1 and 6 months of age. Blood sampling at 12 and 15 months for HBsAg and anti-HBs confirms treatment success. In the newborn nursery, isolation procedures are not required after the infant is washed. The infant need not be isolated from the mother. Breast-feeding is permissible unless the mother's nipples are cracked. Hepatitis B infection in early pregnancy does not cause anomalies, and pregnancy termination is not indicated. As with hepatitis A, premature delivery is associated with hepatitis B.

Little is known about non-A/non-B hepatitis. The diagnosis is one of exclusion as markers for infection are not available. It appears to be transmitted parenterally, and the virus accounts for 85 percent of transfusion-related hepatitis. There is a risk for hepatitis of approximately 1 percent per unit of blood transfused, and a 1 in 5,000 chance per unit infused of death from fulminant hepatitis. A chronic carrier state can develop and chronic hepatitis can occur after non-A/non-B hepatitis. Perinatal transmission is presumed because infants born to mothers with active disease may have persistent elevations of hepatic enzymes. Immune globulin is given to provide passive immunity, although in adults the efficacy of prophylaxis with this agent is not determined.

Delta hepatitis has been discovered more recently. The virus depends on the hepatitis B virus for replication. Its presence can be excluded if hepatitis B can be excluded. A chronic infection can exist as can chronic active hepatitis. Either can progress to fulminant hepatitis. Tests for detection are only available for research purposes at this time. Carriers of HBsAg are at risk for this disease. Perinatal transmission has been documented.

Other viral infections can be responsible for hepatic dysfunction and should be considered in the differential diagnosis of hepatitis. Rubella, herpes, cytomegalovirus, adenovirus, enterovirus, and Epstein-Barr virus may cause elevation of liver enzymes or even fulminant hepatitis. Serologic testing and cultures may help make the diagnosis, along with a high index of suspicion. Many of these agents have greater consequences for the fetus than for the mother. Use of antiviral agents such as acyclovir has been reported for systemic herpesvirus infection, and the drug has been shown to cross the placenta. However, the experience with this drug in pregnancy is extremely limited, and long-term fetal effects are unknown.

Various infections and infestations other than viral agents cause liver disease. *Entamoeba histolytica* causes diarrheal illness, but liver cysts can occur. Treatment of choice is surgical drainage and drug therapy with metronidazole. Portal hypertension has been reported from schistosomiasis. A history of travel to parts of Africa or South America where the disease is endemic should alert the clinician to schistosomiasis. Acute bacterial infections, such as with pyelonephritis, can cause transient elevations of liver transaminases. Disseminated infections with *Mycobacterium tuberculosis* can affect the liver, and granulomatous changes can be seen on liver biopsy. Evidence of pulmonary tuberculosis is present in only 50 percent and skin tests are negative in 20 percent of those tested. Treatment with triple drug therapy, isoniazid, ethambutol, and rifampin, may be necessary for as long as 18 to 24 months. Although rare, fungal infections with *Trichosporon* and *Candida* have also been reported.

INTRAHEPATIC CHOLESTASIS OF PREGNANCY

Intrahepatic cholestasis of pregnancy (IHCP) is the second-leading cause of jaundice in pregnancy, being responsible for 20 percent of cases. High levels of estrogens in pregnancy are implicated as the syndrome can be reproduced in susceptible patients who are taking oral contraceptives. A genetic contribution is suspected because IHCP is more common in some populations in Chile. Severe pruritis, particularly of the palms of the hands and soles of the feet, followed by mild jaundice is the usual presenting symptom. High bile acid levels in serum and skin are responsible for the pruritis. This is usually a disease of the third trimester. Commonly a benign disease, IHCP can be associated with preterm delivery, meconium-stained amniotic fluid, and maternal coagulation problems in some cases. There are reports of a higher incidence of intrauterine fetal demise; therefore, fetal surveillance from 32 weeks should be instituted.

Laboratory findings show elevated serum transaminase levels, particularly alanine aminotransferase. Bilirubin is usually less than 5 mg per deciliter. An increased 5'-nucleotidase distinguishes the elevated alkaline phosphatase caused by hepatic cholestasis. Increased serum cholic acid levels are particularly useful in diagnosing IHCP. Liver biopsy reveals canalicular bile plugs, which are most prominent around the central veins. Liver architecture is intact, and there is little hepatic necrosis. Gallstones are found more often in these patients, and sonography is a useful diagnostic tool. Treatment with cholestyramine is successful in 50 percent of cases. A regimen of 12 to 28 g per day is given in divided doses, before breakfast and lunch. Presumably cholestyramine breaks the intrahepatic circulation of bile salts. This drug causes nausea, and vitamin K absorption is decreased. Supplemental vitamin K, 10 mg per day orally, should be prescribed. If the cholestyramine is ineffective, phenobarbital, 30 mg four times daily, is advocated by some. Symptoms may improve because phenobarbital provides sedation and induces liver microenzymes. Some authors recommend delivery after 37 weeks as the maternal condition greatly improves, often immediately, after delivery. Before elective delivery, fetal maturity should be documented with amniotic fluid studies if gestational age is uncertain. A coagulation profile, including prothrombin time, should be performed prior to delivery. Barrier methods or surgical sterilization rather than oral contraceptives for women with IHCP are recommended.

CHOLELITHIASIS AND CHOLECYSTITIS

Gallbladder disease is the second most common surgical condition of the gravid female in the United States. Inflammation of the gallbladder, cholecystitis, is associated with calculi in 85 to 95 percent of the cases. However, gallstones are a very common finding in pregnancy that occurs in 3.3 percent of asymptomatic pregnant women who undergo sonography of the gallbladder. Hormonal changes in pregnancy are responsible for decreased contractility of the gallbladder, an elevated biliary cholesterol, and an increased residual capacity that favors stone formation. A high-risk group for cholelithiasis is pregnant women of Caucasian race, between ages 35 and 45, with multiparity and obesity. A fetal loss rate of 5 percent is associated with cholecystectomy in the second or third trimester, with the worst prognosis for the fetus when cholecystitis is accompanied by pancreatitis. Perforation of the gallbladder is associated with a substantial increase in morbidity and mortality. Early signs can be nausea following meals and tenderness in the right upper quadrant or epigastrium. A positive Murphy's sign is ellicited by having the patient inspire while the examiner palpates the gallbladder. Pain causes an inspiratory arrest. This sign is almost always present in those with acute cholecystitis, but peritoneal signs are usually absent. Biliary colic signifies obstruction of the common or cystic bile duct.

Laboratory tests show moderate elevations of bilirubin and the serum transaminases. The white blood count is most often normal, but often reveals an increase in band forms if inflammation is present. In the case of common duct stones that result in pancreatitis, the serum amylase rises. Ultrasonography may be the most useful test to confirm the diagnosis and is approximately 95 percent accurate. The study should be performed after a 12-hour fast. Stones can easily be seen in the fluid-filled structure, and marked inflammation is demonstrated by thickening and dilatation of the gallbladder. Rarely is cholecystectomy indicated during pregnancy as conservative management is the first line of therapy. Hospitalization, enteric rest, nasogastric suction, hydration, analgesia, and antibiotics are successful in the majority of cases, with approximately 50 percent of cases resolving at 24 to 48 hours. Morphine increases cholestasis and is not indicated as an analgesic. Broad-spectrum antibiotic therapy (e.g., third-generation cephalosporin) usually obtains adequate levels in the bile and provides coverage for anaerobic bacteria. For recurrent cholecystitis, early cholecystectomy in the second trimester avoids use of anesthetic agents in early pregnancy and decreases the chances of preterm labor that may accompany surgery in the third trimester. Most physicians reserve surgery for those patients (1) who fail medical management, (2) with suspected perforation of the gallbladder, (3) with significant obstruction, (4) with jaundice from a common duct stone, and (5) with pancreatitis.

ACUTE FATTY LIVER OF PREGNANCY

Acute fatty liver of pregnancy (AFLP) is a life-threatening disorder that occurs in approximately 1 in 13,000 pregnancies. Early reports of this disease have noted high maternal (75 to 85 percent) and fetal (85 percent) mortality. Recent studies suggest that earlier diagnosis and prompt treatment can reduce maternal mortality to 33 percent and fetal mortality to 67 percent. The clinical presentation is that of acute hepatic failure after 35-weeks gestation, although this disease can occur as early as 30 weeks. Initially, symptoms include nausea, vomiting, malaise, and fatigue, i.e., signs similar to hepatitis. The presence of abdominal pain should increase the suspicion for AFLP, however, the liver is not palpable. Signs of mild pregnancy-induced hypertension (PIH; minimal hypertension, edema, and proteinuria) may also accompany AFLP. Within a week, the patient's condition deteriorates with jaundice and hypoglycemia, and coagulopathy develops. Mental confusion is usually present late in the process, and hepatic coma occurs in severe cases. Renal failure develops from either lipid infiltration of the kidney or hypoperfusion, with resultant acute tubular necrosis. Portal hypertension can be present, but ascites is not a feature of AFLP. Esophageal varices are usually the cause of gastrointestinal bleeding.

Laboratory studies show an elevation of transaminases, but of less than 500 units. The white blood cell count is increased up to 15,000 per cubic millimeter, whereas the bilirubin is increased, and ammonia levels rise as the disease progresses. The amylase is found to be increased in some cases, but albumin is low. Profound hypoglycemia is commonly present. As disseminated intravascular coagulopathy develops, PT and PTT are prolonged, and fibrin split products are detected; albeit the platelet count is low. Early in the disease process creatinine, uric acid, and blood urea nitrogen may be modestly increased in the absence of renal failure. The most important laboratory finding is from the examination of liver tissue obtained by biopsy. The classic centrizonal microvesicular fatty infiltration confirms the diagnosis. There is an absence of cellular necrosis. Reye's syndrome, alcoholic foamy degeneration, tetracycline toxicity, and valproic acid injury may be confused with AFLP, but the clinical history aids in the diagnosis. A portion of the biopsy should be saved for special stains for lipids, such as the oil red 0 stain. Electron microscopy displays abnormal mitochondria. When liver biopsy cannot be performed because of coagulopathy, ultrasonographic studies or abdominal computed tomography (CT) can be helpful. Ultrasonography shows an increased echogenicity of the liver as compared to the kidney in AFLP, and decreased attenuation ratios on CT scan are evidence of fatty infiltration.

Once the diagnosis is established, prompt delivery is indicated. It is important to distinguish this disease from viral hepatitis, as delivery does not improve the maternal-fetal outcome in viral hepatitis, whereas, in AFLP, one study showed 85 percent of the surviving patients were treated with early delivery. In addition, the fetus is usually mature, and therefore, no fetal benefits are gained with delay, whereas intrauterine fetal death and maternal deterioration are likely if delivery is not expeditious. Induction of labor with oxytocin infusion may be begun as long as delivery can be accomplished in a timely manner and the mother is not in fulminant hepatic failure. However, cesarean delivery may be needed as the condition of the mother or infant can rapidly deteriorate. Uteroplacental insufficiency is thought to be the cause of fetal compromise, and close surveillance with electronic fetal monitoring is essential. After delivery, the neonate has normal liver function, but hypoglycemia is often present and should be detected.

Maternal management of hepatic failure is mainly supportive. Hypovolemia is treated with balanced electrolyte solutions. Supplemental potassium is given for hypokalemia. Hypoglycemia should be treated with 20 percent glucose infusion if necessary. Protein intake is restricted, and a high carbohydrate diet is prescribed. Clotting abnormalities are corrected with fresh frozen plasma, platelets, and packed red cells. If bowel function is adequate, either oral lactulose, 15 to 60 ml every 6 hours, or neomycin, 1 g every 4 to 6 hours, can reduce ammonia levels in those with hepatic encephalopathy. Otherwise, neomycin can be given as a retention enema in a dose of 1 to 2 g in 100 to 200 ml of saline every 8 to 12 hours. Lactulose increases gastrointestinal motility and decreases pH, thereby causing less absorption of ammonia. Neomycin also increases motility and decreases urease-forming bacteria in the intestine, causing the decreased absorption of ammonia. Although little neomycin is absorbed from the gut, cases of renal impairment and ototoxicity have occurred. Cimetidine, 300 mg intravenously every 6 hours, can help to prevent gastrointestinal bleeding from stress ulcers. Esophageal varices may be detected with esophagoscopy, and balloon tamponade with the Sengstaken-Blakemore tube is appropriate should bleeding occur. Operative treatment with portacaval shunt carries a high mortality, thus conservative treatment as previously outlined is the therapy of choice.

HYPEREMESIS GRAVIDARUM AND PREGNANCY-INDUCED HYPERTENSION

Besides AFLP and cholestatic jaundice of pregnancy, two other conditions that affect the liver are peculiar to pregnancy. Transient elevations of transaminases may be noted in hyperemesis of pregnancy. This disorder is usually mild and resolves with time. The important diagnostic consideration with this condition is to differentiate it from early infectious hepatitis by means of an appropriate screen.

Elevated liver enzymes are also found in severe PIH. Right upper quadrant abdominal pain is present in 90 percent of these patients. More severe cases present as the so-called HELLP syndrome of microangiopathic hemolytic anemia, elevated liver enzymes, and low platelets. Microthrombi and fibrin deposition are characteristically noted on liver biopsy. Antithrombin III levels are low in this condition, and there are reports that antithrombin III administration ameliorates the disease. Other studies have revealed spontaneous improvement with bed rest and close observation in the hospital, thus allowing the immature fetus time to mature. Our personal bias is for prompt delivery (within 2 to 3 days) in these cases, either with oxytocin induction or by cesarean birth, if delivery cannot be accomplished readily. The usual treatment for PIH with magnesium sulfate, 4 g given by slow IV followed by a 2 g per hour maintenance infusion, is given with careful monitoring of the serum magnesium level. Marked elevation of diastolic blood pressure above 110 mm Hg should be treated with intermittent doses of hydralazine 5 mg IV. In exceptional cases, plasmapheresis, utilizing a 3-liter exchange, has allowed a 2 to 3 day delay of delivery in order to gain the benefit of corticosteroids, which accelerate fetal pulmonary maturation. Clotting abnormalities are corrected with infusions of platelets and fresh frozen plasma, and anemia is treated with packed red cells. With delivery and meticulous postpartum care, recovery can usually be expected. If clotting abnormalities and liver dysfunction persist beyond 72 hours post partum, consideration to plasmapheresis may again be given.

CIRRHOSIS

Although the fertility of patients with cirrhotic liver disease is decreased, cases of pregnancy with this disorder are reported. The primary risk to the mother is that of gastrointestinal hemorrhage. Additional problems include hepatic coma and postpartum hemorrhage. The fetus is also at risk as 25 percent of patients have intrauterine fetal demise. Esophageal varices result from the increased portal vein pressure in the latter stages of pregnancy, as the added pressure of the gravid uterus on the vena cava increases venous return through the azygos system. It is not surprising that pregnant patients with cirrhosis have problems with esophageal varices, as even healthy pregnant women can have transient esophageal bleeding. Schreyer recommends portosystemic shunting in such cases, as maternal mortality is definitely decreased when affected women have had this procedure performed. Others point out that in nonpregnant individuals survival is not improved and complications can follow shunt procedures; these include encephalopathy and deterioration of liver function.

The use of propranolol has been proposed in nonpregnant patients in order to lower portal pressure. A dose sufficient to lower the resting heart rate by 25 percent is recommended. This drug should be considered with great caution, as hepatic encephalopathy and problems with resuscitation of the bleeding patient can arise. Adverse fetal effects are reported with propranolol; these include fetal bradycardia and a possibility of intrauterine growth retardation. Valsalva maneuvers in the second stage of labor can increase the chance of variceal hemorrhage. Although elective cesarean section is not routinely performed, the use of forceps to shorten the second stage of labor is recommended. The postpartum period is a particularly dangerous time for the patient with cirrhotic liver disease, as postpartum hemorrhage, variceal bleeding, and hepatic coma can occur. As the long-term prognosis for these patients is poor, consideration should be given to permanent sterilization. In alcoholic cirrhosis, the single-most important aspect of therapy is to discontinue alcohol use. In addition, the fetal alcohol syndrome, which includes gross physical retardation, CNS dysfunction, microcephaly, and other minor ocular, facial, and skeletal abnormalities, can occur in up to 32 percent of heavy drinkers.

Primary biliary cirrhosis is a chronic, progressive cholestatic liver disease that presents in middle-aged women, although the range can be from 20 to 80 years. The presence of antimitochondrial antibody is confirmed in 95 percent of these patients. The median 5-year survival is reported to be 63 percent, and associated autoimmune disorders such as thyroiditis, sicca syndrome, calcinosis cutis, and Raynaud's phenomena can be found. Fetal mortality has been markedly increased in this disease, although a few patients have tolerated pregnancy without severe complications. The poor long-term prognosis with this condition should discourage patients from continuing pregnancy.

GENETIC DISEASE

Case reports of various genetic diseases that coexist with pregnancy have been noted. Wilson's disease (hepatolenticular degeneration) is an inherited disorder of copper metabolism. Clinical manifestations include cirrhosis of the liver, central nervous system dysfunction, and corneal copper deposition, which results in the classic Kayser-Fleischer rings. It is inherited as an autosomal recessive trait. Laboratory evaluation shows absent or low serum ceruloplasmin, increased serum nonceruloplasmin copper, a normal or low serum copper level, and increased urinary copper excretion. This disease should be suspected in any diagnosis of cirrhosis of undetermined cause. Before treatment with penicillamine, there were frequent spontaneous abortions in affected women. D-penicillamine is a chelating agent that binds copper and promotes urinary secretion of copper. The usual dose is 1 g per day, and improvement usually parallels depletion of the tissue copper build-up. Abdominal discomfort and nausea are frequently side effects of the medication; more serious side effects include leukopenia and thrombocytopenia. Pregnancy is felt to have an ameliorating effect on Wilson's disease, presumably from increased fetal consumption of copper and a small increase in maternal ceruloplasmin levels. Discontinuation of penicillamine in Wilson's disease on account of pregnancy has resulted in exacerbations of the illness, and therefore this medication should be continued throughout pregnancy. Other than an increase in spontaneous abortions, the fetus seems relatively unaffected by this disease. There are reports of D-penicillamine administration being associated with fetal collagen abnormalities that affect skin and connective tissue. Therefore, the lowest effective dose should be given. In addition, D-penicillamine is a pyridoxine antagonist, and 50 mg of oral maternal pyridoxine should be given each week.

The hepatic porphyrias, which consist of acute intermittent porphyria, varigate porphyria, hereditary coproporphyria, and porphyria cutanea tarda are characterized by an excessive production of porphyrin or porphyrin precursors. Initially, a high maternal mortality had been reported; however, the outlook for successful pregnancy is now considered to be better. It is helpful to remember the five P's in making the diagnosis: onset after puberty, psychiatric abnormalities, pain, polyneuropathy, and photosensitivity. Most patients do quite well normally; however, when aminolevulinic acid synthesis production is increased, the precursor production overwhelms a defective step in heme synthesis. Certain medications, including alcohol, barbiturates, diphenylhydantoin, ergot derivatives, methyldopa, and sulfonamides to name a few, can precipitate an attack of acute intermittent porphyria. A urine sample can be rapidly screened by the Watson-Schwartz test, and 24-hour urine samples can be collected and sent for analysis of aminolevulinic acid, porphobilinogen, and porphyrins.

Therapy consists of providing analgesia and management of electrolyte abnormalities. Administration of large glucose loads seems to suppress aminolevulinic acid synthesis and should be given at approximately 300 g per 24 hours. A second method of treatment involves the use of hematin (hydroxyheme) given intravenously in a dose of 4 mg per kilogram body weight at 12- to 24-hour intervals. Pain relief is provided with meperidine and phenothiazines. If the symptoms do not rapidly improve or if motor neuropathy is present, the patient should be monitored frequently for progressive ventilatory insufficiency. A higher incidence of preterm delivery has been noted in women who experience attacks of acute intermittent porphyria in pregnancy.

Idiopathic hyperbilirubinemia has a variable effect on pregnancy. Gilbert's disease is inherited as an autosomal dominant trait with a variable penetrance. Bilirubin is seldom over 5 mg per deciliter, and almost all of it is unconjugated. During pregnancy, there is a decrease in the unconjugated bilirubin, and mother and fetus remain clinically unaffected. Dubin-Johnson syndrome is characterized by conjugated hyperbilirubinemia and the presence of dark pigment granules in the centrilobar hepatocytes. One study has suggested an increase in fetal wastage with this disease. The maternal prognosis is usually good except that jaundice may increase in the third trimester. In a variant of the Dubin-Johnson syndrome, i.e., the Rotor syndrome, the increased jaundice is not seen. Another genetic disease, Gaucher's disease, is an inherited metabolic disorder of glycolipid metabolism. A chronic, low-grade anemia may be present, and although portal hypertension may complicate the disease, pregnancy is usually uneventful. Hematinics should be prescribed and the pregnancy monitored closely.

AUTOIMMUNE DISEASE

Liver enlargement and mild abnormalities of liver function are occasionally seen in systemic lupus erythematosus. These are usually of little clinical significance. Biopsy changes are nonspecific. Rarely, a chronic hepatitis can occur. Elevations of aminotransferase levels above 400 IU per deciliter are common, and the serum bilirubin may be greater than 3 mg per deciliter. A positive antinuclear antibody test (ANA) and antibodies to smooth muscle are also found. In symptomatic patients, treatment with corticosteroids is indicated. Prednisone, 15 to 20 mg per day, is the usual regimen. A lower dose of 5 to 10 mg per day may be utilized in combination with azathioprine, 50 to 100 mg per day in patients who are unable to tolerate the side effects of prednisone. Clinically asymptomatic patients do not need therapy with corticosteroids. Relapses are common when the immunosuppressant drugs are discontinued.

VASCULAR LIVER INJURY

Injury to the liver from either hemorrhage or thrombosis can produce life-threatening consequences. Rupture of Glisson's capsule, following subcapsular hematoma, is a surgical emergency. Most of these cases are associated with PIH and/or disseminated intravascular coagulopathy, albeit trauma has been implicated in occasional reports. Even minor trauma has caused spontaneous rupture in patients with predisposing conditions. One hypothesis concerning the pathogenesis of the hematoma is that infarction of the liver parenchyma occurs with hypervascularization followed by rupture of the vessel. With intrahepatic hemorrhage, there is destruction of tissue and production of a subcapsular hematoma. Perforation of the liver capsule results in a hemoperitoneum and peritonitis, and could lead to maternal death. The usual site of rupture is in the superior and anterior portion of the right lobe of the liver. The clinical presentation is that of a patient in her late 20's or 30's, multiparous, and in the third trimester of pregnancy. Hypertension is present, which suggests PIH, and there is a constant, progressive pain in the epigastrium or right upper quadrant. As a hemoperitoneum develops, there is evidence of peripheral vascular collapse and shock.

A high index of suspicion is necessary in order to make the diagnosis, and most often the diagnosis is made at the time of laparotomy. There may be mild increases in the aminotransferases, and the hematocrit may be low. A paracentesis may also indicate a hemoperitoneum. Examination of the liver with ultrasonography or with computed tomography helps to localize the area of hemorrhage and to aid in the diagnosis. Selected angiography can also be helpful. If a liver hematoma is identified, serial determinations of hematocrit, blood pressure, heart rate, and urinary output are indicated. In the case of hemoperitoneum, the patient should be rapidly prepared for surgery by expanding the plasma volume with crystalloid and plasma acutely, and then by blood replacement as necessary. As disseminated intravascular coagulation is commonly present in these patients, clotting abnormalities should be corrected with infusions of fresh frozen plasma and platelets. Placing the patient in a MAST (military antishock trousers) suit may be life saving until a laparotomy can be performed. The lowest possible inflation pressure should be used to maintain the patient's blood pressure. Normally a pressure of 40 mm Hg is not exceeded; however, in exceptional cases, pressures up to 100 mm Hg have been used. If the patient is pregnant, a cesarean section is indicated. This removes the fetus from the hostile environment and additionally allows better exposure of the upper abdomen. Most authors recommend unroofing of the laceration and evacuation of the hematoma, taking necessary measures to control bleeding; this usually involves simple suture or application of microvascular collagen as a hemostatic agent. With more extensive lesions, debridement of the devitalized liver tissue is necessary. If these measures are unsuccessful, hepatic artery ligation and, as a last resort, lobectomy have been performed. With the aid of arteriography, Gelfoam pledgets have been embolized by means of a transcatheter technique, and surgery has been avoided. This procedure might be of value in the patient who is relatively stable. In the case of an unruptured hepatic hematoma in the undelivered patient, it is best to proceed with cesarean section as even minor trauma can lead to liver rupture with dire consequences.

In the postpartum patient, larger hematomas should be managed surgically; however, small hematomas of a few centimeters (as diagnosed by ultrasonography) have been managed conservatively without surgery by using blood replacement, following serial hematocrits and by performing serial sonography.

Hepatic vein thrombosis can be equally as dangerous. Thrombosis of the hepatic veins (Budd-Chiari syndrome) may be manifested at term or in the immediate postpartum period. It is characterized by abdominal pain associated with hepatomegaly and ascites. There may be mild elevations of transaminases, but bilirubin is seldom elevated initially. Catheterization of the inferior vena cava may show increased venous pressure and allow contrast venography, which can reveal obstruction of the hepatic veins or inferior vena cava. CT scanning may also demonstrate this condition.

Fetal compromise is rare as most often symptoms occur in the postpartum period. Previous users of the contraceptive pill have been noted to be at high risk, presumably from the hypercoagulable state induced by these drugs. In some patients, the presence of inferior vena cava webbs is amenable to surgery by membranotomy. This condition has been predominantly described in Japanese women. Use of thrombolytic agents has not been of help in this syndrome, and surgical therapy is considered the treatment of choice. Some sort of side-to-side portosystemic decompressive therapy offers the best chance for long-term survival. This procedure is not without hazard as encephalopathy, decreased hepatic blood flow, and hepatic failure can follow. Even with treatment, maternal mortality remains high.

TUMORS OF THE LIVER

Metastatic tumors are the most common tumors of the liver found in pregnancy. In a patient with a previous history of malignancy, a liver biopsy can confirm the diagnosis. These tumors may be from breast, gastrointestinal, or ovarian origin. A quantitative serum human chorionic gonadotropin gives an insight into the possibility of gestational trophoblastic neoplasms. Although uncommon, various cysts and neoplasias of the liver have been reported. Most often, these are incidental findings at the time of abdominal ultrasonography. Helpful parameters in the ultrasound diagnosis include displacement of the hepatic vasculature, an external bulging of the liver capsule, and a posterior shift of the inferior vena cava. In the case of the intrahepatic cyst, the differential diagnosis should include infectious causes. Hepatic cysts may also be seen in association with adult polycystic disease of the kidney.

The most benign hepatic tumor is a hemangioma. These have a characteristic ultrasonographic appearance, and conservative management is appropriate. Tumor size is monitored with serial sonography during pregnancy and, in the postpartum period, the diagnosis is confirmed with bolus-enhanced, sequential computed tomography. A 5 per cent chance of rupture of these tumors with life-threatening hemorrhage exists, but in lesions of less than 10 cm in size complications are rare. Serial determinations of liver transaminases should also be normal if the patient is to be managed conservatively.

Hepatic adenomas and focal nodular hyperplasia, once rare, are being seen more frequently with increased use of oral contraceptives. As there is a great potential for hemorrhage with rupture of Glisson's capsule, most practitioners recommend surgical excision of the tumor once the diagnosis is established. Terminating an early pregnancy in a woman with a new finding of hepatic adenoma has been recommended; however, abrupt necrosis of the adenoma that resulted in emergency partial hepatectomy has been reported following termination of pregnancy. In one series, surgical treatment of focal nodular hyperplasia in the postpartum period resulted in two cases of operative death. A few carcinomatous lesions that arouse primarily in the liver have been reported. These include cholangiocarcinoma of the intrahepatic ducts and primary hepatocellular carcinoma. In these cases, the maternal prognosis is dismal; however, one patient had a successful pregnancy 18 months after complete surgical removal. An increased serum alpha-fetoprotein has been found with hepatocellular carcinoma of the liver. This fact should be kept in mind when no fetal cause for an increased maternal alpha-fetoprotein is determined. Associated hepatocellular carcinoma has also been seen in patients who remain hepatitis B-surface-antigen positive after a hepatitis B viral illness.

DRUG TOXICITY

Many drugs have been associated with elevation of hepatic enzymes in cases in which a toxic level is reached. Besides direct toxicity, a hypersensitivity response may be associated with such drugs as isoniazid, phenyltoin, and the halogenated anesthetics. The beta-agonists, ritodrine and terbutaline, which are commonly used to treat premature labor have been found to cause elevations of the liver enzymes when used intravenously. With discontinuation of the drug, transaminase levels return to normal. Chlorpromazine, used to treat hyperemesis, has been associated with cholestatic jaundice, which rarely progresses to fulminant hepatic failure. Chronic hepatitis has been reported with valproic acid, alpha-methyldopa, and isoniazid. Cimetidine and acetaminophen have also caused hepatic dysfunction. Although intravenous tetracycline is no longer prescribed for postpartum endometritis, this drug was associated with a hepatic toxicity very similar to that found in the acute fatty liver of pregnancy. Tetracycline has been found in the bony matrix of women who took the drug prior to pregnancy and who developed acute fatty liver in late gestation. Erythromycin estolate causes maternal hepatic dysfunction, and other forms of erythromycin should be given in pregnancy. Thiazide diuretics can cause hepatic failure in patients with cirrhosis of the liver. Total parenteral nutrition may cause an enlarged liver and elevated enzyme levels possibly because of an increased carbohydrate load. In addition, a cholestatic reaction that leads to cirrhosis has occurred. When abnormalities of the liver profile develop, the parenteral nutrition should be discontinued in most cases.

It should be remembered that patients with hepatic problems may have lower serum protein, and thus lowered protein binding of certain drugs makes more of the free drug available, thereby increasing the potential for toxicity. In addition, seriously ill patients may have reduced liver blood flow and a decreased ability to metabolize many drugs. The best approach is to avoid multiple agents in the treatment of women with signs of hepatic dysfunction and to monitor serum levels of potentially dangerous substances.

In addition to medical therapies, one should also consider environmental exposures that cause hepatotoxicity. In particular, a history of alcohol abuse and various chemical exposures in the home or workplace should be sought. Residents of some mobile homes and hospital employees working in surgical pathology have been found to be exposed to formaldehyde. Vinyl chloride exposure in industry may predispose to hepatocellular carcinoma.

FETAL CONSIDERATIONS

Although neither hepatitis A nor hepatitis B is associated with teratogenic effects, transplacental infection with rubella or cytomegalovirus can cause anomalies. An increased rate of stillborns and preterm delivery has been seen with HAV and HBV, at least in underdeveloped countries. With intrahepatic cholestasis of pregnancy, intrauterine fetal demise is more frequent and placental changes reported could cause decreased fetal oxygenation. Serial fetal assessments with sonography and bioelectronic fetal monitoring are recommended in such cases. Decreased uterine blood flow can occur with metabolic disturbances from hepatic failure or from hemorrhage enhanced by defective clotting mechanisms often found in liver disease.

Elevations in the fetal bilirubin level have been found in a mother with cirrhosis, and although the levels are seldom high enough to cause fetal neurologic damage, this must certainly be considered when the maternal level of unconjugated bilirubin reaches 15 mg per deciliter. An increased maternal bilirubin also affects the determination of amniotic fluid delta OD 450 (false-positive), which is used to evaluate the fetal condition in the case of maternal antibody-to-red-cell antigens. Maternal and fetal mortality is high in pregnancies with acute fatty liver.

CONTRACEPTION

Oral contraceptive agents may be an acceptable method of birth control for a woman who has fully recovered from a mild viral hepatitis. These drugs should not be given to the patient with a prior history of severe cholestatic problems during pregnancy or from previous use of the pill. Permanent sterilization is better for these women as cholestasis tends to recur with each pregnancy. In most cases, women with gallstones should avoid the pill as stone formation may be enhanced. A history of focal nodular hyperplasia and hepatic adenoma is a contraindication to oral contraceptives. Women with advanced liver disease often have a decreased immune response and coagulation problems and are not candidates for the intrauterine device. The barrier methods of contraception would seem to have the least metabolic effects and are therefore preferred for patients with hepatic disease. In addition, they may prevent the sexual transmission of HBV to the male partner of a hepatitis B carrier. Acute fatty liver has not occurred in subsequent pregnancies. Permanent sterilization is recommended for the patient with cirrhosis as long-term survival is poor.

SUGGESTED READING

Center for Disease Control. Recommendations for protection against viral hepatitis. MMWR 1985; 4:313–335.
Riley CR. Acute hepatic failure at term. Postgrad Med 1980; 68:118–127.
Sherlock S. The liver and pregnancy. In: Sherlock S, ed. Diseases of the liver and biliary system. Boston: Blackwell Scientific Publications, 1985:420.
Steven MM. Pregnancy and liver disease. Gut 1981; 22:592–614.

NEUROLOGIC DISORDERS

WILLIAM PRYSE-PHILLIPS, M.D., F.R.C.P.(C), F.R.C.P.

Eight areas are discussed in this chapter, selected on the grounds of their frequency, seriousness, or susceptibility to treatment. When further details of the clinical entities are desired, reference to a standard textbook is advised.

HEADACHE

Headaches probably represent the commonest single neurologic disorder of pregnancy. A simple classification into muscle tension, vascular, traction, and referred types suffices for understanding.

1. Muscle tension headaches are tight, band-like, or pressing pains felt around the head or over the temporalis or occipitofrontalis muscles, with local tenderness on palpation. They tend to occur for hours or days at a time, to worsen with stress, and to be unaccompanied by other neurologic or physical complaints apart from mild nausea.
2. Vascular headaches (migraine) have various subtypes. Common migraine is that form in which elements of tension headache occur with a throbbing component and sometimes unilaterally; they differ from classic migraine in that there are no preceding or accompanying symptoms or signs, again apart from nausea or vomiting, and in that they may last for days. In classic migraine, the headache is usually unilateral, is preceded by visual, sensory, or other focal neurologic symptoms, and is more acute and severe though usually less prolonged, seldom lasting more than 12 hours. The term complicated migraine refers to this form of headache with prolonged deficits such as ophthalmoplegia, hemiparesis, or dysphasia. Cluster migraine differs greatly from the above; severe pain in and around the orbit is accompanied by miosis, ptosis, rhinorrhea, and lacrimation. Attacks (usually nocturnal) occur in groups over a few weeks, after which they remit for months. The condition is uncommon in pregnancy.

   Vascular headaches also occur with marked elevations of blood pressure (as with eclampsia), alcohol and other drug ingestion, contact with nitrites, fever, and carbon dioxide accumulation.
3. Traction headaches are prolonged, often severe, bursting or pressure pains, poorly localized in the head, and eventually accompanied by focal neurologic symptoms, evidence of raised intracranial pressure, nausea, vomiting, and/or drowsiness. They are caused by traction on pain-sensitive intracranial structures such as the venous sinuses, some of the meninges, and the fifth and ninth nerves by an expanding mass lesion or in the presence of intracranial blood or inflammatory disease.
4. Referred pain from disease of the eyes, sinuses, temporomandibular joints, or neck may also cause diagnostic difficulty unless considered in the differential diagnosis initially.

Treatment of any of these headaches is ideally accomplished without the use of drugs, but this is not always attainable. Muscle tension headaches may respond to the identification and ventilation of any psychopathology present, but often other measures are needed. Biofeedback, muscle relaxation exercises, yoga, and even hypnosis are all preferable to the use of drugs, especially in the first two trimesters of pregnancy, although occasionally a couple of well-placed injections of bupivacaine (Marcaine) or lidocaine 2 percent, 1 to 2 ml into muscle trigger zones, are curative.

Many patients have medicated themselves for so long that they are psychologically if not physically drug-dependent, and elimination of their over-the-counter drugs leads to further intolerable pain; supportive treatment of withdrawal in the hospital is essential in such cases.

In the stage of acute pain, migraine headaches should respond to 100 percent oxygen given at 7 L per minute for 10 minutes, but if this fails an acetaminophen-codeine combination will be needed. The intravenous injection of small (2.5 to 7.5 mg) doses of chlorpromazine is a favored way of terminating migraines in emergency rooms, but hypotension may be a major drawback in pregnant patients. Oral or intramuscular prednisone (e.g., 60 mg repeated once in 24 hours) is also effective but is seldom needed. During pregnancy, about three-quarters of women with vascular headaches claim relief of their severity and/or frequency but, in a few cases, such problems begin during this time, and recurrence of headaches in the postpartum period is common.

Prophylaxis of vascular headaches follows much the same lines as for tension headaches, with two important additions. First, women with migraines should avoid all the foods proscribed in the monoamine oxidase inhibitor diet as well as foods containing nitrites or monosodium glutamate, since all are potent precipitants of headaches. Second, in those uncommon cases in which severe migraines persist in pregnancy, an interval drug such as amitriptyline (25 to 75 mg every night) is usually effective. Unwanted effects include dry mouth, blurred vision, postural hypotension, drowsiness, and occasional urinary retention. Cluster headaches respond to oxygen in the acute phase; prednisone, 75 mg daily for 3 days with subsequent fast reduction, may follow in resistant cases. Interval therapy is difficult, since lithium, methysergide, cyproheptadine, and steroids are usually the mainstays of therapy but are not known to be safe in pregnancy.

The use of ergot and its derivatives for the treatment of vascular headaches (including cluster migraine) is traditional but in this context highly undesirable. In my opinion, ergot is responsible for more side effects than benefits, even in nonpregnant patients.

Traction headaches require intensive and urgent investigation; their treatment is of the cause, as is the case with referred pain.

MULTIPLE SCLEROSIS

Multiple sclerosis is a protean disorder of the central nervous system with a prevalence of between 20 and 100 per 100,000 population in the United States and Canada. Most patients develop the first symptoms of their disease between the ages of 18 and 40, and women are affected more than men in the ratio of about 3 to 2. Thus multiple sclerosis is not an uncommon problem in pregnant women.

Fortunately (but almost uniquely), presumably because of the suppression of maternal cellular immune responses, relapse rates fall in pregnancy, with only 10 percent of women with multiple sclerosis reporting any deterioration. In the remainder, the course is one of general stability or improvement. Only 3 percent of women report the onset of multiple sclerosis symptoms during pregnancy, and these patients have a relatively good prognosis.

Problems that arise include the following:

Use of Drugs for Symptomatic or Suppressive Treatment. The decision to use drugs for multiple sclerosis symptoms that occur or persist in pregnancy is difficult, since almost all have potentially damaging effects on the fetus. At a minimum, diazepam, baclofen, dantrolene, oxybutynin (Ditropan), amantadine, and anticholinergics rate the comment "safety in pregnancy not yet established," whereas adrenocorticotropic hormone and immunosuppressants may be actively toxic to the fetus. In the event of an acute relapse, however, prednisone is the drug of choice after the first trimester (during which time no drug is safe), but to be effective, decreasing doses starting from at least 75 mg per day for 5 days are needed. Use of the other six agents listed above is warranted only when relief of the patient's extreme discomfort is considered to outweigh the potential dangers to the fetus and is an individual clinical decision for which no set rules can be established, except for the need for informed consent.

In patients who have had prior steroid therapy for multiple sclerosis within the previous 2 years, intravenous hydrocortisone, 100 mg, is advised as the patient enters the labor room and thereafter every 8 hours for the next day.

Awareness of Labor Pains. Multiple sclerosis has no overall effect in a given population on labor or delivery, although in women with severe cord involvement and a sensory level, admission well before term is advised because labor pains may not be perceived. The actual stages of labor, however, should proceed normally.

Weakness. Active participation in the second stage of labor may be impossible for a few women with multiple sclerosis, due to pyramidal deficits, and both this problem and maternal exhaustion are indications for an instrument-assisted delivery. When analgesia is required, a general anesthetic is acceptable but spinal epidural block is probably contraindicated.

Fatigability. Fatigability resulting from multiple sclerosis is indistinguishable from that occurring in normal pregnant women. No drug therapy is advised, although much social manipulation may be required.

Infections. For the prophylaxis of urinary tract infection, ampicillin or nitrofurantoin is preferred, since the rate of pyelonephritis is high in the presence of incomplete emptying of a neurogenic bladder, a likely complication of long-standing bilateral pyramidal involvement in multiple sclerosis.

Starting a Family. The decision by a woman with multiple sclerosis as to whether or not to start a family may be helped if it is recalled that the relapse rate in pregnancy is low but definitely raised to between 20 and 40 percent in the first 6 to 12 months following delivery;

that problems in managing the baby are mainly due to gait ataxia and limb weakness, and if these are not marked, mothering should not be physically difficult; that if the woman could manage a baby at her current nonpregnant disability level, she will probably be at the same level following delivery; and that breast-feeding is perfectly safe and that no transmission of multiple sclerosis will occur thereby (although a number of drugs used in treatment of multiple sclerosis may be secreted in the milk). Although there is an increased familial incidence of multiple sclerosis this is only possibly a genetic manifestation.

Fertility. Multiple scerosis does not affect fertility and is not by itself an indication for termination of pregnancy.

CEREBROVASCULAR DISEASE

Subarachnoid Hemorrhage

Subarachnoid hemorrhage is the most serious vascular complication in pregnancy; spontaneous intracerebral hemorrhages have been reported to account for up to 80 percent of maternal deaths and represent the third most common cause of nonobstetric maternal deaths. The differential diagnosis of subarachnoid hemorrhage from eclampsia is not easy, and this figure (80 percent) may be low. Arteriovenous malformations are more common causes of subarachnoid hemorrhage in pregnancy than are aneurysms, which is fortunate since the prognosis is a little better; they commonly bleed, especially between the 16th and 20th and between the 30th and 40th weeks. With aneurysms, the incidence of subarachnoid hemorrhage rises steadily during the pregnancy and is greatest in the third trimester. Subarachnoid bleeding is more common in patients with Marfan's syndrome or with polycystic kidneys and also complicates choriocarcinoma, eclampsia, hematologic disorders, endocarditis, vasculitis, and cerebral venous thrombosis.

The diagnosis of subarachnoid hemorrhage is not difficult in the presence of the typical signs of meningism developing after the abrupt onset of severe headache, with nausea and vomiting, photophobia, drowsiness, and sometimes seizures and focal neurologic signs. A recent "sentinel" headache with neck stiffness may have preceded these acute symptoms. Exclusion of the conditions listed above can be achieved by a review of the obstetric history; consideration of the timing of the event within the pregnancy; general, cardiologic, and neurologic examinations; and examination of the blood and urine. A computed tomographic (CT) scan will detect blood in the subarachnoid space at once, whereas this will only be found at lumbar puncture 4 to 6 hours later. CT scanning will also demonstrate an arteriovenous malformation but seldom an aneurysm. If the CT scan shows blood in the subarachnoid space, lumbar puncture is unnecessary. Lumbar puncture rarely shows blood when CT findings were negative. If the source of the bleeding is not at once apparent from clinical and CT evaluation, as might be the case with cerebral venous thrombosis, angiography should be performed, and this will be necessary in all cases of aneurysm. It should be scheduled as soon as is practicable. The fetus should be screened appropriately from the relatively large amount of radiation consequent upon this procedure. A diagnosis will be achieved by angiography in over 90 percent of cases.

Aneurysms should be attacked by the appropriate neurosurgical technique as soon as practicable, after which the pregnancy may proceed normally to term; ergotamine, antifibrinolytics, and calcium-channel blockers should not be used in pregnant patients with subarachnoid hemorrhage. Patients with aneurysms that rupture at term are best delivered by cesarean section. Arteriovenous malformations may be left until after delivery, although large hematomas need removal. In most cases, delivery should be hastened by the use of low forceps under epidural anesthesia or cesarean section should be employed. When an aneurysm or arteriovenous malformation cannot be obliterated surgically, additional pregnancies will be hazardous.

Cortical Venous Thrombosis

Cortical venous thrombosis occurs mainly in the postpartum period, especially in dehydrated or cachectic women and in those with malignant disease, polycythemia, or hemoglobinopathies. Infective venous thromboses are now less common than aseptic forms. The clinical features include drowsiness, headache, nausea and vomiting, fever, meningism, signs of raised intracranial pressure, paraparesis, and seizures, and the diagnosis is made by CT scanning with or without angiography (which may be IV-digital subtraction angiography). Treatment is directed toward the suppression of seizures with phenytoin (Dilantin) (15 mg per kilogram by slow intravenous infusion, followed if possible by oral phenytoin 300 mg per day or more as determined by blood levels), and the reduction of cerebral edema with steroids and mannitol (although such treatment is not very effective). The use of anticoagulants is controversial; although logical at first sight, they do increase the risk of inducing hemorrhage in the infarcted areas.

Arterial Dissections

Arterial dissections, for example of the carotid arteries, produce the clinical features of migraine-like headaches, often with contralateral neurologic signs and a homolateral Horner's syndrome. Surgery is seldom indicated. Most cases are treated with heparin initially, after which antiplatelet agents are employed. After about 3 months, a repeat angiogram may demonstrate healing of the dissection.

Brain Infarcts

The incidence of embolization or atherothrombotic brain infarcts in pregnancy is also increased by a factor of about 13 compared with nonpregnant women to about 1 in 3,000 pregnancies. About two-thirds of these are embolic arterial occlusions, usually of the middle cerebral artery; they occur mainly after the first trimester and during the first week post partum. Cardiac disease (of the valves or myocardium) or disorders of cardiac rhythm are commonly detectable; endocarditis, paradoxical embolism from deep pelvic or leg vein thrombosis passing through a septal defect, hemoglobinopathies, and thrombotic thrombocytopenic purpura are less commonly associated but require exclusion. Severe hypotension from any cause also can lead to atherothrombotic brain infarcts in the "watershed" areas between the territories of the three major cerebral arteries. The incidence of strokes with mitral valve prolapse is 1 in 6,000, and there is no excess during pregnancy. Intracerebral hemorrhage is usually due to rupture of an arteriovenous malformation (see above), or to bacterial endocarditis, or else it complicates severe hypertension.

Management of the stroke is at first supportive, with particular attention to the correction of hypotension; regarding hypertension, only diastolic values above 110 mm Hg need reduction, and in such cases the management should parallel that of eclampsia, with urgent delivery of the fetus, since the differential diagnosis may be impossible. Anticoagulation with heparin (which unlike warfarin does not cross the placenta) is indicated after cardiogenic embolism as long as there is no intracerebral hemorrhage complicating it and the infarct is not large. A delay of at least 24 hours is usually advised, except in the case of evolving stroke, when heparinization should be begun at once. The use of steroids contributes nothing of value to the management of acute strokes.

Careful general, neurologic and cardiac evaluation is necessary at this time; the pulses must be sought and blood pressures recorded in both arms to exclude aortic arch arteritis. The clinical and laboratory tests chosen must reflect the variety of causative pathologies listed above. CT scanning is desirable to rule out hemorrhage, and cardiac magnetic resonance imaging or at least echocardiography should probably be employed to supplement clinical assessment of the heart. Blood cultures, a complete blood count with estimation of platelets and of clotting factors, erythrocyte sedimentation rate, blood chemistry (e.g., glucose, urea, lipids), immunologic screening to exclude lupus erythematosus, repeat serology, a chest x-ray study, an electrocardiogram, and urinalysis are advisable.

Following the acute stage, during which nursing care and maintenance of fluid and electrolyte status are all the active treatment that can be provided, physiotherapy should be started; at this time, the results of the initial diagnostic work-up should be available, and specific therapy may then be possible.

Transient Ischemic Attacks

Transient ischemic attacks are uncommon in pregnancy, but unless they are due to migraine they will require hospitalization and work-up as above, since they are harbingers of strokes. However, since the benefit of carotid endarterectomy is as yet unproved, there is probably no need for carotid angiography in such cases. Unfortunately, no drug has been shown to reduce either the transient ischemic attacks or subsequent strokes in women, and there is thus little rationale for the prescription of aspirin, let alone more expensive antiplatelet agents. Nevertheless, in the absence of any proven alternative therapy, aspirin is what patients get.

A flurry of transient ischemic attacks in older patients is treated with intravenous heparin to prolong the clotting time by a factor of 1.5; in pregnancy, underlying atherosclerosis is less likely, though quite possible, but because cardiac disease or dissection of the internal carotid artery wall may present in this manner, I advise administering initial heparin in all such cases, proceeding to aspirin 325 mg once daily thereafter, and I do not use warfarin.

SEIZURE DISORDERS

Women with epilepsy represent a high-risk group because of an increased rate of complications during pregnancy and labor and of problems related to the seizure disorder itself.

Complications of Epilepsy

Data indicate that the rates of toxemia, and perhaps antepartum hemorrhage, and of stillbirths, prematurity, reduced intellectual status, primary generalized epilepsy, and congenital malformations are all more common when pregnancy is complicated by epilepsy. Seizures themselves might well damage the fetus, either from direct trauma, through hypoxia, or from the subsequent lactic acidosis, but this point is by no means clear. Postpartum hemorrhage may also be increased, presumably through drug-induced deficiency of vitamin K.

When phenytoin or barbiturates have been used in pregnancy, the risk of hemorrhagic disease of the newborn must be lessened by the injection of vitamin K, 1 mg intramuscularly, soon after birth. If bleeding persists, fresh frozen plasma may be needed to stop it. Infants exposed to benzodiazepines or phenobarbitone in utero may also go through a drug withdrawal phase, usually starting about the 6th day and lasting a week, with yawning, crying, insomnia, myoclonus, hyperexcitability, and restlessness, but not seizures.

Seizure frequency in epileptic women increases in the first and third trimesters of pregnancy in about a third of cases, mainly those with focal (so-called "partial") epilepsy. In the remainder, the frequency stays the same or falls. An increase in seizure frequency could be due to hormonal changes, hemodilution, noncompliance, sleep deprivation, psychological factors, or reduced plasma concentration of antiepileptic drugs due to increased hepatic and renal clearance, decreased absorption, or reduced protein binding. Therefore, the dose of anticonvulsant should be adjusted with particular reference to the clinical state of the patient rather than to the serum levels. Naturally, because of the risk of teratogenesis, the smallest effective dose of a single drug should be used if possible.

The children born to mothers treated for epilepsy during the pregnancy have between a 1.5 and 3 times higher risk of malformations (usually cardiovascular disorders and orofacial clefts) than children of untreated pregnant women. Maternal age and the increased malformation rate occurring in the children of epileptic fathers are also relevant here; drugs are by no means the only factor. However, there is a real increased risk of neural tube defects with sodium valproate (about 1 in 100 cases), which may require amniocentesis for early diagnosis; and trimethadione (Tridione) and other drugs of the dione class induce a large number of malformations and therefore should be avoided. The existence of the fetal hydantoin syndrome (facial and digital abnormalities in about a third of children born of women on phenytoin) is disputed, since these deformities are not drug-specific and other factors may be at least as responsible as the hydantoin drug prescribed. In addition, many of the changes seem to resolve over the years, such as the nail hypoplasia and the relative reduction in the head circumference. The data do not allow proper assessment of teratogenicity of the other anticonvulsant agents used.

Occurrence of Epilepsy

Gestational epilepsy (that present only during pregnancy) occurs in only about 4 percent of epileptic women. Primary or idiopathic epilepsy can occur first at this time, but one should refer all such patients for neurologic assessment, since arteriovenous malformations, ruptured aneurysms, meningiomas, pheochromocytoma, hypoglycemia, water overload, and cortical venous thrombosis are examples of neurologic disorders that may well lead to a first seizure in pregnancy. In all such cases magnetic resonance imaging or at least CT scanning is wise. With the use of appropriate shielding, angiography is not contraindicated by pregnancy, and in cases of arteriovenous malformation it is probably essential. The differentiation between a grand mal seizure occurring as a result of primary generalized epilepsy and that due to eclampsia is only possible when the other features of eclampsia (timing, blood pressure, edema, and urinalysis) are evaluated, since there is nothing different about the actual seizures in the two conditions.

Management of Seizures

The management of seizures occurring for the first time in pregnancy requires first the evaluation of their cause. The conditions mentioned above must be excluded by thorough neurologic examination, supplemented by an electroencephalogram, CT or magnetic resonance image scanning, and appropriate hematologic and biochemical tests. If it is decided to treat the patient with anticonvulsants, the use of one drug is preferable to polypharmacy, and the dose used should be the smallest that is judged clinically effective. Grand mal (major motor) seizures are most likely to need treatment. Either phenytoin, 300 to 400 mg per day, or carbamazepine, 200 mg three to five times daily, is the best agent to employ initially, but the necessary dose is a very individual matter because of the increased metabolism of drugs during pregnancy. In a few cases, doses may have to be much higher than generally used. Serum levels should be checked at least monthly. Phenytoin should be begun at full dose, and carbamazepine at half-dose, increasing by 200 mg per day at weekly intervals.

Unwanted effects of phenytoin include cerebellar signs, drowsiness, hirsutism, macrocytic anemia, and hyperplasia of the gums, all dose-related; rashes, serum sickness, the Stevens-Johnson syndrome, pseudolymphoma, lupus erythematosus, and (rarely) liver or marrow depression are idiosyncratic reactions. Folic acid 5 mg per day and supplemental calcium should be given to pregnant women taking phenytoin to counteract the effects of enzyme induction by this drug.

Carbamazepine typically produces dizziness, nausea, ataxia, and drowsiness initially if not started at a low dose; skin rashes occur occasionally. The only serious idiosyncratic reactions are depression of the bone marrow and hepatic toxicity. Although the usual advice given is that patients should have regular blood counts in order to detect the depression of red or white cell production, such complications can occur at any time and very suddenly; therefore I advise patients who suffer fever, sore throat, or a rash to discontinue the drug and to come to the hospital for a blood test *on the same day.*

Absence seizures are uncommon in pregnancy; when they do occur, ethosuximide, 250 to 500 mg four times daily, is the recommended drug. Unwanted effects include headache, nausea and vomiting, drowsiness, and irritability. Rashes, nephropathy, and marrow depression are idiosyncratic complications of therapy. Sodium valproate is indicated only after the fourth month because of the risk of neural tube defects if ingested early. The benzodiazepine clonazepam, at 0.5 to 1 mg three times daily, may be a reasonable alternative.

When women with preexisting seizures become pregnant (which is common, since most anticonvulsants except valproate induce the enzymes metabolizing the hormones in oral contraceptive pills), the risks are increased, as mentioned above. Women with epilepsy who wish to become pregnant should be helped to achieve maximal seizure control by judicious prescription of those drugs that are acceptable in pregnancy, if possible with substitution of those such as the diones or valproate, which carry risks generally deemed unacceptable. The need for good patient compliance and for a slightly increased frequency of visits for clinical and biochemical evaluation should be stressed. Since there is at least a theoretical risk to the fetus if grand mal seizures should occur, drug therapy, if needed before, will almost certainly be needed during the forthcoming pregnancy, and cessation of treatment is seldom indicated.

Status Epilepticus

Status epilepticus in pregnancy is treated much as in nonpregnant patients, but fetal monitoring is advisable. After blood is taken for hematologic and biochemical screening (urea, glucose, calcium, drug levels, and blood gas readings in particular), bolus doses of glucose and thiamine are given through an intravenous line, and then diazepam 2 mg per minute to total 20 mg or lorazepam

0.5 mg per minute to total 4 mg is injected. This is followed (in the patient who has not been taking phenytoin already) by phenytoin, 15 mg per kilogram body weight, at a rate no faster than 50 mg per minute. Half of this dose should be used if phenytoin has been taken recently, and electrocardiographic monitoring is advisable during the infusion. Phenytoin and diazepam should not flow through the same tubing, nor should they be given in solutions containing glucose, because of the risk of microcrystallization. If seizures persist, intravenous phenobarbital or a diazepam drip may be advised by the neurologic consultant. Diazepam is of no value when given intramuscularly for the prevention of seizures.

Anticonvulsants are not a contraindication to breastfeeding (apart from high-dose benzodiazepines), since they are excreted in the milk in insignificant quantities.

The management of eclampsia is considered in the chapter on *Renal Transplantation in Pregnancy.*

Neoplasms

As mentioned above, meningiomas and arteriovenous malformations may first manifest themselves during pregnancy, the former by increased growth and cortical irritation and the latter by bleeding. This does not necessarily mean that there is an increased incidence of tumors, and in fact the reverse appears to be the case, astrocytomas and meningiomas both presenting less frequently in pregnancy than would be expected in the population at risk. The rate for vestibular schwannomas is close to that expected.

Choriocarcinoma. Commonly preceded by a hydatidiform mole or missed abortion, this tumor of placental tissue may metastasize to the brain, manifesting signs of focal deficits, raised intracranial pressure, intracranial bleeding, or seizures. The diagnosis is suggested by the finding of one or more highly vascular lesions on CT scan. Management is covered in the chapter on *Choriocarcinoma—Gestational Trophoblastic Neoplasia.*

Pituitary Tumors. Pituitary tumors tend to lead to infertility, but if pregnancy occurs, their growth rate is increased. Headache and later visual disturbances (blurred vision and then bitemporal field cuts) are the usual features and are an indication for treatment with bromocriptine (initially at 5 mg per day, rising to 20 mg per day) or for transsphenoidal adenectomy. This operation is certainly indicated when there is obvious growth of the tumor with advancing field cuts and reduction in visual acuity despite treatment with bromocriptine.

Pituitary infarction, which may complicate severe hypotension, for example from postpartum hemorrhage, may also cause acute symptoms resulting from swelling of the ischemic gland; severe headache and visual disturbances are typical, and hypophysectomy may be indicated. More often, the condition (Sheehan's syndrome) presents silently with lactation failure or other evidence of hypopituitarism in the following months.

General Management of Intracranial Masses. For patients presenting in pregnancy with any combination of focal signs, seizures, and evidence of raised intracranial pressure, neurologic assessment is mandatory. There is no place for lumbar puncture in the diagnosis of brain masses. Isotope scanning is not an acceptable screening test, and electroencephalography is not accurate enough to make it worthwhile. Magnetic resonance imaging or CT scanning (with shielding) is necessary for the confirmation of the presence of the tumor, for documentation of its precise site, size, and vascularity, and for a reasonable assessment of its pathology and effect on local intracranial structures. In patients with meningiomas, aneurysms or arteriovenous malformations, arteriography may also be needed to prepare the neurosurgeon for his approach.

Removal of benign tumors may be deferred until after completion of the pregnancy, but masses in the posterior fossa and all malignant tumors should be excised right after diagnosis, mainly because of the risk of herniation as a result of distortion of structures caused by the mass in the presence of an added increase in intracranial pressure during labor. If this occurs, treatment involves giving mannitol 20 percent, 200 ml intravenously in 20 minutes, with intramuscular dexamethasone, 24 mg, while awaiting the arrival of the neurosurgeon.

MUSCLE DISEASES

Myotonic Dystrophy

The clinical course of the pregnancy in a woman with myotonic dystrophy is fraught with hazard. There is an absolute increase in the incidence of abruptio placentae, stillbirth, hydramnios, and fetal death in utero. The first stage of labor is frequently prolonged, and the infant often manifests severe respiratory and feeding difficulties. There is no definitive treatment, but awareness of the nature of the high risks of the pregnancy may allow preparedness.

The remarkable absence of insight in so many patients with myotonic dystrophy leads to frequent noncooperation. Although the disease is inherited as an autosomal dominant, the presence of a maternal nongenetic factor has been postulated to account for the nonmendelian high frequency of infantile involvement. This, and the social and medical disadvantages consequent upon the disease, may make it appropriate for the physician to raise the question of sterilization if informed consent can be obtained.

Polymyositis

Polymyositis is rare in pregnant women, but pregnancy affects its manifestations, usually for the worse. The incidence of spontaneous abortions, of prematurity, and of perinatal deaths is markedly increased, with up to 55 percent fetal loss. About one-quarter of affected patients have the onset of symptoms during pregnancy, and about one-half of those previously affected have an exacerbation during the pregnancy, mainly in the first trimester. In the more severe cases, respiratory as well as other truncal muscle functions are affected so that cooperation in the first and second stages of labor is limited. In such cases, assisted delivery is required. The treatment of the condition normally involves immunosuppression with steroids or methotrexate or azathioprine. The latter agents carry a high risk of teratogenicity, but severe weakness despite steroid therapy may require their use, in which case the question of termination of the pregnancy may be raised if the timing is appropriate.

Myasthenia Gravis

Myasthenia, like multiple sclerosis, occurs more commonly in women and in those between the ages of 20 and 40 years; therefore it is of importance in this context. The course of the disease during pregnancy is so variable that one cannot predict what will happen, but exacerbations are commonest in the puerperium and can be both abrupt and severe, accounting for much of the 3.4 percent maternal mortality reported. Premature labor occurs in about 40 percent of cases, and an increase in the perinatal mortality to some five times the normal rate has also been detected. Up to 20 percent of neonates develop myasthenic signs transiently.

The usual diagnostic test, the intravenous injection of edrophonium, 10 mg, is contraindicated because of an increased chance of abortion with this agent. Single-fiber electromyographic and end-plate electrical studies in the electromyography laboratory are preferable.

Treatment of the disease relies on anticholinesterases such as neostigmine (15 mg by mouth every 3 to 4 hours) or pyridostigmine (60 mg by mouth every 3 to 4 hours), with or (preferably) without the addition of atropine. Unwanted effects include abdominal cramps, diarrhea, nausea and vomiting, and excessive secretions. Overdose leads to excessive end-plate depolarization with girdle weakness and bulbar and ventilatory failure, indistinguishable in most cases from myasthenic crisis.

The role of steroids in pregnancy is under discussion; although they suppress the signs of myasthenia in three-quarters of the patients, the potential for long-term fetal damage makes their use disquieting. However, since relapse is likely in those patients who discontinue steroids after prolonged use, they should be continued in myasthenic women who become pregnant while already taking them for this disorder. Immunosuppressants such as azathioprine and plasmapheresis are employed widely in nonpregnant patients but are undesirable in pregnancy, although the latter has been used without incident. Thymectomy is practiced in many centers as an early treatment option for generalized myasthenia, but there are few reports of its use in the pregnant patient, although there is no theoretical reason why it should not be employed. The favorable remission rate obtained may reduce the patient's reliance on anticholinesterase drugs.

All aminoglycoside antibiotics, magnesium preparations, and narcotic analgesics are contraindicated in myasthenia because of the neuromuscular blockade which they may induce.

For added safety, myasthenic women may be admitted to the hospital 2 or 3 weeks before the expected date of delivery. During this period, baseline studies of cardiac function (ECG), thyroid function, and pulmonary function are advised, and the patient's therapeutic regime is optimized.

During delivery, neostigmine, 0.5 mg intramuscularly, may be given to the symptomatic patient every 4 hours, and regional anesthesia (e.g., epidural anesthesia at T10, using an amide local anesthetic) is commonly recommended, although general anesthesia is sometimes needed; in such cases, nondepolarizing muscle relaxants (curare, succinylcholine) should not be used, since they act as competitive antagonists. Narcotic analgesics also increase the risk of further weakness. If fatigability interferes with the patient's muscular efforts, delivery with low outlet forceps is suggested, but cesarean section should be employed for obstetric rather than for neurologic reasons. The myometrium is not directly affected by myasthenia.

The earliest sign of excessive muscular fatigue is found in measurements of peak flow or forced expiratory volume. Any fall in values is an indication for urgent attention to the patient's neuromuscular status, which may require additional neostigmine (1 to 2 mg intramuscularly, not orally) and assistance with delivery. In pregnant women not yet in labor, consideration will have to be given to plasmapheresis or thymectomy if fatigability becomes severe. In the puerperium, significant worsening of myasthenic fatigability is not uncommon; the patient should have been counseled about such a complication, and the house staff warned that any increase in weakness is best quantitated by repeated estimations of ventilatory function, such as the FEV_1.

Crises of weakness and fatigability occur in myasthenics due both to inadequate and to excessive treatment; these are the myasthenic and cholinergic crises, respectively. The former may be precipitated by labor and are also important complications of severe infections and of medication with aminoglycoside antibiotics, beta-blockers, penicillamine, narcotic and other sedative agents, and divalent cations (Mg^{++}, Li^{++}). The latter usually result from too vigorous anticholinesterase therapy. Intravenous edrophonium (Tensilon), 10 mg in 30 seconds, has traditionally been the method of choice for differentiating the two forms of crisis, but the result is often misleading or at least confusing. Since edrophonium may induce respiratory arrest even in people with rather mild myasthenia, the edrophonium test should not be performed in the office in patients with any significant degree of weakness. If the patient is so weak that crisis is diagnosed, she needs admission to an intensive care unit where there are full facilities for ventilatory support. The condition is truly a medical emergency, which, however, is over when adequate artificial ventilatory support is provided. All drugs can then be stopped and the course of the disease observed for 48 hours, by which time the nature of the crisis will be clear.

Severe weakness at this time may require the use of plasmapheresis, but steroid therapy is another alternative. Such decisions should be made only in consultation with a neurologist experienced in the management of myasthenic patients.

Neonatal myasthenia is caused by passive transplacental transfer of antibodies. It affects about 20 percent of infants born to myasthenic mothers and usually appears within a day of delivery, lasting up to 3 weeks. The infants are listless, with a weak suck and cry; they are in danger of ventilatory failure and must be observed with great care for the first 3 weeks of life, and respiratory support should be at hand in case of need. Anticholinesterases are the mainstay of routine treatment for the first month of life.

There is no absolute contraindication to breast-feeding by mothers with myasthenia, but since both anticholinesterase drugs and antiacetylcholine receptor IgG antibodies are secreted in the breast milk, unwanted effects may be seen in the infant.

NEUROPATHIES

Back Pain

Back pain in pregnancy is usually musculoskeletal and not a result of root compression or irritation. Joint laxity and increased postural lumbar lordosis lead to complaints of moderate aching discomfort in the low back, buttocks, and paraspinal muscles, sometimes with trigger points that are acutely tender. Although the clinical differentiation of root and ligamentous pain may be difficult, the latter seldom radiates below the knee, may be worse at rest and while sitting (as in a car), is unaccompanied by focal neurologic signs, and is not associated with any history of preceding significant trauma. The mainstays of treatment of postural back pain in pregnancy are night-time rest on a firm mattress and 10 minutes daytime spells on the floor with the hips and knees flexed and the calves resting on the seat of a chair, which is inelegant but effective.

Radiculopathy

Root pain from a prolapsed intervertebral disk is managed conservatively, rest in bed or on a sofa being the most important factor; if this is ineffective after a week or 10 days, however, further rest will probably be of no avail. Surgery should be eschewed, unless the deficits are progressive despite rest, or unless there are signs of cauda equina compression such as loss of ankle or knee reflexes, anesthesia in dermatomal distribution, or sphincter involvement. The latter is certainly an indication for investigation and probably for operative relief. The preferred investigations are electromyography and magnetic resonance image scanning, the radiation dose with myelography being excessively hazardous to the fetus.

Nerve Compression

Only three nerve compression syndromes are particularly common in pregnancy. The carpal tunnel syndrome occurs in perhaps 25 percent of all pregnant women. It is manifested by pain, paresthesia, a heavy, swollen, or "dead" feeling without actual anesthesia, and sometimes weakness in one or both hands, worse at night and after use of the hands, and usually without objective physical signs apart from a positive Tinel's sign when the volar aspect of the wrist is tapped. Women who shake or flick their hands when demonstrating what they do when the paresthesia is at its worst almost always have carpal tunnel syndrome. Conservative therapy is preferable except in recurrent cases or in those with significant pain or loss of sleep due to this problem. Such cases may be relieved by decompression of the tunnel under local anesthetic. Otherwise, night splints with 20 degrees of extension of the wrists may provide good relief. Pyridoxine, 25 mg daily, has been reported to help nonpregnant patients, as have local injections of steroids e.g., methylprednisolone (Depo—Medrol), 1 ml, into the carpal tunnel.

The thoracic outlet, tarsal tunnel, and cubital tunnel syndromes are occasionally reported but are relatively rare. Again, conservative management is preferred, as it is with meralgia paresthetica, which affects the lateral cutaneous nerve of the thigh, producing pain, paresthesia, and numbness. This condition frequently resolves untreated after delivery.

The second important nerve compression syndrome is maternal obstetric paralysis, due to direct compression of the L4-L5 nerve roots by the baby's head as they form the upper part of the sciatic nerve on the pelvic brim, or to compression of the iliac artery. The muscles supplied by the peroneal nerve (tibialis anterior, extensor hallucis longus, and peronei) are most affected, but some weakness may be found in the hamstrings, glutei, and adductors, and in the muscles supplied by the tibial nerve. Cephalopelvic disproportion, prolonged labor, and instrument-assisted deliveries make the problem more likely. Treatment is expectant because 75 percent of cases show complete recovery. In the remainder, improvement is not perfect. Pain is a common symptom of this disorder both during and after labor and should be treated with usual doses of non-narcotic analgesics.

Finally, the incidence of Bell's palsy rises sharply in the last trimester. Prednisone, 50 mg at diagnosis, reducing by 10 mg per daily dose, is reportedly safe, but spontaneous remission is highly likely, and in the last 2 weeks no treatment is advised apart from protection of the cornea on the affected side. This can be achieved by taping the eye shut or by an eye patch and methylcellulose eye drops.

Tetany

Pregnancy and lactation act as major drains of maternal calcium, and this may induce symptoms of hypocalcemia, including circumoral and distal paresthesias, positive Trousseau's and Chvostek's signs and, in severe cases, seizures and mental changes. Phenytoin also lowers serum calcium levels. Calcium lactate tablets, 500 mg once daily, are adequate both as prophylaxis and treatment.

Polyneuropathy

Polyneuropathies occurring during pregnancy may be due to vitamin B deficiency, in which case other features of the Wernicke-Korsakoff syndrome must be prevented as well by the administration of intramuscular thiamine, 50 to 100 mg, followed by an oral vitamin preparation. Burning pains, numbness, mild paresthesia distally and clinically, thin-fiber hypesthesia (pain, temperature, and light touch sensations most affected), with hyporeflexia and trophic changes in the skin, are the commonest features. Acute intermittent porphyria may relapse mildly early in pregnancy, and there is an increase in fetal loss in this condition. In the third trimester and the puerperium, relapses are more severe, accompanied by major motor neuropathy, seizures, psychological dysfunction, abdominal pain, and in the most severe cases, ventilatory paralysis. These attacks may have been precipitated by barbiturates and most other anticonvulsants, steroids, rifampin, griseofulvin, benzodiazepines, sulfonamides, or estrogens. Treatment, including the use of propranolol, chlorpromazine, and intravenous hematin, should be coordinated with a hematologic consultant.

Hereditary sensory and motor neuropathies (Charcot-Marie-Tooth disease and variants) may worsen during pregnancy, but the only treatment measures available are orthotic. Acute inflammatory polyneuropathy (Landry-Guillain-Barré syndrome) is most uncommon during pregnancy, but the chronic form may progress. This is a difficult treatment situation, since steroids, plasmapheresis, and immunosuppressants are the only remedies with significant effect, and the last of these is contraindicated, whereas use of the first two may have undesirable effects. Nevertheless, progressive weakness in the limbs may require the use of these therapies.

The incidence of the restless legs syndrome increases in pregnancy; the patient complains that she has to rise from her bed repeatedly in order to overcome the intolerably unpleasant urge to move the limbs. Folic acid, 5 mg per day may be helpful; if symptoms are severe, clonazepam 0.5 to 1 mg at night may also relieve the problem, but the safety of the drug in pregnancy is not established.

Complaints of nocturnal cramps in the calves are even more common. Oral calcium gluconate, 500 mg daily, usually relieves this problem.

MISCELLANEOUS CONDITIONS

Hyperemesis Gravidarum

Severe vitamin B depletion may complicate prolonged vomiting and may lead to the Wernicke-Korsakoff syndrome, manifested by nystagmus, extraocular palsies, delirium ataxia, and neuropathy (although the full-blown syndrome is now seldom seen). Prevention is easy given a high level of suspicion; any woman with vomiting for over 24 hours, and indeed any person requiring intravenous fluids for more than 48 hours, should be given a prophylactic intramuscular injection of thiamine, 50 mg, repeated on alternate days while the emesis or intravenous feeding continues. The slightest hint of nystagmus, or of a complaint of blurred vision in this circumstance, should arouse suspicion, and thiamine should be given. It is not always recalled that many disadvantaged people have little thiamine reserve, and this state is exacerbated during pregnancy.

Management of the clinical syndrome consists of thiamine, this time 100 mg intravenously, repeated intramuscularly daily for two doses and then orally when the vomiting has ceased; for the delirium, intravenous diazepam, 5 to 10 mg, or a phenothiazine such as promazine, 50 to 100 mg intramuscularly, every 4 hours.

Benign Intracranial Hypertension

Since this condition is commoner in women than in men in the ratio of 3:1 and occurs mainly in those between the ages of 20 and 40 years, it is likely to be diagnosed in pregnant women rather often. In pregnancy, it usually appears between the 4th and 28th weeks. The diagnosis of this condition depends on the exclusion of all other likely causes of raised intracranial pressure. Obesity is the commonest associated factor, but ingestion of tetracyclines, indomethacin, nitrofurantoin, vitamin A excess, and both steroids and withdrawal from steroids are other factors, at least in nonpregnant patients.

The presenting features of headache, visual blurring or diplopia, transient visual obscurations, nausea and often vomiting, and tinnitus are unaccompanied by any physical signs other than papilledema and sometimes sixth nerve palsies (a false localizing sign of raised intracranial pressure). The patient appears alert and generally healthy, although she is often obese. Investigation reveals that the cerebrospinal fluid (CSF) is normal but under increased pressure, and the CT scan is also normal except that the ventricles may be small. The electroencephalogram is also normal.

Treatment initially involves repeated lumbar punctures to drain CSF, although the rate of CSF production (about 500 ml per day) should compensate for the removal of 20 ml of CSF within an hour. Perhaps it is the creation by the lumbar puncture needles of a small dural vent for the drainage of CSF into the lumbar spinal tissues that actually results in improvement. Along with this, either steroids (dexamethasone, 10 mg by mouth every 8 hours for 3 days, then 5 mg every 8 hours for 3 days) or acetazolamide (Diamox), 500 mg every 8 hours for 2 weeks, is prescribed. If visual obscurations or headaches persist, consideration must be given to drainage of the CSF; this may be accomplished by a lumboperitoneal shunt or by incision of the optic nerve sheath.

Management should be by a team representing ophthalmology, neurosurgery, and obstetrics. The ophthalmologist should perform repeated testing of visual fields and acuity, because visual function must be protected most carefully.

In labor, the usual large increases in intracranial pressure must be kept to a minimum, so analgesia must be fully adequate; regional or epidural anesthesia has been used.

Chorea Gravidarum

Less commonly seen with the receding incidence of rheumatic fever, chorea still occurs occasionally in the first trimester and should lead to a search for underlying cardiac or autoimmune disease (e.g., systemic lupus erythematosus). The movements may be lessened by acetylsalicylic acid, 325 mg two or three times daily, if they are severe and exhausting, however, haloperidol, 0.5 to 1 mg three times daily, may be necessary. The choreic movements subside after delivery.

Infectious Diseases

Many aspects of infectious disease in pregnancy are covered elsewhere in this book and details of the antimicrobial regimes recommended for AIDS, syphilis, and other infections should be obtained from chapters on *Antepartum Fetal Testing, Heart Disease, Placenta Previa, Prostaglandins,* and *Intrauterine Fetal Demise.*

Meningitis in pregnancy may be of the septic (bacterial) or aseptic (viral) variety. Severe headache and other evidence of raised intracranial pressure and of meningeal irritation, prostration, fever, seizures, rash, and sometimes evidence of infection of non-neural structures such as the throat, sinuses, and blood are the main features of the bacterial forms. These are usually caused by meningococcus or pneumococcus, *Haemophilus influenzae* and *Listeria monocytogenes* being less common infecting agents. Bacterial endocarditis may present with indistinguishable signs. Lumbar puncture is essential for etiologic diagnosis and carries no particular hazard in pregnancy. Treatment employs penicillin for meningococcal infections or cefotaxime, a third-generation cephalosporin effective against all the above microorganisms except for *Listeria*.

Aseptic meningitis is usually viral, although a similar clinical and CSF picture may be found with early meningeal tuberculosis. Polio and other enteroviruses, picorna, coxsackie, and echoviruses, mumps, rubella, and cytomegaloviruses are the commoner infecting agents. Patients with viral meningitis complain bitterly of headache and have mild to moderate signs of meningism but show no focal signs and, within days, the untreated symptoms and signs subside. In all such cases, however, the CSF must be examined to ensure that polymorphonuclear cells are absent, the glucose concentration is normal (except in mumps and lymphocytic choriomeningitis), and the culture is sterile. Where there is doubt (e.g., two or three polymorphs present in the CSF, which is otherwise compatible with a diagnosis of aseptic meningitis), a second sample should be taken 12 hours laters. Parameningeal foci such as otitis and sinusitis produce similar CSF findings.

Benign Encephalopathy of Pregnancy

Mild cognitive dysfunction has been reported to occur in 40 percent of pregnant women, with forgetfulness, drowsiness, disorientation, impaired concentration, and reading difficulties the main symptoms at any stage. Anemia may be an associated factor. No treatment is known, but patients can be reassured that their problems are self-limiting.

SUGGESTED READING

Goldstein PF, ed. Neurological disorders of pregnancy. Mount Kisco, New York: Futuro, 1986.

Noronha A. Neurologic disorders during pregnancy and the puerperium. Clin Perinatol 1985; 12:695–713.

Pryse-Phillips WEM, Murray TJ. Essential neurology. 3rd ed. New York: Elsevier, 1986.

Robertson IG. Epilepsy in pregnancy. Clin Obstet Gynecol 1986; 13:365–384.

THYROID DISORDERS IN PREGNANCY

NeeOo W. CHIN, M.D.
MOON H. KIM, M.D.

Pregnancy-induced hormonal and metabolic alterations result in an array of thyroid function changes. Despite these alterations, the normal pregnant woman remains euthyroid. The thyroid function changes are primarily due to the estrogen-induced increase in the thyroxine-binding globulin concentration and to the declining size of the circulating pool of extrathyroidal iodide that results from the increased renal clearance of iodide. The normal pregnancy state is accompanied by an increase in thyroid size with an extremely active thyroid hormone synthesis and secretion role.

Thyroid diseases generally occur more often in women and are estimated to occur in 0.2 percent of all pregnancies. One of the earliest reports of hyperthyroidism in a female patient was in 1825 by Parry; he described a woman 3 months post partum as having an enlarged thyroid gland with exophthalmos, agitation, and distress. Therapy for thyroid disorders during pregnancy requires an awareness of many fundamental concepts in order to ensure a successful outcome for both the mother and the fetus.

NORMAL THYROID FUNCTION

Iodine is gathered into the thyroid gland against a concentration gradient from the circulation that is primarily regulated by thyroid-stimulating hormone and plasma iodine concentration. About one-fourth of the body's total iodine is found in the thyroid gland. Iodine is organified by a peroxidase enzyme system. Tyrosine rings in 19S thyroglobulin molecules are progressively iodinated and coupled to form the thyroid hormones, triiodothyronine (T_3) and thyroxine (T_4). T_3 and T_4 are maintained in the thyroid gland at a ratio of 1 to 10 or 20, respectively. The thyroid hormone molecules are hydrolyzed off the thyroglobulin molecule and released simultaneously into the circulation. Thyroid-stimulating hormone, (TSH), an anterior pituitary polypeptide hormone, accelerates all steps by binding to specific thyroid surface receptors and activates cyclic adenosine monophosphate (AMP). The pituitary production of TSH is controlled by two factors: thyrotropin-releasing hormone (TRH), which increases TSH synthesis and release, and T_4 and T_3, which exert negative feedback directly by causing a reduction of TRH receptors in the pituitary gland.

THYROID HORMONES

T_4 is 99.5 percent bound to carrier proteins in the circulation, leaving 0.5 percent in the active unbound state. Thyroid hormones are bound to one of three proteins: (1) thyroxine-binding globulin (TBG), an inter-alpha-globulin, binds 60 to 70 percent of the circulating T_4, (2) thyroid binding prealbumin, a prealbumin, binds 20 to 30 percent of T_4, and (3) remaining 10 percent of bound circulating thyroid hormone is bound to thyroid-binding albumin.

T_3 is four to five times more biologically active than T_4. Circulating free T_3 is less affected by changes in the thyroid binding proteins because T_3 is poorly bound to carrier proteins. T_3 constitutes approximately 4 to 5 percent of the total thyroid hormone population in circulation and exerts a greater biologic effect than T_4, since it is so poorly bound. The thyroid gland secretes a small amount of T_3, more so in iodine-deficient states. About 80 percent of circulating T_3 comes from the peripheral deiodination of T_4 by a 5′-monodeiodination occurring in muscles, liver, and other tissues. Therefore T_4 serves as a prohormone for the biologically active T_3.

T_3 and T_4 are probably bound by cell membranes and transferred to the cell nucleus, stimulating protein synthesis by enhancing the transfer of amino acids from soluble RNA to microsomal protein. The significance of mitochondrial and other intracellular binding sites remains to be explored.

MATERNAL THYROID FUNCTION

During pregnancy, the maternal thyroid gland responds to a number of physiologic changes. Iodine turnover is increased because of a higher glomerular filtration rate and renal iodine clearance. This causes a decrease in the amount of iodine sequestered by the thyroid gland and is probably responsible for some degree of glandular hypertrophy.

Placental estrogen synthesis and secretion stimulate an increased hepatic production of thyroxine-binding globulin. Therefore, more T_4 is bound to the increased amount of circulating protein. Even though the total circulating thyroid hormone is increased, the unbound bioactive T_4 is maintained in the euthyroid range. The metabolic clearance rate of T_4 and T_3 is reset at a slightly higher level during pregnancy. The response of TSH to TRH is greater during the 16th to 20th weeks of pregnancy. This finding is partially due to the effect of elevated estrogen levels on the pituitary and probably to higher circulating TRH levels.

Human chorionic gonadotropin (hCG) has thyroid-stimulating activity because of a low affinity interaction at the TSH receptor site. Early in pregnancy, during the time of maximal hCG rise, minimal elevations of free thyroid hormone have been documented. Exaggerated levels of hCG have produced clinical and metabolic pictures of hyperthyroidism in diseases such as hydatidiform moles and choriocarcinoma.

THYROID FUNCTION TESTING IN PREGNANCY

Alterations of thyroid function are seen during pregnancy as a result of a variety of hormone changes. Thyroxine-binding globulin rises to about two times its normal level between 8 and 12 weeks of pregnancy. This rise continues progressively until term, and the level then returns to baseline within 6 weeks after delivery. Total serum T_4 levels can be measured using radioimmunoassay techniques or competitive protein-binding techniques that evaluate the bound as well as the minute fraction of free T_4. The unbound hormone is what produces the biologic activity. Free levels of T_4 and T_3 are not increased throughout gestation. In view of elevated levels of thyroxine-binding globulin, direct measurements of free T_3 and T_4 give the most accurate readings. However, these techniques are not universally available, and therefore the best estimate of free hormonal activity is obtained by the T_3 resin uptake test (T_3RU).

T_3RU provides an indirect evaluation of serum thyroxine-binding globulin levels by measuring the amount of thyroxine-binding globulin saturation by thyroid hormones while measuring the unoccupied thyroid binding sites of thyroxine-binding globulin. It is performed by incubating the patient's serum with radioiodine-labeled T_3 together with ion exchange resin. The resin competes with thyroxine-binding globulin binding sites in the patient's serum for the tracer-labeled T_3. The results are reported as a percentage of tracer hormone that is absorbed onto the resin. During states of elevated thyroxine-binding globulin, such as pregnancy, more unoccupied binding sites are available and therefore the value of the T_3RU test is decreased. In pregnancy that is complicated by hyperthyroidism, the T_3RU test result is higher than normal. This reflects greater saturation of the thyroxine-binding globulin sites with the thyroid hormones, allowing the resin to bind more tracer hormone.

The free thyroxine index (FT_4I, T_7, T_{12}, or adjusted T_4) is calculated from T_4 and T_3RU values. The use of the following calculation in most cases corrects for conditions of altered thyroxine-binding globulin levels:

$$\text{Free thyroxine index } (FT_4I) = \text{Total } T_4 \times \frac{\text{Patient } T_3\text{RU value}}{\text{Mean normal } T_3\text{RU value}}$$

An elevated value is consistent with hyperthyroidism and a low value reflects hypothyroidism.

Calculating the free triiodothyronine index (FT_3I) using the formula

$$\text{Free triiodothyronine index } (FT_3I) = \text{Total } T_3 \times \frac{\text{Patient } T_3\text{RU value}}{\text{Mean normal } T_3\text{RU value}}$$

helps to confirm the diagnosis of thyroid toxicosis in cases with borderline to high FT_4I or in cases of T_3-thyrotoxicosis in which the FT_4I is normal in the presence of hyperthyroidism. The FT_3I cannot help in the diagnosis of hypothyroidism, since it falls within the normal limits of almost 30 percent of hypothyroid patients.

The most helpful test for the detection of primary hypothyroidism is serum TSH concentration, which must be elevated above normal to make the diagnosis. Undetectable values have been reported in almost 30 percent of euthyroid individuals. Serum TSH levels remain in the normal range throughout pregnancy. Elevated TSH levels in light of normal FT_4I values may be indicative of early thyroid failure, even though the patient is clinically euthyroid (subclinical hypothyroidism or latent hypothyroidism). Normal TSH values in the presence of a low FT_4I usually reflect secondary hypothyroidism of central (hypothalamic-pituitary) origin but have been seen in extremely ill individuals (sick euthyroid syndrome).

Antithyroglobulin and antimicrosomes are serum thyroid autoantibodies that are helpful in the diagnosis of chronic autoimmune thyroiditis or Hashimoto's thyroiditis. Some women with these antibodies during pregnancy or post partum may develop transient hyperthyroidism or hypothyroidism. Patients with euthyroid goiter or a positive family history of thyroid disease should be screened for these autoantibodies and should be followed closely if they are present. Positive autoantibodies are not specific for Hashimoto's thyroiditis or Graves' disease. Low autoantibody titers have been found to occur with multinodular goiter, silent or painless thyroiditis, and subacute thyroiditis.

HYPERTHYROIDISM

The frequency of hyperthyroidism in pregnancy has been reported with an incidence that approximates two cases per 1,000 pregnancies. Graves' disease is the most common form and is characterized by a diffuse goiter and at times exophthalmos and pretibial myxedema. Toxic nodular goiters found in thyroid hyperfunction from excessive pituitary TSH secretion are very uncommon. It is necessary to rule out trophoblastic disease when biochemical signs of hyperthyroidism appear during early pregnancy. The signs and symptoms of thyroid hyperactivity include nervousness, tachycardia, weakness, increased appetite, heat intolerance, and shortness of breath. These symptoms may be difficult to distinguish from similar complaints of normal pregnancy.

Most women with mild to moderate hyperthyroid disease appear to tolerate pregnancy well. There is no clear evidence that pregnancy worsens the disease or makes it more difficult to treat. However, thyroid storm is a complication that may be encountered in undiagnosed or undertreated patients. Adequate control of hyperthyroidism is essential for both fetal and maternal well-being. In situations in which maternal hyperthyroidism is untreated, stillbirth rates have been reported to increase to 8 to 15 percent and premature delivery is considered to be increased to 11 to 25 percent.

Therapy is necessary to avoid serious maternal and fetal complications. Many patients may become more symptomatic and develop thyrotoxicosis, which can be considered a medical emergency during labor and delivery. A goiter with hyperthyroidism in the fetus may occur when stimulated by a long-acting thyroid stimulator of the IgG type that crosses the placenta from the maternal circulation. Serum T_4 values above 16μg per deciliter with a normal T_3 resin uptake are helpful in diagnosing hyperthyroidism during pregnancy.

After the diagnosis of hyperthyroidism in the pregnant woman, a decision must be made whether to treat the patient medically or surgically. Radioactive iodine therapy (^{131}I) has no place in the treatment of hyperthyroidism during pregnancy because of its damaging effects on the fetal thyroid after placental transfer. Fetal synthesis of thyroid hormone begins at approximately 10 to 12 weeks, when colloid and follicle formation may be demonstrated and the gland begins to concentrate iodine. Inadvertent exposure to radioactive iodine around the time of the missed menstruation, does not usually propose a specific risk to the fetal thyroid gland prior to the 10th week of gestation.

A subtotal thyroidectomy is reserved for patients who fail to respond to medical management because of poor compliance, severe disease, or the need for excessive amounts of antithyroid medication. Postoperative complications may include hypothyroidism, hypoparathyroidism, airway obstruction, recurrent laryngeal nerve paralysis, and infection.

Medical treatment of hyperthyroidism is the primary form of treatment during pregnancy. The thiourea derivatives are intended to decrease the amount of circulating thyroid hormones and to decrease the excessive thyroid symptoms. Hyperthyroidism is best treated during pregnancy by using the minimal effective dose regardless of treatment. A small number of infants with a birth weight less than the 25th percentile, goiter, and premature delivery can be anticipated when the mother has hyperthyroidism. Propylthiouracil (PTU) is usually prescribed in three or four divided doses starting between 200 and 400 mg per day with maintenance doses in the 50 to 100 mg range. Since PTU has a relatively short duration of action, frequent doses each day may be necessary. Patients should be followed closely for improvement of their symptoms, including weight gain and normalization of pulse as well as decline in serum T_4 levels. The response of hyperthyroidism to therapy depends on the lengthy period needed to deplete thyroid stores, which may persist until 3 to 6 weeks after the initiation of treatment. At that time, if the free T_4 is falling, the dose of PTU may be reduced. Subsequent monitoring of thyroid activity is done every 2 weeks to avoid hypothyroidism and to minimize the effective dose necessary. Serum free T_4 levels should be maintained within an upper limit of normal or slightly elevated range during pregnancy. Reducing the dose and even discontinuing the drug are possible and desirable, especially late in pregnancy. Daily doses exceeding 300 mg should be avoided because of potential effects on the fetus.

Minor side effects for the mother, such as nausea, headaches, or jaundice during PTU therapy, are infrequently found and are usually well tolerated. Agranulocytosis is the most serious complication and occurs in about one in 500 cases; therefore a leukocyte count should be determined before therapy and regularly thereafter. A blood count needs to be performed immediately if fever, sore throat, or diarrhea develops. Minor allergic reactions such as mild purpuric rashes may resolve spontaneously without discontinuing the drug. Arthralgias involving the hands and wrist are infrequently seen.

Transplacental passage of antithyroid drugs and their effects on the fetus have been a great concern when using this medication during pregnancy. Fetal goiters and neonatal hypothyroidism appear to be rare complications of maternal therapy, however. In the past, thyroid replacement was given to mothers receiving PTU in the hope that it would protect the fetus from developing hypothyroidism. This practice should be discouraged because transplacental passage of T_3 and T_4 is minimal. Also, administration of thyroid hormones may make maternal thyrotoxicosis more difficult to control. Transient mild hypothyroxemia and elevated TSH values have been observed in neonates exposed to antithyroid medications in utero. It is therefore quite important to reevaluate abnormal neonatal blood studies several days after birth in this group of infants. Thyroxin and TSH levels usually revert to normal in approximately 5 days. In previous studies, the intellectual development of children whose mothers received PTU during gestation was compared with that of siblings not exposed to antithyroid medication, and it was found that long-term intellectual development was not impaired.

Careful evaluation of the neonate for hyperthyroidism is equally important. It has been estimated that 1 percent of women with Graves' disease give birth to infants with neonatal hyperthyroidism. Thyroid stimulation of the fetus is believed to result from maternal passage of a thyroid-stimulating immunoglobulin, formerly referred to as LATS. Most cases of neonatal hyperthyroidism are usually transient, but some may progress and, if they remain unrecognized, central nervous system development may be impaired. It has been shown that infants born with toxic goiters may demonstrate significantly retarded intellectual development.

Methimazole (Tapazole) is another thiourea derivative that prevents the iodination of tyrosine by inhibiting the oxidation of iodide to iodine. Methimazole offers no advantages over PTU during pregnancy and may have more adverse side effects for the fetus. Recommended dosage range varies between 20 and 40 mg per day in divided doses, with maintenance doses of 5 to 15 mg per day. In comparable dosage ranges, methimazole lacks the ability to inhibit peripheral monodeiodination of T_4 to T_3. Methimazole is metabolized more slowly and transferred more rapidly across the placenta than PTU. A maldevelopment of the fetal scalp, aplasia cutis, has also been described with methimazole use. In light of this rare but severe anomaly, PTU has been the recommended standard antithyroid drug for use during pregnancy.

Propranolol, a beta-adrenergic blocking drug, has been successfully used when the symptoms of hyperthyroidism are found to be severe. Tachycardia, tremors, hyperreflexia, and palpitations are related to enhanced sympathomimetic activity and are readily controlled by beta-blocking agents. Although it is not intended to correct the altered metabolism, propranolol may also decrease the peripheral conversion of T_4 to T_3. Oral dosages of 10 to 30 mg three to four times daily are usually adequate for symptomatic relief. An intravenous dose of 1 to 3 mg may be given slowly, either during severe thyrotoxicosis or to avoid thyrotoxicosis before or during an operation or delivery. Prolonged use of propranolol should be avoided, and the dose should be titrated to maintain a maternal pulse above 80 beats per minute and to control tremors and nervousness.

Adverse maternal symptoms from propranolol use are uncommon and are usually dose-dependent. Bradycardia, hypotension, and congestive heart failure may result. These adverse side effects are more common if a preexisting heart condition is present. Bronchial spasm is possible with propranolol therapy, and therefore caution should be taken with its use in a patient with a history of asthma. Propranolol may compete with $beta_2$-adrenergic agents used to inhibit premature labor and may actually increase uterine muscle tone.

Propranolol does cross the placenta, but no congenital anomalies have been associated with its use. A higher incidence of growth-retarded neonates has been seen with propranolol use, which may be attributed to the underlying metabolic condition. Intermittent mild bradycardia of the fetal heart rate may be seen during the antepartum and interpartum periods. The fetal serum propranolol concentration is approximately 20 percent of the maternal concentration. Glucose and calcium levels and electrolyte balance are usually not impaired in the neonate. On occasion hypoglycemia may be encountered. Intravenous propranolol use prior to administration of anesthesia for cesarean section has been associated with transient neonatal respiratory depression. At present, the recommendation for propranolol during pregnancy is for severe thyrotoxicosis or preoperative management when antithyroid drugs are contraindicated. When used, it should be discontinued approximately 24 to 48 hours prior to delivery in order to minimize the risk of neonatal metabolic or respiratory side effects.

LABOR IN HYPERTHYROIDISM

The majority of gravid hyperthyroid women are under good control with antithyroid medications at the onset of labor. A euthyroid patient usually experiences no increased risk of complications of labor or of exacerbated hyperthyroidism. For the patient in whom hyperthyroidism was not detected prior to the onset of labor, more drastic measures are necessary to avoid the risk of severe accelerated hyperthyroidism precipitated by the stress of labor and delivery. The untreated woman should be started on blocking doses of antithyroid medication at the onset of labor and begun on intravenous sodium iodide (1 g) therapy to block the release of preformed thyroid hormone from the thyroid gland. The beta-blockers such as propranolol may be used carefully in the event of tachycardia and circulatory distress. Oral or parenteral corticosteroids such as dexamethasone, 2 mg four times a day for 24 hours, should be added because evidence exists that they may decrease circulating T_3 levels and may reduce the morbidity of what is often termed thyroid storm. Steroid medication may alter thyroid hormones by decreasing cellular prostaglandin action at the level of the thyroid and reducing hormonal release. It may also inhibit peripheral deiodination to T_3. This combination drug regimen reduces maternal morbidity without undue danger to the fetus. Accelerating degrees of hyperthyroidism remain a significant complication, although this deterioration has not been known to be common in the pregnant hyperthyroid patient.

THYROID STORM

Thyroid storm is an infrequent emergency that may occur in the undiagnosed as well as the partially treated hyperthyroid patient. It is more likely to occur when there is some precipitating factor such as infection, surgery, or labor and delivery. The clincial symptoms of exaggerated hypermetabolism are characterized by hyperprexia (>103° F), tachycardia, agitation, prostration, and severe dehydration. The fatality rate can be as high as 25 percent despite good medical management. Hypotension and cardiovascular collapse may ensue if the condition is not recognized and promptly treated. Peripheral catecholamine-mediated effects from thyroid excess are responsible for the presentation of this disorder. Treatment with propranolol is usually successful in counteracting the catecholamine overload. Propranolol can be administered orally or intravenously in association with careful cardiac monitoring. After stabilization of the patient's pulse, an oral maintenance dose of 20 to 80 mg every 6 hours can be given. There is a great deal of insensible water loss from perspiration, and therefore aggressive intravenous hydration is important in the therapy during thyroid storm.

Precipitating factors should be alleviated if possible, and specific therapy should also include sodium iodide, 1 g intravenously, to block the secretion of thyroid hormone. An oral solution of saturated potassium iodine (5 to 10 drops of potassium iodide oral solution [SSKI], three times a day in water) can also be used. It should be noted that these iodinated compounds may cross the placenta and block fetal thyroid hormone synthesis. PTU should be started immediately in doses up to 1,800 mg per day and then tapered to a maintenance dose. This is to block the formation of thyroid hormone and the deiodination of T_4 to T_3. Dexamethasone should also be considered at 8 mg per day to further block the deiodination of T_4 to T_3. If malignant pyrexia is present, then hypothermia therapy should be instituted. When hyperthyroidism is diagnosed early in a pregnant woman and adequate therapy is initiated, this potentially fatal complication of thyrotoxicosis can be virtually eliminated.

HYPOTHYROIDISM

Hypothyroidism is often not seen in pregnancy because women with markedly reduced thyroid gland function may experience subfertility. Hypothyroidism in such cases is usually due to Hashimoto's disease, thyroid gland ablation by ^{131}I, previous surgery, or antithyroid medications. Hypothalamic or pituitary failure causing secondary hypothyroidism is rare, and only a few cases have been described in adults.

Symptoms of hypothyroidism include decreased energy, hyporeflexia, and lethargy. Sensitivity to cold may be an early manifestation. Patients often complain of hair loss, brittle nails, and dry skin. The voice may become husky and periorbital edema may become evident, especially during early morning hours. Stiffness and aching muscles along with muscular cramping may be found. Multiple symptoms associated with pregnancy may overlap with these classic hypothyroid symptoms, making the diagnosis of the disease difficult.

Diagnosis is made by the measurement of T_4 along with a binding measurement, thyroxine-binding globulin or T_3 resin uptake, and an elevated TSH. Autoimmune thyroiditis is usually diagnosed with significantly elevated thyroglobulin and microsomal antibody titers and perhaps a family history of autoimmune endocrine disorders. Any significant increase in TSH concentration (>6 μU per ml) during pregnancy signifies thyroid insufficiency and requires therapy.

The effect of hypothyroidism on pregnancy outcome has been widely debated. In untreated patients, the rate of first trimester fetal loss may approach 50 percent with a 20 percent stillbirth and neonatal death rate. However, more recent studies have shown that good obstetric practice is as important as treating the hypothyroid mother with replacement therapy.

Thyroid preparations are used to supplement low serum concentrations of free thyroid hormone. The two most commonly used preparations, thyroid extract and synthetic levothyroxin sodium, contain thyroxin (T_4). Additionally, thyroid extract contains levotriiodothyronine (T_3) in variable concentrations. Levothyroxine or Synthroid is the preferred drug during pregnancy, since patients seem to tolerate this therapy better than thyroid extract. The patient is usually begun on 0.05 to 0.1 mg per day, with the dose increased to a maximum of 0.2 mg per day over several weeks. Ideal replacement may be titrated by following the serum TSH concentration, which may take up to 2 months to return to baseline. Thyroid extract has been held in disfavor because of the unpredictability in the preparation contents and, in particular, the high serum T_3 levels that patients may develop.

Thyroid hormone supplementations do not traverse the placental barrier in any appreciable amount and should have no effect on the fetal thyroid pituitary function. The major complication with thyroxine therapy is overdose, and signs of excessive thyroid hormone replacement may range from subclinical to overt. The response to thyroid supplementation should therefore be determined by the standard thyroid tests. The dosage of levothyroxine should be such that the TSH level is less than 6 μU per milliliter.

POSTPARTUM THYROID DYSFUNCTION

Occurrence of subclinical thyroid disease may be seen in the postpartum period. Physiologic and immunologic changes associated with pregnancy may ameliorate autoimmune thyroiditis during gestation. During the postpartum time period, however, the autoimmune thyroiditis may intensify and transient thyrotoxicosis may develop, followed by transient hypothyroidism. Patients who are often seen have a previous history of goiter with the development of thyroid enlargement between 1 to 4 months post partum. When they are examined, transient thyrotoxicosis is found, followed by hypothyroidism with spontaneous recovery in approximately 90 percent of the cases at 5 to 10 months post partum. These patients usually have antithyroid microsomal antibodies and high tiers, with the persistence of a small goiter. Patients with previous postpartum hypothyroidism tend to develop similar episodes with the same severity of hypothyroidism in subsequent pregnancies.

Hypothyroidism may last for several months. Although it is transient, it is reasonable to treat the patient as if she has classic hypothyroidism. After approximately 3 months of therapy, the administration of thyroid hormones can be stopped and thyroid function reevaluated.

CHRONIC LYMPHOCYTIC THYROIDITIS (HASHIMOTO'S DISEASE)

Chronic thyroiditis is a common autoimmune disorder that occurs in women of all age groups. The histologic features in the goiters demonstrate lymphoid follicles, diffuse round cell infiltration, connective tissue formation, and changes in the acinar epithelium. The cause of chronic lymphocytic thyroiditis is not known, but the disease is associated with serum antibodies directed against thyroglobulin and microsomal fractions of the thyroid gland. Hashimoto's disease is frequently associated with patients who have insulin-dependent diabetes, Addison's disease, Down syndrome, and Turner's syndrome.

In most pregnant patients, the only indication of Hashimoto's disease is the finding of an asymptomatic goiter on physical examination. The thyroid gland has an irregular contour and is typically firm in consistency. There is usually no tenderness associated with the enlargement. The patient may be euthyroid, hyperthyroid, or hypothyroid. In pregnant women, the symptoms of mild hypothyroidism may be masked by the normal metabolic changes of gestation.

Thyroid autoantibodies are almost always present. The hypothyroidism is confirmed by a low serum T_4 value (usually <8 μg per deciliter) and an elevated serum TSH level (>6 μU per milliliter). During the hyperthyroid phase of Hashimoto's disease, it is difficult to distinguish it from Graves' disease, although the ophthalmologic signs of Graves' disease are not found in Hashimoto's disease. If the serum T_4 level is higher than 20 μg per deciliter and the FT_4I, FT_3, and FT_4 levels are elevated, a low dosage of PTU (25 to 50 mg every 8 hours) may be initiated. In patients with mild symptoms and normal maternal weight gain with normal fetal growth and normal ultrasonographic findings, treatment may not be necessary. Evaluation of the fetus should include serial ultrasonography to detect possible intrauterine growth retardation and close measurements of the fetal heart for tachycardia or bradycardia.

A small group of hyperthyroid patients have clinical features of both Graves' disease and Hashimoto's thyroiditis. This combined picture has been named "Hashitoxicosis." The histologic examination from these goiters demonstrates abnormalities from both disease processes. Infants born to affected mothers may be at risk for either neonatal hypothyroidism or hyperthyroidism.

SOLITARY THYROID NODULE

The development of a single thyroid nodule during pregnancy is quite rare, but the concern is a possible malignancy. Thyroid biopsy is usually recommended, along with routine thyroid function tests. Radioisotope scanning is contraindicated during pregnancy; ultrasonography is the preferred method for evaluating a solitary thyroid nodule. A cystic lesion is usually benign. In the case of a suspicious malignancy, surgical evaluation should be undertaken. If the biopsy is benign and the nodule is enlarging, then an attempt at thyroid hormone treatment for suppression can be started without any risk to the fetus.

MULTINODULAR GOITER

The etiology of multiple nodular formation of the thyroid gland is not well understood. Speculations include hypersensitive TSH receptors in clones of thyroid cells along with innate hyperactivity of the follicular cell at the postreceptor level. The follicular heterogeneity of the normal thyroid gland has been well documented, proving the potential for nodular development in all thyroid tissues. If a patient had previously been placed on thyroid hormonal suppression therapy in hopes of suppressing further enlargement, this should be continued throughout the pregnancy. Stopping this medication may reveal permanent hypothyroidism due to an associated autoimmune thyroiditis and is not recommended during the pregnancy. If the patient is euthyroid, observation is all that is required.

SUBACUTE THYROIDITIS

Subacute thyroiditis is thought to be a viral-like inflammation of the thyroid gland that can manifest with either painful or painless enlargement associated initially with the release of thyroid hormone from damaged glandular tissue followed by thyroid failure when cellular demise occurs. The transient appearance of thyroid antibodies in low titers can occur, along with increased T suppressor cells. The majority of patients have total recovery of normal thyroid function. Thyroid hormone supplementation may be needed for the hypothyroid phase. Low-dose steroid therapy for the pain is contraindicated because of the possible effects on the fetus. The acute onset of painful subacute thyroiditis in pregnancy is extremely rare.

HYDATIDIFORM MOLE AND CHORIOCARCINOMA

Hydatidiform moles have been noted to elevate the total serum T_4 concentration two- to three-fold above that in normal pregnancy. Interestingly, the symptoms and signs of maternal hyperthyroidism are not overt. The high levels of T_4 can be correlated with the size of the mole and essentially reflects the secretion of the thyroid-stimulating beta subunit of hCG.

It has also been found that patients with choriocarcinoma have increased thyroid function without clinical hyperthyroidism. In this group of patients, the plasma level of hCG may be greatly elevated but is refractory to the effects of the hormone, with a desensitization at receptor and postreceptor sites. Normalization of thyroid function has been found after excision of moles. In addition, surgical removal of or chemotherapy for the choriocarcinoma has resulted in euthyroid hormone levels. When a pregnant woman has elevated thyroid hormone levels with little or no evidence of hypermetabolism, the diagnosis of molar gestation or choriocarcinoma should be pursued.

THYROID CARCINOMA

Carcinoma of the thyroid has not been found to affect the course of pregnancy, nor has pregnancy had any significant effects on the course of thyroid carcinoma. Multiple studies have not demonstrated any alteration in the growth of the tumors or metastasis in these women.

In the evaluation of solitary nodules or very firm goiters during pregnancy, ultrasonography and fine needle biopsy have been extremely important diagnostic tools. Surgical evaluation of a suspicious nodule during the second trimester may be indicated in patients who have previously received irradiation of the face or neck (for acne or thymic enlargement) or who have firm nodules with regional lymphadenopathy or a family history of medullary thyroid carcinoma. Usually, however, TSH suppression with exogenous thyroid hormone and a delay in further diagnostic evaluation and therapeutic procedures until after delivery are reasonable.

The diagnosis of carcinoma during pregnancy is not an absolute indication for terminating the pregnancy, nor is pregnancy a contraindication to the necessary thyroid surgery. However, radioactive iodine therapy (which is rarely indicated) should be withheld until after delivery.

SUGGESTED READING

Burrow GN. Thyroid disease. In: Burrow GN, Ferris TF, eds. Medical complications during pregnancy. Philadelphia: WB Saunders, 1982:187.

Gibson M, Tulchinsky D. The maternal thyroid. In: Tulchinsky D, Ryan KJ, eds. Maternal-fetal endocrinology. Philadelphia: WB Saunders, 1980:115.

Rayburn WF, McNulty RM, O'Shaughnessy RW. Endocrine disorders during pregnancy. In: Rayburn WF, Zuspan FP, eds. Drug therapy in obstetrics and gynecology. Norwalk, CT: Appleton-Century-Crofts, 1986:93.

HEART DISEASE

KENT UELAND, M.D.

Our knowledge of basic cardiovascular physiology in general and as it pertains to pregnancy in particular has improved considerably during the past 2 decades. New research techniques, along with noninvasive methods for evaluating cardiac function and anatomy, have provided us with the opportunity to assess hemodynamic competence carefully and improve our ability to manage even the most critically ill patient with cardiovascular disease.

The changing pattern of heart disease in pregnancy has also become apparent during the last 3 decades. Rheumatic fever and its sequela, rheumatic heart disease, have declined dramatically and are infrequently encountered in the United States except in the South American or Southeast Asian immigrant. Congenital heart disease, on the other hand, is encountered more frequently in the woman of child-bearing age. This is mostly the result of the fact that more children born with congenital heart defects are surviving into adulthood because of cardiac surgery and to a lesser extent because of improved medical management. As a result, more children are born to women with congenital heart disease who, because of heredity, are at greater risk of having congenital heart disease themselves, frequently the same lesion as the parent. Another challenging problem now encountered with increasing frequency is the pregnant woman who underwent palliative or partly corrective surgery during childhood and presents with an altered hemodynamic state with which there is little if any experience. Last are the groups of young women with valvular prostheses who frequently need long-term anticoagulation therapy, and the drug abuser with the occasional devastating tricuspid valve bacterial endocarditis.

Fortunately, our capacity to manage even the most difficult problems has improved with the help of modern technology, and most women with heart disease can negotiate pregnancy safely. However, there are still women with a few cardiovascular lesions in whom pregnancy is exceedingly dangerous and contraindicated. These individual lesions, their pathophysiology and risk factors as they relate to pregnancy, and the therapeutic alternatives will be discussed in detail.

THERAPEUTIC ALTERNATIVES

Ideally, women with correctable cardiovascular lesions should have surgery prior to becoming pregnant. However, frequently the woman is seen by a physician for the first time after she has become pregnant. There are certain general guidelines in management that should be followed in caring for all pregnant patients with heart disease. In order to minimize fear and anxiety for both potential parents, it is important not to overdiagnose heart disease. Therefore, unless the diagnosis is firm, consider the cardiovascular system normal and avoid extensive testing that can create unnecessary anxiety. When treating a pregnant patient with heart disease, prioritize maternal health and safety. Use whatever diagnostic and therapeutic modalities are necessary for optimal maternal care while utilizing a form of therapy that is least hazardous to the fetus. The obstetrician should be the primary physician, but consultants should be used freely as part of a management team, including a cardiologist, anesthesiologist, and neonatologist.

The therapeutic goals are to improve or prevent deterioration in cardiovascular function, to prevent complications, and to prolong life. Optimal hemodynamic status can be maintained by appropriate medication, by dietary restriction, by limitation of physical activity, and by appropriate counseling and reassurance. In selected at-risk individuals, antibiotic prophylaxis against rheumatic fever is indicated. In others, prophylaxis against endocarditis is mandatory at delivery or for dental or surgical procedures. In some, long-term anticoagulation therapy is required to prevent or reduce the risk of thromboembolism. All of these issues need to be addressed, and appropriate application can significantly improve the outcome for both mother and fetus and ensure a safer pregnancy.

Medical Therapy

The mainstay of management of the pregnant cardiac patient is medical, in order to achieve optimal health. A delicate balance among regular exercise and rest and good nutrition in order to prevent obesity and anemia is an important aspect of management. In some women with certain forms of cardiovascular disease, strict limitation of all physical activity is required. In others, prohibition of certain forms of activity may be necessary. Since exercise during pregnancy exerts a greater demand on the heart, some women may find that certain forms of activity that were tolerated without symptoms prior to pregnancy may result in symptoms during pregnancy. One should use clinical indications such as fatigue, dyspnea, palpitations, and excessive tachycardia to titrate the amount of physical exercise of which a patient is capable. The symptoms produced by exercise should disappear within 10 minutes of stopping. If they persist beyond this time, some modification of activity becomes necessary.

Another factor that increases the demand on the heart is emotional stress. Counseling and firm reassurance are important in order to allay the patient's fears about her heart disease. Counseling and educating the patient's family are equally important, so that they have a full understanding of the patient's special problem and the interaction of her heart disease with pregnancy, including the prognosis for the health of the baby.

Other conditions that increase the cardiac burden include obesity and anemia. Caloric adjustment may be necessary in order to prevent excessive weight gain. In the average sized woman with appropriate weight for stature, a 25-pound weight gain for pregnancy seems ideal. Since all pregnant women develop a "physiologic" anemia during pregnancy regardless of the status of their iron stores, the routine use of iron and folate supplements is mandatory. The iron demands of pregnancy cannot be met by diet alone during the second and third trimesters, and the iron supplement modifies the total fall in hemoglobin, especially in women with low hemoglobin levels and deficient iron stores prior to pregnancy.

Medical conditions that increase the demand on the heart include hyperthyroidism, infection, and tachyarrhythmia. Although it is not a frequent complication associated with pregnancy, hyperthyroidism has been reported to cause heart failure. Prompt evaluation and therapy are important in order to decrease the cardiac output and heart rate associated with the hypermetabolic state. If the patient has severe clinical manifestations, therapy with a beta-blocker may be necessary until propylthiouracil therapy becomes effective several weeks after initiation of treatment. Infections of all kinds during pregnancy in women with heart disease should be treated promptly. The increase in cardiac burden caused by fever and, in those women with respiratory infection, by the work of coughing, can be substantial. Prevention of many viral infections can be achieved through appropriate immunizations before pregnancy is contemplated. This should include influenzal immunization. Most authorities also recommend vaccination against pneumococci because pneumococcal pneumonia can be a serious problem in pregnant women with cardiovascular disease.

Although acute rheumatic fever is rarely encountered during pregnancy, prophylaxis against streptococcal infections is advisable for women who have had documented rheumatic fever in the past and for those who have rheumatic heart disease. Prophylaxis against bacterial endocarditis is also recommended for most women with cardiovascular disease at the time of delivery and during dental procedures or any invasive diagnostic or therapeutic procedure. Three doses 8 hours apart of ampicillin (1 g IM or IV) and gentamicin (1.5 mg per kilogram IM or IV) are suggested because of the broad spectrum of coverage provided.

Tachyarrhythmia can precipitate pulmonary edema, especially in women with mitral stenosis. Prompt recognition and treatment are important, and women with intrinsic abnormalities of rhythm or a history of recurrent problems need long-term antiarrhythmic therapy.

The treatment of cardiovascular complications during pregnancy, such as pulmonary edema and congestive heart failure, is similar to that for a nonpregnant individual. However, readjustment of the dose of certain drugs, i.e., digitalis, is frequently necessary because of the increased blood volume and glomerular filtration rate and the passage of the drug into the fetal compartment. The use of cardiovascular drugs in pregnancy is discussed in more detail in the section dealing with the fetus and neonate.

Cardiovascular Surgery

Although there are many reports in the literature

regarding cardiac surgery during pregnancy for a variety of lesions, it is infrequently indicated. Pregnancy is not an optimal time to perform surgery because basal conditions do not prevail and the cardiac burden is substantially higher than in the nonpregnant state. Furthermore, there is suggestive evidence of anatomic changes in the media of the aorta associated with pregnancy that may or may not be related to vessel strength. It is also possible that there are subtle changes in the heart that could conceivably interfere with postoperative healing. Nonetheless, cardiac surgery in pregnancy should be offered only as a management choice in those few women with life-threatening disease in whom surgery would improve outcome. In exceedingly rare cases, a combined approach of cesarean section and open heart surgery may be considered. This unusual combination must be well timed in order to optimize neonatal and maternal outcomes. It circumvents the risk to the fetus if cardiopulmonary bypass is required and allows the mother to receive the best surgical procedure.

Mitral commissurotomy, both open and closed, has been performed in numerous pregnant patients in the past with an excellent maternal and perinatal outcome. Unfortunately, the procedure is only palliative, and the benefits of the operation are temporary. Again this operation is best performed under basal conditions, and most women with predominant mitral stenosis respond well to strict medical management. Fortunately, severe rheumatic mitral valve stenosis is now infrequently encountered in this country and the need for surgery has markedly diminished.

The need for surgery for congenital cardiovascular disease in pregnancy is exceedingly limited. Pregnancy in most women with congenital lesions can be undertaken safely, and surgical correction is rarely justified. Nonetheless, there are several reports in the literature documenting successful repair of atrial septal defects, coarctation of the aorta, patent ductus arteriosus, pulmonic stenosis, tetralogy of Fallot, and ventricular septal defect.

There are now several case reports in the literature of the use of cardiopulmonary bypass during open heart surgery in pregnancy. Older data reported fetal loss at 33 percent when using a variety of oxygenators and with a gestational age range from 2 to 18 weeks. Most now feel that open heart surgery should be delayed until the fourth month, following completion of organogenesis. More recent data reported in the literature show a fetal survival rate in excess of 80 percent. However, several reports have documented the occurrence of sustained fetal bradycardia during the bypass, which at times was partially corrected by increasing the flow rate. Current opinion would seem to favor maintaining extracorporeal pump flow at a high level, in the range of 3.0 L per minute per square meter of body surface area. With adequate hypothermia, a rate of 2.0 L per minute per square meter of body surface area seems adequate. The latter has been used successfully in over 20 cases during pregnancy with maternal rectal temperature ranging between 26.5 and 32° C.

In summary, cardiovascular surgery during pregnancy plays a very small but definitive role in the management of the cardiac patient. Strict medical management remains the mainstay of therapy.

Contraception, Therapeutic Abortion, and Sterilization

The two main reliable and relatively safe contraceptive techniques currently being used worldwide are oral contraceptives and the intrauterine device (IUD). However, in the United States, because of problems with pelvic inflammatory disease, the use of the IUD has virtually ceased. Only the progestin-releasing devices are in use in this country at the present time because they appear to carry a lower risk of infection. IUDs are not recommended for use in women with cardiovascular disease at high risk of developing bacterial endocarditis, i.e., those with coarctation of the aorta, patent ductus arteriosus, aortic valve disease, ventricular septal defect, or mitral regurgitation. They are relatively contraindicated in women with significant arrhythmias or cardiac disease that predisposes to them. In all cases, a small-diameter device is indicated, i.e., Progestasert. Birth control pills are the most reliable means of preventing pregnancy. The complications that have been reported with the use of oral contraceptives in the past have been minimized with the introduction of low-dose preparations. When they are prescribed in women with cardiac disease, a low estrogen tablet (20 to 50 μg) should be used.

However, in some women with certain forms of cardiovascular disease oral contraceptives are contraindicated, e.g., in those with prosthetic heart valves, pulmonary hypertension, cardiomyopathy, Marfan's syndrome, and hypertensive cardiovascular disease. Birth control pills appear safe in women with uncomplicated congenital heart disease such as atrial septal defect, ventricular septal defect, and patent ductus arteriosus and in women with most valvular disease as long as they have a normal sinus rhythm.

Barrier contraception can also be safely used in women with cardiovascular disease. However, unless the individual using a condom, diaphragm, or sponge and spermicidal foam is sufficiently motivated, pregnancy rates are unacceptable. In reliable and intelligent hands, a diaphragm and spermicidal foam or jelly are as effective as IUDs or birth control pills.

The long-acting injectable progestins are the last form of contraception to be considered. Over 3 million women in the world currently use this form of contraception, but it has not been approved for use in this country by the Food and Drug Administration. These agents are as effective as birth control pills and seem to have no cardiovascular side effects. In the future, this form of contraception may supplant all others in the cardiac patient.

Permanent contraception or sterilization such as vasectomy or bilateral tubal ligation is indicated when a women has a nonreparable and life-threatening cardiovascular lesion. Although vasectomy is now an acceptable means of sterilization, it makes little sense to sterilize the male partner when it is the female who suffers from heart disease. Therefore, under most circumstances it seems inappropriate to sterilize the man who will outlive his wife and who may, in the future, wish to have children with another partner. Bilateral tubal ligation is reserved for those few women who have certain forms of high-risk cardiovascular diseases such as dilated cardiomyopathy, Eisenmenger's syndrome, Marfan's syndrome, and primary pulmonary hypertension. These conditions are life-threatening to a woman undertaking pregnancy and are similarly hazardous to the woman taking birth control pills. In women with surgically correctable heart disease or in those with a lesion such as mitral stenosis for which palliative surgery can temporarily improve their cardiac status, some form of contraception is recommended until surgery can be performed. Pregnancy can then be carefully timed and undertaken when there is maximum cardiovascular reserve.

Therapeutic abortion is recommended during the first trimester in those women with high-risk cardiovascular disease as outlined in the previous paragraph. This also applies to any woman whose cardiac status exposes her to unacceptable risks. To be safe, early interruption is necessary prior to the time when maternal hemodynamic demands are evident and when the procedure itself is safe.

CARDIOVASCULAR DISEASE CLASSIFIED ACCORDING TO MATERNAL RISKS

Pulmonary Hypertension

This is a strong contraindication to pregnancy regardless of etiology. In primary pulmonary hypertension a maternal mortality rate in excess of 50 percent has been consistently reported in the literature. In the Eisenmenger's syndrome the maternal mortality again approaches 50 percent. The most common cause of this syndrome is a ventricular septal defect. It also carries the highest maternal mortality as compared with an atrial septal defect and a patent ductus arteriosus. The prognosis for the fetus in those mothers who survive is also unfavorable, with over a 50 percent prematurity rate and a 30 percent incidence of intrauterine growth retardation.

The current recommendation for nonpregnant women with documented pulmonary hypertension is sterilization by a bilateral tubal ligation. Early therapeutic abortion is recommended for those who are already pregnant.

Although early therapeutic abortion appears safer than continuing the pregnancy, any surgical intervention can be dangerous and should be performed under continuous invasive hemodynamic monitoring.

Maternal death may occur at any time during pregnancy, but the risk is greatest during labor, delivery, and the early puerperium. The mortality risk increases with increasing pulmonary pressures. Management in those women who choose to continue the pregnancy against medical advice is aimed at maintaining pulmonary blood flow and perfusion of vital organs, maintaining venous return, preventing increases in pulmonary vascular resistance, and maintaining peripheral vascular resistance. The latter is particularly important in patients with Eisenmenger's syndrome, in which right-to-left or bidirectional shunting exists.

Antepartum weekly physician visits are suggested, along with limited physical activity, use of elastic support hose, home oxygen administration, and monthly platelet counts. In preparation for labor and delivery, Swan-Ganz catheter monitoring is imperative, along with continuous rhythm monitoring in an intensive care unit. Blood should be available, prophylactic antibiotics should be given, and hypovolemia and hypotension should be strictly avoided. Postdelivery continuous hemodynamic monitoring must be maintained, and elastic support hose used with early and supervised ambulation. Most now recommend a scheduled cesarean section for delivery under inhalation anesthesia in order to have all necessary personnel with expertise available. Long-term management should include tubal ligation along with a trial of vasodilator therapy and chronic low-flow oxygen administration. The use of chronic anticoagulation therapy is controversial.

Marfan's Syndrome

Marfan's syndrome is associated with several significant risks during pregnancy. The most important cardiovascular hazards are acute aortic dissection or rupture or the development of intractable aortic regurgitation. Some past studies have reported a maternal mortality rate of 50 percent. Other more recent studies have shown a much smaller risk. It does appear, however, that the women at risk are those with a dilated aortic root. It has been recommended by some that women with an aortic diameter in excess of 40 mm as shown by echocardiography should not entertain pregnancy. Currently, however, most would counsel all women who fulfill the diagnostic criteria of Marfan's syndrome to avoid pregnancy.

In women who undertake pregnancy and in whom interruption is not acceptable, prompt limitation of physical activity is important, as is the administration of a beta-adrenergic blocking agent, although it is not clear whether or not the latter effectively decreases complications. For delivery, cesarean section under inhalation anesthesia with a negative inotropic agent such as halothane is suggested. This circumvents the repetitive and cumulative hemodynamic demands of labor and vaginal delivery. Antibiotic prophylaxis is recommended in women with aortic regurgitation. In women with Marfan's syndrome, life expectancy is approximately half that of normal. Therefore, affected women who desire a pregnancy despite medical advice to the contrary should complete their reproduction early in life. The hereditary aspects of the disease are discussed later.

Peripartum Cardiomyopathy

The diagnosis is suspected when clinical manifestations of cardiomyopathy appear near the end of pregnancy or in the puerperium. It is not distinguishable from other forms of dilated cardiomyopathy. If it exists prior to pregnancy, pregnancy is contraindicated because of the high risk of congestive heart failure and death. Maternal mortality as high as 50 percent has been reported. If a patient had cardiomyopathy with a prior pregnancy but without cardiomegaly, the risk of recurrence is substantial and pregnancy should be avoided. If the cardiomegaly persisted for 6 months or more, the risk of recurrence with a subsequent pregnancy is 50 percent, and the maternal mortality approaches 100 percent.

The rate of occurrence of peripartum cardiomyopathy

varies in different geographic areas. It is also more common in black, older, multiparous women or following a twin pregnancy or one complicated by toxemia. The etiology remains a mystery, but perhaps it is an exaggerated response to the decrease in myocardial contractility that is normally encountered in the puerperium.

Management consists of bed rest, restriction of sodium intake, and diuretics. Digitalis is used to improve myocardial contractility. If this is unsuccessful, afterload reduction is indicated with vasodilator therapy. If myocarditis is suspected, an endomyocardial biopsy should be performed. If the biopsy results are positive, immunosuppressive therapy is suggested. The two most common cardiovascular complications are arrhythmia (usually atrial fibrillation) and systemic arterial embolization. Prompt cardioversion is indicated in the former and anticoagulation therapy for the latter. In the puerperium, some recommend the use of warfarin (Coumadin) as long as the cardiomegaly persists.

The long-term prognosis for patients with peripartum cardiomyopathy is poor, especially in women with persistent cardiomegaly. Eighty-five percent die in just over 5 years, compared with 14 percent of those whose heart size returns to normal. It is clear that pregnancy should not be undertaken by anyone who has experienced a congestive or dilated cardiomyopathy, and early therapeutic abortion should be offered to those who do become pregnant.

Tetralogy of Fallot

The hazard to maternal life in women with tetralogy of Fallot is not as high as in those with pulmonary hypertension. Nonetheless, the maternal mortality rate has been reported in excess of 10 percent. The frequency of pregnancy in women with uncorrected tetralogy of Fallot is low and is probably related to subnormal fertility and sexual development. There is a high incidence of fetal loss, low birth rate, and congenital heart disease in the offspring. Pregnancy is therefore discouraged in these women, especially in those who have repeated syncopal attacks, high hematocrit values ($>$60 ml per deciliter), and a high right ventricular pressure ($>$120 mm Hg). The results of pregnancy in women who have had corrective surgery are much more favorable.

Management of patients with uncorrected tetralogy of Fallot includes limitation of physical activity, prompt treatment of arrhythmia, wearing of elastic hose support when they are ambulatory, and administration of low-flow oxygen, especially at night. Venesection for polycythemia is rarely necessary because of the normal hemodilution that accompanies pregnancy. During labor and delivery prophylactic antibiotics are recommended, along with continuous hemodynamic monitoring. Patient comfort is best maintained with conduction anesthesia (segmental epidural).

Strict maintenance of venous return is important in order to minimize right-to-left shunting by maintaining systemic vascular resistance. Blood loss must be carefully monitored and replaced if excessive. A forceps delivery in the second stage of labor is indicated when deemed safe obstetrically.

In patients who have had a palliative surgical procedure, the chances of having a successful pregnancy are good. In women with high hematocrit values, spontaneous abortion, preterm delivery, intrauterine fetal demise, and fetal growth retardation are common. Corrective surgery is, therefore, strongly recommended prior to contemplating a pregnancy. Following complete repair, long-term prognosis also improves substantially.

Coarctation of the Aorta

It is rare for women to have coarctation as an isolated lesion. It is frequently associated with a bicuspid aortic valve. Other cardiovascular congenital defects that may accompany it include patent ductus arteriosus, ventricular septal defect, mitral valve deformity, and aneurysms of the circle of Willis. The most common complication of coarctation of the aorta is sytemic arterial hypertension, but other complications can include left ventricular failure, rupture of the aorta, dissection of the aorta, rupture of a cerebral aneurysm, and endocarditis.

Maternal mortality has been reported to vary between 3 and 9 percent in coarctation of the aorta. Most commonly the deaths occur before labor and delivery. Intrapartum and puerperal deaths are rare. Although maternal mortality is relatively low compared with that for other high-risk cardiovascular lesions, the maternal complication rate is extremely high, and fetal mortality can reach 40 percent. The latter is attributed to reduced blood flow to the uterus and placental bed because of poor collateral circulation. Pregnancy following repair is relatively safe for the mother; however, the danger from associated cardiovascular anomalies still exists. Repair of the lesion in childhood is indicated and results in the best long-term prognosis. When the lesion is repaired in an adult, the operative mortality is much higher.

Control of blood pressure during pregnancy, labor, and delivery is important. A cardioselective beta-adrenergeric blocker seems most appropriate to use during pregnancy. In the author's opinion, surgical correction during pregnancy is not indicated. Segmental epidural anesthesia is recommended, along with a forceps delivery, in order to circumvent maternal bearing-down efforts in the second stage of labor. Antibiotic prophylaxis is strongly recommended at delivery. Cesarean section should be reserved for patients who have past evidence of an actual arterial rupture. Since the risks of aortic dissection and rupture are increased during pregnancy, an alternative approach to management would be an early termination of pregnancy, followed by corrective surgery in the nonpregnant state, and a subsequent safer pregnancy following recovery. This would be a more meaningful approach, especially in patients who exhibit cardiac failure or uncontrolled hypertension or have a history of a vascular accident.

Prosthetic Heart Valves

Artificial heart valves were introduced over 30 years ago. Current overall experience with pregnancy in women with artificial valves involves over 200 cases. One must keep in mind that the insertion of a prosthetic valve is never curative. However, the improved design and function of the newer prostheses have reduced the magnitude of the difficulties associated with them, although substantial problems still exist. The increasing use of tissue prostheses has also influenced the outcome of pregnancy in women with artificial valves and reduced the need for anticoagulation. This valve is preferred for young women who are contemplating pregnancy, even though it does not have the durability of mechanical prostheses.

The data in the literature support the contention that the fetal loss is two to three times as high in pregnant women with mechanical prostheses who are taking oral anticoagulants as in women with tissue prostheses who are not on anticoagulants. In the author's experience, women with mechanical valve prostheses on anticoagulant therapy run a high risk of hemorrhage and embolization during pregnancy. On the other hand, women with tissue valves run the risk of congestive heart failure due to valvular degeneration. However, the dangers of oral anticoagulation to the fetus would argue strongly for the use of tissue prostheses in young women. The alternative would be to switch to heparin anticoagulation prior to a contemplated pregnancy.

During pregnancy, limitation of physical activity is warranted, as are frequent visits for cardiac evaluation. Women on long-term anticoagulation therapy need to be warned about the potential fetal and maternal problems inherent in such therapy and informed about possible alternatives. Since these women are fully anticoagulated, conduction anesthesia during labor is contraindicated. With the onset of labor, heparin therapy can be temporarily discontinued and restarted soon after delivery. Prophylaxis against bacterial endocarditis is warranted at delivery, and if the prosthesis replaced a valve damaged by rheumatic fever, prophylaxis to prevent streptococcal infections should be continued. With improvement in design and function and the development of new and safer forms of anticoagulation therapy, the outcome of pregnancy in women with artificial valves should continue to improve.

Rheumatic Heart Disease

Rheumatic fever and its sequela rheumatic heart disease is encountered with decreasing frequency in developed Western countries. In addition, the severity of the disease has also diminished, and complications such as pulmonary edema, atrial fibrillation, heart failure, and systemic embolization are now rarely encountered. In spite of this, rheumatic heart disease is still sufficiently common to be discussed in this chapter and can be sufficiently severe to contribute to a serious risk during pregnancy. Interestingly, new cases of rheumatic heart disease are being encountered in Southeast Asian immigrants and in the Mexican-American population in whom past medical care has been poor or nonexistent.

In managing the pregnant patient with rheumatic heart disease, two basic principles must be kept in mind. First, continuous antibiotic prophylaxis against recurrence of rheumatic fever is necessary for all patients. Second, antibiotic prophylaxis against bacterial endocarditis is indicated in all patients with rheumatic valvular heart disease.

Since mitral stenosis is the dominant valve lesion in 90 percent of patients with rheumatic heart disease, this lesion will be discussed in detail. The outcome of pregnancy in women with mitral stenosis is directly dependent on the severity of the disease (functional classification) and whether or not atrial fibrillation is present. If the latter complicates rheumatic mitral stenosis, the maternal mortality rate can reach 15 percent.

Limitation of cardiac output both at rest and during exercise is encountered during pregnancy in all women with mitral stenosis, even those who are asymptomatic or mildly symptomatic. Careful and close medical management is indicated in these women during pregnancy, and most negotiate pregnancy safely. In general, symptoms provide a fairly accurate estimate of the severity of the disease, but not uniformly so. Some women with asymptomatic or mildly symptomatic disease (functional grades I and II) can develop pulmonary edema and even die. It is, therefore, important to stress that the effect of pregnancy on the cardiac status of women with mitral stenosis can be unpredictable. The time of maximum risk in these women is in the second half of pregnancy. This is a time when maximum cardiac output is maintained and when heart rate increases progressively. Data in the literature clearly support that contention, as pulmonary edema occurs with increasing frequency from 21-weeks gestation to term. Currently the most common cause of death in pregnant women with mitral stenosis is acute pulmonary edema. This is caused by mechanical obstruction to flow through the tight mitral valve.

Since the severity of stenosis is at times difficult to predict based on a patient's symptoms, careful hemodynamic evaluation prior to pregnancy is indicated in all women with confirmed disease. Doppler echocardiography is probably sufficient and reduces the need for an invasive study. In an occasional asymptomatic patient, severe mitral stenosis may be documented.

Guidelines for management are found in the section on Medical Therapy earlier in the chapter. Additional recommendations include the use of prophylactic digitalization in women who have an enlarged left atrium and in those with a past history of atrial fibrillation. This therapy prevents a rapid ventricular response, in the event that atrial fibrillation occurs, and decreases the maternal risk from such an event. If atrial fibrillation does occur, it constitutes a medical emergency, and prompt cardioversion is recommended.

In the occasional woman with severe mitral stenosis who develops pulmonary edema that is unresponsive to strict medical management in the hospital, uncontrollable hemoptysis, or significant pulmonary hypertension, mitral valvotomy should be considered. A closed mitral valvotomy is the preferred procedure, and in carefully selected patients this can be lifesaving. Much preferred is mitral valve surgery prior to pregnancy in patients with severe mitral stenosis. If this palliative surgery is successful, it is recommended that patients wait 1 year before becoming pregnant. Even though these patients may become asymptomatic, careful supervision during a subsequent pregnancy is mandatory, as they are still at risk of developing pulmonary edema. Maternal mortality as high as 3 percent has been reported.

There is no evidence that pregnancy has a long-term

detrimental effect on health in women with rheumatic mitral stenosis. In the past their life spans were substantially shorter than normal. However, with decreasing severity of the disease and diminishing incidence and severity of complications, long-term prognosis for these women has improved. This, in addition to major advances in medical and surgical care, has improved long-term survival in women with mitral stenosis.

CARDIOVASCULAR DISEASE AND ITS EFFECT ON THE FETUS AND NEONATE

The intrauterine fetal environment is optimized in several ways. Good maternal health habits prior to pregnancy, including good nutrition, regular exercise, and appropriate rest, improve pregnancy outcome. Surgical correction of remediable congenital heart lesions is an important consideration before pregnancy, as this has been shown to decrease the recurrence risks of some congenital heart lesions. This is especially true in women with cyanotic congenital cardiovascular disease because cyanosis has a deleterious effect on fetal growth and development. The outcome of pregnancy appears to be directly related to the level of the hematocrit, i.e., the severity of the cyanosis. Avoidance of cigarette smoking and excessive alcohol and caffeine ingestion also affects fetal well-being, as does abstinence from street drugs and most prescription drugs. Limitation of heavy physical activity in order to decrease the total burden on a diseased heart also seems important not only for maternal safety but also for fetal growth and development. This may be particularly important in women with mitral stenosis, as these women cannot increase their cardiac output to meet the normal needs of pregnancy. This discrepancy is substantially increased with exercise. However, mothers with asymptomatic or mildly symptomatic heart disease in general, whether it is congenital or rheumatic, have twice the prematurity rate of normal women, and when their babies are carried to term, they are smaller than those of normal women.

Fetal evaluation is begun at the first prenatal visit in women with cardiovascular disease. An ultrasound scan is performed to confirm gestational age and to serve as a baseline measurement for future scans used to evaluate fetal growth. The next ultrasound examination at 20 to 22 weeks is performed to evaluate fetal cardiac anatomy, particularly in women with congenital heart disease. Fetal echocardiography is also carried out. Fetal growth is evaluated at 4- to 6-week intervals beginning at approximately 26 weeks. If growth continues to be appropriate, no further fetal testing is deemed necessary. However, if there is evidence of fetal growth retardation, the ultrasound scans are repeated at 2-week intervals, along with a nonstress test or a contraction stress test weekly and a biophysical profile if necessary. Occasionally a preterm delivery is indicated if there is convincing evidence of fetal compromise. If such a delivery is being considered, fetal lung maturity should be defined by amniocentesis and determination of either a lecithin-sphingomyelin ratio or a phosphatidylglycerol test. A lecithin-sphingomyelin ratio of two-to-one or greater and the presence of phosphatidylglycerol indicate fetal lung maturity and would place the newborn at minimal risk of developing respiratory distress.

Cardiovascular Drugs

Cardiovascular drugs and drugs with cardiovascular effects are frequently used in managing patients with cardiac disease. The potential fetal and maternal complications from these drugs are described briefly in the following paragraphs.

Antiarrhythmics

In pregnancy most experience with this group of drugs has been with quinidine. Even though it crosses the placenta, there are no reports of teratogenicity. Since it is chemically related to quinine, a concern about preterm labor has been expressed but never validated.

Procainamide has been used to treat maternal arrhythmias, but it has been associated with the formation of antinuclear antibodies and development of psychosis and should probably be avoided. Disopyramide has been suggested to cause uterine hyperactivity and is, therefore, not recommended during pregnancy. Phenytoin, an effective drug for treating ventricular arrhythmias, should not be used, especially in the first trimester of pregnancy, because of its teratogenicity (fetal hydantoin syndrome). Its fetal effects in the second and third trimesters may include mental deficiency.

Anticoagulants

Warfarin derivatives in general are contraindicated at any time during pregnancy. These drugs readily cross the placenta and are teratogenic when given during the first trimester. Warfarin embryopathy occurs in approximately 15 to 20 percent of exposed embryos. The use of these agents later in pregnancy increases the risk of fetal hemorrhage and can cause excessive bleeding during labor and delivery.

Heparin, on the other hand, is the anticoagulant of choice during pregnancy in spite of the inconvenience of long-term parenteral administration. It does not cross the placenta and hence is not teratogenic. Prolonged administration can occasionally cause thrombocytopenia or osteoporosis.

The role of antiplatelet agents in pregnancy has not been established, but these agents cross the placenta and affect fetal as well as maternal clotting mechanisms. At this time their use must be considered experimental.

Beta-Adrenergic Blockers

These agents have not been shown to be teratogenic; however, some have been shown to have an oxytocic effect on the uterus. In fact, propranolol has been used to treat abnormal labor successfully. Potential fetal effects include intrauterine growth retardation. Neonatal complications reported include respiratory depression, decreased Apgar scores, hypoglycemia, hyperbilirubinemia, and polycythemia. These adverse effects should preclude frequent use of these agents during pregnancy. These remarks are directed at the nonselective beta-blockers. The newer, more selective beta-blockers, such as atenolol and metoprolol, do not appear to be associated with many of these adverse effects and have been successfully used to treat hypertension in pregnancy.

Calcium-Channel Blockers

These agents are effective in treating supraventricular tachycardia. Nifedipine has been successfully used as an antihypertensive agent and has also been shown to be an effective tocolytic agent. Little information is available about the fetal-neonatal effects of these agents, but preliminary animal work suggests that uterine blood flow decreases substantially when the drugs are given to the mother. Caution must be exercised regarding their use in pregnancy.

Diuretics

In the past these agents were extensively used to treat dependent edema of pregnancy, a condition now considered physiologic. There is little experience with the use of all but the thiazide diuretics in pregnancy. Fetal and neonatal complications reported with their use include hyponatremia, hypokalemia, hypoglycemia, and jaundice. Diuretic use in pregnancy should be reserved for cardiac patients who exhibit persistent pulmonary edema that is unresponsive to bed rest and sodium restriction. Potassium-sparing agents such as triamterene or spironolactone may be better alternatives.

Inotropics

Digitalis therapy in pregnancy has been proved safe, but the dose of the drug must be increased because of its rapid excretion by the kidney, the hypervolemia of pregnancy, and its transfer into the fetal compartment. None of the inotropic agents has been shown to be teratogenic.

Beta-agonists such as ritodrine, terbutaline, and hexoprenaline have been used extensively as tocolytic agents. Arrhythmia, myocardial ischemia, pulmonary edema, and maternal death have been reported with their use. They are absolutely contraindicated in the pregnant patient with any form of cardiovascular disease.

Vasodilators

These agents have seen extensive use in the past and are still used currently for the treatment of hypertension, and more recently they have been employed as afterload reducers. There is a great deal of experience with the use of hydralazine in the treatment of hypertension in pregnancy. No teratogenicity has been reported with its use, but it is infrequently used in the first trimester of pregnancy. Clonidine has seen little use in pregnancy and hence cannot be recommended at this time. Alpha-methyldopa has been used in pregnancy without any evidence of teratogenicity, but its effectiveness alone in treating hypertension is limited, and hence it should not be used as a front-line drug. Captopril has not been used a great deal in pregnancy. Preliminary animal and human data of potential teratogenic effects as well as reduced litter size in animals indicate that caution should be exercised with its use in pregnancy. Nitroprusside has been used in acute treatment of severe hypertension for the stabilization of patients prior to delivery. Short-term use, for 4 to 6 hours, has demonstrated no deleterious fetal effects. Long-term use may be harmful, and animal studies have shown fetal cyanide accumulation with its use.

GENETIC COUNSELING

The risk in the general population of a child's being born alive with congenital heart disease is 0.8 percent in the United States. It is more than twice as high in children who are born to fathers with congenital heart disease, a figure that is similar to when a sibling has congenital heart disease. If there are two affected first-degree relatives, the risk is two to three times greater than when one sibling is affected. If the mother has congenital heart disease, the risk to the child is nearly ten-fold over that of the general population. It then appears that the intrauterine environment created by a mother with congenital heart disease is not optimal for fetal development. Further supporting evidence is the fact that the incidence of congenital heart disease in newborns of mothers with surgically corrected congenital heart disease is lower. This effect is even more dramatic when comparing mothers who have surgically corrected cyanotic heart disease with those with uncorrected disease. In the majority of cases, the congenital defect of the child is similar to that of the mother.

Earlier data on the incidence of congenital heart disease in the infant would support a polygenic mode of transmission, whereas more recent data showing a much higher incidence would not. An explanation for the dramatic rise is probably attributed to a combination of two facts; a general change in the environment and improved ability to make the diagnosis.

It is of interest to note that certain forms of congenital cardiac lesions have an especially high risk of transmission. They include left ventricular outflow obstruction, e.g., aortic stenosis and atrioventricular defects, and right ventricular outflow obstruction, e.g., pulmonary stenosis. Overall the rate of risk to the child if either parent has congenital heart disease ranges between 3 percent (older data) and 10.4 to 16.1 percent (recent data). This wide range of estimated risk makes genetic counseling more difficult. The true risk probably lies somewhere in-between. Nonetheless, genetic counseling is an important aspect of overall management and should begin before pregnancy.

SUGGESTED READING

Elkayam U, Gleicher N, eds. Cardiac problems in pregnancy. New York: Alan R. Liss, 1988.

Metcalfe J, McAnulty JH, Ueland K. Heart disease and pregnancy: physiology and management. 2nd ed. Boston: Little, Brown, 1986.

Szekely P, Snaith L. Heart disease and pregnancy. Edinburgh: Churchill Livingstone, 1974.

Ueland K. Cardiovascular diseases in pregnancy. Clin Obstet Gynecol 1981; 24:691–861.

CHRONIC HYPERTENSION IN PREGNANCY

FREDERICK P. ZUSPAN, M.D.

Hypertensive disorders in pregnancy are the most common, serious medical complications seen by the obstetrician. The incidence of hypertension complicating pregnancy in the United States approaches 8 to 10 percent; two-thirds of the cases involve acute hypertension or preeclampsia, and the remaining third represents chronic hypertensive disease that antedates pregnancy. Although maternal mortality from all causes has declined over the past two decades, the complications of hypertension in pregnancy continue to remain the most common cause of maternal death in the United States today.

Data from a study of pregnancies complicated by hypertension at the Chicago Lying-In Hospital revealed that 51 percent of 7,093 of these patients had chronic hypertension; 46 percent had preeclampsia; 1.7 percent had eclampsia; and the remainder had a clinical diagnosis of chronic renal disease.

Chronic hypertension is usually seen in the older gravida, but this does not exclude the young primigravida, who also have chronic hypertension. It is known that approximately 8 percent of adolescents have chronic hypertension, and these same women also become pregnant.

DEFINITION

Chronic hypertension implies a disease state that antedates pregnancy or occurs prior to the 20th week of gestation. The nonobstetrician tends to be concerned about blood pressures that are much higher than those encountered by the obstetrician. Hypertension is diagnosed with the patient in the lateral recumbent position if the sustained elevation of arterial blood pressure is greater than 140/90 mm Hg in both the pregnant and nonpregnant state. The phase four Korotkoff sounds, i.e., when the point of muffling is heard, is the most desired diastolic pressure reading, since pregnancy is a high output state. The fourth Korotkoff sound and not the fifth, should be used which is generally recorded by most obstetricians. The woman should be lying on her side at a 15 to 30 degree tilt when the recording of the blood pressure is done on at least two consecutive measurements. The calculation of the mean arterial blood pressure is complicated and does not significantly add to the prognosis. The absolute level is more important than a rise in blood pressure in the chronic hypertensive patient. A diastolic blood pressure of 90 mm Hg corresponds to approximately three standard deviations from the mean in the midtrimester of pregnancy as well as to the rise observed with increased perinatal mortality as reported by Friedman.

Recommended standard methods for the measurement of the blood pressure by sphygmomanometry are:

1. *Preparation*: All clothing should be removed from the upper body so the sphygmomanometer cuff can be applied easily to the right upper arm. Have the patient lie comfortably on her left side on a couch or bed at a 15 to 30 degree tilt, with the right arm well supported at the same level as the heart, horizontal with the sternum, at the fourth intercostal space. It is important that the patient rest comfortably on her left side for at least 3 minutes before the blood pressure is taken.
2. *Application of cuff*: The position of the cuff should be at the center of the bladder and the sphygmomanometer cuff should be directly over the brachial artery on the inner side of the right arm, with the connecting tubes pointing toward the hip. Apply the cuff evenly and firmly, but not too tightly, around the arm, leaving the antecubital fossa free. The cuff size should fit comfortably around the arm. If the circumference of the arm is greater than 35 cm, a thigh cuff should be used to avoid a spurious blood pressure recording.
3. *Taking the blood pressure*: Palpate the brachial artery in the antecubital fossa, and place the stethoscope directly over the artery without undue pressure. The initial cuff pressure should be increased rapidly 20 to 30 mm above the point at which pulsation in the brachial artery ceases or the first Korotkoff sound disappears. (The rate of the inflation of the cuff with the air out of the cuff without delay so that the mercury falls steadily at least 3 mm per second.) The systolic pressure is recorded to the nearest 2 mm of mercury, at the point when the first tapping sound is heard at the top of the mercury meniscus. The diastolic blood pressure is the point at which the sound first becomes muffled (phase 4); this likewise is read at the top of the mercury meniscus and recorded to the nearest 2 mm of mercury. Release the cuff pressure completely to allow free flow of blood to the arm and repeat the process. It is known that two individuals taking the blood pressure will vary in their reading by as much as 5 mm Hg.

To avoid confusion in recording, it is advisable to record the systolic blood pressure and both the fourth Korotkoff sound (diastolic blood pressure) and the fifth Korotkoff sound when the sound disappears. Interpretation of the three readings will avoid confusion as to whether or not the fourth or fifth Korotkoff sound was used.

Studies have been done that use the mean arterial pressure as a guidepost for fetal prognosis. In general, a mean arterial pressure greater than 90 mm Hg during pregnancy is associated with a higher rate of fetal loss. A persistent diastolic blood pressure in excess of 84 mm Hg merits consideration for both chemical and nonchemical therapy. This is not based upon science but an empiric figure.

Examples of rather modest blood pressure readings that achieve a reading of 90 mm Hg mean arterial pressure would be 110/80, 120/74, or 130/70; to the untrained observer, these are all within normal limits, but they may be significant for the pregnant patient. Systolic hypertension with a diastolic pressure of less than 80 mm Hg in early pregnancy may be associated with anxiety, thyrotoxicosis, or other similar conditions. It is now known that an elevated systolic blood pressure is also correlated with an increase in fetal morbidity and mortality.

CLASSIFICATION

There are a number of classifications for chronic hypertension in pregnancy. Through its council, the International Society for the Study of Hypertension in Pregnancy has recommended the following classifications:

1. Women found to have hypertension and/or proteinuria at the first prenatal visit before the 20th week of pregnancy are presumed to have chronic hypertension of undetermined cause. Causes include chronic renal disease, renovascular disorders, lupus erythematosus, and hyperaldosteronism.
2. Women with unclassified hypertension and/or proteinuria may be reclassified after delivery.
   a. If the hypertension and/or proteinuria disappear, as in gestational hypertension without proteinuria, gestational proteinuria without hypertension, or gestational proteinuria with hypertension (preeclampsia).
   b. If hypertension and/or proteinuria persists after delivery, or if other tests confirm the diagnosis, there may be chronic hypertension (usually without proteinuria), chronic renal disease (usually proteinuria with or without hypertension), or chronic hypertension of other causes.

A useful and more simplified classification of hypertensive disease in pregnancy is as follows:

I. Preeclampsia-eclampsia (acute hypertension, toxemia, pregnancy-induced hypertension)
II. Chronic hypertensive disease:
   1. Primary (essential, idiopathic), the most common form of hypertension
   2. Secondary (related to a known cause)
      a. Renal: Parenchymal disease such as chronic pyelonephritis, interstitial nephritis, polycystic kidney, renovascular disease, lupus erythematosus
      b. Adrenal gland: cortical—Cushing's disease, hyperaldosteronism; medullary—pheochromocytoma
      c. Other: thyrotoxicosis
III. Chronic hypertensive disease with superimposed preeclampsia can be a catastrophy for the patient and may result in a cerebrovascular accident.
IV. Transient hypertension occurs during labor and/or in the immediate postpartum period, and most likely is associated with either preeclampsia or chronic hypertension or both, but it is not of long-term significance.

The classification of disease on clinical grounds appears to be easy and straightforward. However, the accuracy of such clinical diagnoses have been challenged by renal biopsy studies done at Chicago Lying-In Hospital. Although in clinical practice approximately 1 percent of pregnant women are diagnosed to have chronic renal disease, renal biopsy confirms the diagnosis in between 15 and 17 percent of women. Renal disease does not necessarily occur in only the multiparous patient; likewise, these studies by renal biopsy underscore the difficulty in making a definitive diagnosis based only on clinical findings.

The current role of renal biopsies is somewhat guarded in that they are only done under very special circumstances, no longer routinely during or after pregnancy. The ideal time for performing a renal biopsy is 2 to 5 days following delivery in selected patients. There is some long-term predictive value of the findings of the renal biopsy following pregnancy, especially as regards future pregnancy and specific etiology of the problem.

MATERNAL PHYSIOLOGY AND PATHOPHYSIOLOGY

The pathophysiology of chronic hypertension in pregnancy is not well understood. However, there are alterations in many organ systems. The organ system predominantly involved may well be the largest clue to the underlying severity of the problem and its effect upon the fetus. The pregnant woman retains between 800 and 900 mEq of sodium throughout pregnancy and has a commensurate retention of water amounting to 6 to 7 L. Fluid is retained in the body as physiologic saline that is distributed throughout the maternal organism and products of conception. There is at least a 1.5 L increase in plasma volume, which is 40 to 50 percent above normal.

Many factors contribute to this volume expansion, including an increase in the sex steroids and in prostaglandin, aldosterone, and other salt-retaining hormones as well as the posture and the arterial venous shunt-like effects of the placenta. The increase in plasma volume parallels the increase in cardiac output, which begins as early as 8 to 10 weeks of gestation and is near its peak by 20 to 22 weeks of gestation; it reaches its true peak around the 28th week and plateaus until after delivery.

Vascular Resistance

There is a gradual decline in mean arterial blood pressure during the second trimester of pregnancy, with a commensurate decrease in peripheral resistance. The familiar fall in mean arterial blood pressure during the second trimester of pregnancy is largely a recording artifact that is eliminated if the patient is placed in the lateral recumbent position when the blood pressure is recorded at the level of the heart in the upper arm. The dynamic increase in uteroplacental perfusion is mediated by the vasodilating capability of various gestational substances, including progesterone and members of the prostaglandin E series. Arteriolar tone decreases and the vasculature becomes refractory to pressor agents, specifically infusion of angiotensin II and catecholamines. The blood pressure tends to return to prepregnancy levels during the third trimester, coincidental with an increase in vascular resistance as well as an increase in blood volume.

Blood Volume

Attempts have been made to divide essential hypertension into those types that may be volume- or vasoconstriction-dependent. Although this is done in the nonpregnant state, it is not applicable to pregnancy. The subdivision is based on concentrations of peripheral blood renin in the nonpregnant woman. Therefore, it is not applicable for investigation of essential hypertension in pregnancy because estrogen induces an increase in plasma renin and angiotensin concentrations in normal pregnancy. Plasma volume increases 40 to 50 percent above the prepregnant level in normal pregnancy. On the other hand, the patient with chronic hypertension behaves differently in that on occasion there is failure of the plasma volume to increase, and this is associated with poor perinatal outcome. In general, it can be stated that the blood volume expansion in patients with hypertensive disease is reduced, and this reduction is still greater if the patient has superimposed preeclampsia or is on chronic diuretic therapy.

Adrenergic Nerves

The smooth muscle of the uterus is innervated by the short adrenergic neurons whose neural plexus lies adjacent to that organ in contrast to the long adrenergic neurons. These neurons are unique in that their transmitter content of *norepinephrine* decreases during pregnancy under the influence of exogenous sex hormones.

The uterine adrenergic transmitter in the human dramatically decreases during pregnancy and becomes functionally denervated when the pregnancy is near term. Studies that measure enzyme content have demonstrated tyrosine hydroxylase and dopadecarboxylase levels to be markedly reduced near term, which parallels the reduction of norepinephrine concentration. On the other hand, the level of choline acetyltransferase, the synthesizing enzyme of acetylcholine, is unchanged, which indicates that the adrenergic system is selectively affected. Additionally, women who develop preeclampsia have an increase in tissue norepinephrine concentrations in uteroplacental bed biopsies. Women who have chronic hypertension do not have an increase in uterine tissue norepinephrine values unless they develop preeclampsia. They have values similar to those found in normal pregnancy.

Uteroplacental Bed

The hemochorial placenta in the human has a separate but intimate association with maternal blood vessels. Fetal and maternal circulations are separated by as little as one layer of cells. The intimacy of this association is highlighted by the migration of nonvillous trophoblasts into the spiral arteries for replacement of muscular and elastic tissue that begins at the time of implantation. As pregnancy progresses, this trophoblastic tissue migrates farther down the spiral arteries to as far as the myometrial segment, where the radial arteries begin.

The migration of trophoblastic tissue into the spiral arteries results in a loss of reactive smooth muscle and vascular tissue, leading to a decrease in resistance and a dilation of the spiral arteries. Physiologically, this converts the high resistance system of the radial arteries to a low resistance system, as found in the spiral arteries, and permits maximum interchange of nutrients and gases between the fetus and the mother. This progressive migration of trophoblastic tissue takes place in two phases: the first is from the time of implantation until approximately 10 weeks of gestation, and the second or later invasion is completed by the 24th week.

Patients who have essential hypertension at times have hyperplastic arteriosclerotic changes in the myometrial segment of the radial and low spiral arteries that extend into the myometrium. The extent of this vessel wall modification is probably related to the degree of hypertension, i.e., the worse the hypertension the greater the magnitude of vascular involvement. If preeclampsia develops in either a normotensive or a hypertensive woman, acute atherosis and necroarteriopathy occur in the small muscular arteries of the placental bed. This causes constriction of the spiral arteries at their base near the myometrium, which leads to less dilation of the spiral arteries and results in a decrease in the placental perfusion.

We have described an adrenergic innervation in the uterine musculature at the base of the spiral arteries and the myometrium. Functional denervation of the adrenergic nervous system most likely is incomplete in the patient who has preeclampsia, since tissue norepinephrine concentration is significantly elevated. On the contrary, in patients with essential vascular hypertension in the absence of preeclampsia, tissue norepinephrine levels are not elevated. As previously mentioned, the vascular volume of the patient with essential hypertension may be smaller than that of the normotensive woman.

Likewise, when the weight and the volume of placentas are evaluated, the hypertensive patient may have a smaller placenta than her normotensive counterpart and these women tend to have babies that are small for gestational age. The functional size of the placenta relates to the degree of hypertension, which is significant for the outcome of the fetus.

A thorough understanding of the pathologic changes in the uteroplacental bed is necessary before therapy is instituted in the patient with chronic hypertension. It is unlikely but as yet unproved that drugs can alter the pathologic changes in the uteroplacental bed, especially if preeclampsia develops in the hypertensive patient.

FETAL EFFECTS

The fetal effects seen in mothers who have chronic hypertension are varied. The degree of hypertension is the dependent variable, and the quality of the placenta determines whether the most overt effect (a stillbirth) or minimal effects will be noted. Fetal effects basically relate to the blood flow through the uteroplacental bed and the ability of the spiral arteries to dilate in order to provide nutrition and exchange of gases to the fetus. Disturbances of fetal growth and development are seen if hypertension is more profound. Fetal growth retardation is defined as a birth weight less than the 10th percentile for any gestational age, and this is usually not recognized prior to the 30th week of gestation. The most common causes of intrauterine growth retardation are chronic maternal hypertension and smoking. The following factors correlate in a positive manner with the degree of fetal growth retardation: (1) severity of maternal hypertension, (2) contraction of blood volume, and (3) plaque formation in the radial or low spiral arteries of the uteroplacental bed with inability to dilate.

Uterine blood flow (UBF) is a critical issue for the fetus. The formula for calculations is as follows: UBF = Blood Pressure/Resistance (Extrinsic + Resistance). Evaluation of the formula indicates that if blood pressure is reduced and resistance remains unchanged, uterine blood flow will decrease. Most investigators feel that there is no autoregulation in the pregnant uterus and that the placental perfusion is maximal at all times. Generalizations that equate severity of the hypertension with the size of the placenta and the degree of intrauterine growth retardation are basically correct. The fundamental issue for the fetus is the amount of placental reserve remaining. Vascular changes below the spiral arteries and the myometrium in the chronic hypertensive patient includes plaque formation and impediment to flow. The more profound the hypertension and the greater the physical changes that take place in the vessels, the greater the risk of perinatal mortality, which increases as much as eightfold in some with compromised infants.

The most devastating event that can take place for a fetus whose mother has chronic hypertension is the superimposition of preeclampsia, which causes necrosis of the spiral artery, plaque formation, and plugging of the vascular spaces. Fetal morbidity and mortality are at least five times greater than that expected in patients who do not have preeclampsia. Additional factors affecting maternal mortality are the presence of coexisting renal and vascular disease.

Another problem for the fetus is the occurrence of abruptio placentae, which further compromises fetal circulation. This has greater significance in women who have chronic hypertension because, in all probability, the placental function is less than in a normal patient. Our experience at Chicago Lying-In Hospital indicates that in a nontoxemic patient the incidence of abruptio placentae is 0.8 percent, whereas in mild hypertensive patients it is 3 percent, and in severe hypertensive patients it is 6.3 percent. The diagnosis of abruptio placentae is made by history, clinical findings, and occasionally it may be helpful to do an ultrasound examination.

DIAGNOSIS AND MANAGEMENT

The blood pressure in all pregnant patients should be taken in the lateral recumbent position with the arm at the level of the heart. The blood pressure is recorded as systolic when the muffled sound changes (fourth Korotkoff sound), and when the blood pressure sound ends (fifth Korotkoff sound); hence, three readings are recorded for each patient. A persistent diastolic blood pressure of greater than 90 indicates chronic hypertension in pregnancy in the absence of preeclampsia. The lowest blood pressure is seen when the patient is asleep and the next lowest when the patient first awakens before she gets out of bed. As the day progresses, the highest blood pressure reading is noted in the afternoon.

We teach our pregnant patients who have chronic hypertension to monitor their own blood pressures. We begin by using a two-headed stethoscope—one for the nurse and one for the patient—and instruct the patient on how to record the first, fourth, and fifth Korotkoff sounds, with all three numbers being recorded.

The patient is instructed to take her blood pressure three times each week, twice during the week when she is working and on Sunday. The reading should be recorded twice during the day: on awakening, which will be the lowest reading, and in the afternoon before the patient rests on her side in bed. For the past 9 years we have utilized this method in instructing patients who have chronic hypertension. Our studies have shown that *only one-third of the blood pressures taken in the office are similar to the home blood pressures;* hence, erroneous conclusions can frequently be drawn from office blood pressure recordings. These serial home blood pressure readings are important. One of the benefits of having the patient take her own blood pressure is to teach her about her own environmental situation and work habits and how her blood pressure responds to these stimuli. The patient is asked to record any unusual events that would be associated with an elevation of blood pressure, and if the increase is excessive to immediately report it to the physician. The patient, when instructed properly, can identify trends in blood pressure elevation that suggest preeclampsia as well as the necessity to alter her antihypertensive medications.

One additional fact that emerged is that only 46 percent of patients who were on self blood pressure determinations required antihypertensive medications compared with 76 percent of the patients who did not take their blood pressures.

There are times when hospitalization is necessary for evaluation of the patient with chronic hypertension. In this study, 11 percent of those who took their own blood pressure, in contrast to 76 percent of those who did not, required admission to the hospital. This represents a major savings in health care costs brought about by the simple procedure of self blood pressure determinations.

Guidelines for maternal and fetal evaluation follow.

Maternal Evaluation

1. General physical examination
2. Funduscopic examination with dilated pupils
3. Self-determination of blood pressure (use first, fourth, and fifth Korotkoff sounds)

History

1. Family history of hypertension
2. History of renal disease in childhood
3. History of repeated urinary tract infections
4. History of sibling and mother having hypertension during pregnancy

Laboratory Diagnosis

1. Urine: 24 hour protein or protein/creatinine ratio of spot urine
2. Urine culture and sediment
3. Blood urea nitrogen and serum creatinine tests
4. Creatinine clearance measurement
5. Serum electrolyte measurement
6. Ultrasound renal evaluation*
7. Electrocardiogram*
8. Chest x-ray film*
9. Urine catechols, vanillylmandelic acid)

* Depends upon severity of blood pressure level.

Antenatal Fetal Assessment Tests

1. Ultrasound examination—first determination at 10 to 20 weeks; second at 20 to 26 weeks; third at 32 to 34 weeks; thereafter as needed
2. Amniocentesis for fetal maturity studies
3. Biophysical testing
4. Nonstress testing, nipple stimulation test (start at 30 to 32 weeks)
5. Contraction stress tests
6. Fetal kick counts (start at 34 weeks)—six per hour indicate fetal health

MANAGEMENT OF THE NONPREGNANT PATIENT

Ideally, the hypertensive nonpregnant patient should visit the obstetrician prior to conception for evaluation of her hypertension. The obstetrician may feel uncomfortable in evaluating such a patient but by using the aforementioned guideposts, the majority of the work-up can be done without referral, although in consultation with an internist or cardiologist. It is important for the patient to come away from the consultation with a degree of guarded optimism, regardless of her experience with previous pregnancies. A woman who has lost a baby or has almost died because of hypertension during pregnancy has a good deal of anxiety. It is important to rule out any genetic component or the possibility of recurrent preeclampsia, and this is done by taking a careful genetic history and individually evaluating the patient. The interval between the last pregnancy and conception should be at least 6 months, to allow adequate time for work-up and perhaps psychotherapy in order for the patient to better understand her problem prior to conception. Before she begins a pregnancy, the woman should understand her own emotional and physical makeup, how to take her blood pressure, and what the warning signs are regarding her pregnancy, so that the anxiety reaction can be largely confined to the nonpregnant state rather than occur during gestation. It is essential to tell the patient that she will probably need to be seen every 2 weeks throughout her pregnancy, which may reassure her about counseling and guidance. If consultation is needed from a nephrologist for a renal biopsy, the best time for this to be done is before pregnancy occurs. All problems that the patient has should be corrected, i.e., if she is overweight, she should try to achieve her normal height-wieght ratio prior to conception as closely as possible. If she has a history of chronic urinary tract infections, the cause should be carefully evaluated and a urologic consultation considered. Discussion should include counseling in regard to a diet containing 1 g of protein per kilo of body weight a day, with adequate minerals and vitamins. If anemia is present, iron should be prescribed to assure adequate iron stores prior to conception. It might be wise to teach the patient that a half-hour of bed rest at noontime and an hour after return from work are desirable, even though she is not pregnant, in order to help her understand the importance of this simple method to help achieve increased uterine blood flow, which will assure adequate growth of the fetus during pregnancy. It is important that this interview be conducted in a very serious manner, since the outcome of the pregnancy is of the greatest emotional concern for the patient and her spouse. After all the data are available, it is highly desirable to invite the spouse for at least one visit for a serious discussion and to verify that there is a joint supportive role between the couple. A form of barrier contraception should be used prior to conceiving, since oral contraceptives are inappropriate for use by the patient with chronic essential hypertension.

MANAGEMENT OF THE PREGNANT PATIENT

Once the patient has missed the first period, it is essential to document as carefully as possible the date of the last period and when conception took place. An early visit is essential to achieve this goal. If the patient who is pregnant early is on some form of a diuretic agent, it should gradually be reduced and ideally discontinued by 16 weeks. If necessary, she can be placed on antihypertensive therapy prior to conception and the drug dosage adjusted in early pregnancy. An intense relationship develops between the patient and her obstetrician, and this should be effectively utilized to the patient's advantage for support and guidance during the pregnancy. The first visit should include the customary prenatal test battery as well as the baseline laboratory tests for blood urea nitrogen, serum creatinine, urine protein, and serum electrolyte levels and urine culture. A creatinine clearance test should be done early in pregnancy, preferably before the 12th week, to establish a baseline value. If significant hypertension is present, an electrocardiogram is in order, although there is a difference of opinion as to whether or not a chest x-ray film is needed. An ultrasound examination should be done prior to the 12th week of gestation for dating of the pregnancy and to reassure the patient that everything appears normal. She should consult the dietitian either on the first or second visit for a complete evaluation of the adequacy of her diet and an estimation of her sodium and calcium intake. It is best when the patient is first seen to ask her to keep a diet calendar for at least 1 week so the dietitian will have adequate information with which to counsel the patient. If the patient has chronic renal disease and spills a considerable amount of protein, more than 1 g of protein per kilo of body weight per day will be needed in her diet. During normal pregnancy, salt restriction is not advised; however, we instruct the patient who has chronic hypertension to curtail salt intake and to cook without salt. We do not advise salt-free foods. The total role of sodium intake and excretion in the patient with chronic hypertension during pregnancy has yet to be clarified.

Bed Rest

One and one-half to 2 hours of bed rest per day is the single most important modality in the management of the patient who has chronic hypertension during pregnancy. I request that the patient have 1 hour of bed rest at noontime and another hour after she returns home from work. This request may pose a problem for the working woman, but with the realization of the importance of increasing uterine blood flow to the fetus along with the compensatory increase in gaseous and nutrient exchange, the patient will most likely comply. Your nurse must reinforce this periodically when the patient returns on each visit and find out how much she is resting. We instruct the patient to bring her lunch to work and to lie on her side at lunchtime and to have an additional hour of rest when she arrives home. This bed rest, coupled with the patient's home determinations of blood pressure, permits her to be actively involved in the health care of her pregnancy and the growth of her fetus. She has more energy, less fluid retention, and a sense of well-being. Bed rest increases renal blood flow and glomerular filtration, which results in the excretion of more sodium and mild diuresis. This in turn decreases or stabilizes the cardiovascular reactivity and helps maintain a stable or lowered blood pressure. Additionally, bed rest diminishes endogenous secretion of amines, namely, epinephrine, and norepinephrine, which in turn further decreases cardiovascular reactivity with the net end result of an increase in uterine blood flow and enhanced fetal well-being (Fig. 1).

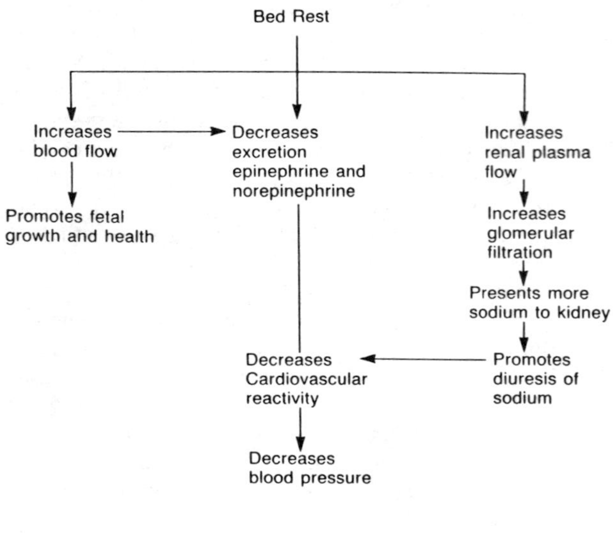

Figure 1 The role of bed rest in fetal-maternal health.

Antihypertensive Drugs

Antihypertensive drugs should be utilized if the diastolic blood pressure is persistently elevated above 84 mm Hg. There are a variety of drugs to choose from, and there is sparse information on most. Antihypertensive drugs do not prevent the onset of preeclampsia. There have been no randomized, prospective, large series of patients on antihypertensive therapy who have chronic hypertension in pregnancy studied in the United States. Our limited experience requires we learn from the randomized studies of others, namely, those in Europe and Australia. The magnitude of the difficulty to which the mother and fetus are subjected depends on the presence or absence of superimposed preeclampsia, and the end organ involvement dictates the degree of morbidity and mortality they will experience. Pregnancy wastage is frequently encountered in those patients with superimposed preeclampsia. For a number of years, the drug of choice for chronic gestational hypertension has been methyldopa (Aldomet), a false neurotransmitter blocker. This is a soft antihypertensive drug that requires a gradual increase in dosage in order to achieve the desired results. If the desired response is not accomplished by 2 g of methyldopa a day, another therapeutic agent should be selected. Two randomized prospective studies in Great Britain have utilized methyldopa, and both showed a beneficial effect for the mother, but neither demonstrated a benefit for the fetus.

The primary objective for antihypertensive therapy in pregnancy is to prevent maternal obstetrical complications. There is still a question, however, as to whether or not the fetus derives any benefit from this treatment. The problem encountered in evaluating the outcome in these studies is that there have been no comparative investigations with all the variables controlled, such as self blood pressure determinations. We know that only 31 percent of patients who take their own blood pressures have a home blood pressure equal to that in the office; hence, many patients are placed on antihypertensive medication when they really don't need it, and this influences the final result. Previous studies have not controlled the position in which the blood pressure is taken, nor have they utilized the fifth Korotkoff sound instead of the fourth, as should be done in a high output physiologic condition such as pregnancy. Hence, despite many anecdotal and retrospective studies, none has satisfied the above criteria. In the absence of reliable information, we must treat our patients in a rational manner using the facts that are known. The drugs in Table 1 have been useful in the treatment of chronic hypertension in pregnancy. None have Federal Drug Administration approval for use in pregnancy, but that does not mean that they cannot be used.

Propranolol was the first beta-blocker to have extensive use in the treatment of hypertension in nonpregnant women. There is currently a debate as to whether propranolol should be used in pregnancy; however, the preponderance of available information indicates that it is acceptable and useful in pregnancy when needed. Some have suggested that it is associated with intrauterine growth retardation, but this is probably related to the underlying disease and not to the drug. If a patient takes propranolol

TABLE 1 Drugs Used in the Treatment of Chronic Hypertension in Pregnancy

Drug	*Action*	*Average Dose*
Methyldopa	Inhibition of vaso-constricting impulses from vasoregulating center in medulla oblongata, inhibition of impulses from hypothalamus, false neurotransmitter	250–500 mg t.i.d.
Propranolol	Beta-adrenergic blockade usually associated with decreased cardiac output	20–40 mg q.i.d.
Labetalol	Alpha- and beta-adrenergic blockade (stronger beta component)	100 mg b.i.d. to t.i.d.
Hydralazine	Direct relaxation of arterioles, action on vascular smooth muscle. Tachyphylaxis seen in pregnancy	20–40 mg q.i.d.
Atenelol	Beta-adrenergic blockade	50 mg q.d. to b.i.d.

Diuretics are not indicated in and have no beneficial effect on pregnancy.

for mitral valve prolapse, we usually continue the low doses of propranolol and add a second drug such as methyldopa to the therapeutic regimen. If methyldopa does not achieve the necessary control of blood pressure, two avenues of therapy are available. Labetalol may be added at a dosage of 100 mg twice a day or hydralazine may be prescribed in the amount of 20 to 40 mg four times a day. The combination of methyldopa and one of these agents is often all that is needed to control blood pressure. Labetalol has been used extensively in the United Kingdom and Australia, but there is limited experience with this agent in the United States, despite the fact that it has been available for more than 3 years. Its principal mechanism of action is a blockade of the alpha-adrenergic receptors of the arteriolar smooth muscle, along with concurrent blockade of beta-adrenergic receptors.

Protocol

The protocol for chronic hypertension in pregnancy is as follows:

1. Do a work-up to rule out renal disease and pheochromocytoma. Start home blood pressure determinations. Hopefully, all of this can be done prior to pregnancy. Obtain baseline laboratory studies.
2. Advise 2 hours of bed rest daily with the patient recording her blood pressure before rest periods.
3. Self blood pressure should be taken three times a week on the side,—using the first, fourth, and fifth Korotkoff sounds.
4. Start antihypertensive drug therapy if the diastolic blood pressure is consistently above 84 mm Hg. Methyldopa should be started at 250 mg twice or four times a day. See the patient on a weekly or biweekly basis thereafter. If blood pressure shows no decrease after 5 to 7 days on therapy and it is 140/90 mm Hg or greater, increase the dose of the antihypertensive drug and increase bed rest.
5. If organ systems deteriorate in spite of adequate therapy, hospitalize the patient and then reevaluate
6. Start biophysical testing at 32 weeks and repeat it weekly or biweekly.
7. Rule out incipient preeclampsia, which will be shown by increased blood pressure and proteinuria. Ask the patient to do a dipstick urine protein determination at least twice a week.
8. Evaluate fetal growth by ultrasound examination and clinical fundal height measurements.
9. Do not permit the pregnancy to go beyond term and induce labor for fetal growth retardation or if organ failure occurs.
10. Suspect incipient preeclampsia in all patients with chronic hypertension.

Home blood pressure measurements should be taken in the lateral recumbent position with the arm at the height of the heart. Suspicion of preeclampsia in a woman who has chronic hypertension comes mostly from clinical data and minimally from laboratory data. The most solid indications for the diagnosis of preeclampsia follow:

1. An increase in baseline blood pressure can be detected most easily if the patient is doing home blood pressure determinations, and she may well be the first to alert you that there has been a gradual increase in her basal blood pressure; believe it when she tells you.
2. Edema is normal for pregnant women, but if edema is more than dependent or if there is a sudden weight increase in a period of a week, then there is indication to suspect incipient preeclampsia. Edema, we feel, is the least reliable of all observable signs.
3. Symptoms such as blurred vision, headache or epigastric pain should alert the clinician to rule out preeclampsia and are late symptoms of disease.
4. If the patient does not have proteinuria, she should utilize protein dipsticks on a weekly basis, and if protein is present, it should be suspected that preeclampsia is developing.
5. An antithrombin III test result of less than 70 percent should make you suspicious of impending preeclampsia.

When Delivery Should Be Performed

The chronic hypertensive patient, in the absence of preeclampsia, should undergo delivery no later than term. On the second or third visit, I talk to the patient about mode of delivery and tell her that, instead of the conventional 20 percent incidence of cesarean sections in this country, she probably has a chance closer to 40 percent of having an abdominal delivery if her cervix is not properly prepared or if some form of fetal distress occurs. The careful surveillance of the fetus by growth measurements, utilizing a tape measure and augmenting this with ultrasound and clinical hands-on evaluation, is most useful. It is emphasized that testing is done on a weekly basis beginning at 30 to 32 weeks of gestation, and if any abnormalities are found in the fetus, serious consideration is given to terminating the pregnancy. If it is necessary to terminate the pregnancy prior to 34 weeks of gestation, amniocentesis may be required to see whether or not lung maturity is present. In the absence of pulmonary maturity, consideration should be given to administering glucocorticoid therapy utilizing 12 mg of betamethasone on two occasions 12 hours apart. We have treated more than 150 women with this protocol, and there has been no evidence that betamethasone worsens the hypertension. Prior to consideration for delivery, usually around 34 weeks, the patient is placed on kick counts in which she lies on her side for two 1-hour periods and records fetal movement; if it is greater than six per hour, this usually indicates good fetal health. The nonstress test is satisfactory for evaluation of the majority of these patients; however, if intrauterine growth retardation is present, it may be necessary to resort to nipple stimulation or contraction stress testing.

Once a decision has been made that the patient should undergo delivery, there are times when the obstetrician is confronted with a woman whose cervix is unfavorable for induction of labor. Ripening of an unfavorable cervix can be achieved by the use of a prostaglandin gel. It is unfortunate that products of this nature are not commercially available in the United States. Prostin E2 suppositories are available, however, and these can be used to make a solution (20 mg Prostin plus 40 mg KY Jelly) that is effective in ripening the cervix. Four milliliters of this solution may be placed in a diaphragm that is then inserted in the vagina in apposition to the cervix. In Europe, stable prostaglandins are available for insertion into the cervical canal to bring about ripening. It is hoped that preparations such as these will be available in the United States in the future, since they are valuable clinical tools that may lower our cesarean section rate. A reference for the preparation of prostaglandin E_2 solution is included in the Suggested Reading.

Following delivery, the patient continues her antihypertensive medication and is instructed to monitor her own blood pressure and to readjust the dose as it seems most appropriate. As a general rule, her dismissal dose is considerably less than that required during the pregnancy.

Therapy for the Patient Who Has Superimposed Preeclampsia and Chronic Hypertension

Preeclampsia superimposed on chronic hypertension poses a major problem for both mother and fetus, since a large number of neonatal deaths, stillbirths, and intrapartum deaths have been observed in this condition. There are also individuals in whom maternal mortality is seen in this particular group of patients, most notably from cerebrovascular accidents. This patient requires all the seriousness of acute health care and must be hospitalized. The degree of preeclampsia and the suddenness of its onset determine the need for an urgent delivery and care for the mother.

Primary Therapy for Preeclampsia/Eclampsia

The woman who has chronic hypertension with superimposed preeclampsia should be treated primarily as a patient who has severe preeclampsia, with special concern for her blood pressure. We have advocated the use of magnesium sulfate given intravenously as the principal agent to provide temporary control of the patient and to prevent seizures. Its use in preeclampsia is not to control the blood pressure but to prevent convulsions. Magnesium sulfate in therapeutic amounts most likely will increase uterine blood flow and act as a protective mechanism for the fetus. It is excreted principally by the kidneys and is administered intravenously. Magnesium and calcium have a complex interdependent influence on the excitability of the components of the neuromuscular junction, and calcium can be utilized if an overdose of magnesium occurs. Magnesium in pharmacologic doses has a curare-like action on the neuromuscular junction and presumably interferes with the release of acetylcholine for motor and nerve terminals. Magnesium can be administered either intramuscularly or intravenously in the regimen that we have recommended. We utilize 4 to 6 g given initially over a period of 5 minutes, then 1 to 2 g per hour, depending on the clinical condition and the size of the patient. The secondary drug utilized in these patients is hydralazine, given in 5-mg boluses, followed by a controlled intravenous infusion utilizing 100 mg of hydralazine in 200 ml of saline in a plastic bag and administered by a controlled infusion mechanism. A Dynamap ultrasound blood pressure monitor is placed on the opposite arm and utilized to help determine the flow rate needed to stabilize the diastolic blood pressure at a level that is not critical for the patient. The patient who has chronic hypertension should not have the blood pressure lowered to a level less than that of the patient who has acute hypertension. One should use external fetal monitoring to make sure that the lowering of the blood pressure does not create fetal distress. The major target organs for preeclampsia are the cardiovascular system, the kidneys, and the uteroplacental bed. The secondary shock organs, which are often more significant, are the liver with hepatocellular damage, the reticuloendothelial system with decrease in platelets, and the brain with edema and hemorrhage. The objective is to control the blood pressure at a level that prevents a stroke but is sufficient to permit the kidneys to continue to function.

PROGNOSIS

Ninety percent of patients who have chronic hypertension in pregnancy can be managed by the general obstetrician-gynecologist, and 10 percent probably need referral because of the intensity and complexity of their hypertension. No matter where they are sent, the results are not good. The salvage rate for women who have chronic hypertension is not higher than that for women with a normal pregnancy and is primarily dependent upon the degree of diastolic blood pressure and the presence or absence of complications interfering with the pregnancy, most notably the onset of preeclampsia with resulting prematurity and its complications for the mother.

SUGGESTED READING

Chesley LC. The renin-angiotensin system in pregnancy. J Reprod Med 1975; 15:173–176.

Chesley LC. Hypertensive disorders in pregnancy. New York: Appleton-Century-Crofts, 1978:237.

Curet LB, Olson RW. Evaluation of a program of bed rest in the treatment of chronic hypertension. Obstet Gynecol 1979; 53:336–340.

Friedman ED. Progressing clinical and biological research. Vol. 7. Blood pressure, edema in pregnancy. New York: Allan R. Liss, 1976.

Gauger LJ. Extemporaneous preparation of a dinoprostone gel for cervical ripening. Am J Hosp Pharm 1983; 40:2195–2196.

Gibson HM. Plasma volume and infiltration rate in pregnancy and their relation to the difference in fetal growth. J Obstet Gynaecol Br Commonwealth 1973; 80: 1067–1074.

Iams JD, Semchyshyn S, O'Shaughnessy RW, Moynihan V, Zuspan FP. Blood pressure response in hypertensive pregnancies treated with cortisol. Clin Exp Hypertens 1980; 2:923–932.

Lopez-Llera M, Linarez GR. Factors that influence maternal mortality and eclampsia. In: Lindheimer MD, Katz AI, Zuspan FP, eds. Hypertension in pregnancy. New York: John Wiley, 1976:41.

Lund CJ, Donovan JC. Blood volume during pregnancy; significance of plasma and red cell volumes. Am J Obstet Gynecol 1967; 98:393–403.

MacGillivray I, Campbell DM. A prospective study of factors affecting intrauterine growth retardation. In: Lindheimer MD, Katz AI, Zuspan FP, eds. Hypertension in pregnancy. New York: John Wiley, 1976:23.

Matthews DD, Agarwal V, Shuttleworth TP. A randomized controlled trial of complete bed rest versus ambulation in the management of proteinuric hypertension during pregnancy. Br J Obstet Gynaecol 1982; 89:128–132.

O'Shaughnessy RW, Zuspan FP. Uterine catecholamines in normal and hypertensive human pregnancy. Clin Exp Hypertens 1982; B1(2 and 3):183.

Owman C, Alm P, Rosengren, Sjoberg NO, Thorbert G. Variations in the level of uterine norepinephrine during pregnancy in the guinea pig. Am J Obstet Gynecol 1975; 122:961–964.

Gant NF, Dailey GL, Chan DS, et al. A study of angiotensin to pressor response throughout primigravid pregnancy. J Clin Invest 1973; 52:2682–2689.

Pruyn SC, Phelan JP, Buchanana GC. Long term propranolol therapy in pregnancy: maternal and fetal outcome. Am J Obstet Gynecol 1979; 135: 485–489.

Rayburn WF, Zuspan FP, Biehl EJ. Self blood pressure monitoring during pregnancy. Am J Obstet Gynecol 1984; 148:159–162.

Redman CWG, Beilin LH, Bonnar J, et al. Fetal outcome in trial of antihypertensive treatment in pregnancy. Lancet 1976; 2:753–756.

Reiss RE, O'Shaughnessy RW, Quilligan EJ, Zuspan FP. Retrospective analysis of blood pressure course during preeclamptic and matched controls. Am J Obstet Gynecol 1987; 156:894–898.

Robertson WB, Brosens I, Dickson G. Maternal uterine vascular lesions and the hypertensive complications of pregnancy. In: Lindheimer MC, Katz AI, Zuspan FP, eds. Hypertension in pregnancy. New York: John Wiley, 1976:115.

Sibai BM, Abdella TN, Anderson GD. Pregnancy outcome in 211 patients with mild chronic hypertension. Obstet Gynecol 1983; 61:571–576.

Stamler J. Hypertension screening in one million Americans. JAMA 1976; 235:2299–2306.

Talledo OE, Chesley LC, Zuspan FP. Renin-angiotensin system in normal and toxemic pregnancies. Am J Obstet Gynecol 168; 100:218–221.

Thorbert G, Alm P, Bjorklund AB, Sjoberg NO. Adrenergic innervation of the human uterus—disappearance of a transmitter and transmitter-forming enzymes during pregnancy. Am J Obstet Gynecol 1979; 135:223–226.

Zuspan FP, O'Shaughnessy RW. Maternal physiology and diseases; chronic hypertension in pregnancy. In: Pitkin RM, Zlatnik FJ, eds. 1979 Yearbook of obstetrics and gynecology. Chicago: Year Book Medical Publishers, 1979:11.

Zuspan FP, O'Shaughnessy RW, Vinsel J, Zuspan MF. Adrenergic innervation of uterine vasculature in human term pregnancy. Am J Obstet Gynecol 1981; 139:678–680.

DIABETES IN PREGNANCY

MARK B. LANDON, M.D.
STEVEN G. GABBE, M.D.

The past 60 years have seen a remarkable improvement in the prognosis for pregnancies complicated by diabetes mellitus. The understanding of the pathophysiology of diabetes in pregnancy, as well as the development of techniques to prevent complications, have helped to reduce fetal and neonatal mortality from approximately 65 percent before the discovery of insulin to 2 to 3 percent at the present time. If one excludes deaths caused by major congenital malformations, the perinatal mortality rate in diabetic women receiving optimal care is similar to that observed in normal pregnancies.

The overall incidence of insulin-dependent diabetes in pregnancy has been found to be approximately 0.1 to 0.5 percent. Gestational diabetes, which accounts for

90 percent of the cases of diabetes in pregnancy, occurs in 3 to 5 percent of the obstetric population; albeit, this depends upon the patients screened and the diagnostic criteria utilized.

Controversy still exists regarding the management of pregnancy complicated by diabetes. Although careful regulation of maternal glycemia is generally well accepted, questions remain regarding the etiology of intrauterine death and congenital malformations, as well as the most predictive techniques to use in the assessment of antepartum fetal condition and maturity. This chapter attempts to review some of these controversies and to present the therapeutic strategies that have reduced morbidity and mortality for the pregnant diabetic and her infant.

CLASSIFICATION AND RISK ASSESSMENT

A program of patient care may be best developed if the risks to the patient and her infant are considered first. The quality of maternal glucose control is probably the most important consideration in assessing perinatal risk.

In 1949, Priscilla White pointed out that the age at onset of diabetes, its duration, and the severity of vascular disease have an influence on perinatal outcome. This classification has assumed tremendous importance and wide application because it has enabled obstetricians to focus on those diabetic patients who are at greater risk during pregnancy (Table 1).

Pregnancies that are complicated by diabetes mellitus may be simply divided into three groups: (1) those women with recent onset of pregestational diabetes (White's classifications B and C), (2) patients with pregestational diabetes who have vascular complications (White's classifications D, F, R, and H), and (3) women with gestational diabetes. Nephropathy, particularly if associated with hypertension, appears to affect perinatal outcome most adversely by increasing the risk for superimposed, pregnancy-induced hypertension and fetal growth retardation. On the other hand, women who have gestational diabetes, but maintain a normal fasting glucose level, rarely experience an intrauterine death. However, serious neonatal morbidity can occur in any pregnancy complicated by diabetes mellitus.

Pedersen et al observed that unfavorable prognostic signs in pregnancy, specifically ketoacidosis, pyelonephritis, pregnancy-induced hypertension, and poor clinic attendance or neglect, were more often associated with unfavorable perinatal outcomes.

THE INSULIN-DEPENDENT PATIENT

Maternal Assessment

Evaluation of the insulin-dependent patient should begin prior to gestation (Table 2). The patient must be assessed as to her suitability for pregnancy. She should undergo an ophthalmologic evaluation, an electrocardiogram, and have a 24-hour urine collection performed for creatinine clearance and protein excretion.

At present, the most frequent cause of perinatal loss in pregnancies that are complicated by insulin-dependent diabetes is fatal congenital malformation. Infants of diabetic mothers have an increased incidence of severe malformations that involve major organ systems. The frequency of major congenital malformations observed in the offspring of insulin-dependent diabetics is 6 to 8 percent, whereas infants of women with gestational diabetes have a 2 to 3 percent rate; this is the same figure observed in the normal population. The caudal regression syndrome, and cardiac, renal, and central nervous system anomalies arise during the first 7 weeks of gestation, a time when it is most unusual for patients to seek prenatal care.

With the increasing evidence that poor metabolic control at conception and during embryogenesis is responsible for the greater number of congenital malformations seen in pregnancies that are complicated by insulin-dependent diabetes, it is essential that preconception counseling that involves both the patient and her partner be instituted. The obstetrician should explain the techniques for self blood glucose monitoring as well as the need for proper dietary management to the nonpregnant patient. Other physicians who care for young women with diabetes must also be aware of the importance of such counseling. Questions should be answered regarding the risk factors for fetal complications and the plan for general management of the patient's diabetes in pregnancy. Two European studies performed in hospitals with special diabetes clinics have shown a reduced rate of major congenital malformations in patients with optimal glucose control before conception.

TABLE 1 White's Classification of Diabetes in Pregnancy

Class	*Age at Onset (yr)*		*Duration (yr)*	*Vascular Disease*	*Insulin*
A	Any		Any	None	Diet only
B	>20		<10	None	+
C	10–19	or	10–19	None	+
D	<10	or	>20	Benign retinopathy	+
F	Any		Any	Nephropathy	+
R	Any		Any	Proliferative retinopathy	+
H	Any		Any	Heart disease	+

+ = insulin required.

TABLE 2 Prepregnancy Care

Procedure
Discuss contraceptive program
Assess patient's vascular status
Obtain optimum glucose control
Determine immune status against rubella
Evaluate psychosocial well-being

Detection of Fetal Malformations

Glycosylated hemoglobin serves as an index of long-term glucose control. It has been observed that elevated hemoglobin A_{1c} concentrations early in pregnancy correlate with an increased incidence of malformations. Because problems may arise in the laboratory with the determination of glycosylated hemoglobin, it is important to have a reliable assay and to establish control values before using these results to counsel patients. In general, we do not recommend that termination of pregnancy be advised on the basis of an elevated glycosylated hemoglobin value. However, these women may have as much as a 20 to 25 percent chance of having a malformed infant. Therefore, evidence of poor glycemic control during embryogenesis, as reflected by an elevated first trimester glycosylated hemoglobin level, warrants a maternal serum alpha-fetoprotein (AFP) level at 16 weeks, a detailed ultrasonographic examination of the fetus at 18 weeks, and an assessment of fetal cardiac structure by echocardiography at 20 weeks. At the present time, it is our practice to evaluate all patients with insulin-dependent diabetes in this manner.

Regulation of Maternal Diabetes

Maternal plasma glucose levels during a normal pregnancy rarely exceed 100 mg per deciliter, ranging between fasting levels of 60 mg per deciliter and postprandial levels of 120 mg per deciliter. These values should be the therapeutic objectives in pregnancies complicated by diabetes mellitus (Table 3).

The ability to achieve normoglycemia requires that patients evaluate their blood glucose levels frequently. In the past urine testing was traditionally employed. However, these results fail to reflect maternal glycemia. During pregnancy, the increase in the glomerular filtration rate is not accompanied by an increase in the tubular reabsorption of glucose. Glycosuria may be present even at low blood glucose levels. Therefore, it is essential that the pregnant diabetic rely on self monitoring of capillary blood glucose in order to achieve optimal control. Frequent monitoring provides an early warning of hypoglycemia and allows for appropriate adjustments in insulin dosage.

Self glucose monitoring, combined with aggressive insulin therapy, has made the maintenance of maternal normoglycemia a therapeutic reality. Patients should monitor their glucose control using glucose-oxidase impregnated reagent strips and a glucose reflectance meter. Glucose determinations are made in the fasting state and before lunch, dinner, and bedtime. Postprandial values, as well as the periodic assessments of glycosylated hemoglobin, can also be helpful. With this data, the clinician can formulate an insulin regimen to meet the patient's individual requirements.

During pregnancy, most insulin-dependent patients require multiple insulin injections. A combination of intermediate-acting and regular insulin before breakfast and at dinner time is the most commonly employed regimen. As a general rule, the amount of intermediate acting insulin taken in the morning exceeds that of regular insulin by a 2:1 ratio. Patients usually receive two-thirds of their total insulin dose at breakfast and the remaining third at supper time. In an alternative regimen, the patient may take separate injections of regular insulin at dinner time and intermediate-acting insulin at bedtime in order to reduce the risk of nocturnal hypoglycemia. The latter may occur when the mother is in a relative fasting state while placental and fetal glucose consumption continues. As the third trimester approaches, maternal insulin requirements may increase by 30 to 100 percent. Ketoacidosis is most common at this time; for this reason, patients with evidence of a respiratory or urinary tract infection should be promptly evaluated.

The effectiveness and safety of the continuous subcutaneous insulin infusion pump have been demonstrated in selected pregnant patients. However, in a randomized prospective study, the pump has not been shown to improve control or reduce complications in pregnancy. In general, this therapy should be reserved for highly motivated women whose diabetes cannot be controlled despite a program of multiple insulin injections. However, it must be remembered that ketoacidosis and fetal death have occurred in association with pump failure. Serious hypoglycemic reactions have also been reported.

The average diet for a pregnant, insulin-dependent, diabetic patient includes 20 percent of the calories derived from protein, 35 percent from fat, and 45 percent from carbohydrate. In terms of caloric distribution, 25 percent of the calories are provided with breakfast, 30 percent with lunch, 30 percent with dinner, and 15 percent with a bedtime snack. Some patients are more prone to hypoglycemia and may require snacks in the midmorning and/or midafternoon. In such cases, 5 percent of the calories are subtracted from breakfast and lunch respectively. The average daily caloric intake for the pregnant diabetic woman ranges from 2,200 to 2,400 calories. Patients who are restricted in activity or who demonstrate

TABLE 3 Target Glucose Levels in Pregnancy*

Time	*Levels (mg/dl)*
Before breakfast	60–90
Before lunch, supper, bedtime snack	60–105
Two hours after meals	≤120
2 AM to 6 AM	>60

* Mean capillary glucose levels should be maintained at ≤110 mg/dl. Glycosylated hemoglobin levels should be within the normal range for the individual laboratory.

early excessive weight gain may necessitate a lower caloric prescription. Obese patients are advised against weight loss during pregnancy.

Program of Care

Most pregnant women with insulin-dependent diabetes can be managed successfully as outpatients. In selected cases, hospitalization may be required early in gestation to assure optimal control through intensive patient education.

Outpatient visits are usually scheduled at 1-to 2-week intervals. The log of glucose values kept by the patient should be reviewed at each visit. Patients are encouraged to contact their physician if they experience episodes of hyper- or hypoglycemia. In patients found to have benign retinopathy during the first trimester, follow-up ophthalmologic examination is scheduled for the second and third trimesters. Proliferative retinopathy usually requires monthly examinations. Renal function studies are performed at least once during each trimester.

Fetal Assessment

Biophysical techniques have proven most valuable in assessing fetal well-being (Table 4). Ultrasonography is an extremely important tool that may be used to evaluate fetal growth, detect anomalies, and diagnose hydramnios. As previously mentioned, determination of maternal serum AFP should be employed in an attempt to detect anomalies.

During the third trimester, when the risk of sudden intrauterine death may be increased, a program of fetal surveillance is initiated. Because normal tests are rarely associated with intrauterine demise, the primary value of such surveillance has been to allow the clinician to delay delivery and await fetal maturation. Excellent control of maternal diabetes also reduces the risk of fetal death and the frequency of abnormal test results.

A negative contraction stress test (CST) in a well-controlled patient should predict fetal survival for 1 week. A positive CST, observed in approximately 10 percent of insulin-dependent diabetic patients, has been associated with an increased perinatal mortality rate, late decelerations during labor, low Apgar scores, respiratory distress syndrome (RDS) and growth retardation. The CST does have a significant false-positive rate of up to 60 percent.

In recent years, the nonstress test (NST) has become the preferred antepartum heart rate screening test, which is used to follow patients with diabetes mellitus. Heart rate monitoring is begun in the third trimester and should probably be performed twice weekly at 32-weeks gestation and thereafter. If the NST is nonreactive, a CST must then be performed.

Some clinicians now prefer to use the biophysical profile as a primary screening technique to evaluate the fetus or after a nonreactive NST. Such sequential fetal evaluation is probably necessary in less than 10 percent of cases, and it appears from several recent studies that intervention for abnormal test results is actually a rare event.

Maternal monitoring of fetal activity is an easy and practical method that has proven to be a helpful screen for fetal compromise. Maternal assessment of fetal activity has been used in monitoring a variety of high-risk pregnancies. Although this technique has not been studied solely in pregnancies complicated by diabetes, it appears that assessment of fetal activity is comparable to heart rate testing with the NST. Beginning at 28-weeks gestation, patients are asked to record fetal activity over a 12-hour period, usually from 9 o'clock in the morning until 9 o'clock in the evening. Ten movements should be noted in this time period. If the length of time is found to increase before this number of movements is appreciated, or if less than ten movements are recorded, heart rate testing is performed as soon as possible. Patients may also count fetal movement at several designated time periods each day.

The Timing of Delivery

With techniques now available to maintain normoglycemia, several less vigorous protocols have been adapted. Physicians are now comfortable about following a select group of pregnant diabetics as outpatients until term. The assessment of maternal glycemia by means of self glucose testing, as well as the availability of outpatient heart rate testing, have made this possible. Perinatal outcome does not appear to be compromised by this management, and the likelihood for the spontaneous onset of labor and vaginal delivery is increased. Inpatient care is reserved for patients with poor glycemic control, severe vascular complications, or those who require more intensive fetal surveillance.

Delivery should be delayed until fetal maturation has taken place, provided that the patient's diabetes is well controlled and that antepartum surveillance remains normal. Before most elective deliveries, an amniocentesis should be performed in order to document fetal pulmonary matu-

TABLE 4 Fetal Evaluation

Midpregnancy	*Weeks*	*Late Pregnancy*
Maternal serum alpha-fetoprotein	16 weeks	Maternal assessment of fetal activity
Ultrasonography	16-18 weeks	Nonstress test
Fetal echocardiography	20 weeks	Contraction stress test
		Fetal biophysical profile
		Ultrasonography
		L:S ratio, lung profile

rity. Although the value of the lecithin:sphingomyelin ratio (L:S) has been questioned in pregnancies that are complicated by diabetes mellitus, many series report a low incidence of RDS with a mature ratio. In one large study, L:S ratio of 2.0 or greater was associated with a 3 percent risk of hyaline membrane disease, a result no different from that observed in the nondiabetic population.

The presence of the acidic phospholipid, phosphatidylglycerol (PG), is the final marker of fetal pulmonary maturation. Several authors have suggested that hyperinsulinemia may be associated with delayed appearance of PG and an increased incidence of RDS. There are numerous reports of RDS in infants of diabetic patients with mature L:S ratios in the absence of PG. Therefore, should the amniotic fluid analysis fail to reveal fetal pulmonary maturity and if the antepartum fetal assessment remains reassuring, elective delivery is postponed and an amniocentesis is repeated in approximately 1 week.

Most importantly, the clinician must be familiar with the laboratory analysis of amniotic fluid in his or her institution and the neonatal outcome at various L:S ratios in the presence or absence of PG.

When antepartum fetal testing suggests fetal compromise, immediate delivery must be considered. An amniocentesis should be performed, and in the presence of a lecithin:sphingomyelin ratio of or greater than 2.0, delivery should be accomplished. If the lecithin:sphingomyelin ratio is immature, clinical management must be individualized. If the patient develops pregnancy-induced hypertension, rapidly worsening retinopathy, or renal failure, delivery may be necessary.

Labor and Delivery

The route and timing of delivery must be individualized. With excellent control, no evidence of hypertension or vasculopathy, reassuring fetal testing, and normal fetal growth, the obstetrician may elect to await the onset of spontaneous labor. Expectant management beyond 40-weeks gestation has not been widely adopted. With adverse factors such as maternal hypertension, a prior stillbirth, or poor control, elective induction or cesarean section may be planned after pulmonary maturity has been documented. In most institutions, the cesarean section rate for diabetic pregnancies approaches 50 percent.

A skilled neonatal team should be present at delivery. If adequate neonatal care cannot be provided, the patient should be transferred to a hospital with an appropriately equipped nursery.

During labor, continuous fetal heart rate monitoring is mandatory. Labor is allowed to progress as long as normal rates of cervical dilation and descent are documented. Elective cesarean section is advised with an estimated fetal weight of 4,000 g or more as the incidence of shoulder dystocia in this group exceeds 20 percent. Despite attempts to select patients with obvious fetal macrosomia for delivery by elective cesarean section, an arrest pattern in labor should alert the physician to the possibility of cephalopelvic disproportion. About 25 percent of macrosomic infants who are delivered after a prolonged second stage have shoulder dystocia. Patients who fail to demonstrate significant cervical change after 6 to 8 hours of oxytocin stimulation are best delivered by cesarean section. In general, serial inductions of labor are discouraged since maternal control may deteriorate.

The goal of maintaining euglycemia during pregnancy is also important during labor and delivery. Intrapartum, mean maternal capillary glucose values that exceed 120 mg per deciliter significantly increase the frequency of neonatal hypoglycemia. Such morbidity may occur despite the presence of excellent control before the onset of labor. Therefore, the intrapartum management of the diabetic patient requires careful attention to maternal glucose values, the glucose infusion rate, and insulin dosage. In general, glucose determinations are made at the bedside every 1 to 2 hours with self blood glucose monitoring techniques. A flow sheet to summarize these data is essential. Several approaches have been utilized to maintain maternal euglycemia during labor and delivery: a continuous infusion that combines insulin and glucose is often employed, or 5 units of regular insulin are added to 500 ml of a 5 percent dextrose solution. Albumin may be added to decrease the adherence of insulin to the infusion line or the infusion line may be purged with a washout solution of insulin in saline before starting the infusion. An infusion rate of 100 to 125 ml per hour usually results in good glucose control. Another simplified regimen has been devised by Jovanovic. In well-controlled patients, the usual dose of NPH insulin is given at bedtime and the morning insulin dose is withheld. Once active labor begins or glucose levels fall below 70 mg per deciliter, the infusion is changed from saline to 5 percent dextrose and delivered at a rate of 2.5 mg per kilogram per minute. Glucose values are recorded, and the infusion rate is adjusted accordingly. Regular insulin is administered if glucose values exceed 140 mg per deciliter. Why insulin requirements fall during labor is poorly understood. This fall may reflect decreasing maternal levels of anti-insulin hormones, which are produced by the placenta.

In patients who undergo elective cesarean section, the procedure is scheduled for the early morning in order to simplify glucose control and maximize the neonatal resources. The patient is given nothing by mouth, and the usual morning insulin dose is withheld. Epidural anesthesia is preferred because it enables the anesthesiologist to evaluate the mental status of the patient and to detect potential hypoglycemia. After surgery, glucose levels are monitored every 2 hours, and an intravenous solution of 5 percent dextrose is administered.

After delivery, insulin requirements are usually significantly reduced. Because of the changing hormonal milieu, a regimen of multiple subcutaneous injections is the preferred form of therapy. The objective of strict control used in the antepartum period is relaxed. Patients who deliver vaginally and who are able to eat a regular diet are given one-half of their prepregnancy dose of NPH insulin on the morning of the first postpartum day. Frequent capillary glucose determinations help to guide insulin dosage. If a patient has been given supplemental regular insulin in addition to the morning NPH dose, the amount of NPH insulin given on the following morning is increased by an amount equal to two-thirds of the additional regular insulin. With this method, most patients are stabilized within a few days of delivery.

Patients who deliver by cesarean section receive regular insulin during the first 24 to 48 hours postoperatively in order to maintain glucose values below 200 mg per deciliter. As their diet is advanced, NPH insulin is administered based on the regular insulin requirement of the preceding day.

All patients are encouraged to breast-feed. Insulin requirements may be somewhat lower in lactating women.

THE PATIENT WITH GESTATIONAL DIABETES

During pregnancy, abnormal carbohydrate metabolism must be detected and precisely defined. Gestational diabetes has been characterized as a state that is restricted to pregnant women in whom the onset or recognition of diabetes or impaired glucose tolerance occurs during pregnancy. Patients with gestational diabetes represent a group with significant risk for developing glucose intolerance later in life. Therefore, detection of these women is an important diagnostic challenge.

Gestational diabetes is a result of inadequate pancreatic reserve in response to the "diabetogenic stress" of pregnancy and is most often encountered in late pregnancy. These patients, although a heterogeneous group in terms of body weight and insulin kinetics, will exhibit postprandial hyperglycemia.

Because, in most cases, women with gestational diabetes have a normal fasting glucose value, some challenge of glucose tolerance must be undertaken. In the past, the obstetrician would assess glucose tolerance in patients thought to be at increased risk for gestational diabetes. This group included patients with a family history of diabetes, an unexplained stillborn, a prior malformed infant, or a macrosomic baby. Obesity, hypertension, glycosuria, and maternal age over 25 were other indications for screening.

Interestingly, over half of all patients who develop gestational diabetes lack the above mentioned risk factors. Therefore, it is recommended that *all* pregnant women be screened by administering a 50-gram oral glucose load followed by a glucose determination 1 hour later (Table 5). Patients need not be fasting for this test. Few false-negative results are obtained when this test is performed at 24- to 28-weeks gestation. An abnormal screening test must be followed by a 3-hour oral glucose tolerance test (GTT), the "gold standard" for the diagnosis of gestational diabetes (see Table 5). One can expect approximately 15 percent of all patients to have an abnormal screening value and about 15 percent of this group to have an abnormal 3-hour oral GTT.

Women with a positive 50-gram screen who initially exhibit a normal GTT, but who have significant risk factors that include a previous history of gestational diabetes, obesity, or advanced maternal age, should undergo a repeat oral GTT at 32- to 34-weeks gestation. Glycosylated hemoglobin has not proved to be helpful in detecting gestational diabetes.

Often the question arises as to the benefit of screening for diabetes at term. Poorly compliant patients or those without historical clues who exhibit fetal macrosomia or polyhydramnios should be tested, even in late pregnancy, to establish this diagnosis. Glucose testing in the post partum period is unreliable, although elevated fasting values indicate overt diabetes. Similarly, glycosylated hemoglobin, if markedly elevated, suggests that gestational diabetes may have been present.

Women with gestational diabetes generally do not require hospitalization. Once the diagnosis is established, patients are begun on a dietary program of 2,000 to 2,200 calories daily. Complex carbohydrates from foods high in soluble fiber provide 50 to 60 percent of total calories, 10 to 20 percent of protein, and 25 to 30 percent of fat. Simple sugars as found in concentrated sweets are eliminated from the diet. Fasting and 2-hour postprandial glucose levels are monitored at each weekly visit. If the fasting plasma glucose level exceeds 105 mg per deciliter and/or postprandial values are greater than 120 mg per deciliter, insulin is begun. If insulin is used, highly purified porcine insulin or human insulin should be administered to decrease the likelihood of antibody formation. Although insulin treatment may be associated with a reduction in fetal macrosomia, routine insulin therapy in all cases of gestational diabetes is not recommended.

Gestational diabetic patients may be safely followed until 40 weeks as long as fasting and postprandial glucose levels remain normal. If labor cannot be safely induced at 40 weeks, fetal surveillance should be initiated with twice weekly NSTs. Patients with gestational diabetes should be delivered by 42 weeks. The risk of intrauterine death and perinatal morbidity is greater in those gestational diabetics who have had a prior stillbirth, who develop pregnancy-induced hypertension, whose diagnosis is delayed until late in pregnancy, or who have required insulin therapy in a prior gestation. In these patients, a program of fetal surveillance similar to that employed in insulin-dependent patients should begin at 34-weeks gestation. As in women with insulin-dependent diabetes, clinical assessment of fetal size and ultrasonographic monitoring should be used to select those patients best delivered by cesarean section.

All women with a history of gestational diabetes should undergo a 75-gram oral GTT several months after delivery to determine if they still demonstrate carbohydrate intolerance (see Table 5).

POSTPARTUM CARE

Contraception remains an important consideration in the care of the young diabetic woman. Family planning is used to optimize the best timing for pregnancy after consultation with the couple. As previously mentioned, optimizing preconceptional control may significantly reduce the risk of congenital malformations in the offspring of insulin-dependent women. Women with diabetes should also be informed that the risks of pregnancy may increase with the duration and the severity of the disease.

It appears that thromboembolic and vascular occlusive disease may be increased in insulin-dependent diabetic women who take combined oral contraceptives. For this reason, many practitioners are reluctant to prescribe

TABLE 5 Screening for Gestational Diabetes Mellitus*

Method

Administer a 50-g oral glucose load between the 24th and 28th week, without regard to time of day or time of last meal, to all pregnant women who have not been identified as having glucose intolerance before the 24th week
Measure venous plasma glucose 1 hr later
Value of 140 mg/dl or above in venous plasma indicates the need for a full diagnostic glucose tolerance test

Diagnosis

Administer a 100-g oral glucose load the morning after an overnight fast (≥ 8 hr; < 14 hr) and following at least 3 days of unrestricted diet (≥ 150 g carbohydrate) and physical activity
Measure venous plasma glucose fasting and at 1, 2, and 3 hr; subject should remain seated and not smoke throughout the test
Positive diagnosis is if two or more of the following venous plasma concentrations are met or exceeded:

Fasting	105 mg/dl
1 hr	190 mg/dl
2 hr	165 mg/dl
3 hr	145 mg/dl

*Postpartum Evaluation***

Administer a 75-g oral glucose load under conditions described for the 100-g oral test
Measure venous plasma glucose fasting and at 30-minute intervals for 2 hr

	Normal	*Impaired Glucose Tolerance*	*Diabetes Mellitus*
Fasting	< 115 mg/dl and	< 140 mg/dl and	≥ 140 mg/dl or
½, 1, 1½ hr	< 200 mg/dl and	1 value ≥ 200 mg/dl and	1 value ≥ 200 mg/dl and
2 hr	< 140 mg/dl	≥ 140 – < 200 mg/dl	≥ 200 mg/dl

* Data from the Proceedings of the second international workshop-conference on gestational diabetes mellitus. Diabetes 1985; 34(Suppl 2):125.
** Data from the National Diabetes Data Group. Classification and diagnosis of diabetes mellitus and other categories of glucose intolerance. Diabetes 1979; 28:1049.

these preparations for diabetic patients. However, low dose contraceptive pills have been used in young women with diabetes who have no evidence of hypertension or vasculopathy.

The progestin-only pill has been recommended for diabetic women. Its failure rate is approximately 1.25 pregnancies per 100 women-years of use. The absolute effects of these preparations on the cardiovascular system are unknown. Some progestogens have been shown to lower high density lipoprotein (HDL)-cholesterol levels. When increased, HDL-cholesterol levels appear to represent a risk factor for the development of atherosclerosis.

Screening for lipid levels should be done prior to instituting oral contraceptive therapy. Obese women with a history of gestational diabetes often have elevated serum triglycerides. These patients should not receive hormonal contraception. Several studies from Sweden suggest that lean women with a history of gestational diabetes who use certain triphasic oral contraceptives do not exhibit carbohydrate intolerance or abnormal lipid profiles.

The diaphragm is a simple, easy, and effective way to prevent conception. Failure seems to occur with inconsistent use. Undoubtedly, the diaphragm and other barrier methods pose the least risk to the diabetic patient.

Surgical sterilization may be appropriate after the couple has completed their family. This issue should be frankly discussed. In the patient with significant vasculopathy, postpartum tubal ligation is frequently performed after appropriate counseling.

SUGGESTED READING

Gabbe SG. Management of diabetes mellitus in pregnancy. Am J Obstet Gynecol 1985; 153:824–828.

Jovanovic L, Peterson CM. Optimal insulin delivery for the pregnant diabetic patient. Diabetes Care 1982; 5(Suppl 1):24–37.

Landon MB, Gabbe SG. Glucose monitoring and insulin administration in the pregnant diabetic patient. Clin Obstet Gynecol 1985; 28:496–506.

Steel JM, Johnstone FD, Smith AF, Duncan LJP. Five years' experience of "prepregnancy" clinic for insulin-dependent diabetics. Br Med J 1982; 282:353–356.

IMMUNOLOGY OF PREGNANCY AND SPONTANEOUS ABORTION

STEVEN S. WITKIN, Ph.D.

The fetus receives half of its genetic material from its father. Expression of these paternal genes during fetal development leads to the appearance on fetal cell surfaces of antigens recognized as "foreign" and thus subject to attack by the maternal immune system. However, both the mother and the fetus contribute to the elaboration of factors that protect the fetus from immunologically mediated destruction. This chapter focuses primarily on recent human studies that have sought to delineate the various immunosuppressive factors, how they are induced, and their mechanism of action. Based on these reports, some women with a history of spontaneous recurrent abortion and who are deficient in one or more of these factors have been identified. Novel clinical treatment of these patients are currently being undertaken at several institutions. The use of immunizations to boost the concentration of factors that suppress maternal immune rejection of the fetus and the theoretic and actual negative consequences of these treatments are described.

The recent explosion in the number of obstetrics and gynecology departments and of private clinicians who perform in vitro fertilizations greatly intensifies the need for an awareness of the immunologic aspects of pregnancy. The term "chemical pregnancy," describing a rise in maternal B chorionic gonadotropin levels indicative of pregnancy followed by its decrease and the onset of menstruation, is becoming an everyday component of our medical vocabulary. Subtle alterations in fetal antigen expression, influenced by in vitro conception and early embryonal development, undoubtedly play a role in these apparent early stage pregnancy losses. An awareness of the immunologic constraints placed on the preimplantation stage embryo will lead to the development of protocols that increase chances for survival following the implantation of an embryo conceived in vitro.

ALLOGRAFT REJECTION

The immune system is able to differentiate between "self" and "nonself," and it selectively attacks and destroys cells and tissues transplanted from one individual to another (allografts). The chromosomal region containing genes primarily responsible for distinguishing foreign from self antigens is known as the major histocompatibility complex. In humans, the genes contained within this complex are known as HLA genes (for human leukocyte gene region A). Relevant to reproductive immunology are three class I genes; HLA-A, HLA-B, and HLA-C, and the class II gene, HLA-DR. Many different alleles of each of these genes exist, so that most individuals differ in the composition of the glycoproteins encoded for by these genes. The HLA class I gene products, present on the surfaces of most cells, are the primary determinants by which "foreign" cells are recognized and destroyed. HLA class II gene products are only present on the surface of a small number of cell types—macrophages, B-lymphocytes, and Langerhans'-dendritic cells. These cells, which function as antigen-presenting cells, impose a further limit on immune recognition. T-lymphocytes initiate an immune response to a foreign antigen when the antigen is present on the surface of an antigen-presenting cell in conjunction with a class II HLA antigen. Different alleles of class II antigens vary in their ability to facilitate immune recognition of any given antigen. Thus, individuals will differ in the quantity of their immune responses because of the restriction imposed by their inheritance of a specific HLA class II gene.

The fetus has long held a unique fascination for the immunologist, since it appears to be the one allograft that defies the laws of HLA-bearing transplanted tissue rejection. Development of an intact cellular immune system capable of rejecting foreign tissue grafts predates the appearance in evolution of placental mammals. Thus, one of the selective influences guiding evolution of the placenta and embryo gene expression undoubtedly has been the need to develop means of preventing maternal immune system recognition of paternal HLA antigens on fetal cells.

MAJOR HISTOCOMPATIBILITY COMPLEX ANTIGEN EXPRESSION

A layer of trophoblastic tissue encases the fetus, separating it from the maternal uterus. Until recently, it was generally believed that trophoblast cells, which are derived from the fetus, did not express paternal histocompatibility gene products and that the fetus was passively shielded from immune recognition by this barrier. If this was the sole protective mechanism, then the developing fetus would not be analogous to a successful allograft that is able to persist despite the *presence* of HLA incompatibility. More recent data, however, give this notion only partial validity. Although trophoblast populations closest to the fetus (syncytiotrophoblast, villus trophoblast) lack class I and class II major histocompatibility complex–derived antigens, nonvillus cytotrophoblast adjacent to the mother does express class I but not class II HLA antigens. However, the HLA antigen present on these cells appears to be an incomplete or modified class I gene product. Some monoclonal antibodies specific for classic HLA class I determinants fail to react with the HLA class I antigen on trophoblast. This apparent modification or partial expression of a major histocompatibility locus gene product may be sufficient to minimize direct attack by the maternal cellular immune system while still stimulating the production of blocking antibodies (see below).

The evidence is clear that the maternal immune system comes into contact with paternal antigens on the fetus and mounts an immunologic response to these determinants. Many pregnant women have readily detectable antibodies to class I HLA antigens. It is generally assumed that this maternal recognition of paternal HLA antigens is beneficial to the fetus. The antibodies produced are believed to function as blocking factors that inhibit maternal lymphocytes from recognizing paternal HLA determinants on fetal cells. This could occur by the masking of these antigens by maternal anti-HLA antibody or by antibody blocking of HLA antigen recognition sites on maternal lymphocytes. Second, the lymphokines produced by the maternal immune system in response to paternal antigen recognition may actually be stimulatory to placental growth. The experimental destruction of lymphocytes in pregnant mice results in a diminution of placental proliferation. The HLA-bearing trophoblastic cells, which, as already stated, are in contact with maternal circulation, may also function as immunoadsorbents, binding anti-HLA antibodies and HLA-primed lymphocytes. This would lower the circulating concentration of these immune reactants and lessen the likelihood of their passage to the fetal circulation. The efficiency with which trophoblasts perform this function is apparent from observations documenting the rapid reappearance of new paternal HLA antigens on trophoblast following digestion of HLA antigen-maternal antibody complexes.

It is clear that incompatibility between husband and wife at HLA loci has no negative effect on pregnancy outcome (and, in fact, is probably beneficial). However, in those cases in which both parents have identical alleles at one or more major histocompatibility complex loci, the fetus and pregnant mother may be at increased risk for developing graft versus host disease or immunodeficiency. Graft versus host disease occurs when there is a successful transfer of immunocompetent cytotoxic T-lymphocytes into a host. When the host's immune system does not obliterate the foreign lymphocytes, they are able to successfully engraft and produce a population of cells that attack foreign host cells. Lymphocyte transfer between mother and fetus is normally prevented by the lack of vascular continuity between the two circulations and by the trophoblastic and extraembryonic membrane physical barriers. However, in those instances in which maternal lymphocytes penetrate the fetal circulation through leaks in the placental barrier, HLA sharing between mother and fetus decreases the likelihood that maternal lymphocytes are recognized as foreign and destroyed by fetal lymphocytes. An additional factor fostering maternal lymphocyte engraftment is the placental passage from mother to fetus of IgG antibodies reactive with paternal antigens on fetal lymphocytes. A similar situation can evolve from migration of fetal cells into the maternal circulation.

Some investigators also claim that maternal-paternal major histocompatibility complex antigen sharing increases the probability for spontaneous abortion. Decreased ability of maternal lymphocytes to recognize paternal major histocompatibility complex antigens could result in inadequate generation of those immunologic blocking factors and lymphokines that enhance prospects for fetal survival.

UTERINE HLA CLASS II GENE EXPRESSION

In response to blastocyst implantation, there is a transformation of the uterine endometrial stroma into decidua. Of major interest from an immunologic standpoint is the observation that some decidual cell populations at the maternal-fetal interface possess class II major histocompatibility complex antigens. This is significant since, as noted above, HLA class II molecules function as codeterminants, allowing T-lymphocytes to initiate an immune response to foreign protein antigens. Decidual cells, through their ingestion, degradation, and presentation of adjacent paternal HLA class I–containing fetal trophoblastic cells to maternal T-helper lymphocytes, appear to contribute to the specificity and quantity of the immune response to paternal HLA determinants.

The extent of decidual cell involvement in the induction of paternal immune recognition appears to be regulated by the production of prostaglandin E_2 (PGE_2) by decidual cells. PGE_2 is an inhibitor of HLA class II gene expression and, thus, ultimately inhibits T-lymphocyte recognition of foreign proteins. It appears that a dynamic equilibrium exists between HLA class II antigen expression and PGE_2 biosynthesis to allow for the generation of an immune response sufficient to induce immunosuppressive molecules while preventing development of a destructive antifetal immune response.

ANTIBODY EFFECTS ON PREGNANCY

Maternal antibody responses are largely unaltered by pregnancy. This is undoubtedly beneficial, since the production of antibodies that block cytotoxic maternal cell-mediated immune responses promotes fetal survival and maturation. The best characterized blocking antibody produced during pregnancy is known as antitrophoblast-lymphocyte cross-reactive (TLX) antibody, so named because it reacts with a cell surface determinant present on both trophoblasts and lymphocytes. It is commonly believed but still not established that maternal antibody formation to TLX antigens on trophoblasts elicits production of complement-dependent antibodies that are cytotoxic for maternal lymphocytes and, thus, limits the lymphocyte response to paternal antigens on fetal cells. A problem hindering more widespread acceptance of the purported role of anti-TLX antibodies in pregnancy has been the failure to detect these antibodies in primiparous serum. More recent studies, however, have revealed that pregnant women also produce another type of antibody, known as an anti-idiotypic antibody, which specifically reacts with anti-TLX antibodies and hinders their detection in vitro. Newer methodologies that are able to assay for anti-TLX antibodies in the presence of anti-idiotype antibodies have provided evidence that anti-TLX antibodies are, indeed, present in normal first pregnancies. The potency of this blocking factor to suppress lymphocyte responses to HLA cell surface determinants in vivo is evident from the observation that administration of blocking factor-containing gamma globulin significantly improves the success of kidney transplants. Some women with a history of recurrent spontaneous first trimester abortions were shown to be deficient in anti-TLX antibody production during their pregnancies. Unlike the sera of women with successful pregnancies, their sera did not block the ability of their own lymphocytes to recognize and be activated by their husband's lymphocytes.

Antibodies reactive with the receptors for IgG present on the surface of maternal B-lymphocytes and phagocytic cells have also been identified in maternal serum. In experimental animals, administration of these antibodies prolonged the survival time of histoincompatible allografts. They may similarly enhance fetal survival by dampening immune responses.

Not all antibodies produced during pregnancy are protective. Women with autoimmune disease who become pregnant produce antoantibodies to self components such as phospholipids or thyroid antigen, which results in an increased rate of first or second trimester pregnancy loss. In women with lupus erythematosus, antibodies to cardiolipin are correlated with early abortion and fetal distress or fetal death.

Continued elaboration of antibodies to one's own cell components leads to the persistence in the circulation of immune complexes (noncovalent conjugates of antigen and its specific antibody). These complexes, through activation of the complement system and release of factors chemotactic for macrophages and polymorphonuclear leukocytes, initiate inflammatory responses. The subsequent damage to placental tissue or trophoblast could expose new antigenic sites to maternal lymphocyte attack and thereby negatively affect the fetus.

The vast majority of pregnant women with no history of autoimmune disease lack circulating immune complexes capable of activating the complement system. Occasionally, significant levels of these complexes are identified in maternal serum and may indicate an early stage infection. Detection of immune complexes in cord blood has been shown to be a sensitive predictor of infection in the newborn. Several studies have implicated circulating immune complexes in the etiology of preeclampsia. Immune complex deposition in the kidneys was offered as a possible immunologic mechanism for the observed hypertension. However, the incidence of immune complexes in sera of these patients is low. Currently there appears to be a consensus that immune complex–mediated effects are not involved in the etiology of that disorder.

HORMONAL AND PROTEIN SUPPRESSOR FACTORS

Fluctuations in hormone levels and new proteins synthesized during pregnancy have also been purported to suppress the maternal cellular immune response to paternal antigens present on cells of the fetus. In most cases, however, the body of data is conflicting, and the immunologic role of these products (if any) in the pregnant woman still remains to be definitively established. The trophoblast initiates synthesis of the protein hormone, chorionic gonadotropin, shortly after conception; maximal levels are reached before the end of the first trimester. Until recently, it was widely believed that this hormone was strongly immunosuppressive to maternal immune responses. However, it now appears that chorionic gonadotropin-related immunosuppression was due to a contaminant that was coisolated with the hormone. Purified human chorionic gonadotropin appears to be devoid of antilymphocyte activity.

The circulating levels of estradiol and progesterone also become markedly elevated during pregnancy. These hormones inhibit the activation of cell-mediated immune responses in vitro by altering the production of lymphokines, such as interleukin 1 and interleukin 2. Whether or not they contribute to in vivo immune suppression in the pregnant woman is still uncertain.

Alpha-fetoprotein has been postulated as contributing to the suppression of maternal lymphocytes that have gained access to the fetal circulation. Levels of this protein are highest in fetal serum and amniotic fluid during the first trimester, whereas maternal serum levels progressively rise throughout gestation. In vitro, alpha-fetoprotein inhibits helper T-lymphocyte functions and activates suppressor cells. Another protein with immunosuppressive properties that increases in concentration during pregnancy is pregnancy-associated alpha$_2$-glycoprotein. Estrogen stimulates peripheral blood leukocytes to produce this protein, which inhibits lymphocyte activity.

EMBRYO-PRODUCED SUPPRESSOR FACTORS

Within 24 hours of conception, the fertilized ovum produces an inducer for the synthesis of a molecule known as early pregnancy factor (EPF). Produced first by the corpus luteum and then by the blastocyst itself, EPF has been postulated to inhibit immune destruction of the fertilized ovum prior to its implantation in the uterus. EPF is suppressive for T-lymphocyte functions in vitro and, recently, a diminution of EPF activity has been correlated with spontaneous abortion.

Interferon alpha, a lymphokine with immunomodulating properties, is present in high levels in the fetal circulation and placenta but absent from maternal serum. In contrast, fetal lymphocytes are markedly deficient in the production of a second form of interferon, interferon gamma, which is a potent activator of natural killer cells and cytotoxic lymphocytes. In addition, interferon gamma has now been shown to also function as a potent inducer of class I HLA antigen expression. Depression of its synthesis, therefore, would also minimize trophoblastic HLA expression. This overproduction of interferon alpha and underproduction of interferon gamma are further contributing mechanisms to the maintainance of immune tolerance to the fetal allograft.

CONSEQUENCES OF IMMUNE SUPPRESSION DURING PREGNANCY

Although there appears to be little or no alteration in numbers of B-lymphocytes or in antibody concentration during pregnancy, the various cell-mediated suppressor factors enumerated above do affect selected aspects of T-lymphocyte functions. Some studies, but not all, have shown fluctuations during pregnancy in the ratio of total numbers of helper to suppressor T-lymphocytes. These differences were due to a decrease in the T-helper subset or an increase in the T-suppressor subset or both. The validity of these findings is strongly reinforced by clinical observation of pregnancy-associated infections.

Infections caused by microorganisms defended against primarily by the cellular immune system may have exacerbated sequelae during pregnancy. Diseases induced by protozoa, such as malaria or amebiasis, are more virulent in pregnant women. Similarly, viral diseases such as poliomyelitis, hepatitis, influenza, varicella, and herpes-associated lesions often manifest more severe clinical symptoms during pregnancy. The greatly increased incidence in pregnant women of vulvovaginal candidiasis also reflects the role of the cellular immune system in defending against colonization by this organism.

SPONTANEOUS ABORTIONS DUE TO IMMUNOLOGIC MECHANISMS

Application of the technology allowing for the detection of pregnancy within 1 to 3 days of conception has established that approximately 50 percent of pregnancies abort within the first several weeks. In addition to pregnancy loss due to such genetic factors as the expression of recessive lethal genes, immunologic factors are also responsible for a significant number of early stage abortions. The various mechanisms leading to immune-mediated pregnancy rejection are listed in Table 1. Inappropriate expression of paternal major histocompatibility complex genes on fetal trophoblastic cells, specifically the elaboration of classic complete class I HLA antigens, leads to the rapid recognition and destruction of these cells by maternal cytotoxic T-lymphocytes. Similarly, failure of the maternal immune system to generate blocking antibodies, such as anti-TLX antibodies, or synthesis of inappropriate quantities of anti-idiotypic antibodies will, in the former case, result in insufficient suppression of maternal antifetal lymphocyte responses and in the latter situation to the production of unrestrained antibody-mediated attack on fetal and maternal lymphocytes. Misregulation in the transformation of the uterine lining, leading to inappropriate PGE_2 elaboration or class II major histocompatibility antigen expression on decidual cells, would also result in insufficient fetal antigen presentation to maternal lymphocytes and decreased production of immunologic blocking factors. Insufficient production of EPF by the preimplantation stage embryo similarly increases the probability of its destruction by the maternal immune system.

TABLE 1 Categories of Immune-Mediated Pregnancy Rejection

Failure in regulation of gene expression in fetal cells, leading to the synthesis of complete paternal HLA class I antigens that increase vulnerability to maternal lymphocyte attack.
Failure of the maternal immune system to generate blocking factors or their anti-idiotypic antibodies, leading to inadequate suppression of maternal cytotoxic T-lymphocytes.
Failure in the relative proportion of HLA class II antigens and PGE_2 in uterine decidua, leading to quantitative errors in the presentation of fetal antigens to the maternal immune system and inappropriate production of suppressor factors.
Insufficient production of early pregnancy factor by the preimplantation stage embryo, resulting in its increased susceptibility to attack by maternal cytotoxic T-lymphocytes.

An intriguing clinical observation is that a woman may be a habitual aborter with one sexual partner but not with another. This appears to be related to the differing capacity of paternal antigens from the two spouses to evoke in the female an immune response that triggers the synthesis of paternal antigen-specific blocking factors. Dissimilarity, especially, of histocompatibility antigens between husband and wife appears to favor elaboration of the requisite maternal immune response. Although the sharing of histocompatability antigens does not preclude a viable pregnancy, there is some evidence suggesting an increased probability of premature pregnancy termination among couples with shared HLA antigens.

IMMUNOLOGIC CONSEQUENCES OF COITUS DURING PREGNANCY

Trophoblast and spermatozoa appear to share an antigenic determinant. Some monoclonal antibodies to spermatozoa also react with trophoblast. In laboratory mice, immunization of females with spermatozoa prior to mating leads to a greatly increased rate of postimplantation pregnancy loss. Similarly, there is poor survival of mouse embryos when transferred to pseudopregnant recipients that were previously immunized with spermatozoa. Several investigators have reported an association in women between antisperm antibodies and a high rate of spontaneous abortion. Women diagnosed as infertile due to the presence of antisperm antibodies and who then conceive following temporary reduction of antibody levels with prednisone treatment subsequently abort at a higher rate than do women who lack these antibodies. Apparently, antisperm antibody binding to trophoblast renders these cells susceptible to complement-mediated lysis. Exposure to semen in sensitized women will also induce local inflammatory responses and complement depletion in the genital tract, thereby increasing vulnerability to maternal or fetal infection.

IMMUNIZATION AS TREATMENT FOR IMMUNOLOGICALLY MEDIATED RECURRENT SPONTANEOUS ABORTION

For women with a history of recurrent first trimester spontaneous abortions in whom chromosomal, infectious, hormonal, autoimmune, and gynecologic etiologies have been ruled out as much as possible and an abnormal in vitro maternal immune response to paternal lymphocytes

TABLE 2 Potential Complications of Immunization as a Treatment for Recurrent Abortion

Antibodies induced in females to paternal lymphocytes can cross the placenta, enter the fetal circulation, and reduce the activity of paternal antigen-containing fetal lymphocytes. This can increase susceptibility to graft versus host disease or immunodeficiency.
Possible transmission or activation of cytomegalovirus can induce fetal malformation.
The artificial enhancement of blocking factors may allow development of a genetically flawed embryo.
An increased incidence of intra-uterine growth-retarded infants has been reported.

has been observed, an increasing number of clinical centers are attempting to overcome immune-mediated pregnancy loss by immunization of the mother with paternal or third-party lymphocytes or lymphocyte or trophoblast membrane fractions. The aim of the immunization, usually performed prior to attempts to achieve pregnancy, is to induce the formation of protective antibodies that will suppress immune rejection of the fetus.

Most of the investigators who have reported the results of maternal immunization claim it to be an effective procedure for inducing blocking factors that allow spontaneous abortion–prone women to deliver term infants. With future improvements in methodology to identify those women who will truly benefit from this procedure and optimization of the immunization protocol, improved success rates are anticipated. Patient selection must be stringent in order to avoid the unnecessary immunization of immunologically competent women.

The possible negative complications of maternal immunization with paternal lymphocyte antigens are listed in Table 2. Since IgG antibodies are readily transferred from the maternal to the fetal circulation, immunization of the mother to paternal antigens may inhibit fetal lymphocytes and thereby increase susceptibility to graft vs host disease, or immunodeficiency. For reasons yet to be explained, some women with probable immune-mediated spontaneous abortions also have impaired immunity to cytomegalovirus but not to other herpesviruses, such as herpes simplex virus and Epstein-Barr virus. Cytomegalovirus is the most common infectious cause of fetal malformations; it is able to cross the placenta and infect the fetus. Since this virus can exist in a latent form in lymphocytes and become activated following blood or lymphocyte transfusion, women with deficient immunity to cytomegalovirus may be less than ideal candidates for immunization. There have been reports of congenital abnormalities in infants born to lymphocyte-immunized mothers due to either a cytomegalovirus infection or (by correcting an innate deficiency) to allowing the development of a genetically flawed embryo. In addition, the incidence of intrauterine growth retardation in pregnancies achieved after immunization has been estimated to be as high as 10 percent.

IMMUNOLOGIC ASPECTS OF IN VITRO FERTILIZATION

It is estimated that about one-half of morphologically normal in vitro fertilized eggs that are returned to the uterus are lost prior to or at the implantation stage. Immunologic processes are suspected as playing a major role in rejection of these embryos. It is postulated that in vitro manipulations and development of the early embryo lead in subtle ways to inappropriate trophoblast antigen expression. These alterations result in enhanced fetal cell recognition by maternal lymphocytes or to an inability to generate adequate levels of suppressor factors. Attempts are now being initiated to improve the success of in vitro fertilization by prepregnancy immunization of the mother with paternal lymphocytes.

A rejection response would also be anticipated if the in vitro fertilized and developing embryo was rendered deficient in the production of EPF. In fact, EPF has been detected in sera of women who underwent a successful pregnancy following in vitro fertilization and embryo transfer, but it was absent in those women with failed in vitro pregnancy attempts. Investigators have also assayed supernatants obtained from in vitro embryo cultures for soluble components (probably EPFs) that could inhibit lymphocyte activation and proliferation. A significant correlation was observed between an embryo's ability to produce measurable quantities of immunosuppressive factor and a subsequent successful pregnancy. Since EPF is produced 24 hours after conception and embryos fertilized in vitro usually are not transferred until the four to eight cell stage, the quantity of this factor available to function in vivo would be expected to be significantly less for in vitro as opposed to in vivo fertilization. Perhaps this is one of the factors responsible for the increased rate of success of gamete intrafallopian transfer over in vitro fertilization. In such transfer, spermatozoa and ova are transferred to the fallopian tubes, and fertilization occurs in vivo.

SUGGESTED READING

Clark DA, Croy BA, eds. Reproductive immunology 1986. New York: Elsevier Science, 1986.

Hearn JP, ed. Immunological aspects of reproduction and fertility control. Baltimore: University Park Press, 1980.

Weinberg ED. Pregnancy-associated depression of cell-mediated immunity. Rev Infect Dis 1984; 6:814–831.

RENAL TRANSPLANTATION IN PREGNANCY

HAMID A. HADI, M.D.

With advancement in medical science and improvement in transplant surgery, pregnancy in renal transplant recipients is no longer an uncommon occurrence. Among the 4,000 to 5,000 renal transplants per year in the United States, until recent recorded pregnancies exceed 760 cases. Although pregnancy in renal transplant recipients was once considered a frightening experience for patients as well as for obstetricians, it no longer presents an insurmountable barrier to successful pregnancy. Current statistics reported by the Advisory Committee of the Renal Transplant Registry indicate an average 5-year survival rate after transplantation of between 61 percent and 78 percent with related living donor and of 42 percent to 51 percent with cadaver organs.

The pregnancy outcomes in these patients have considerably altered with perinatal advances throughout the years. Originally, the Registration Committee of the European Dialysis and Transplant Association in 19 countries reported 120 successful pregnancies in renal transplant recipients. More recent data substantiate this fact. Since pregnancy outcome is dependent upon numerous factors prior to conception and prenatal care, obstetricians should be aware of the following potential problems in the course of such pregnancies.

REPRODUCTIVE FUNCTION

Reports regarding menstrual pattern in renal transplant recipients are conflicting. There is no single specific pattern relating to renal transplants in female individuals. In one series of 144 patients on chronic renal dialysis, 105 were in the reproductive age group; of these 53 had irregular menses and 52 were amenorrheal, suggesting a variable menstrual pattern in these patients. It is reported in one study that patients with chronic renal failure had low serum levels of pituitary follicle-stimulating hormone (FSH) and luteinizing hormone (LH) and that with hemodialysis, levels of both hormones became elevated. It was suggested that dialysis was associated with removal of gonadotropin inhibitors from the circulation. Other studies in patients with hemodialysis found elevated basal LH level, hyperprolactinemia, galactorrhea, and low basal 17-beta estradiol, testosterone, and progesterone levels suggestive of deranged ovarian function. Sexual dysfunction, i.e., loss of libido, is not uncommon in renal transplant recipients. Patients with chronic renal disease may have menstrual abnormalities. These abnormalities range from menorrhagia and irregular menses to amenorrhea and infertility. A recent European registry reported 28 pregnancies among 25,000 patients receiving dialysis. Therefore, it is important to note that patients on dialysis may ovulate and may conceive if they engage in active sexual intercourse. There are sporadic reports of successful pregnancy outcomes in women on dialysis. In the latest report from the registry of the European Dialysis and Transplant Association on 25,310 patients, 28 pregnancies occurred in patients on hemodialysis. Half of the pregnancies in dialyzed patients ended in spontaneous abortions, and one infant had a congenital anomaly. In another report among 350 dialyzed patients, three pregnancies occurred, one of which ended in spontaneous abortion, and the other two patients underwent termination of their pregnancies because of medical complications. Although prenatal care of such patients has improved, the optimism for a 25 percent chance of a normal full-term fetus in a pregnant patient undergoing hemodialysis remains to be confirmed. In addition, patients who receive immunosuppressive therapy may have normal ovarian function and become pregnant. Reports from the American College of Surgeons/National Institute of Health Renal Transplant Registry and the author's institution as well as various other reports substantiate favorable pregnancy outcome in renal transplant recipients in a proper perinatal set-up (Fig. 1).

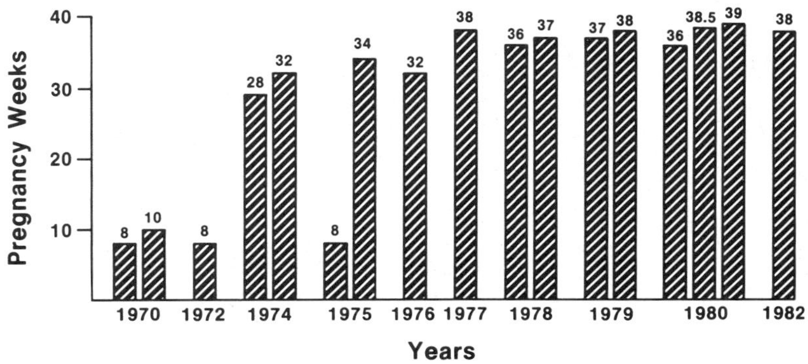

Figure 1 Outcome in 17 pregnancies in 13 renal transplant patients between 1970 and 1982. (From Hadi HA, Stafford CR, Williamson JR, Fadel HE, Devoe LD. Pregnancy outcome in renal transplant recipients: experience at the Medical College of Georgia and review of the literature. South Med J 1986; 79:960, reprinted by permisson.)

FUNCTION OF TRANSPLANTED KIDNEY DURING PREGNANCY

During normal pregnancy, glomerular filtration rate (GFR) increases in the first trimester and is maintained thereafter. In pregnant renal transplant patients, although the allograft is immunologically different, the GFR assumes a rising pattern. A transient reduction in glomerular filtration rate has been reported in these patients, which is similar to that in women with normal near-term pregnancies. However, in 15 percent of cases, a significant decline in renal function is reported in transplant recipients that may persist in the postpartum period. It should also be noted that significant renal failure may result in death. Proteinuria in renal transplant recipients near term associated with decreased glomerular filtration rate is reported in 40 percent of the patients. In the absence of hypertension, this proteinuria is not considered significant. It has been reported that pregnancy outcome improves if the interval between transplantation and pregnancy exceeds 2 years. However, previous experience has shown that if pregnancy occurs 5 or more years after transplantation, renal function deteriorates during pregnancy in most cases and does not return to prepregnancy levels in the postpartum period. A stable renal function prior to conception and a waiting period of 1 year or more before planning a pregnancy are important factors for smoother renal adaptation during pregnancy and an optimal maternal and fetal outcome. Reports from this author's institution indicate a mild reduction in creatinine clearance in renal transplant recipients, which returns to prepregnancy levels in the postpartum period (Table 1).

Although pregnancy is considered to be an immunologically privileged state, rejection episodes can occur during pregnancy in about 9 percent of cases. The fetus is an allograft that contains antigenic properties derived from the father (paternal human leukocyte antigen [HLA]). This antigen may provoke greater reactivity against the transplacental kidney and result in rejection. Rejection episodes are characterized by oliguria, deterioration of renal function, organ enlargement, and tenderness commonly associated with fever. It is difficult to distinguish a rejection process from acute pyelonephritis. Renal biopsy can differentiate between the two episodes and is recommended prior to initiation of antirejection therapy. Traditionally, renal transplants from unrelated donors were superior to cadaveric transplantation for various reasons. However, there has been tremendous improvement in the outcome of cadaveric renal transplantation as a result of advances in immunology, HLA matching, blood transfusion, and immunosuppressive therapy. Therefore it has been suggested that cadaveric transplantation be routinely considered for most young and middle-aged patients with renal failure, and transplantation from an unrelated living donor is indicated for those for whom neither a living related donor nor a cadaveric donor is available. It is well known that stressful situations of pregnancy termination or the stress of labor may increase the risk of kidney rejection. Rejection may occur in the postpartum period as a rebound phenomenon from the immunosuppressed state of pregnancy. Therefore, it is strongly recommended that the corticosteroid dose be increased during labor and early puerperium.

TABLE 1 Blood Pressure and Renal Function

	Before Pregnancy			*During Pregnancy*			*Post Partum*		
Patient No.	*Blood Pressure (mm Hg)*	*Creatinine Clearance (ml/min)*	*Urine Protein (g/L/day)*	*Blood Pressure (mm Hg)*	*Creatinine Clearance (ml/min)*	*Urine Protein (g/L/day)*	*Blood Pressure (mm Hg)*	*Creatinine Clearance (ml/min)*	*Urine Protein (g/L/day)*
1a	110/70	82	0.1	150/100	70	0.15	120/70	80	0.1*
1b	115/60	67	Trace	180/120	50	1.2	110/80	70	Trace†
2a	105/70	62	0.12	110/60	63	0.3	115/76	68	0.1
2b	110/62	72	Trace	128/60	65	0.2	125/70	60	Trace
3	120/70	80	0.15	118/75	54	0.2	120/70	68	0.03
4a	115/76	58	Negative	130/80	53	0.2	110/63	62	Negative
4b	108/68	72	Trace	120/82	65	Trace	150/72	71	Negative
5	118/76	65	Negative	130/70	60	Trace	125/60	74	Negative
6	120/75	78	Trace	130/68	70	0.1	118/70	79	Negative
7	110/60	72	Trace	145/90	58	0.3	120/80	64	0.1‡
8	130/80	66	0.1	132/70	60	0.1	118/74	72	Trace
9	110/60	75	Trace	120/75	70	Trace	115/66	74	Trace
10	115/70	80	Trace	160/105	57	0.35	125/85	64	Trace*
11	120/60	70	Negative	130/75	75	Trace	120/64	80	Negative‡
12	118/65	80	Trace	140/90	65	0.25	130/80	70	Negative‡
13a	120/70	72	Negative	120/60	70	Negative	110/75	85	Negative
13b	110/70	75	Trace	150/100	55	0.420	115/80	70	Trace§

* Severe preeclampsia.
† Eclampsia.
‡ Chronic hypertension with superimposed preeclampsia.
§ Mild preeclampsia.
From Hadi HA, Stafford CR, Williamson JR, Fadel HE, Devoe LD. Pregnancy outcome in renal transplant recipients: experience at the Medical College of Georgia and review of the literature. South Med J 1986; 79:961, reprinted by permission.

PRETERM LABOR

Urinary tract infections and chronic renal disease are considered important causes of preterm labor. Premature rupture of the membranes occurs in between 20 percent and 40 percent of cases. In some series, the incidence of preterm labor is as high as 45 percent in renal transplant recipients. Experience at the author's institution shows that with advances in perinatology and with increasing physician awareness of the potential problems in these patients, maternal and fetal prognoses have dramatically improved. Outcome of such pregnancies as well as of other complications is shown in Table 2.

INFECTIONS AND MALIGNANCIES

Various viral infections such as hepatitis, cytomegalovirus, herpes simplex, and herpes zoster are not infrequent in renal transplant recipients because of the maternal immunosuppressed state. The incidence of urinary tract infections in such patients during the early weeks after transplantation and later (3 months after transplantation or later) is reported to be 73 to 88 percent and 61 percent, respectively. This high rate of infection could be due to an indwelling urethral catheter and/or the use of immunosuppressive agents. Other infections, e.g., bronchopneumonia, infection with *Aspergillus fumigatus,* and even lung abscess, have also been reported in these patients. Since the incidence of bacteriuria in renal transplant recipients far exceeds that in the general population (6.5 percent), careful screening of patients during pregnancy is mandatory. It should be noted that a higher incidence of viral infection, e.g., herpes simplex, warrants more frequent evaluation.

Use of immunosuppressive drugs has been reported to be associated with increased risk of malignancies in

TABLE 2 Data on Outcome of Pregnancy in Patients with Renal Transplants

Patient No.	*Age/Parity*	*Onset of Renal Disease (year)*	*Onset of Pregnancy After Transplantation (months)*	*Renal Donor*	*Prednisone (mg/day)*	*Azathioprine (mg/day)*	*Duration of Pregnancy (weeks)*	*Complications*
1a	26/1	1974	30	Cadaver	40	100	32	Severe preeclampsia, urinary tract infection
1b	28/2	1974	54	Cadaver	40	100	82	Eclampsia, carcinoma in situ of the cervix post partum
2a	21/1	1970	36	Sister	30	100	8	Therapeutic abortion
2b	26/2	1970	10	Sister	60	100	10	Therapeutic abortion, urinary tract infection
3	20/0	1972	5	Brother	30	100	8	Therapeutic abortion
4a	20/0	1975	12	Mother	40	100	8	Therapeutic abortion, class A diabetes
4b	24/1	1975	36	Mother	60	100	34	Preterm labor, urinary tract infection
5	21/1	1980	24	Sister	20	100	38.5	None
6	26/1	1980	28	Sister	40	100	39	None
7	24/1	1978	22	Brother	30	100	37	Chronic hypertension, superimposed preeclampsia urinary tract infection
8	23/1	1980	28	Brother	20	100	36	Preterm labor
9	25/1	1979	16	Cadaver	40	100	37	Premature
10	20/1	1977	15	Sister	20	100	38	Severe preeclampsia
11	26/1	1978	23	Cadaver	40	100	36	Class A diabetes chronic hypertension with superimposed preeclampsia
12	28/2	1979	18	Mother	40	100	38	Chronic hypertension, superimposed preeclampsia, urinary tract infection
13a	23/1	1972	96	Cadaver	30	100	32	Preterm labor
13b	28/2	1976	20	Cadaver	40	100	38	Mild preeclampsia

From Hadi HA, Stafford CR, Williamson JR, Fadel HE, Devoe LD. Pregnancy outcome in renal transplant recipients: experience at the Medical College of Georgia and review of the literature. South Med J 1986; 79:960, reprinted by permission.

renal transplant patients. The combination of an immunosuppressive state and a high incidence of herpes simplex infections may provide the conditions for the development of cervical carcinoma in renal transplant recipients. Gynecologic cancers account for 9 percent of all malignancies in these patients. Since the incidence of squamous cell carcinoma of the uterine cervix is as high as 13-fold in renal transplant recipients, pelvic evaluation and periodic cervical smears should be obtained during pregnancy and afterward.

LOCATION OF TRANSPLANTED KIDNEY AND POTENTIAL OBSTRUCTION OF LABOR

The schematic drawing of Figure 2 illustrates the location and type of vascular anastomosis of transplanted kidney. The transplanted kidney is usually placed in the iliac fossa within the false pelvis. Renal blood supply is established by end-to-end anastomosis between renal and hypogastric arteries and between the renal and external iliac veins. Because of the location of the kidney in the false pelvis, mechanical obstruction of labor is an infrequent occurrence. A single shot intravenous pyelogram is recommended by some authors. Careful pelvic examination as well as evaluation of the transplanted kidney by ultrasonography is extremely useful in assessing renal compression or obstruction of labor. In this author's institution, the location of the transplanted kidney is determined by ultrasonography before vaginal delivery. None of the patients had dystocia and all delivered vaginally. It appears that cesarean section is indicated in these patients for obstetric reasons only. Although rarely reported, previous urologic surgery may make the exposure of the lower uterine segment difficult.

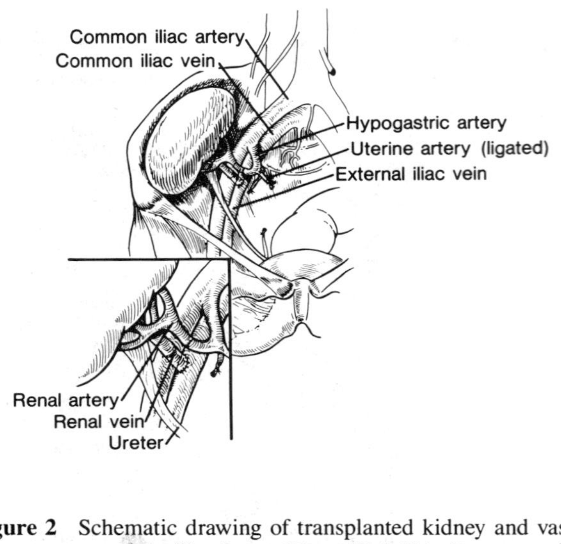

Figure 2 Schematic drawing of transplanted kidney and vascular anastomosis in iliac fossa. (From Hadi HA. Pregnancy in renal transplant recipients. A review. Obstet Gynecol Surv 1986; 41:267, reprinted by permission.)

HYPERTENSION, DIABETES MELLITUS, AND METABOLIC CHANGES

Preeclampsia, chronic hypertension, superimposed preeclampsia, and eclampsia are significantly higher in renal transplant patients (fourfold increase over nontransplant pregnant women). The reported incidence of preeclampsia in these patients is 30 percent, which concurs with our findings of 29.4 percent. Compression of the blood supply to the kidney and increased retrograde pressure by a gravid uterus may play a role in the development of hypertension. It has also been reported that renin-angiotensin-aldosterone activity is increased in renal transplant recipients. However, the pathogenesis of this phenomenon remains unclear.

Abnormal glucose metabolism (hyperglycemia, glycosuria), abnormal glucose tolerance, overt diabetes, and/or diabetic ketoacidosis has been reported in renal transplant recipients. Earlier glycosuria following transplant could rarely be as a result of fever. However, a prolonged course of steroid therapy or acute tubular necrosis may also be the cause of such change. It is also noted that steroid therapy may predispose such patients to become diabetics when there is a history of diabetes in the family. Abnormal cholesterol-rich and triglyceride-rich lipoprotein and high basal insulin levels are also reported in transplant patients. There is some speculation that these lipid changes are similar to those occurring in patients with type II hyperlipidemia, and therefore such patients may be at higher risk for premature development of cardiovascular disease. In the author's experience of 17 pregnancies in 13 renal transplant patients, no significant changes in serum cholesterol or triglyceride levels were noted. Tables 1 and 2 illustrate the data on outcome of pregnancy and post partum in 13 renal transplant recipients.

OTHER REPRODUCTIVE ISSUES

Ectopic pregnancy may occur in renal transplant recipients. Whenever culdocentesis is required for diagnostic purposes, it should be done with caution to avoid injury to the kidney. Laparoscopy carries with it the risk of trauma to the kidney and should be replaced by laparotomy. It is recommended that the abdomen be opened through a vertical incision. This minimizes the risk of injury to the kidney in the presence of adhesions.

Azathioprine can be transferred to the neonate through breast-feeding, and its effect on the neonate depends on the drug concentration in milk. Additional studies are needed regarding the drug's metabolism in milk.

Aseptic necrosis of the femur head is a common problem following prolonged therapy with steroids in renal transplant recipients.

NEONATAL PROBLEMS

The risks of preterm labor and respiratory distress syndrome are the immediate problems that the neonates of renal transplant recipients may face. It appears that use of prednisone in these patients, unlike betamethasone or dexamethasone, does not protect the neonates from respiratory distress syndrome. This may be because of inadequate maternal-fetal transfer of prednisone.

Renal transplant recipients receive prednisone and azathioprine for suppression of their immune systems. It has been suggested that treatment with prednisone in humans as well as in rats has resulted in fetal growth retardation. It is believed that immunogenic disparity between the fetus and the mother results in apparent reproductive advantages. Such disparities facilitate growth of the fetoplacental unit. It has been suggested that suppression of the maternal immune system by immunosuppressive drugs could result in fetal growth retardation. Scott examined this issue by treating a group of pregnant rats with either cyclophosphamide (Cytoxan) or azathioprine (Imuran) in doses similar to human therapeutic doses and compared his results with those from a group of control rats. He found an increased incidence of fetal death and neonatal growth retardation in the drug-treated group. He also found small placentas and decreased cell numbers in the affected group. Analysis of maternal weight, spleen weight assays, and changes in the lymph nodes draining the uterus indicated that the detrimental effect of the drug on fetuses was primarily due to immunosuppressive and cytotoxic mechanisms. Although species variability exists in regard to immunosuppressive agents, this study conveys a significant message that immunosuppressive drugs should be kept to the minimum dose required to control the maternal condition.

Follow-up of infants of mothers who received azathioprine and prednisone during pregnancy revealed a reduction in lymphocyte count and chromosomal aberrations (gaps, breaks, and deletions). Studies in mice have shown that the ovaries of female offspring of mothers treated with 6-mercaptopurine (the principal metabolite of azathioprine) contained fewer oocytes and ovarian follicles compared with those who did not receive the drug during pregnancy. It is important to note that since the fetal germ cells are exposed to immunosuppressive agents, their effects may not be manifest until they produce children much later on. It is also conceivable that since the synthesis of deoxyribonucleic acid ceases when the germ cells are arrested in the prophase of the first meiotic divison in utero and no deoxyribonucleic acid is synthesized until after fertilization, the effects of such drugs can be irreversible. Therefore continuing follow-up of the children of such mothers is recommended.

Depressed neonatal hematopoiesis, lymphopenia, lymphoid hypoplasia, adrenocortical insufficiency, and increased incidence of maternally transmitted viral infections (cytomegalovirus and hepatitis) have also been reported.

High doses of corticosteroids in various species have resulted in resorption of embryo, decreased fetal size and cleft palate. The use of azathioprine during pregnancy, has also been reported to be associated with fetal chromosomal aberrations, skeletal and central nervous system anomalies, cleft palate, hematopoietic depression, and hydrops fetalis. Azathioprine is metabolized to 6-mercaptopurine in animals and results in decreased body weight and sterility. Inosinate pyrophosphorylase enzyme is required to convert azathioprine to its active form, and the fetus lacks this necessary enzyme. There are sporadic reports of neonatal lymphopenia, adrenocortical insufficiency, premature closure of the fontanelle, and umbilical hernia in neonates of renal transplant recipients treated with prednisone and azathioprine during pregnancy.

CONCLUSIONS

It is important to note that as pregnancy progresses, certain physiologic changes such as an increase in intravascular volume or an increase in glomerular filtration rate occur that are necessary for an optimal outcome. If renal function is impaired by 50 percent prior to conception, these physiologic changes will not occur, and subsequently the goal of achieving a viable fetus and a low maternal complication rate will be impeded.

Pregnancy can occur in women who undergo dialysis or in those who have had renal transplants. Menstruation returns to normal on an average of 6 months following successful renal transplantation. Therefore, women should be protected by barrier contraceptives for at least 1 year after the transplantation of a kidney from a related donor and for 2 years following cadaver transplant. If pregnancy occurs, the outcome depends on preconceptional counseling, or close follow-up of the patient, and on the physician's awareness of the potential problems that may arise in the course of pregnancy. Good prognostic criteria include patients who have had good health for 2 years following transplantation, absence of hypertension, proteinuria, signs of graft rejection, and pelvicalyceal distention, a serum creatinine level of less than or equal to 2 mg per deciliter, a prednisone requirement of less than or equal to 15 mg per day, and an azathioprine requirement of less than or equal to 2 mg per kilogram per day.

Pregnancy termination is indicated in the presence of significant deterioration of renal function. Penn and associates reported 56 pregnancies in 37 women following renal transplantation. In their series, only seven patients terminated their pregnancies, and 43 had live births with a neonatal survival rate of 90 percent. More recently, these results have been confirmed by our report. It is apparent that since 1970, both more patients and physicians have elected not to terminate such pregnancies. The incidence of preterm labor has significantly decreased in transplant patients in recent years (see Fig. 1).

The major decline in maternal-fetal complications in these patients is the result of improved technology, awareness of the problems, and better perinatal care. It is recommended that these patients be followed in a high-risk obstetric service. Electronic and ultrasonographic modalities should be used to monitor fetal well-being and growth. Frequency of occurrence of abnormal cervical cytology and of certain viral infections, e.g., herpes simplex and cytomegalovirus, requires periodic testing. Evaluation of other reports suggests that vaginal delivery is not contraindicated in these patients. Cesarean section should be reserved for cases in which labor is obstructed by a renal homograft. Other obstetric indications for cesarean section include fetal distress, cephalopelvic disproportion,

TABLE 3 Treatment Recommendations for Women Regarding Renal Transplant and Pregnancy

Preconception recommendations:	Barrier contraceptive for 2 years. Routine urinalysis for proteinuria, serum blood urea nitrogen, and creatinine—24-hour urinary protein measurement. Treatment of hypertension or other medical complications if present. Adjust medications, routine antenatal work-up. Intravenous pyelogram.
Recommendations for pregnancy and delivery:	First prenatal visit, evaluation for proteinuria randomly; blood urea nitrogen and creatinine clearance tests.
	Close observation for signs of pregnancy-induced hypertension.
	Periodic assessment of Pap smear.
	Observe for signs of allograft rejection; periodic ultrasonographic assessment of transplanted kidney.
	Follow-up of fetal growth by ultrasound examination. Nonstress test and/or contraction stress test from 32 weeks onward.
	Assessment of the kidney's location at labor.
Neonatal recommendation:	Immediate and continued assessment and follow-up of the child by a pediatrician.

previous cesarean section, fetal malpresentation, and in those patients who have avascular necrosis of the femur head that impairs abduction. Because of the stresses of labor and delivery, additional doses of corticosteroid during this period of time are logical (hydrocortisone 100 mg every 6 hours during labor).

Davison and Lindheimer have proposed the following criteria for identifying those patients who are good candidates for pregnancy following renal transplantation:

1. Two years of good, stable health of the renal transplant recipient.
2. Anatomic status compatible with good obstetric outcome.
3. Absence of proteinuria.
4. Absence of significant hypertension.
5. No evidence of active allograft rejection.
6. No renal or calyceal distention as revealed by a recent intravenous pyelogram.
7. A recent serum creatinine measurement of less than 2 mg per 100 ml.
8. Dose of prednisone of 15 mg per day or less and of azathioprine of no greater than 3 mg per kilogram per day.

Table 3 is a summary of treatment recommendations for pregnant women with renal transplants.

Multidisciplinary follow-up of renal transplant recipients during pregnancy and post partum by a perinatologist, neonatologist, nephrologist, and immunologist provides the best care.

SUGGESTED READING

Davison KM, Lindheimer MD. Pregnancy in renal transplant recipients. J Reprod Med 1982; 27:613–621.

Hadi HA. Pregnancy in renal transplant recipients. A review. Obstet Gynecol Surv 1986; 41:264–271.

Hadi HA, Stafford CR, Williamson JR, Fadel HE, Devoe LD. Pregnancy outcome in renal transplant recipients: experience at the Medical College of Georgia and review of the literature. South Med J 1986; 79:959–964.

Penn I, Makowski E, Harris P. Parenthood following renal transplantation. Kidney Int 1980; 18:221–223.

INFECTION

INFECTIOUS DISEASE THERAPY IN PREGNANCY

YOGESH G. SHAH, M.D.
RICHARD K. MILLER, Ph.D.

In treating patients for any disease process, the therapy must be tailored to the patient and the disease itself. Unfortunately for the pregnant patient, most drugs are tested only in males or nonpregnant females. Thus, our collective experience with drug use during pregnancy is based on postmarketing or phase IV testing. For some agents, especially those for infectious disease therapy, a substantial literature has developed because these infectious diseases are often quite prevalent in pregnant patients. Yet the actual therapy administered is based on the pharmacokinetics in the male and nonpregnant female.

Of major consideration in this review are two points: (1) Are dosages of chemotherapy given to a pregnant patient appropriate for treating the infection in either mother or conceptus? (2) Are mother or conceptus or both at increased risk for toxic insult at the dosages used? The pharmacokinetic issue is not a simple one. Is treatment specifically for a maternal infection, a fetal infection, or both? The separate treatment of the organism within an organism, i.e., conceptus within mother, presents multiple difficulties because of inaccessibility. Yet with sophisticated ultrasonographic techniques, it is possible to remove fluids from the conceptus as well as to introduce drugs directly into different compartments of the conceptus. Thus, maternal chemotherapy is not mandatory, even though it is a more convenient and accessible form when treating the conceptus.

As with nonpregnant patients, many common factors must be considered with therapeutic intervention: (1) the chemical characteristics of the drug: molecular weight, ionic strength, lipid solubility, and degress of protein binding; (2) dose, mode of administration, and time interval between doses; (3) distribution, metabolism, and excretion of the drug; (4) other concurrent medications; and (5) intercurrent disease processes. For the pregnant patient, many of the factors in (3) through (5) may be substantially different, depending on the stage of gestation and the sensitive period of embryonic and fetal development. Physiologic changes in the pregnant patient during pregnancy can affect the disposition of the drug. Because of changes in gastrointestinal absorption, decreased gastric motility can lead to increased transit times for drugs. Subcutaneous absorption may be erratic because of increased vasomotor instability. Maternal blood volume is increased by 40 to 50 percent, which can lead to greater volumes of drug distribution. Plasma proteins are selectively increased (e.g., thyroid binding-globulin) or decreased (e.g., serum albumin). Blood flow redistribution occurs, leading to increased blood flow to the uterus by 70 to 80 percent. Nutrient metabolism undergoes changes: the carbohydrate consumer (mother) is converted to a fatty acid consumer. Xenobiotic metabolism occurs in that there is selectively increased or decreased production of metabolites to either inactive or active products in two different organisms. In renal function, there is increased glomular filtration rate and excretion of water-soluble metabolites. Thus to a large degree, pregnant and lactating patients are unique.

To explore these issues of pharmacokinetics, the class of penicillins is used as an example, since it is among the best studied and most frequently used of all antibiotics during pregnancy. Ampicillin and dicloxacillin are examined. Typically, one can monitor adult levels of a drug by measuring blood and urine samples at multiple times throughout the exposure period without substantial difficulty. Unfortunately, access to the conceptus is limited, except during labor and delivery. Sources for monitoring the conceptus for concentration of drugs, which do not change functional parameters in the conceptus, are amniotic fluid and blood (often from the fetal scalp). With advances in magnetic resonance imaging and spectroscopy, it may be possible to monitor drug distribution based on labeling the drug with ^{13}C or a paramagnetic ion to examine its distribution within the conceptus.

It is essential in deciding on the appropriate drug that the following considerations be reviewed: (1) use approved drugs rather than new agents, (2) use the lowest effective dose to the site of action for the minimal amount of time, and (3) examine in detail the exact stage of gestation for which the drug will be administered.

Ampicillin is rapidly absorbed and excreted in the nonpregnant patient, as noted in Table 1. However, in the pregnant patient, the plasma levels of ampicillin are about one-half of the concentrations in the same patient when she is not pregnant. Such reductions in plasma levels during pregnancy are attributed to increased renal clearance and increased volume of distribution, as noted in Table 1.

TABLE 1 Pharmacokinetic Comparisons Following Intravenous Administration of Ampicillin in Women During and After Pregnancy

Assessment	*Nonpregnant*	*Pregnant*
Half-life, B-phase (min)	44 ± 7	39 ± 8*
Peak level (μg/ml)	44 ± 15	45 ± 36
Volume of distribution (L/kg)	0.41 ± 0.20	0.55 ± 0.29*
Area under the curve (cm^2)	28 ± 10	18 ± 6*
Dose recovered (%)†	80 ± 31	79 ± 25
Plasma clearance (ml/min)	394 ± 165	613 ± 302*
Renal clearance (ml/min)‡	228	323*

* Significantly different at least at $p<0.05$.
† Up to 8 hours after dosing.
‡ Between 0 and 3 hours after dosing.
(Modified from Nau H. Clinical pharmacokinetics in pregnancy and perinatology. II. Penicillins. Dev Pharmacol Ther 1987; 10:174–198. Based on original data of Phillipson A. J Infect Dis 1977; 136:370; Clin Pharmacokinet 1979; 4:297.

Such alterations result in an increase in plasma clearance. As a consequence of the increased plasma clearance of ampicillin, the area under the plasma concentration-time curve was notably decreased during pregnancy. As noted in Table 1, the dose of ampicillin recovered was not different in pregnancy. Such information indicates that absorption of ampicillin is not impaired in pregnant patients and that excretion and distribution may have the greatest impact on circulating levels of the drug.

At different stages of gestation, there may be differential pharmacokinetics. This is especially true during labor. The absorption of amoxicillin from patients in labor is dramatically reduced to the point of not being effective for therapy of gram-negative infections.

Besides distribution within the mother, distribution of the agent to the conceptus has equal importance. The appearance of ampicillin in amniotic fluid can be variable, depending on the stage of gestation. During the first two trimesters, little ampicillin is present in the amniotic fluid compared with the third trimester. The stage-dependent changes are partially attributed to the increased exchange of drug between amniotic fluid and maternal blood early in gestation and the decreased activity of the embryonic-fetal kidneys in the first two trimesters. Other maternal factors are of particular importance for the movement into the conceptus, as noted in the case of ampicillin and dicloxacillin. Even though ampicillin rapidly appears in the conceptus following maternal administration, little dicloxacillin appears. Such differences in distribution have been partially attributed to the high degree of plasma protein binding for dicloxacillin (greater than 90 percent). Such differences can provide important therapeutic advantages, depending on which patient is being treated—mother or conceptus.

During lactation, neonatal development and drug therapy must be considered prospectively. As with exposures during pregnancy, concerns are especially relevant to an immature functioning organism. Now, with the capability of maintaining the very premature infant, the impact of an immature liver, kidney, and other organs raises critical issues concerning the ability of the neonate to appropriately biotransform and eliminate chemotherapeutic agents. Therefore, at issue is not simply whether the compound appears in the milk, but rather how much may be consumed in a day relative to body mass, and how well the neonate can eliminate this agent.

As with placental transfer, the same chemical factors apply; however, there is a major difference in pH between milk and blood. In addition to the many proteins, including immunoglobulins in milk, there are substantial amounts of lipids and lipoproteins. These constituents make the milk and the mammary gland itself sites for concentrating lipid-soluble substances compared with serum. Thus, these factors can modify the ability of drugs to appear, to be retained in the milk, and then to be presented to the neonate.

Table 2 reviews not only the issues of exposure during pregnancy and the critical nature of the actual exposure but also lists known effects of drugs on the neonate based on exposure through breast-feeding. The comments listed in this table emphasize the benefits of breast-feeding, but concern is raised when certain medications are required for the mother.

In examining the issues of infectious disease therapy or in fact other chemotherapy during pregnancy, a number of references are suggested at the end of this chapter as a means of exploring the issues of principles in pharmacology or catalogs of information concerning specific agents. If the reader is interested in having a computer link for evaluating both therapeutic and environmental exposures, on which the information is summarized and current references listed, he or she is referred to REPROTOX, a computer service of the Reproductive Toxicology Center, in Washington, DC. The remainder of this chapter explores specific forms of infectious disease therapy.

PENICILLINS AND CEPHALOSPORINS

Penicillins have proven to be the safest antibiotics for use during pregnancy. There are no known contraindications to the use of this group of drugs, except drug sensitivity. There have been no major reports associating antibiotic use during the first trimester of pregnancy with

TABLE 2 Effects of Infectious Disease Therapy on the Conceptus or Neonate*

Category/Agent	*First Trimester*	*Second and Third Trimesters*	*Labor/Delivery*	*Lactation*
Antibiotics				
Penicillin	U maternal allergic responses	U	U	S fungus GI tract
Ampicillin	U maternal allergic responses	U	U	S fungus GI tract
Chloramphenicol	U	K neonatal gray baby	K neonatal gray baby	K bone marrow K GI tract
Streptomycin	K 8th nerve damage, micromelia,	K 8th nerve damage	U	U
Gentamicin	S 8th nerve damage			
Kanamycin	S 8th nerve damage	S 8th nerve damage	U	U
Nitrofurantoin	U/A mutagen	S 8th nerve damage	U	U
		K hyperbilirubinemia	K hyperbilirubinemia	S hemolysis G-6 PD
Sulfonamides	U	K hemolytic anemia	K hemolytic anemia	S hemolysis G-6 PD
Tetracycline	K inhibition of bone growth S micromelia S syndactyly	K hyperbilirubinemia K stain deciduous teeth K inhibition of bone growth S enamel hypoplasia	K hyperbilirubinemia K stain deciduous teeth	S hemolysis G-6 PD
Sulfamethoxazole	Q/A malformation	U	K hyperbilirubinemia	K hyperbilirubinemia
Trimethoprim	Q/A malformation	U	U	U
Metronidazole	U/A tumors	U	U	U
Methenamine mandelate	U	U	U	U
Cephalosporins	U	U	U	U
Nalidixic acid	U/NR	U	U	U
Erythromycin	U	U	U	U
Clindamycin	U	U	U	U
Antihelmintic Drugs				
Mebendazole	U/NR/A	U	U	U
Piperazine	U	U	U	U
Antimalarial Drugs				
Quinine	S malformations, abortions, 8th nerve damage	S deafness, thrombocytopenia	Q thrombocytopenia	U
Primaquine	U	U	U	U
Pentaquine	U	S 8th nerve damage	U	U
Chloroquine	S 8th nerve damage A malformations	S hemolysis G-6 PD	S hemolysis G-6 PD	U
Pyrimethamine	U/A/D/NR	S hemolysis G-6 PD	S hemolysis G-6 PD	U
Antitubercular Drugs (usually combinations)				
Ethambutol	U/A malformations	U	U	U
Rifampin	U/A CNS	U	Q hypoprothrombinemia	U
Isoniazid	Q CNS	U	U	U
Leprostatic Drugs				
Dapsone	U	U	K hyperbilirubinemia	U
Thalidomide	K micromelia, phocomelia multiple anomalies	U	U	U
Antiviral Drugs				
Amantadine	U/A malformations	U/NR	U/NR	U/NR
Vidarabine	U/A malformations	U	U/NR	U/NR
Acyclovir	U/NR	U	U/NR	U/NR
Azidothymidine	U/NR	U/D/NR	U/D/NR	U/D/NR
Antiparasitic Drugs				
Hycanthone	U/A malformations, NR	U/NR	U/NR	U
Suramin sodium	U/A malformations, NR	U/NR	U/NR	U
Metronidazole	U/A carcinogen	U	U	K lactose intolerances K diarrhea
Vaccine Drugs				
Allergy/desensitization	U	U	U	U
Inactivated	U	U	U	U
Live virus	K malformation, abortion	U/NR	U/NR	U
Gamma globulin	U	U	U	U
Antifungal Drugs				
Nystatin	U	U	U	U
Miconazole	U	U	U	U
Amphotericin B	U	U	U	U
Flucytosine	U/A malformations	U/NR	U/NR	U
Griseofulvin	U/A malformations, NR	U/NR	U/NR	U

* This partial list of drugs used during pregnancy and lactation is divided into therapeutic classes. The statements made reflect the need for treatment. If there are no currently known effects on the conceptus or a lack of studies, these drugs are listed as unknown (U). Since long-term follow-ups of progeny have not been completed, caution should be considered with all therapy. In some instances the drug has been associated with an increase in abnormalities in the conceptus and neonate and is therefore also listed as disease-related (D). If no human data are available and animal data indicate abnormalities, A is used. Symbols: K, known effects; S, suspected effects; Q, questionable effects/sporadic case report(s); U, unknown effects or no reported adverse effects; NR, unknown effects, however, not recommended based upon adult toxicity information; D, maternal disease-related effects; A, animal-documented effects.

(Modified from Miller RK, Kellog C, Saltzman R. Reproductive and perinatal toxicology. In: Haley T, Berndt WO, eds. Handbook of toxicology. Washington, DC: Hemisphere Press, 1987.)

induction of congenital abnormalities in humans. All penicillin derivatives rapidly cross the placenta. These agents have a low degree of lipid solubility and a high degree of ionization, requiring high doses of administration when therapeutic levels are to be achieved in the fetus. Penicillins with high protein binding, i.e., greater than 90 percent (oxacillin, cloxacillin, dicloxacillin, and nafcillin), reach lower levels in tissues than those with moderate protein binding, i.e. 40 to 60 percent (penicillin G, methicillin, carbenicillin). Ampicillin and amoxicillin have the lowest protein binding (less than 20 percent). Fetal drug concentrations are almost nil during the first trimester and are highest at term. Amoxicillin, a semisynthetic penicillin, resembles ampicillin chemically and antimicrobiologically. Azidocillin is structurally similar to ampicillin. Concentrations of the drug in the maternal plasma are higher than those of ampicillin after oral or intramuscular administration. Fetal and amniotic fluid levels are lower than those of ampicillin. The concentrations of benzylpenicillin (penicillin G) in fetal blood are lower than those of ampicillin or carbenicillin, both early in pregnancy and at term. The limited transfer of penicillin G across the placenta may be the result of high polarity, rapid clearance, and its low pKa.

Most cephalosporins are well tolerated during pregnancy, and their pharmacokinetics are similar to those of the penicillins. Levels in maternal serum are lower and elimination half-lives are shorter than in nonpregnant patients, whereas renal clearance is higher. The safety of second- and third-generation cephalosporins during pregnancy has not been thoroughly tested, but they appear to provide the same margin of safety as their predecessors. Most penicillins and cephalosporins are excreted into the breast milk.

AMINOGLYCOSIDES

Included here are streptomycin, kanamycin, and amikacin. They appear to be safe when given for short periods. Fetuses are susceptible to the ototoxic and nephrotoxic effects of the drug, and in the mother it may exaggerate the action of neuromuscular blocking agents (magnesium sulfate, succinylcholine, *d*-tubocurarine).

TETRACYCLINES

Oxytetracycline, demethylchlortetracycline, and tetracycline all cross the placenta readily and appear in cord blood. They produce adverse effects in the pregnant mother and the fetus, and hence are contraindicated for use during pregnancy. Dose-related hepatotoxicity with fatty infiltration of the liver may occur when a pregnant woman is given parenteral tetracycline, especially if there is an underlying renal impairment or pyelonephritis. It is associated with a high mortality related to liver and renal failure. There have also been reports of fatty degeneration in the renal tubular cells and of nephrogenic diabetes insipidus in pregnant women. The latter is probably related to interference by tetracyclines with the activity of antidiuretic hormone on the kidney. Administration of tetracyclines in the first and second trimesters may lead to discoloration and severe dysplasia of the teeth and inhibition of bone growth. Damage to growing bones and teeth by tetracyclines is due to chelation of calcium (dose-dependent) interference with protein synthesis. Congenital limb abnormalities and cataracts have also been observed in infants of mothers who received tetracycline during the first trimester. Hypoplasia of the deciduous and permanent teeth with discoloration may occur up to 6 to 8 years of age if drug exposure is continued postnatally. Absorption of tetracycline by the infant via ingestion of breast milk is negligible because of chelation with milk calcium.

CHLORAMPHENICOL

The use of chloramphenicol during pregnancy is not indicated because of potential aplastic anemia and blood dyscrasias. Chloramphenicol given to neonates may produce the "gray syndrome" characterized by pallor, cyanosis, tachypnea, and vascular collapse. It is caused by accumulation of toxic levels of the drug, particularly in the preterm infant who lacks the enzyme responsible for glucuronyl conjugation and the functionally mature renal system required for effective excretion. The drug's serum half-life is prolonged, with a mortality of 40 percent associated with this syndrome. Serum levels of chloramphenicol are similar in pregnant and nonpregnant individuals. It crosses the placenta, and fetal serum levels reach 30 to 150 percent of maternal levels. It is secreted into breast milk, but levels are too low to induce the "gray syndrome."

MACROLIDES

Included here are erythromycin base and its salts. Absorption of this drug from the gastrointestinal tract during pregnancy is erratic. It crosses the placenta, but fetal and amniotic fluid levels are low and subtherapeutic. Erythromycin base produces no known deleterious effects in the mother or fetus, whereas estolate salts have been associated with subclinical and reversible cholestatic hepatitis in 10 to 15 percent of women when given this during the third trimester. This is a hypersensitivity reaction, and it rapidly recurs if the drug is administered again.

LINCOSAMIDES

This group consists of lincomycin and clindamycin. Lincomycin has become obsolete and has been replaced by clindamycin. Serum clindamycin levels in nonpregnant and pregnant patients are identical, but the serum half-life is shorter during pregnancy. It crosses the placenta easily. As of the present, fetal toxicity due to clindamycin has not been documented. The potential serious complication of pseudomembranous enterocolitis must be considered in the mother.

SULFONAMIDES

Sulfonamides are a large class of antibacterial agents commonly used for treatment of asymptomatic bacteriuria and cystourethritis during pregnancy. They readily cross the placenta and enter both the fetal circulation and amniotic fluid during all stages of pregnancy. Equilibrium with maternal plasma is achieved after 2 to 3 hours, with fetal levels averaging 70 to 90 percent of maternal ones.

Direct toxic effects of sulfonamides on the fetus are not well documented. Because of a relative deficiency of fetal glucose-6-phosphate dehydrogenase (G-6-PD) and glutathione, there is a theoretical risk of hemolysis. Sulfonamides bind to serum albumin and may competitively displace bilirubin from its binding sites on the same molecule. In the fetus this competition is not worrisome, since the placenta is capable of clearing unconjugated bilirubin. However, in the neonatal period, the protection offered by the placenta is no longer available, and the presence of long-acting sulfonamides predisposes the infant to hyperbilirubinemia with diffusion of free bilirubin into the central nervous system, potentially causing kernicterus. Hence, long-acting sulfonamides, such as sulfamethoxydiazine, should not be administered at term because levels may remain significant in the fetus for 4 to 6 days after maternal ingestion. Most reports of sulfonamide exposure during gestation have failed to demonstrate a significant teratogenic risk.

Sulfonamides are excreted in breast milk in low concentrations but do not appear to pose a significant risk for the healthy, full-term neonate. However, the premature neonate and infants with hyperbilirubinemia and G-6-PD deficiency should not be exposed to sulfonamides through breast milk.

Trimethoprim-sulfamethoxazole (TMP/SMZ) inhibits folate synthesis and is best avoided during pregnancy, especially during the first and third trimesters. TMP/SMZ has induced cleft palate in rats, although no similar case of human birth anomaly related to maternal ingestion of TMP/SMZ has been documented. Both components of the drug readily cross the placenta and reach similar levels in maternal and fetal circulations. The theoretical risk exists of hemolysis and kernicterus from relative G-6-PD and glutathione deficiency in the fetus. TMP/SMZ may induce megaloblastic anemia during pregnancy as a result of its antifolate effects. However, this reaction can be prevented by concomitant administration of folinic acid, which does not inhibit the bacteriostatic action of TMP/SMZ.

Nitrofurantoin readily crosses the placenta and achieves a high fetal-to-maternal serum concentration ratio. Therapeutic levels are not maintained in the cord serum, probably because of rapid renal clearance. Nitrofurantoin is excreted into breast milk in very low concentrations. It should be used cautiously in early pregnancy because there is evidence of mutagenesis in mammalian cells. There is again a theoretical risk of hemolysis in the fetus and neonate, with relative G-6-PD deficiency.

Nalidixic acid inhibits deoxyribonuclease in bacteria, and hence theoretically it could affect DNA synthesis in pregnancy and should be avoided during the first trimester. It also crosses the placenta and is highly protein-bound. It occasionally may induce toxic psychosis and convulsions, and should be avoided in patients with seizure disorders. Nalidixic acid has been reported to cause increased intracranial pressure, papilledema, and bulging fontanelles in the newborn infant. It is excreted into breast milk in insignificantly low concentrations and is not contraindicated in nursing mothers.

Methenamine mandelate is rapidly absorbed following oral administration, but its distribution in maternal and fetal tissues and in amniotic fluid is not well known. However, its use appears to be safe during pregnancy, and no increased risk to the fetus has been reported. It is excreted into breast milk in insignificant amounts.

TUBERCULOSTATIC AND LEPROSTATIC AGENTS

Untreated tuberculosis can have serious consequences, and the course of infection may be aggravated by pregnancy. Isoniazid, ethambutol, and rifampin are first-line antituberculosis agents used during pregnancy. Isoniazid appears to be the safest and most effective of the available antituberculosis agents. It crosses the placenta and is also excreted in breast milk. It is potentially hepatotoxic, and this risk is increased in rapid acetylators (e.g., Orientals, Eskimos) and in pregnant women. Ethambutol has been widely used during pregnancy, although congenital anomalies such as cleft palate, exencephaly, and vertebral defects have been reported in mice. No increased risk of toxicity or teratogenicity has been established in humans given this drug. At present there are no adequate data available regarding the penetration of ethambutol into amniotic fluid, fetal tissues, or breast milk.

Rifampin rapidly crosses the placenta, and appreciable amounts of the drug reach fetal blood and amniotic fluid, whereas only trace amounts are detected in human breast milk. The reported incidence of birth defects, e.g., limb reduction, is not different from the expected background rate. A theoretical risk of hypoprothrombinemia and bleeding during the perinatal period resulting from hepatic enzyme induction or from drug interaction with rifampin has been suggested.

The increased risk of ototoxicity in infants of mothers who receive prolonged courses of streptomycin during pregnancy has been discussed (see section on aminoglycosides). Streptomycin is no longer considered a first-line antituberculosis agent.

Dapsone, a sulfone, is the drug of choice for treatment of all forms of leprosy. It has no significant adverse effects on the fetus except near the time of delivery, when it may displace bilirubin from albumin. Clofazimine, used in dapsone-resistant infection, has not been associated with any teratogenicity. Pigmentation of the skin has been observed in some infants, suggesting that placental transfer may occur.

Thalidomide used for treatment of erythema nodosum leprosum may be difficult to use in pregnancy because of its known teratogenic effects.

ANTIVIRAL AGENTS

In the last four decades only a few major advances in antiviral chemotherapy have developed. These few include the use of amantadine and its derivatives for the prophylaxis and treatment of influenza, the use of vidarabine and acyclovir for the treatment of life-threatening herpes simplex and varicella-zoster infections, and the use of acyclovir for the treatment of genital herpes simplex infection. Idoxuridine and cytarabine are too toxic for systemic use and are reserved primarily for topical treatment of herpes keratitis.

Amantadine in high doses has been found to be embryotoxic and teratogenic in laboratory animals. Hence its use during pregnancy is contraindicated. There has been a case report of cardiovascular malformation in the offspring. It is excreted in breast milk in low concentrations. Although there have been no reported adverse effects in breast-fed infants, it is recommended that the drug not be used in nursing mothers.

Vidarabine has not been studied in human pregnancy but the drug is teratogenic in some animal species, and its use in pregnant women should be reserved for life-threatening herpes infections. No data are currently available regarding the pharmacokinetics of vidarabine in maternal and fetal tissues or breast milk.

Acyclovir in laboratory animals is neither embryotoxic nor teratogenic. Nevertheless, its safety in pregnancy has not been established. Human embryonic lung cells in culture show minimal growth effects when exposed to acyclovir. Its use during human pregnancy has not been frequent. However, those cases reported do not suggest particular fetal toxicity of the drug. Acyclovir has been found in breast milk at concentrations equal to or greater than those in maternal plasma. It has been estimated that a nursing infant would attain subtherapeutic and subtoxic levels of acyclovir from breast milk exposure.

At present there are no published reports concerning the teratogenicity of azidothymidine in humans.

Even though there has been no published association between antiviral drug therapy in pregnancy and congenital malformation, systemic antiviral drug therapy should not be used in pregnancy, particularly in the first trimester, except in cases of life-threatening maternal infections.

ANTIMALARIALS

Antimalarial agents may be necessary during pregnancy for prevention and treatment of malaria. The classic drugs used in malaria therapy are chloroquine and its congeners, inhibitors of dihydrofolate reductase—primaquine and quinine. Other antimalarials include pyrimethamine, dapsone, and a combination of pyrimethamine and sulfadoxine.

Chloroquine is the drug of choice for all forms of malaria except that caused by resistant strains of *Plasmodium falciparum.* Chloroquine in high doses is fetotoxic in the rat and produces anophthalmia and microphthalmia in the offspring. Present studies suggest that antimalarial doses of chloroquine during pregnancy do not demonstrate any teratogenic effects. The possibility of hemolysis related to G-6-PD deficiency in mother or fetus must be considered whenever this drug or any of the other quinine derivatives, such as primaquine, are administered. Chloroquine crosses the placenta and accumulates in the fetal uveal tract, and it produces cochleovestibular damage if administered on a long-term basis in high doses. Hydroxychloroquine, a quinine derivative, is slightly more potent than chloroquine, and its pharmacologic properties are similar to those of chloroquine. Since chloroquine is the more widely used and studied compound, its use in pregnancy is preferable to that of hydroxychloroquine.

Treatment of exoerythrocytic stages of *Plasmodium vivax* and *Plasmodium ovale* with primaquine should be withheld until after the completion of pregnancy because it can precipitate hemolysis in patients with a deficiency of G-6-PD. Pregnant women for whom primaquine is indicated should receive only chloroquine once weekly until delivery. Primaquine can then be administered after delivery.

Treatment and prophylaxis of chloroquine-resistant malaria require the combined use of pyrimethamine, a folic acid antagonist, and a long-acting sulfonamide, namely, sulfadoxine. Pyrimethamine is teratogenic in laboratory animals, and its safety in human pregnancy has not been established. If pyrimethamine must be used during pregnancy, then folinic acid should be given to prevent the possibility of folate deficiency. Reproductive effects specific to sulfadoxine have not been reported, but the monitored use of other sulfonamides during pregnancy does not suggest that this group of drugs poses a significant teratogenic risk. However, use of long-acting sulfonamides late in pregnancy may be associated with neonatal jaundice and kernicterus. In short, women who are pregnant or are likely to become so should not travel to areas where the presence of chloroquine-resistant malaria requires prophylaxis with pyrimethamine and sulfadoxine. Pregnant women who cannot avoid exposure to these malarial strains should be informed of the possible risks of fetal teratogenicity and neonatal jaundice before they take this medication.

Dapsone is also used with pyrimethamine in malaria prevention. A rare hypersensitivity reaction called "sulfone syndrome" has been reported. This potentially fatal syndrome consists of fever, malaise, hepatitis with hepatic necrosis, exfoliative dermatitis, lymphadenopathy, and hemolytic anemia. Treatment consists of withdrawal of dapsone and early use of corticosteroids. Like pyrimethamine-sulfadoxine, pyrimethamine and dapsone are not recommended for use during prgnancy.

Chloroquine is the drug of choice for prevention and treatment of sensitive malaria species during pregnancy. Therefore, pregnant women traveling in malarial regions are advised to follow current recommendations to avoid exposure to malaria whenever possible and to receive prophylaxis with chloroquine, if needed, since the risks of the disease often outweigh the risk of exposure to the antimalarial drugs.

MISCELLANEOUS ANTIPARASITICAL DRUGS

Few drugs described in this group have shown teratogenic potentials in animals. The antischistosomal drug, hycanthone, is teratogenic in laboratory animals. This drug is potentially toxic to both the mother and fetus. Therapy should be avoided in pregnancy. The antifilarial trypanosomicide, suramin sodium, has induced multiple malformations (26 percent frequency) in mice but was not teratogenic in rats at higher dosages. Because of the absence of human data, this agent currently cannot be recommended for use during pregnancy or lactation.

Metronidazole, a trichomonacide, has been associated with induction of birth defects in human pregnancy. Carcinogenicity in rodents and mutagenicity in bacteria have been observed, and because of this, one publication has suggested that metronidazole is potentially dangerous and should not be used in humans The teratogenic and carcinogenic risk, if it exists, is small, and hence the drug can be safely administered during pregnancy when therapy is indicated. Treatment of asymptomatic infection should be withheld during pregnancy. Metronidazole is excreted into breast milk. Diarrhea and secondary lactose intolerance have been reported in a nursing male infant whose mother was taking the drug. Although other reports of untoward effects in the breast-fed infant have not been documented, three problems may exist for the infant: modification of bowel flora, direct effects of the drug on the infant, and interference with the interpretation of culture results if a work-up for fever is required.

VACCINES

This group includes experimental and marketed vaccines of human origin. Immunotherapy in general has not been associated with congenital malformations in the human. Allergy desensitization vaccines have shown no association between use in pregnancy and congenital malformations. Inactiviated vaccines such as those for influenza, typhoid fever, diphtheria, tetanus, pertussis, rabies, poliomyelitis, cholera, plague, and Rocky Mountain spotted fever have not been shown to be harmful to either mother or fetus. Live virus vaccines demonstrate a varying ability and potential to produce placental infection, transplacental passage of the agent, and fetal infection. Of the common live-virus vaccines such as measles, mumps, and poliomyelitis, only rubella seems to retain teratogenic potential.

Inadvertent rubella vaccination during the first trimester of pregnancy carries a risk of fetal infection. Since 1971, the Centers for Disease Control have maintained a register to monitor and quantitate the risk to the fetus of exposure to live attenuated rubella vaccine virus. Data collected so far show that RA 27/3 rubella vaccine, like other vaccines (Cendhehill and HPV-77), has not caused defects compatible with congenital rubella syndrome. While no congenital rubella syndrome–like defects have been noted, it is clear that rubella vaccine viruses, including RA 27/3 strain, can cross the placenta and infect the fetus. Approximately 1 to 2 percent of infants born to susceptible vaccinees had serologic evidence of subclinical infection, regardless of vaccine strain. On the other hand, although the rubella virus isolation rate from the products of conception of women who have received RA 27/3 vaccine is only 3 percent, the rate of virus isolation from the products of conception of those receiving Cendehill and HPV-77 vaccines is 20 percent. Thus, the risk of placental or fetal infection from RA 27/3 vaccine is low. Pregnancy remains a contraindication to rubella vaccination because of the theoretical risk of congenital rubella syndrome. Reasonable precautions should be taken to rule out pregnancy before vaccination. Because the risk of congenital rubella syndrome is so small as to be negligible, rubella vaccination of a pregnant woman should not ordinarily be a reason to consider termination of pregnancy, even if vaccination does occur within 3 months of conception.

Even though no data are available at present concerning the teratogenicity of measles, mumps, or poliomyelitis virus vaccine, they must be viewed as potentially hazardous and should not be used during pregnancy. With live, oral (Salk) polio vaccine, increased abortion rates have been observed in several studies. The risk of infection to pregnant patients from children immunized with measles, mumps, or rubella is minimal.

Yellow fever vaccine uses a live attenuated virus. A retrospective study found no association between use of this vaccine during pregnancy and birth defects in the offspring. It is recommended that pregnant women avoid travel to areas where yellow fever is a risk. If travel is unavoidable, vaccination is recommended, since morbidity and mortality from yellow fever are significant.

Hepatitis B vaccine is made of formalin-inactivated surface units of the hepatitis virus or of antigen produced through recombinant technology in yeast. The nature of the vaccine suggests that vaccination during pregnancy should not have greater consequences for the conceptus than infection with hepatitis B virus. Since it is likely that vaccination during pregnancy is preferable to hepatitis B infection, vaccination should be considered in women at risk of acquiring the disease.

Tetanus toxoid is inactivated toxin from *Clostridium* tetanus. In developing countries, tetanus neonatorum is an important complication of delivery under nonhygienic conditions, and a number of studies have shown that immunization of pregnant women with tetanus toxoid is an important public health measure. Treatment with tetanus and diphtheria toxoids in adults who have had primary immunization is recommended every 10 years.

Gamma globulins are antibodies given therapeutically to people who cannot make antibodies or who require passive immunization to disease. The Collaborative Perinatal Project found no association between gamma globulin administered early in pregnancy and abnormalities in the offspring.

ANTIHELMINTICS

Treatment of helminth infections during pregnancy is not uncommon. There are three common drugs for such treatment: piperazine, niclosamide, and thiabendazole. These drugs actually affect different functions in the worms.

Piperazine blocks acetylcholine at the neuromuscular junctions of roundworms, creating paralysis and release of the worms in the feces. Piperazine is primarily eliminated in the urine following oral administration. Currently, caution is primarily suggested in using this drug in women with renal or hepatic failure.

Niclosamide kills worms by inhibiting their anaerobic metabolism. The worms are then digested by enzymes in the gastrointestinal tract. Niclosamide is poorly absorbed from the gastrointestinal tract and is therefore used during pregnancy.

Thiabendazole is an antihelmintic agent, yet its mechanism of action is not fully appreciated. However, it is known to inhibit the helminth-specific fumarate reductase. Thiabendazole is hydroxylated and excreted as a glucuronide or sulfate in the urine. Currently there are no case reports of congenital defects associated with this agent; however, its safe use during pregnancy or lactation has not been established.

Antifungal Agents

There have been no reports of human malformations associated with the use of amphotericin, nystatin, flucytosine, and miconazole. Unfortunately, however, only case reports exist. The largest series evaluated is for nystatin with 142 cases and candicidin with 69 cases.

Since nystatin is poorly absorbed following oral administration, little would be expected to be found in the serum or milk. However, no studies have been reported as to transfer across the mammary gland. The drug is widely used for treatment of vulvovaginal candidiasis.

Another agent used for vulvovaginal candidiasis is miconazole. Miconazole can be detected in the serum following vaginal treatment; however, there are no reports of an increased incidence of malformations following topical use. Hyponatremia and itching may be a problem for the mother with continued use.

Amphotericin B is an important therapy for candidiasis, coccidioidomycosis, and sporotrichosis; in multiple studies, no increased incidence of malformations or fetal effects was noted when the drug was administered at different stages of gestation.

Flucytosine can be metabolized to 5-fluorouracil, a cancer chemotherapy, following oral administration. Insufficient human studies have been performed to assess risk. It is known that flucytosine can be teratogenic in laboratory animals.

Griseofulvin is teratogenic at high doses in laboratory animals. Because of this observation, the fact that its use in pregnant patients has not been thoroughly investigated, and it crosses the term human placenta, caution has been recommended in its use.

OTHER ANTIBACTERIAL AGENTS

Among the premier antibacterial agents is hexachlorophene. Its use in surgery and on neonates has reduced bacterial infections, especially with *Staphylococcus aureus*. However, concern has increased involving the potential teratogenicity of this agent. Animal studies have shown birth defects in some species (rats and rabbits), but not in others (hamsters and mice). In the late 1970s, two studies raised the association of hexachlorophene use during pregnancy with malformations. However, three larger series of investigations could not confirm any association with use of this agent and birth defects.

SUGGESTED READING

Briggs G, Freeman R, Yaffe S. Drugs in pregnancy and lactation. Baltimore: Williams & Wilkins, 1986.

Fabro S, Scialli A, eds. Drug and chemical action in pregnancy. New York: Marcel Dekker, 1986.

Kuemmerle H, ed. Clinical pharmacology in pregnancy. New York: Thieme-Stratton, 1984.

Miller RK, Kellogg C, Saltzman R. Reproductive and perinatal toxicology. In: Haley T, Berndt WO, eds. Handbook of toxicology. Washington, DC: Hemisphere Press, 1987:195.

Nau H. Clinical pharmacokinetics in pregnancy and perinatology. II. Penicillins. Dev Pharmacol Ther 1987; 10:174–198.

Schardein JL. Chemically induced birth defects. New York: Marcel Dekker, 1985.

Shepard T. Catalog of teratogenic agents. Baltimore: Johns Hopkins University Press, 1985.

GESTATIONAL HERPESVIRUS INFECTIONS

BISHARA J. FREIJ, M.D.
JOHN L. SEVER, M.D., Ph.D.

The human herpesviruses are a group of enveloped double-stranded DNA viruses that include herpes simplex virus types 1 and 2, cytomegalovirus, varicella-zoster virus, and Epstein-Barr virus. Herpesvirus infections are very common and are associated with a spectrum of clinical manifestations that range from asymptomatic infection to severe, and sometimes fatal, disseminated disease. The human host continues to harbor these viruses in latent form following recovery from primary infection. Periodic reactivation leading to recurrent disease is a characteristic shared by all herpesviruses.

The concurrence of pregnancy and herpesvirus infections significantly complicates the management of either condition. Infections that may be benign for the majority of immunocompetent pregnant women can have devastating effects on the developing fetus (e.g., with cytomegalovirus). Genital herpes simplex virus infection is commonly associated with premature labor, and cesarean section is usually needed if active lesions are present at delivery. Acyclovir and other antiviral agents are not approved for use during pregnancy because of potential adverse fetal effects. Optimal management of gestational herpesvirus infections hinges on establishing an accurate etiologic diagnosis, the judicious use of antiviral chemotherapeutic or immunotherapeutic agents, relief of symptoms, counseling of the mother as to the fetal and neonatal risks associated with these infections, and intervention strategies.

HERPES SIMPLEX VIRUS

Overview

All herpes simplex virus (HSV) strains can be grouped into one of two serologic subtypes, HSV-1 and HSV-2. Primary HSV-1 infections most commonly manifest as gingivostomatitis or pharyngitis. The virus may also cause from 7 to 50 percent of primary genital herpes infections in the United States and as many as 90 percent of those diagnosed in Japan. The most common clinical manifestation of primary HSV-2 infection is genital herpes, but pharyngitis, urethritis, proctitis, and aseptic meningitis also may be encountered. Infections with either HSV-1 or HSV-2 are commonly subclinical, especially when they are recurrent in nature. Compared with recurrent disease, primary genital HSV infection is associated with more systemic symptoms and signs. In addition, the local symptoms are more prolonged and severe, virus concentrations from lesions are 100- to 1,000-fold higher, and the likelihood of extragenital spread is greater.

The clinical manifestations of genital HSV infections are essentially unaffected by pregnancy, although there may be a slightly greater risk of dissemination. Primary genital herpes occurring during the first 20 weeks of gestation is associated with an increased frequency of spontaneous abortions and stillbirths as well as an increased risk of congenital malformations in the offspring. Primary infections later in pregnancy are associated with premature onset of labor. Most herpes infections in pregnancy represent recurrent disease, however, and it has been estimated that asymptomatic shedding of HSV occurs in from 0.2 to 7.4 percent of pregnant women and in from 0.2 to 4 percent of those at or near term. Genital HSV-2 infection is more likely to reactivate than that caused by HSV-1. The recurrence rate is also slightly higher during the third as compared with the first trimester of pregnancy.

Transmission of HSV from mother to fetus may occur through hematogenous spread via the placenta, as an ascending infection (particularly in the presence of ruptured membranes), or through intimate contact of the fetus with infected secretions during vaginal delivery. The risk of intrapartum transmission is higher if the infection is primary, if there are cervical lesions, if there are multiple lesions, and if the delivery is complicated by prematurity, prolonged rupture of membranes, and instrumentation. It is estimated that the risk of intrapartum transmission of HSV to neonates is approximately 40 to 50 percent for those with primary genital herpes and about 5 percent for mothers with recurrent disease.

The diagnosis of HSV infection is best established by virus isolation. The recovery rate is greatly enhanced if cultures are obtained by swabbing the base of a suspicious lesion or, in the case of inapparent lesions, in an area where the patient may be experiencing symptoms suggestive of recurrent disease such as pruritus, paresthesias, or numbness. The swabs should be placed in special viral transport media and sent to the laboratory immediately. Specimens that cannot be transported promptly to the laboratory should be kept refrigerated at 4°C but not frozen, as this will significantly reduce the virus yield. If large quantities of the virus are present, one can expect a positive culture result within 24 to 48 hours. More rapid methods of diagnosis are currently available, such as direct detection of HSV antigens in exfoliated cells by immunofluorescent staining or enzyme-linked immunosorbent assay, but they are less sensitive and specific than viral isolation. Cytologic examination using Tzanck's and Papanicolaou's smears is useful but not very sensitive or specific. Serologic tests are usually of limited usefulness in the diagnosis of HSV infections.

Antepartum Management

The management of primary or recurrent genital HSV infection during pregnancy is aimed at alleviating symptoms in the mother and preventing viral transmission to her unborn child.

Pain is often severe, requiring analgesics for relief, including codeine-containing preparations. Lesions should be kept clean by washing with plain soap and water and drying thoroughly. Dysuria is a common complaint, and women may get partial relief by sitting in a warm bathtub and voiding in the water. If urinary retention develops, catheterization and hospitalization may be necessary. Oral and intravenous acyclovir preparations are effective in shortening the duration of symptoms and viral shedding and in reducing the severity of symptoms, but the drug is not approved for use during pregnancy. However, pregnant women who develop disseminated HSV infections should be treated with acyclovir, since this complication is associated with a mortality rate in excess of 50 percent for the mother or her fetus. The dosage schedule is 5 mg per kilogram intravenously every 8 hours for as long as clinically warranted. Acyclovir therapy may not prevent fetal infection. This drug has also been recently shown to be teratogenic in rats, and accumulation in human breast milk has been documented.

Based on the concept that most cases of neonatal herpes are preventable if contact with and acquisition of the virus during passage through an infected birth canal is avoided, it has become standard obstetric practice to identify women at high risk for genital herpes and to monitor them with weekly viral cultures during the last trimester of pregnancy in order to deliver their infants by cesarean section in the event that they are found to be shedding HSV at or near the time of delivery. This approach has numerous limitations, as outlined below.

Screening all pregnant women for genital herpes just prior to term is currently impractical because of the poor yield expected. The yield would be anticipated to improve if high-risk groups such as women with a history of genital herpes or those whose sexual partners have a history of this infection are targeted. The value of this selective screening process is limited by the fact that both primary and recurrent genital herpes may be asymptomatic and that approximately two-thirds of neonates who develop HSV infection are born to mothers who are asymptomatic at the time of delivery. Approximately two-thirds of these asymptomatic mothers have no history of herpetic infections themselves, nor do their sexual partners.

Monitoring women at high risk with viral cultures is usually started at 32 to 36 weeks of gestation. Women are allowed to deliver vaginally if their last one or two cultures prior to delivery are negative, and there are no symptoms or visible lesions on examination. However, an estimated 15 percent of neonates with HSV infections are born between 28 and 32 weeks of gestation. In addition, a single genital sample will not identify all HSV-positive women if there are no visible lesions present. The length of time available to isolate HSV from tissue cultures may not be sufficient if the interval between sampling and onset of labor is short. The use of Papanicolaou's smears to screen women at the time of delivery has been suggested, but this technique lacks adequate sensitivity or specificity. An additional problem with weekly viral cultures is that women whose last cultures were positive may have stopped shedding virus by the time of delivery and, conversely, those whose last cultures were negative may subsequently reactivate and shed HSV at delivery. It has been estimated that weekly viral cultures for women with recurrent genital herpes can diagnose only one-fourth of those with asymptomatic infection at delivery, and that the cost of such a screening program would be about two million dollars per case of neonatal HSV infection that is prevented. The inability of antepartum maternal viral cultures to correctly identify women who are shedding HSV at onset of labor has been well documented in recent prospective studies.

Because of the limitations of antepartum monitoring, women with a history of recurrent genital herpes who are asymptomatic at onset of labor and have no prodromal symptoms or suspicious lesions on examination should be allowed to deliver vaginally.

Cesarean section is recommended for women with signs or symptoms suggestive of HSV infection at the onset of labor. This method is most effective when the fetal membranes have been ruptured for 4 hours or less prior to surgery. Cesarean section should not be performed if the membranes have been ruptured for 12 or more hours, since the risk to the neonate is probably the same if delivery is vaginal. Women whose membranes had been ruptured for 4 to 12 hours are usually delivered by cesarean section, although the benefits of this approach are not well defined.

Patients should be informed that cesarean sections do not prevent cases of infection that result from the transplacental transmission of HSV to the fetus. Women who develop genital herpes during pregnancy, especially those with primary infections in the first trimester, should be informed that they are at increased risk for spontaneous abortion or stillbirth and that there is a small risk of congenital defects that cannot be quantitated at present. Therapeutic abortions are not recommended for women with genital herpes during pregnancy.

Postpartum Management

Contact isolation precautions should be observed for mothers with active genital lesions. Breast-feeding is permitted as long as careful handwashing is followed and any infected sites are covered to prevent postpartum transmission of the virus to the neonate.

Infants delivered through an infected birth canal should be isolated for the purpose of protecting other infants in the nursery. Cultures of exposed mucous membranes such as in the eyes and nasopharynx should be obtained at 24 to 48 hours of age. Cultures obtained at an earlier time may represent transient contamination if positive. If any of the cultures obtained is positive for HSV, acyclovir therapy should be initiated even in asymptomatic infants.

Fetal and Neonatal Disease

HSV infections are estimated to occur in one to six neonates per 10,000 deliveries per year. These infections may be localized to one body site or disseminated to involve multiple organs, but only rarely are they asymptomatic.

Congenital malformations following intrauterine HSV infections include cutaneous vesicles, scars, and calcifications, cerebral atrophy, hydranencephaly, intracranial calcifications, hepatosplenomegaly, chorioretinitis, microphthalmus, cataract, retinal dysplasia, short digits, and other anomalies. Most reported cases have been associated with primary maternal genital herpes during the first trimester of pregnancy. However, these malformations have also been noted to occur following primary infection in the third trimester and, rarely, following recurrent disease during the first trimester. Most of these cases have been caused by HSV-2.

Neonatal disease resulting from the intrapartum acquisition of HSV may not manifest before 9 to 17 days of age. Infection may be localized or disseminated in nature. Disseminated disease is associated with a mortality rate of 80 percent without antiviral therapy. However, the mortality rate is reduced to 15 to 20 percent with acyclovir or vidarabine therapy, but an estimated 40 to 55 percent of survivors have long-term neurologic residual. Clinical manifestations of acute neonatal HSV infections may include vesicular rash, chorioretinitis, keratoconjunctivitis, pneumonia, hepatitis, seizures, shock, and disseminated intravascular coagulation. Postinfectious complications may include microcephaly, hydranencephaly, porencephalic cysts, seizures, psychomotor retardation, blindness, spasticity, hearing defects, and recurrent mucocutaneous herpes.

VARICELLA-ZOSTER VIRUS

Overview

Varicella-zoster virus (VZV) infects most people during their lifetime. About 95 percent of women of childbearing age in the United States have serologic evidence of past VZV infection.

Varicella is a highly contagious childhood disease. Less than 2 percent of cases occur in adults 20 years of age or older. The incidence of gestational varicella has been estimated at one to seven per 10,000 pregnancies. Zoster results from reactivation of latent VZV and is usually encountered in elderly or immunocompromised patients. Its incidence in pregnancy is not known, but one estimate places this at about 0.5 per 10,000 pregnancies.

Less than 5 percent of primary VZV infections are asymptomatic. Varicella usually manifests 10 to 20 days following exposure of susceptible individuals to VZV. The illness is characterized by fever, malaise, and a pruritic rash. The rash is primarily truncal in distribution and manifests as crops of maculopapules that rapidly progress to form vesicles, which eventually crust over. Newer lesions continue to appear for 3 to 5 days, leading to the typical finding of lesions in various stages of development. Complications include pneumonia, encephalitis, arthritis, bacterial cellulitis, and a variety of bleeding manifestations. The risk for varicella complications in otherwise normal adults may be 9- to 25-fold greater than that for normal children. Pregnancy does not seem to further increase this risk. Immunity following varicella is long-lasting.

Zoster is characterized by pain localized to the area of distribution of one or more sensory nerve roots. The skin lesions are unilateral in the vast majority of patients and follow the same evolutionary pattern as those of varicella but remain localized to the radicular lines.

The diagnosis of varicella or zoster is usually based on the clinical findings only, and laboratory confirmation is seldom needed. If necessary, the virus can be isolated from vesicular fluid by inoculating freshly collected specimens onto human diploid cell lines. VZV-specific antigens can be detected in vesicular fluid by countercurrent immunoelectrophoresis or by immunofluorescence staining of smears of cell scrapings collected from the base of fresh vesicles.

Several serologic assays are currently available for the detection of antibodies to VZV. These include complement fixation (CF), neutralization, indirect hemagglutination, immune adherence hemagglutination (IAHA), fluorescent antibody against membrane antigen (FAMA), and enzyme-linked immunosorbent assay (ELISA). These tests can be used to diagnose VZV infections or to determine the susceptibility status of an individual.

CF antibodies develop within 10 days after onset of varicella and reach a peak by 2 to 3 weeks. These antibodies appear earlier in zoster. CF antibodies tend to disappear with time, and by 1 year after infection about two-thirds of individuals do not have detectable antibody titers. This test is insensitive compared with FAMA or ELISA. FAMA is more sensitive but more difficult to perform and is not readily available. ELISA is rapidly becoming the test of choice for measuring VZV-specific antibodies. Two serum samples collected 1 to 2 weeks apart can provide a retrospective diagnosis of VZV infection if a four-fold or greater rise in antibody titer is demonstrated. If the first sample is collected late in the course of the illness, a single high titer indicates a recent primary or a reactivated VZV infection.

Detection of VZV-specific IgM antibodies can be used to document a recent infection with this virus. The antibody can be detected for several weeks following varicella. It may also be present for a brief period following zoster. False-positive results may be encountered in patients positive for rheumatoid factor.

Antepartum Management

Proper management of individuals exposed to VZV is critical, since varicella is a highly communicable infection that can adversely affect pregnant women and their offspring. Exposed susceptible persons can be protected by passive immunization with pooled immune serum globulin, zoster immune globulin, or varicella-zoster immune globulin. Zoster immune globulin is obtained from herpes zoster patients during their convalescent stage, whereas varicella-zoster immune globulin is prepared from plasma of normal blood donors who are found to have high IgG antibody titers to VZV. Zoster immune globulin and varicella-zoster immune globulin are comparable products, but the latter is available in greater supplies. Immune serum globulin contains less than one-tenth of the anti-VZV antibodies found in zoster immune globulin or varicella-zoster immune globulin and should not be used unless the other two preparations are unavailable. Zoster immune globulin and varicella-zoster immune globulin can prevent or modify clinical varicella in susceptible individuals if given shortly after exposure.

The first step in managing a pregnant woman exposed to VZV is to determine whether or not she is susceptible to the virus. A carefully elicited history of a previous varicella infection is considered sufficient evidence of immunity. Clinical reinfections can occur but are rare. The second step is to decide if exposure is likely to result in infection. Situations involving prolonged contact with varicella patients, as within a family, place susceptible adults at a very high risk (90 percent) of contracting the infection.

Pregnant women exposed to varicella who have negative or uncertain prior histories of this infection should be tested for VZV susceptibility provided that sensitive assays are available and the results can be obtained rapidly. About 80 to 95 percent of these women are found to be immune to varicella, as indicated by a positive CF, IAHA, FAMA, or ELISA test result. Negative CF test results may not necessarily imply susceptibility to VZV, since these antibody assays are not very sensitive. The significance of low anti-VZV antibody titers detected by sensitive tests is unclear, since some of these individuals have developed clinical varicella following exposure.

Once it is determined that a pregnant woman with significant exposure to varicella is susceptible, or if the laboratory test results cannot be obtained in a short time period, zoster immune globulin or varicella-zoster immune globulin should be administered for the purpose of preventing or modifying the infection in the mother to avoid complications. It is not known whether passive immunization of mothers will prevent fetal VZV infection. Zoster immune globulin and varicella-zoster immune globulin are most effective when given as soon as possible after exposure but not later than 96 hours. The dosage is 125 U per 10 kg of body weight (maximum, 625 U). Varicella-zoster immune globulin can be obtained from regional offices of the American Red Cross.

For uncomplicated varicella, symptomatic treatment with antipruritics and cleansing of lesions is adequate. Analgesics are needed for pain control in zoster. Antiviral agents such as acyclovir are used in immunosuppressed patients but are not indicated for otherwise normal adults. Pregnant women should not be treated with this drug unless they develop life-threatening primary varicella pneumonia. Acyclovir is not useful for varicella encephalitis. The use of varicella-zoster immune globulin in the treatment of varicella is of no benefit.

Prenatal diagnosis by detection of VZV-specific IgM in fetal blood has been successful in one fetus evaluated at 32 weeks' gestation, about 12 weeks after the mother developed chickenpox. The sensitivity of this method is unknown at the present time.

Postpartum Management

Women with varicella at parturition need to be isolated from their newborns until all vesicles are crusted. On the other hand, neonates with varicella lesions should be isolated from other infants but not from their mothers.

Fetal and Neonatal Infection

VZV is transmitted to the fetus primarily via the placenta following maternal viremia. Intrauterine transmission of VZV is estimated to occur in about one-fourth of mothers with varicella and in almost none of those with gestational herpes zoster.

Gestational varicella is not associated with an increased risk of prematurity or fetal death. However, when infection occurs between 8 and 20 weeks of gestation, there is an estimated 5 percent risk of congenital malformations in the offspring. These include cicatricial skin lesions, denuded skin, limb hypoplasia, muscular atrophy, rudimentary digits, clubfoot, intrauterine growth retardation, microcephaly, seizures, intracranial calcifications, psychomotor retardation, autonomic dysfunction, microphthalmia, cataract, chorioretinitis, optic atrophy, herpes zoster, and other anomalies. Management of these patients is supportive.

One of four newborns becomes infected when maternal varicella occurs during the last 3 weeks of pregnancy. The most important determinant of the severity of neonatal disease is the time of onset of maternal varicella relative to delivery. When maternal infection occurs within 4 days before and 2 days after delivery, varicella lesions in neonates will usually appear at 5 to 10 days of age. The illness may be mild with only a few cutaneous lesions, or it may become severe with fever, hemorrhagic rash, and generalized visceral involvement. The mortality rate is about 30 percent, and death is usually due to severe pulmonary disease. When maternal varicella occurs 5 to 21 days before delivery, lesions in newborns typically appear in the first 4 days of life, and the prognosis is good with no associated mortality. The mild course is probably due to the production and transplacental passage of maternal antibodies that modify the course of the illness in newborns.

Infants born to mothers who develop varicella within 5 days before and 2 days after delivery should receive 125 U of varicella-zoster immune globulin as soon as possible. Zoster immune globulin and varicella-zoster immune globulin do not reduce the clinical attack rate in treated newborns, but they develop milder infections when compared with those in untreated neonates. Although a few cases of severe varicella in neonates exposed to infected mothers who develop the infection more than 2 days after delivery have been described, routine zoster immune globulin or varicella-zoster immune globulin administration is not currently recommended, since this group of infants is not generally considered to be at increased risk of complications from this disease.

Newborns with varicella should be kept in strict isolation if hospitalization is required. Acyclovir or vidarabine should be used to treat neonates with severe disease, although neither drug is currently approved for this purpose.

CYTOMEGALOVIRUS

Overview

Epidemiologic surveys conducted in the United States have indicated that about 50 to 60 percent of pregnant middle class women and 70 to 85 percent of those from lower socioeconomic groups have serologic evidence of past cytomegalovirus (CMV) infection. Two to two and one-half percent of susceptible women acquire primary CMV infection during pregnancy, a risk similar to that of nonpregnant susceptible women. Seropositive women can develop recurrent disease either from reactivation of a latent CMV infection, or occasionally, from reinfection with an exogenous CMV strain. The virus is usually acquired by kissing, sexual contact, or from young children in the household, especially those attending day care centers. More than 90 percent of primary CMV infections are asymptomatic and the remaining 10 percent typically consist of a mononucleosis-like illness. Rare complications may include interstitial pneumonia, thrombocytopenia, aseptic meningitis, and Guillain-Barré syndrome.

CMV shedding from multiple sites such as saliva, tears, urine, semen, cervical secretions, and breast milk usually follows the initial infection and can persist for prolonged periods. The rate of CMV shedding among pregnant women is about 8 percent from the cervix, 4 percent from the urinary tract, 2 percent from the throat, and 14 percent from breast milk in the postpartum period. CMV shedding is the result of recurrent infections in the majority of these women.

Diagnosis of active CMV infection can be achieved by isolating the virus from body fluids such as urine, saliva, cervical secretions, or buffy coat. Recovery of CMV from these sites cannot distinguish primary from recurrent infections. A number of sensitive serologic tests for measuring antibody to CMV are currently available. These include CF, anticomplement immunofluorescence, indirect immunofluorescent antibody, immune adherence hemagglutination, and enzyme immunoassays. ELISA is the most commonly used test in diagnostic laboratories. Demonstration of either seroconversion or a fourfold or greater rise in antibody titer is usually considered proof of a recent infection. However, fourfold fluctuations in CMV antibody titers may occur in seemingly healthy seropositive individuals, and CMV infections are not always accompanied by significant rises in antibody titers. The detection of CMV-specific IgM antibody serves as a useful marker for a recent primary infection. This antibody may persist for 4 to 8 months following a primary infection, and problems in interpretation may arise if recurrent disease occurs within this period. Rapid diagnosis of CMV infection is also possible using either nucleic acid hybridization techniques or centrifugation culture assays, but these methods are not widely available at the present time.

Antepartum Management

There are no universal guidelines for the detection and follow-up of CMV-susceptible women during pregnancy. Routine serologic screening of all pregnant women is expensive and of limited usefulness. Maternal CMV antibodies do not prevent recurrent infections in the mother or hamper the transplacental passage of the virus, but fetal infection is rarely severe in such instances. It is also difficult for susceptible pregnant women to reduce their risk of exposure to CMV, since the virus is ubiquitous and most infected individuals are asymptomatic. Good personal hygiene, especially frequent handwashing, should be encouraged, particularly if these women work closely with infants and children at schools or hospitals. Therapy for symptomatic CMV infection is only supportive at the present time. For immunocompromised patients with serious CMV infection, the use of acyclic nucleoside DHPG may be warranted, but there is no experience with the use of this drug in pregnancy.

Termination of pregnancy is one option for women who develop primary CMV infection. These patients should be informed that their risk of delivering an infant with symptomatic congenital CMV infection is only about 5 percent. Prenatal diagnosis by recovering the virus from amniotic fluid is of limited value. If CMV is isolated, it indicates fetal infection but does not necessarily imply severe disease. On the other hand, failure to recover the virus from amniotic fluid does not rule out fetal infection.

Fetal Infection

CMV can be transmitted to the fetus following either primary or recurrent maternal infection. This occurs in an estimated 40 percent of pregnancies complicated by primary CMV infection. Although transmission may occur at all stages of pregnancy, the risk of severe congenital disease is probably higher when the infection is acquired during the first half of gestation. CMV acquisition during passage through an infected birth canal occurs in about half these infants, but CMV excretion by these patients is not apparent before 4 to 12 weeks of age. Infants with symptomatic congenital CMV are usually born to women with primary CMV infections. Recurrent infections only rarely result in symptomatic congenital disease.

One to two percent of all newborns in the United States are infected with CMV. Of these, 10 percent are symptomatic and the remaining 90 percent have subclinical infection. Symptomatic infants have a mortality rate of 20 to 30 percent, and the vast majority of survivors develop long-term serious sequelae such as hearing loss, mental retardation, and visual impairment. In infants who are asymptomatic at birth, serious sequelae such as hearing loss or ocular abnormalities develop in 5 to 15 percent by 2 years of age.

The clinical features of congenital CMV include hepatosplenomegaly, hyperbilirubinemia, petechiae, microcephaly, cerebral atrophy, periventricular calcifications, prematurity, intrauterine growth retardation, chorioretinitis, microphthalmia, cataract, deafness, hemolytic anemia, and other abnormalities. Asymptomatically infected neonates may develop a number of late-appearing abnormalities such as microcephaly, sensorineural hearing loss, mental retardation, optic atrophy, chorioretinitis, hypotonia, spasticity, and dental defects.

The diagnosis of congenital CMV infection is best established by isolating the virus from urine, saliva, or other body fluids within the first 2 weeks of life. Viral isolation at a later time may represent either congenital or perinatal infection. Immunofluorescent staining of cells after 24 hours of culture may provide a rapid diagnosis in some instances. More rapid detection of urinary CMV can be achieved by electron microscopy, ELISA for CMV-specific antigens or antibodies, and DNA hybridization, but these methods are not readily available and are not as sensitive as viral cultures. Serologic diagnosis of congenital CMV can be difficult. Detection of CMV-specific IgM antibodies by ELISA or radioimmunoassay is useful, but these tests may be falsely negative or positive. It has been suggested that the serologic diagnosis of congenital CMV infection can be enhanced by simultaneous measurements of CMV-specific IgM and IgE antibodies by ELISA. IgG antibodies cross the placenta, and consequently detection of CMV-specific IgG antibodies is not helpful. Maternally derived antibodies disappear within a few months. Persistence of elevated anti-CMV titers is serial serum samples therefore confirms CMV infection. This method, however, cannot distinguish infants congenitally infected from those who acquired the virus in the perinatal period.

There is no effective therapy for congenital CMV. A variety of agents have been tried, including cytosine arabinoside, adenine arabinoside, acyclovir, leukocyte interferon, and transfer factor, but none has proved useful.

EPSTEIN-BARR VIRUS

Overview

Epstein-Barr virus (EBV) infections are very common during childhood. Epidemiologic surveys of pregnant women indicate that at least 95 percent have serologic evidence of past EBV infection. Primary EBV infection during pregnancy is rare, and more than half of these infections are subclinical. Infectious mononucleosis is the most common clinical manifestation and is usually self-limited. Complications are uncommon but may include airway obstruction, meningoencephalitis, splenic rupture, and Guillain-Barré syndrome.

Laboratory diagnosis of EBV infections is most commonly based on serologic testing. The detection of heterophil antibodies in patients with infectious mononucleosis is considered diagnostic of a primary EBV infection, although there is a small frequency of false-positive reactions. EBV-specific serology can be used in those with a negative heterophil antibody test. Antibodies against several EBV antigens are produced at different times during the course of an infection. Typically, antibodies to EBV viral capsid antigen and early antigen appear during the acute phase of the infection, whereas those against EBV nuclear antigen develop weeks to months later. Primary infections can be diagnosed by detecting IgM antibodies to viral capsid antigen, but this serologic test may be falsely positive if the serum contains rheumatoid factor. If no IgM antibodies are detected, then the presence of IgG antibodies to viral capsid antigen and early antigen and none against EBV nuclear antigen is suggestive of either a primary or a postacute infection. IgG antibodies to viral capsid antigen and early antigen are usually at their peak very early in the illness in 80 to 90 percent of patients. Fourfold or greater increases in antibody titers between acute and convalescent sera are therefore only occasionally documented. EBV isolation using lymphocyte transformation assays, genome detection using DNA hybridization, and detection of EBV nuclear antigen in tissues by anticomplement indirect immunofluorescent staining are useful for diagnosis, but these methods are mostly employed in research studies and are not widely available.

Antepartum Management

The treatment of infectious mononucleosis is supportive. Antipyretics are needed for fever reduction. Fluid intake should be encouraged. If dehydration develops because of reduced oral intake secondary to anorexia, sore throat and increased insensible water losses from fever, intravenous hydration becomes essential. A topical anesthetic can be sprayed on the pharynx to reduce the discomfort associated with pharyngitis. Patients should be advised to avoid exertion. Corticosteroids are usually used only in patients with severe airway obstruction, severe thrombocytopenia, or hemolytic anemia. Oral acyclovir reduces the duration of EBV salivary excretion but has only minimal effects on the course of the acute illness. The drug is not approved for use during pregnancy at the present time.

Specific preventive measures are not available. Susceptible pregnant women should avoid contact with infectious mononucleosis patients to reduce their risk of infection, although intimate contact is usually needed for transmission to occur.

Fetal Infection

Transplacental transmission of EBV is believed to occur, but very rarely. Cervical EBV shedding has recently been demonstrated, but its significance for infants born through infected birth canals is unknown.

A few published case reports have described an association between gestational infectious mononucleosis and the occurrence of congenital malformations in the offspring. However, no specific pattern has emerged. Reported defects include low birth weight, micrognathia, low-set ears, myositis, congenital heart disease, biliary atresia, cataract, microphthalmia, hip dysplasia, and central nervous system defects.

Because of uncertainty as to whether EBV is truly teratogenic, women who develop primary EBV infection during pregnancy are not candidates for therapeutic abortions but should be made aware of the rare cases describing the association of congenital malformations with maternal EBV infection. Pregnant women with EBV reactivation are probably not at increased risk for an adverse pregnancy outcome.

SUGGESTED READING

Freij BJ, Sever JL. Herpesvirus infections in pregnancy: risks to embryo, fetus, and neonate. Clin Perinatol 1988, in press.

Watts DH, Eschenbach DA. Sexually transmitted diseases in pregnancy. Infect Dis Clin North Am 1987; 1:253–275.

Webb DH, Fife KH. Genital herpes simplex virus infections. Infect Dis Clin North Am 1987; 1:97–122.

TRICHOMONIASIS DURING PREGNANCY

W. SOYINI POWELL, M.D.
MICHAEL R. SPENCE, M.D., M.P.H.

Trichomonas vaginalis is one of three trichomonads that inhabit humans. It is pathogenic to the lower urogenital tract, causing an infection that is sexually transmitted. An estimated 2.5 million women in the United States contract trichomoniasis annually, making it one of the most frequently encountered sexually transmitted diseases. The prevalence of infection depends on the population studied. It ranges from 7 to 32 percent among women attending sexually transmitted disease clinics and from 50 to 75 percent in prostitutes. The prevalence of trichomoniasis in pregnancy is also varied and has been reported as low as 3.7 percent to as high as 61 percent. Abnormal vaginal discharge and pruritus are the most common symptoms. Diagnosis is made by documenting the presence of the organism on wet mount preparation, Papanicolaou smear, or by culture.

METRONIDAZOLE

Metronidazole is the drug of choice for the treatment of trichomoniasis. It has been used effectively to treat trichomonal infections for the past 28 years. Chemically it is classified as a nitroimidazole [1-(2-hydroxyethyl)-2-methyl 5-nitro imidazole]. Metronidazole is bactericidal to anaerobic bacteria and is also effective therapy for giardiasis and amebiasis.

The drug's mechanism of action is not clearly understood, although in its unreduced form it is nontoxic to cells. It is thought than an intracellular reduction reaction facilitated by electron transport proteins (doxins) generates biologically active intermediate products. The mechanism of action of these reduced products is also not well understood. Two stable reduction products, *N*-(2-hydroxy-ethyl)-oxamic acid and acetamide, are formed as metronidazole is completely reduced. However, five intermediates of nitro reduction are possible, and it is believed that the drug's toxic effects are due to these unstable intermediate compounds. These compounds may also be responsible for the mutagenicity and carcinogenicity associated with the drug that has been noted in bacterial and animal studies. The mutagenic activity in bacteria suggests interaction of metronidazole's metabolites with bacterial DNA. In vitro studies have shown that metronidazole interacts with DNA if the drug is reduced in the presence of DNA. It is not certain if this interaction with DNA is a major or important mechanism for the drug's microbiocidal action. However, this is the currently held theory of its mechanism of action.

Pharmacokinetics

Metronidazole is completely absorbed after oral intake and is widely distributed in all tissues throughout the body. Approximately 1 hour after ingestion peak serum levels are achieved, although a delay is seen when the drug is taken postprandially. However, postprandial ingestion is often encouraged to avoid gastrointestinal intolerance.

The drug is eliminated primarily by hepatic metabolism and is excreted by a renal pathway with 70 percent unchanged and 30 percent in metabolite form. Although excretion is primarily renal, the drug has been found in small amounts in feces. The elimination half-life values vary between 6 and 12 hours, with an average of 7 hours in nonpregnant patients with normal renal function. Elimination values for pregnant women are not significantly different.

Adverse Effects

Gastrointestinal disturbances, including nausea and a bad taste in the mouth, are the principal side effects. Headache, ataxia, vertigo, sleepiness and depression are central nervous system symptoms that have been reported at low dose levels. With long-term use (i.e., as a radiosensitizer), moderate to severe nausea, vomiting, and anorexia can occur. High doses used to treat nonpregnant women with documented resistant infection have been associated with peripheral neuropathies. Also reported at higher doses are myalgia, transient encephalopathy, and persistent paresthesia. Other side effects reported even at low doses are dark urine and disulfiram-like intolerance to alcohol. The majority of these effects resolve with discontinuance of the drug.

TREATMENT IN PREGNANCY

Gestational age at the time of diagnosis of *Trichomonas vaginalis* infection is the principal determinant of treatment choice. During the first trimester alternate treatment modalities (discussed below) should be used, as this is the period of organogenesis. Metronidazole has been used extensively during pregnancy with no reports of adverse effects. Most sources, however, still advise restricting its use to after the first trimester.

Metronidazole is the drug of choice for *Trichomonas* infection during pregnancy in the second trimester or later. It is given as a 2-g single oral dose. Metronidazole passes freely through the placental barrier, with high drug levels found in fetal tissues, cord blood, and amniotic fluid. Embryonic and teratogenic effects have been evaluated in mice, rats, rabbits, and guinea pigs. The only reported toxic effects came from studies performed by a single laboratory. No other laboratories have confirmed these findings.

Treatment of symptomatic infections during pregnancy is consistent with standard medical practice. The organism, however, can be harbored asymptomatically. Treatment of an asymptomatic *Trichomonas* infection during pregnancy is controversial. Supporters of withholding treatment unless symptoms occur cite the exposure of the fetus to a potentially toxic drug (although still unproven) as a primary concern. Advocates for treatment consider *Trichomonas vaginalis* a sexually transmitted pathogen that has been associated with abnormal Papanicolaou cervical cytology. The inflammatory changes induced by an infection can confuse the identification of dysplasia. The etiology of cervical carcinoma is not known; however, it has been linked to various sexually transmitted diseases. The role of *Trichomonas vaginalis* infection in pregnancy outcome has not been extensively investigated, but there have been some studies linking it to low birth weight infants and maternal puerperal febrile morbidity. Further studies in this area of adverse pregnancy outcome are needed.

There are no alternative treatment options. Palliative therapy relieves the pruritus associated with infection but does not eradicate the organism. Clotrimazole vaginal cream applied once or twice daily has been successfully used, particularly during the first trimester of pregnancy. It should be kept in mind that asymptomatic infections eventually become symptomatic, although the duration of time in which this occurs is variable. From an epidemiologic point of view, treating a sexually transmitted disease whenever it is diagnosed eliminates the infection's reservoir and decreases its prevalence.

TREATMENT DURING LACTATION

Of special concern is the use of metronidazole for the treatment of trichomoniasis in the postpartum breast-feeding patient. Studies have demonstrated that the drug is secreted in breast milk. Erickson and associates measured the amount of drug in breast milk by 2-hour intervals for up to 24 hours after the mother's ingestion of a 2-g metronidazole dose. The highest concentrations were measured in the samples obtained during the first 2 to 4 hours. If breast-feeding were discontinued for a 24-hour period, a 3-month-old infant consuming 1 L of milk per day would receive a lower (3.5 mg) dose during the first 48 hours after maternal drug ingestion.

Immaturity of the newborn's renal and hepatic systems could result in slower drug elimination, particularly in the case of the premature infant. Exposure to a lower dose would therefore be more acceptable. Thus, the recommendation for treating trichomoniasis in the lactating woman is cessation of breast-feeding for at least 48 hours after a single 2-g dose is given.

SUGGESTED READING

Erickson SH, et al. Metronidazole in breast milk. Obstet Gynecol 1981; 57:48–50.

Holmes K. Trichomonas vaginalis. In: Holmes K, ed. Sexually transmitted diseases. New York: McGraw Hill, 1984:525.

VACCINATION IN PREGNANCY

MARVIN S. AMSTEY, M.D.

The need for active and passive immunization in pregnancy is becoming greater as travel expands, distances contract, and infectious agents find rapid and easy means of dissemination. The number of available products both for active and passive immunization has increased dramatically in the last 30 years. Except for rabies, polio, and yellow fever vaccines, there were no other viral vaccines before 1964. Now there are at least five more products for active immunization and two for passive immunization. Within the area of bacterial vaccine products, there are now seven or eight for active and at least three for passive immunization. In addition, there are products for several toxins and rickettsial infections that are used for vaccination. Therefore continued updating of knowledge about availability and use of various vaccines is essential. Their use in pregnancy is a special area with limited information. Because the effects of many infectious diseases and toxins in pregnancy and on the fetus are unknown, this current information is subject to change with increasing information. The best example of the on-going change is the frequent updates provided by the Centers for Disease Control (CDC) about the inadvertent use of rubella vaccine during pregnancy. When the vaccine product (a live virus) was first available in 1967, great fear surrounded the exposure of the fetus to this vaccine-virus. At this time, it has become clear that there may be little or no harm to the fetus, although the use of this vaccine in pregnancy still is interdicted.

THERAPEUTIC ALTERNATIVES

There are no alternatives to vaccination against any viral infection. Currently, chemotherapy against any virus infection is not effective enough to recommend its routine use. An effective drug—amantadine—exists as a means of *preventing* (not treating) influenza type A. However, its use in pregnancy is contraindicated, except in those women with severe chronic cardiopulmonary disease, because of toxic and teratogenic effects in animal models.

Chemotherapy exists for a wide variety of bacterial infections. However, by the time effective therapy is instituted for such infections as typhoid, meningococcus, or tetanus, serious consequences to the pregnant woman and/or fetus have occurred. There are no other means of *preventing* these infections other than by immunization.

CRITERIA FOR VACCINATION

The accepted criterion for vaccination is susceptibility to the infectious agent as determined by the absence of antibody protective against the organism or its toxin. In most situations, it is not possible to determine this absence. Routine antibody testing for tetanus antitoxin or polio antibody simply is not available. Therefore, a history and record of previous vaccinations and history of infections in previous years are helpful. In the United States, most women of child-bearing age should be immune to measles, mumps, polio, rubella, tetanus, and diphtheria because of state requirements for school admissions. However, among these infections, antibody testing is available for rubella. Immunity to tetanus and diphtheria is assumed only if the last booster injection of vaccine was less than 10 years ago; otherwise susceptibility to the toxins of these bacteria must be presumed.

The first and foremost principle that should serve as a guide is avoidance of vaccination in pregnancy whenever possible. However, as noted previously, this principle cannot always be followed. During pregnancy, a live vaccine, either viral or bacterial, should be avoided because of risk of infection not only to the mother but to the fetus. When vaccination is required, an inactivated (killed) organism or toxoid should be used. None of these products has been reported to cause harm in pregnancy. Using this as a base for all vaccination in pregnancy reduces the concern for disease risk to mother or fetus versus risk from vaccine to a negligible level. Only in the rare situation of having to administer live, attenuated rabies vaccine or live, attenuated yellow fever vaccine do these concerns become real. In either of these cases, the known disease is far worse than the possible unknown risks associated with the vaccines.

The CDC maintains a registry of women who receive live virus vaccines 3 months prior to or following conception. Physicians are urged to report such cases to the CDC (404–329–3091) so the pregnancy can be followed prospectively.

In the United States the only immunizing agents recommended for routine administration *during* pregnancy are tetanus and diphtheria toxoids. Pregnant women should receive primary vaccination against polio only when the risk of exposure is high. Such a situation is rare in this country. Physicians should vaccinate pregnant women with influenza vaccine, using the same criteria for use of this vaccine in the nonpregnant individual.

MODES OF IMMUNIZATION

Active Immunization

Some understanding of how active immunization results in antibody response is helpful before tabulating those agents currently available for use in practice. When using an immunizing antigen—either portions of organisms or the whole organism—the vaccine must be administered from 1 to 3 weeks in advance of exposure in order to allow protective antibodies to develop. After an antigen is injected, inhaled, or swallowed, it enters a regional lymph node. Macrophages process this antigen in a complex way, thereby resulting in stimulation of T- and B-lymphocytes. This stimulation is recognized by the transformation of cells into large blast cells within the lymph node. When these blast cells divide, clones of differentiated T and B cells are produced. The first antibody production is usually of the IgM class followed shortly by an IgG antibody response. Reexposure to the same antigen elicits a memory found in both the T and B cells so that there is an expansion of the lymphocyte clones, thus producing the antibody that is now only of the IgG class. One can find numerous examples of prolonged or "lifetime" antibody responses after vaccination with a live organism (oral polio vaccine), but only a short-lived humoral antibody response after vaccination with a killed or inactivated vaccine (Salk polio vaccine).

In general, the maternal antibody response to commercially available vaccines is the same as that of a nonpregnant individual. That means that the dose of vaccine and the interval of administration (if multiple doses are necessary) are the same whether pregnant or not. Table 1 is modified from the American College of Obstetricians and Gynecologists (ACOG) and lists the known information relative to pregnancy for each available vaccine. The table is organized into live bacterial, live viral, inactivated viral, inactivated bacterial, and toxoid vaccines.

Passive Immunization

Passive immunity is conferred on an individual when exposure to an infectious agent does not allow time for the patient to develop an appropriate antibody response by active immunization. As mentioned in the section on active immunization, time is needed for the processing of antigens, stimulation of the blast cells, and differentiation of clones of T and B cells. This primary production of antibody requires 1 to 3 weeks. If this time is not available, as for example after accidental inoculation of hepatitis-containing blood, then actual introduction of circulating antibody is required. This process is passive immunization. Since heterologous antibody has a finite half-life, the protection provided by passive immunization is finite and short—usually less than 30 days.

Antibody is injected directly usually in the form of purified immunoglobulins or as whole serum, which contains the appropriate immunoglobulins (Table 2). Several preparations that are noticeably absent from this list include polyvalent horse serum against clostridia, human immunoglobulins against pertussis, mumps and rubella, and pooled human immunoglobulin against hepatitis B. None of these preparations has any clinical efficacy. In general only human preparations should be used if at all possible, in order to avoid serum sickness and hypersensitivity leading to subsequent fatal anaphylaxis. (For the commonly used human, hyperimmune preparations see Table 1).

TABLE 1 Immunization During Pregnancy

Immunizing agent	*Risk from disease to pregnant female*	*Risk from disease to fetus or neonate*	*Type of immunizing agent*	*Risk from immunizing agent to fetus*	*Indications for immunization during pregnancy*	*Dose schedule*	*Comments*
			LIVE BACTERIAL VACCINES				
BCG (tuberculosis)	Significant morbidity and mortality, worse in puerperium	No direct effect		Unknown	Contraindicated. Inefficient vaccine. Therapy is preferable to prophylaxis.		
Tularemia	Significant morbidity; not altered by pregnancy	Unknown		Unknown, but has been used without effect	Same indications as non-pregnant; for exposure	Consult public health officials	Scarification of skin under several drops of vaccine
			LIVE VIRAL VACCINES				
Measles	Significant morbidity, low mortality; not altered by pregnancy	Significant increase in abortion rate; may cause malformations	Live attenuated virus vaccine	None confirmed	Contraindicated (See immune globulins)	Single dose 0.5 ml	Vaccination of susceptible women should be part of postpartum care
Mumps	Low morbidity and mortality; not altered by pregnancy	Probable increased rate of abortion in 1st trimester Questionable association of fibroelastosis in neonates	Live attenuated virus vaccine	None confirmed	Contraindicated	Single dose 0.5 ml	
Poliomyelitis	No increased incidence in pregnancy, but may be more severe if it does occur	Anoxic fetal damage reported; 50% mortality in neonatal disease	Live attenuated virus (OPV) and inactivated virus (IPV) vaccine*	None confirmed	Not routinely recommended for adults in US, except persons at increased risk of exposure	Primary: 3 doses IPV (1.0 ml each) at 4–8 wk intervals and a 4th dose 6–12 mo after the 3rd dose; 2 doses OPV (0.5 ml each) with a 6–8 wk interval and a 3rd dose at least 6 wk later, customarily 8–12 mo later Booster: Every 5 yr until 18 yr of age for IPV	Vaccine indicated for susceptible pregnant women traveling in endemic areas or in other high-risk situations
Rubella†	Low morbidity and mortality; not altered by pregnancy	High rate of abortion and congenital rubella syndrome	Live attenuated virus vaccine	None confirmed	Contraindicated	Single dose 0.5 ml	Teratogenicity of vaccine is theoretic, not confirmed to date Vaccination of susceptible women should be part of postpartum care
Yellow Fever	Significant morbidity and mortality; not altered by pregnancy	Unknown	Live attenuated virus vaccine	Unknown	Contraindicated except if exposure unavoidable	Single dose 0.5 ml	Postponement of travel preferable to vaccination, if possible

* inactivated polio vaccine (IPV) recommended for unimmunized adults at increased risk
† measles, mumps, and rubella are available mixed as a single subcutaneous injection of 0.5 ml

TABLE 1 Immunization During Pregnancy *(Continued)*

Immunizing agent	*Risk from disease to pregnant female*	*Risk from disease to fetus or neonate*	*Type of immunizing agent*	*Risk from immunizing agent to fetus*	*Indications for immunization during pregnancy*	*Dose schedule*	*Comments*
			INACTIVATED VIRAL VACCINES				
Influenza	Possible increase in morbidity and mortality during epidemic of new antigenic strain	Possible increased abortion rate; no malformations confirmed	Inactivated type A and type B virus vaccines	None confirmed	Usually recommended only for patients with serious underlying diseases; public health authorities to be consulted for current recommendation	Consult with public health authorities since recommendations change each year	Criteria for vaccination of pregnant women same as for all adults
Rabies	Near 100% fatality; not altered by pregnancy	Determined by maternal disease	Killed virus vaccine	Unknown	Indications for prophylaxis not altered by pregnancy; each case considered individually	Public health authorities to be consulted for indications and dosage	
			INACTIVATED BACTERIAL VACCINES				
Cholera	Significant morbidity and mortality; more severe during 3rd trimester	Increased risk of fetal death during 3rd trimester maternal illness	Killed bacterial vaccine	Unknown	Only to meet international travel requirements	2 injections, 4–8 wk apart of 1.0 ml each	Vaccine of low efficacy
H. influenzae, type B	Low morbidity in adults, unchanged by pregnancy	Leading cause of meningitis in infants; no fetal effects reported	None		No current indications	Single dose 0.5 ml	May enhance immunity if given during pregnancy
Meningococcus	No increased risk during pregnancy; no increase in severity of disease	Unknown	Killed bacterial vaccine	No data available on use during pregnancy	Indications not altered by pregnancy; vaccination recommended only in unusual outbreak situations	Public health authorities to be consulted	
Plague	Significant morbidity and mortality; not altered by pregnancy	Determined by maternal disease	Killed bacterial vaccine	None reported	Very selective vaccination of exposed persons	Public health authorities to be consulted for indications and dosage	
Pneumococcus	No increased risk during pregnancy; no increase in severity of disease	Unknown	Polyvalent polysaccharide vaccine	No data available on use during pregnancy	Indications not altered by pregnancy; vaccine used only for high-risk individuals	In adults 1 dose only of 0.5 ml	
Typhoid	Significant morbidity and mortality; not altered by pregnancy	Unknown	Killed bacterial vaccine	None confirmed	Not recommended routinely except for close, continued exposure or travel to endemic areas	Primary: 2 injections, 4 wk apart Booster: single dose 1.0 ml, each containing 8 units of vaccine	

TABLE 1 Immunization During Pregnancy *(Continued)*

Immunizing agent	*Risk from disease to pregnant female*	*Risk from disease to fetus or neonate*	*Type of immunizing agent*	*Risk from immunizing agent to fetus*	*Indications for immunization during pregnancy*	*Dose schedule*	*Comments*
			TOXOIDS				
Tetanus-Diphtheria	Severe morbidity; tetanus mortality 60%, diphtheria mortality 10%; unaltered by pregnancy	Neonatal tetanus mortality 60%	Combined tetanus-diphtheria toxoids preferred: adult tetanus diphtheria formulation	None confirmed	Lack of primary series, or no booster within past 10 years	Primary: 2 doses at 1- to 2-mo interval with a 3rd dose 6–12 mo after the second Booster: single dose every 10 yr, after completion of the primary series, each dose 0.5 ml	Updating of immune status should be part of antepartum care
			IMMUNE GLOBULINS: HYPERIMMUNE				
Hepatitis B	Possible increased severity during 3rd trimester	Possible increase in in abortion rate and prematurity Neonatal hepatitis can occur if mother is a chronic carrier or is acutely infected	Hepatitis B immune globulin (HBIG)	None reported	Postexposure prophylaxis	0.06 ml/kg immediately and 1 mo later of HBIG	Infants born to HBsAg-positive mothers should receive 0.5 ml of HBIG as soon after birth as possible and the same dose repeated 3 and 6 mo later
Rabies	Near 100% fatality; not altered by pregnancy	Determined by maternal disease	Rabies immune globulin (RIG)	None reported	Postexposure prophylaxis	20 IU/kg in one dose of RIG	Used in conjunction with rabies killed virus vaccine
Tetanus	Severe morbidity; mortality 60%	Neonatal tetanus mortality 60%	Tetanus immune globulin (TIG)	None reported	Postexposure prophylaxis	250 units in one dose of TIG	Used in conjunction with tetanus toxoid
Varicella	Possible increase in severe varicella pneumonia	Can cause congenital varicella with increased mortality in neonatal period; very rarely causes congenital defects	Varicella-zoster immune globulin (VZIG)	None reported	Not routinely indicated in healthy pregnant women exposed to varicella	1 vial/kg in one dose of VZIG, up to 5 vials	Only indicated for newborns of mothers who developed varicella within 4 days prior to delivery or 2 days following delivery Approximately 90-95% of adults are immune to varicella
			IMMUNE GLOBULINS: POOLED				
Hepatitis A	Possible increased severity during 3rd trimester	Probable increase in abortion rate and prematurity Possible transmission to neonate at delivery if mother is incubating the virus or is acutely ill at that time	Pooled immune globulin (IG)	None reported	Postexposure prophylaxis	0.02 ml/kg in 1 dose of IG	IG given as soon as possible and within 2 wk of exposure Infants born to mothers incubating the virus or acutely ill at delivery should receive 1 dose of 0.5 ml as soon as possible after birth

TABLE 1 Immunization During Pregnancy *(Continued)*

Immunizing agent	*Risk from disease to pregnant female*	*Risk from disease to fetus or neonate*	*Type of immunizing agent*	*Risk from immunizing agent to fetus*	*Indications for immunization during pregnancy*	*Dose schedule*	*Comments*
			IMMUNE GLOBULINS: POOLED *(Continued)*				
Measles	Significant morbidity, low mortality; not altered by pregnancy	Significant increase in abortion rate; may cause malformations	Pooled immune globulin (IG)	None reported	Postexposure prophylaxis	0.25 ml/kg in 1 dose of IG, up to 15 ml	Unclear if it prevents abortion Must be given within 6 days of exposure

Modified from ACOG Technical Bulletin No. 64, 1982.

TABLE 2 Materials Available Currently for Passive Immunization

Disease	*Antibody source*	*Comment*
Black widow spider	Antivenom (horse serum)	Risk of serum sickness and other hypersensitivity reactions from horse serum
Botulism	Polyvalent antitoxin (horse serum)	Same
Diphtheria	Antitoxin (horse serum)	Same
Hepatitis A	Pooled human immunoglobulins	Modifies but does not prevent disease
Hepatitis B	Anti-hepatitis B human immunoglobulin	Persons should be tested for hepatitis B antigens and antibodies
Measles	Pooled human immunoglobulins	
Rabies	Anti-rabies human immunoglobulins	
Rh isoimmunization	Anti-Rh-D human immunoglobulin	For nonimmune women only Effective for D-antigen antibody prevention
Snakebite	Antivenom (coral and crotolid snakes—horse serum)	Same as other horse serum prophylaxis
Tetanus	Anti-tetanus human immunoglobulin	
Varicella—Zoster	Anti-V-Z human immunoglobulin	For immunosuppressed individuals and neonates

Modified from ACOG Technical Bulletin No. 64, 1982.

One must not forget to follow-up passive immunization with active immunization—either simultaneously or at some more convenient later time.

FUTURE CONSIDERATIONS

The preceding discussion is directed toward protection of the mother against infection before or after exposure to hazardous infectious agents during pregnancy. No consideration has been given to protection of the fetus since the infectious diseases against which one would protect the mother are not pertinent to the fetus, per se. The concern for the fetus must be addressed from the standpoint of protection against those infectious diseases that are more likely to affect the neonate soon after birth. Any maternal vaccination confers passive immunity to the fetus or neonate because the IgG antibodies produced by the mother in response to active immunization cross the placenta. This should provide protection for the neonate at least for several half-lives of the isologous immunoglobulins.

Therefore, purposeful immunization of pregnant women may be helpful to neonates. The best example of this is tetanus toxoid booster immunization of pregnant women in underdeveloped countries in order to prevent neonatal tetanus. Recent data has demonstrated that the same thing is possible with *Haemophilus influenzae,* type B vaccine. A plan to immunize pregnant women actively in order to protect their infants passively may be the future of vaccination in pregnancy. If this is so then it is important for practicing physicians to learn about the effects of vaccines and the response to vaccines during pregnancy.

SUGGESTED READING

Albrecht R, Cefalo R, O'Brien W. Tularemia immunization in early pregnancy. Am J Ob Gyn 1980; 138:1226–1227.
Amstey MS. Vaccination in pregnancy. Clin Ob Gyn 1983; 10:13.
Amstey M, Insel R, Munoz J, et al. Fetal/neonatal passive immunization against *H. influenzae,* type B. Am J Ob Gyn 1985; 153:607–611.
Immunization in pregnancy. ACOG Technical bulletin. 1982; No. 64.
Preblud S, Stetler H, Frank J, et al. Fetal risk associated with rubella vaccine. JAMA 1981; 246:1413–1417.
Varner M, McGuiness G, Galask R. Rabies vaccination in pregnancy. Am J Ob Gyn 1982; 143:717–718.

PROPHYLACTIC ANTIBIOTICS IN OBSTETRICS

ALAN S. BERKELEY, M.D.

The decision to employ prophylactic antibiotics in obstetrics involves a risk-benefit evaluation not only for the mother but often also for the fetus or neonate. Because all antibiotics are transported across the placenta to some degree, it is imperative that the disease theoretically being prevented by the prophylactic antibiotics poses a distinct threat to the pregnant woman and, therefore, to the fetus. Although organogenesis is virtually complete by the end of the first trimester, the practitioner must remember that antibiotics given after the first trimester still have the potential to cause subtle untoward effects on the rapidly growing fetus.

Ledger has proposed that certain criteria be met in order to justify the use of prophylactic antibiotics for surgery. The operation should carry a significant risk of postoperative infectious morbidity and that morbidity should be serious enough to justify the use of systemic antibiotics (or operative drainage). It is important to emphasize that morbidity rates for the same operation may vary greatly from hospital to hospital, depending on patient population, operative technique, and surgical experience. Sweet and Gibbs have pointed out that obstetric patients are generally healthy and that, although postoperative infection may be common in some groups, the incidence of serious or life-threatening infection is low. Second, the operation should cause significant bacterial contamination of the traumatized tissues. Third, a short-term, low-toxicity drug regimen should be used. Finally, antibiotics needed for the treatment of resistant bacteria should not routinely be used for prophylaxis. Looked at from the perspective of cost containment, one might argue that an additional criterion would be that the cost of the treatment of the infections being prevented by the prophylactic antibiotics should be greater than the cost of the antibiotics themselves.

The exact mechanism by which prophylactic agents prevent postoperative infection remains unclear. A decrease in bacterial colony count at the time of surgical trauma may allow host defense mechanisms to work more effectively. In addition, the antibiotics may decrease the concentration of organisms that are vital to the development of synergistic infections, although it is clear that, in order to be effective, a prophylactic agent need not have activity against all potential contaminating microorganisms. In his classic work, Burke has demonstrated that the most important factor in the success of prophylaxis is the presence of the antibiotic in the tissue at risk before or at the time of the surgical incision; antibiotic given as little as 1 hour later was less effective than pre- or periincisional dosing, and antibiotic given more than 3 hours later was no more effective than placebo in decreasing wound infection. It is clearly important to establish tissue levels of antibiotics before clamping and suturing cause decidual and myometrial necrosis; devitalized tissue is usually required for the development of endomyometritis. Bacterial contamination alone, as in vaginal delivery with uterine exploration, rarely causes infection.

CESAREAN SECTION

The incidence of cesarean section in the United States now approaches 20 percent of all deliveries. The incidence of postpartum endomyometritis varies from as low as 10 to 15 percent at some community hospitals to as high as 85 to 90 percent of all operative deliveries at hospitals that serve indigent populations; a postcesarean infection rate of 30 to 40 percent would be quite common. Fortunately, the occurrences of pelvic abscess and septic pelvic thrombophlebitis, the most serious forms of postpartum infection, are rare events, with a frequency of less than 1 percent on most services. However, endomyometritis itself can cause significant discomfort for the mother, interfere with maternal-infant bonding, increase the length of the hospital stay (and therefore increase its cost), and be a precursor to the more serious forms of infection.

Strategies for reducing the incidence of endomyometritis have focused on identifying those women undergoing cesarean deliveries who have a high risk of developing postpartum infection; those at low risk (variably defined as an endomyometritis rate of less than 15 to 20 percent) would not require prophylaxis. Yonekura, Duff, Mead, Cartwright, Swartz, Cunningham, and Sweet and Gibbs have all attempted to identify high-risk factors for postoperative infection. Those factors most often evaluated include (Table 1):

1. socioeconomic status of the patients,
2. the presence and duration of labor,
3. the presence and duration of ruptured membranes,
4. the presence and duration of internal fetal monitoring,
5. the number of vaginal examinations during labor,
6. whether the cesarean section was emergent or elective,
7. the presence of group B *Streptococcus* and other bacteria in the cervicovaginal secretions,
8. the presence of neutrophils and/or bacteria in amniotic fluid or endometrium,
9. obesity, and
10. surgical experience of the operator.

It is often difficult to identify the specific contribution of each factor, since more than one is almost always present in a given patient. The following is an analysis of the relative importance of the various factors in causing endomyometritis.

Socioeconomic Status

Although most clinicians agree that the rate of postoperative infection is highest in indigent populations, the mechanism of this increased risk is less clearly defined. The terms "decreased nutritional status" and "lowered host defense mechanisms" are often used to summarize the complex interaction of a patient's immune system, endogenous bacterial flora, and the environment. Indigent patients are more likely to be anemic and have had suboptimal or no prenatal care. In addition, once in labor, these patients are more likely to be cared for by residents and students and therefore have multiple vaginal examinations with internal monitoring, and their cesareans are performed by less experienced surgeons. Race alone, independent of socioeconomic status, does not appear to be a risk factor.

Labor

It is well documented that women who are not in labor and have intact membranes also have sterile amniotic fluid; as the duration of labor increases, the bacterial count in the amniotic fluid increases as the bacteriostatic properties of the amniotic fluid decrease. This effect may be more pronounced in premature labor or in the presence of meconium, since the amniotic fluid in both these situations has decreased bacteriostatic activity. In his stepwise analysis of peripartum events, D'Angelo determined that the duration of labor alone was the primary determinant of postpartum morbidity. The duration of monitoring and the number of vaginal examinations were only markers of the length of labor. In his review, Swartz found that the presence of labor increased febrile morbidity from 24 to 57 percent without prophylaxis and from 6 to 22 percent with prophylaxis. The exact duration of labor required to cause this increased morbidity cannot be clearly defined, but most authorities demonstrate the increased rate of endomyometritis after 6 to 12 hours in most cases.

Rupture of Membranes

Gilstrap and Bobitt have demonstrated virtually 100 percent bacterial contamination of the amniotic fluid in indigent populations after 6 and 12 hours of ruptured membranes, respectively. Despite these findings, it remains controversial whether or not the presence of ruptured membranes infers increased risk for endomyometritis.

D'Angelo found ruptured membranes to be a poor predictor of postoperative infection, as did Moro and Itskovitz. However, it would be well to remember that many if not most of the studies concerning risk factors and postcesarean infection have too few subjects to identify a small or moderate statistically significant difference in infection

TABLE 1 High-Risk Factors For The Development Of Postcesarean Section Endomyometritis

Independent variables:
Indigent patient population
Presence of labor
Dependent or associated variables:
Presence of ruptured membranes
Multiple vaginal examinations in labor
Internal fetal monitoring
Emergency cesarean section
Obesity
Laboratory markers:
Presence of group B *Streptococcus*, *Neisseria gonorrhoeae*, *Chlamydia*, *Gardnerella*, or *Trichomonas* in cervicovaginal secretions
Vaginal pH greater than 5, with decreased *Lactobacillus*
Neutrophils or bacteria in amniotic fluid
Leukocytic infiltration of endometrium and chorioamniotic membrane
Amniotic fluid phosphorus-to-zinc ratio >200:1
Surgical factors:
Inexperienced surgeon
Long operating time
Excessive blood loss
Breaks from sterile technique

rates. Again, the pooled data from Swartz strongly support the role of ruptured membranes. Gibbs has suggested that increasing length of time of rupture of membranes is associated with increased infection rates; Apuzzio found that those who had ruptured membranes longer than 8 hours developed endomyometritis 54 percent of the time compared with 36 percent with a shorter duration. Cunningham feels that, in indigent populations, having ruptured membranes for longer than 6 hours is a high-risk factor.

Vaginal Examinations

It would seem logical that increasing numbers of vaginal examinations during labor would increase the bacterial contamination of the cervix and lower uterine segment, thereby increasing the postoperative infection rate. In fact, Apuzzio found that the number of examinations in labor was the most important single factor in the development of endomyometritis; Gibbs and Morrison also cited the number of examinations as having an etiologic role in infection. Yonekura reported that the incidence of isolation of high-virulence organisms from amniotic membrane specimens was increased with more than seven pelvic examinations. However, D'Angelo and Kreutner both found the number of examinations to reflect the length of labor rather than being a separate risk factor.

Internal Fetal Monitoring

Patients who require internal monitoring in labor represent a particularly high-risk group for postpartum infection, since they usually have long labors, always have ruptured membranes, and often require multiple vaginal examinations for equipment placement and evaluation, frequently in the presence of meconium-stained amniotic fluid. Despite all these factors, although some studies have found increased infection rates with internal monitoring, the preponderance of evidence suggests that, in and of itself, internal monitoring is not a risk factor for endomyometritis. Both D'Angelo and Gibbs found internal monitoring not to be an independent variable in identifying those at risk for postcesarean infection. In most studies it is not clear what is meant by "internal monitoring," whether it signifies the placement of scalp electrode, of an internal pressure transducer, or of both. One might consider the insertion of the pressure catheter to carry more risk of infection than the placement of the scalp electrode alone. Collected amniotic fluid becomes progressively unsterile as the time after placement of a pressure catheter increases. Indirectly, Haverkamp showed that the incidence of postcesarean endomyometritis was the same whether auscultation alone, internal monitoring, or monitoring with scalp sampling was utilized to evaluate labor and fetal status.

Elective Cesarean Section

Because of the increase in the incidence of cesarean delivery over the last 20 years, coupled with the relatively low incidence of a trial of labor before repeat operative delivery, nearly one-third of all cesareans are now repeat procedures. It is clear that a repeat, elective cesarean section, defined as a procedure performed on a patient who is not in labor and with intact membranes, carries a much lower chance for endomyometritis than does a cesarean following labor, with or without intact membranes. In addition, some primary cesarean sections are performed on an elective basis (breech presentation, for example). These also have a lower infection rate than those on patients in labor. The majority of studies do not make clear the proportion of patients who underwent primary procedures and/or repeat elective procedures and the proportion of each of these groups that became infected. Hagglund found a 25 percent infection rate with emergency section compared with 9 percent for an elective procedure. In indigent populations, postcesarean infection rates can be quite high even with repeat, elective procedures, justifying the use of prophylactic antibiotics. In addition, most studies actually reveal a decrease in postoperative infectious morbidity for repeat, elective cesarean section patients given prophylactic antibiotics, but the numbers in the studies have been too small to show statistically significant differences.

Obesity

Because obese women are more likely to carry a macrosomic fetus, sometimes on the basis of abnormal glucose tolerance, they are at greater risk for cephalopelvic disproportion and thus for longer, more complicated labors. However, obesity itself does not seem to be a risk factor for endomyometritis. On the other hand, obesity is a significant risk factor for wound infections following all operations; since it is likely that prophylactic antibiotics decrease the incidence of wound infection, obesity alone may be an indication for their use.

Other Factors

Many investigators have identified risk factors for postoperative infection that, when present, are very specific markers of risk for endomyometritis; the problem with most of these markers is that they are relatively nonsensitive (may be present in the absence of infection) and are often available to the clinician hours or days after the operative procedure. Duff has shown that women with amniotic fluid bacterial cultures positive for high-virulence organisms, with positive Gram's stains of that fluid, and with histologic leukocytic infiltration in chorioamniotic membrane and endometrium are more likely to develop endomyometritis. Cunningham has shown that those with high bacterial counts and multiple organisms develop their postcesarean infections sooner than those with less bacterial contamination, a finding confirmed by Blanco. Hagglund suggests that the presence of *Staphylococcus aureus* in the nares of the mother is a risk factor. Minkoff shows a higher infection rate in the presence of group B *Streptococcus* and in the presence of an elevated phosphorus-to-zinc ratio in amniotic fluid. There is also evidence that cervical carriage of *Neisseria gonorrhoeae* and *Chlamydia trachomatis* is a factor that identifies an at-risk subgroup. Faro has suggested that even such "benign" findings as a vaginal pH greater than 5, decreased concentration of lactobacilli, the presence of *Gardnerella* or *Trichomonas*, or the presence of clue cells and white cells in the vaginal secretions all identify a patient at high risk for infection.

Patients may also be at high risk for infection based on certain operative events that often reflect the level of training of the surgeon and thus the service assignment of the patient. Miller recently demonstrated that, even after controlling for other variables, endomyometritis was more likely to develop following surgery performed by a junior resident than following surgery by a chief resident or attending staff member. Cesarean sections that take longer than 60 minutes, are followed by significant falls in the patient's hematocrit, and are associated with breaks in sterile technique all have increased chance for development of postoperative morbidity.

Controversies in Cesarean Prophylaxis

Given the diversity of risk factors enumerated above, it is mandatory that every obstetric service know its postoperative infectious morbidity rate for cesarean section in labor and repeat elective section. Strong consideration should be given to the routine use of prophylactic antibiotics for either indication if its associated infection rate is above 15 percent.

Once the decision to employ antibiotics has been taken, there are still several areas of controversy concerning the manner of their use. Among these are (1) the timing of administration, (2) the duration of administration, (3) the choice of antibiotic, and (4) the route of administration. Each of these problems is addressed individually.

Influenced by Burke, all the original investigators of antibiotic prophylaxis efficacy administered the drug prior to the start of the operation. Because all these antibiotics cross the placenta, the neonate was exposed to serum levels of the drug. This exposure had the potential of triggering a toxic reaction in the newborn, altering the neonatal bacterial flora, and, most importantly, masking or delaying diagnosis of neonatal infection. Cunningham has shown that nearly double the number of infants (28 versus 15 percent) are given a sepsis evaluation in the nursery if they have been exposed to antibiotics in utero. Wong and Gordon have both demonstrated that administration of antibiotic after cord clamping is just as effective as a preoperative dose in preventing postoperative infection. It seems clear that antibiotics used for prophylaxis (not treatment) of endomyometritis should be given following cord clamping.

The trend for the last 10 years has been toward a shorter course of prophylaxis. The original studies of prophylaxis really were studies of the early treatment of infection, with patients receiving 2 to 5 days of antibiotic therapy. This was followed by studies of perioperative antibiotic treatment, usually consisting of a dose of drug administered at cord clamping followed by two more doses within 12 to 16 hours. However, Apuzzio, Harger, and Cunningham have all reported that as the intensity of the risk for endomyometritis increases, the failure rate of the shorter prophylactic regimens also increases. In several series, Cunningham describes a 4-day course of early treatment for his particularly high-risk population, with a resulting dramatic decrease in infectious morbidity. This decrease was more dramatic with the 4-day regimen than with the three-dose perioperative use of cefamandole. It is important to note that the incidence of serious complications (abscess and septic pelvic thrombophlebitis) was equal in both groups, leading to the recommendation that the short course of antibiotic therapy be used. De Palma also reported that three doses of cefamandole were equal in efficacy to a 4-day regimen of the same agent. Elliott was one of the few to demonstrate an advantage for a longer treatment schedule, 3 days of ampicillin being better than three doses; both were better than placebo.

More recently, Gonik, Krotec, Saltzman, Robichaux, and Read and Duff have all demonstrated that a single dose of a variety of agents has efficacy equal to three-dose regimens. All of these studies used second- or third-generation cephalosporins or one of the newer penicillins as the single-dose agent; the comparative agent was almost always three doses of cefoxitin. The question is therefore raised whether all antibiotics are equally efficacious in preventing postoperative infection, especially when used as a single dose. Stiver found that cefoxitin and cefazolin (both given in three doses) were distinctly and equally superior to placebo. However, those who did develop infection following cefazolin on average had a longer hospital stay than those who developed infection following cefoxitin. Hawrylyshyn found no statistical difference between one dose and three doses of cefoxitin (9.4 and 5.0 percent), but this may be a matter of small numbers rather than no difference. O'Leary found the combination of ampicillin plus gentamicin to be superior by any measure to ampicillin alone (both were used for 2 days). On the other hand, Louie found both cefazolin and ampicillin to be equal to cefotaxime, and Rayburn demonstrated cefazolin to be equal to moxalactam. Although it appears that ampicillin or cefazolin as single doses are adequate for prophylaxis in most cases, there may be certain cases that warrant the longer-acting or more broad-spectrum agents (extreme high-risk groups) or cases in which the initial dose needs to be repeated (when the cesarean section lasts longer than 60 to 90 minutes).

Uterine Lavage

Long suggested that delivery of antibiotic to the tissue directly at risk for infection by uterine and peritoneal lavage at the time of surgical closure would be an effective way to decrease endomyometritis with a single drug administration; he reasoned that a single lavage application had little chance of a dosing or compounding error, would be less expensive than multiple dosing regimens, and would achieve only low serum levels of antibiotic, thus minimizing the risk of allergic reactions and lessening the pressure toward the selection of resistant organisms in the cervicovaginal flora. His initial and expanded reports of success with this method led to several confirming placebo-controlled studies, most using either cefamandole or cefoxitin. At our own center we demonstrated equal efficacy with lavage or with three intravenous doses of cefotaxime; Donnenfeld found the same result with cefazolin.

Lavage was particularly attractive when compared with multiple dosing regimens of intravenous antibiotics. This attraction has decreased with the demonstration of the efficacy of single-dose intravenous prophylaxis. Read and Duff most recently found a single intravenous dose of either cefamandole or cefotaxime equal to lavage with the same agent. One report, by Conover, found lavage to be inferior to intravenous dosing; both he and Duff also reported serum levels of antibiotic from lavage patients that were above the minimum inhibitory concentration for many of the microorganisms that commonly cause postcesarean infection, suggesting that a systemic effect was at least partly responsible for the efficacy of the method. This finding also suggests that anaphylactic reactions are not eliminated by lavage. In short, there appears to be little reason to employ the lavage method of prophylaxis when a single dose of intravenous antibiotic accomplishes the same purpose with less effort.

Prophylaxis And Other Infections

The efficacy of prophylactic antibiotics in preventing wound infection and urinary tract infection is open to debate. As stated earlier, most studies included too few patients to detect a significant difference in attack rates considering the low baseline incidence of these infectious complications. It should be noted that Swartz did find a significant reduction in wound infection (10 to 3 percent) and urinary tract infection (13 to 6 percent) with prophylaxis when the data from multiple studies were pooled.

Possibly the most controversial point about routine prophylaxis is whether or not it reduces the incidence of serious, life-threatening infectious complications. No one study has a high enough incidence of pelvic abscess or septic thrombophlebitis for any differences to become statistically significant. Mead summarized the data from multiple studies; prophylaxis reduced the incidence of these two complications from 1.1 to 0.5 percent.

Risks of Prophylaxis

The greatest concern centers around allergic or anaphylactic reactions to the antibiotic. Two cases of anaphylactic shock followed by death are always quoted from the orthopaedic literature. No study thus far published reports a similar death in obstetrics. Although allergic reactions of a mild nature may be common, fatal reactions must be extremely rare events. Single-dose regimens may also decrease the opportunities for local and systemic reactions.

A more practical worry is that the widespread use of prophylactic antibiotics will alter bacterial flora, with the emergence of resistant organisms. Endomyometritis, when it does occur, will then be more difficult to treat. It is for this reason that agents whose major purpose is the treatment of serious infections should not be used for prophylaxis and that all agents should be used for as short a course as possible. Most studies that have evaluated bacterial shifts have found increased recovery of resistant enterococci and Enterobacteriaceae. In addition, when cephalosporins are used for prophylaxis, postoperative urinary tract infections are more commonly associated with enterococci. Organisms recovered from patients infected postoperatively are more commonly resistant to the prophylactic agents than are the same species of organisms recovered from control patients.

Costs of Prophylaxis

Since most studies demonstrate at least a 50 percent reduction in postcesarean infection rates with prophylaxis, any service with an infection rate somewhere above 10 to 20 percent will show financial savings compared with no use of prophylaxis. The degree of savings is increased as the attack rate rises, since the savings from increased hospital room, pharmacy, and nursing charges far outweigh the cost of single doses of antibiotic used for prophylaxis. In addition, using ampicillin or a first-generation cephalosporin rather than a newer, more expensive antibiotic increases the amount of savings. Duff has estimated that 100 patients receiving prophylaxis with a first-generation drug at his institution will decrease pharmacy costs by approximately $17,000, assuming a 40 percent infection rate without and a 20 percent infection rate with antibiotics.

Table 2 summarizes current guidelines for the use of prophylactic antibiotics in women undergoing cesarean section.

CERVICAL CERCLAGE

The need for prophylactic antibiotics with cerclage placement has never been scientifically evaluated in either a randomized or a prospective manner. Charles reported a 15 percent postoperative amnionitis rate without prophylaxis for procedures performed between 14 and 18 weeks and a 40 percent rate for those performed between 19 and 32 weeks. Sixty percent of the infections occurred more than 4 weeks after the procedure. He concluded that the risk of infectious morbidity for cerclages placed after 18 weeks was high enough to warrant prophylaxis. On the other hand, Harger reported that only one per 202 elective cerclage placements was followed by acute amnionitis; even with emergency placements, only two in 49 patients had this complication. In a review of our own experience, Kessler reported that four out of 40 patients with cerclages placed between 12 and 18 weeks developed amnionitis postoperatively; interestingly, all four were treated with antibiotics without delivery being necessary. When complications necessitating delivery did occur, it was at a mean time of 8 to 10 weeks from the procedure. Although we are not underestimating the potential for serious postplacement infection (both fetal and maternal deaths from sepsis have been reported), there is no evidence that antibiotic prophylaxis reduces the incidence of either immediate or delayed complications in elective procedures.

A recent fascinating report by Goodlin describes the placement of modified Wurm and McDonald sutures at

TABLE 2 Guidelines For Cesarean Section Antibiotic Prophylaxis

Prophylaxis is indicated for all women with either of the major high-risk factors (labor or indigent population)
Prophylaxis is probably indicated in the presence of one or more of the associated or dependent factors listed in Table 1
Prophylaxis for repeat, elective cesarean section is indicated only on those services with high baseline rates of infectious morbidity
In most cases, a single dose of a first-generation cephalosporin after cord clamping is adequate prophylaxis
Extended-spectrum antibiotics should be reserved for the treatment of serious infections
Infections that develop following prophylaxis should be fully evaluated for the presence of resistant organisms
For patients with penicillin allergy, a single dose of the combination of clindamycin and gentamicin suffices

18 to 24 weeks in women with hourglass membranes and cervical dilation greater than 3 cm. The procedure was accompanied by transabdominal amniocentesis with suction withdrawal of amniotic fluid in order to decompress the bulging membranes. One gram of either ampicillin or a cephalosporin was injected into the amniotic cavity following the amniocentesis; in addition, antibiotics (not specified) were given for 2 to 4 days following the procedure. One-fifth of patients with a singleton pregnancy and five-sixths with multiple pregnancies ruptured their membranes at the time of or shortly after the procedure; one patient with triplets delivered immediately with no infant survival, but all the rest delivered at least one viable infant. If delayed membrane rupture occurred, a second 5-day antibiotic course was given; outcome was uniformly good in these cases. Goodlin stressed that seven out of 11 patients had excessive vaginal drainage despite documented intact membranes. Again, it is difficult to attribute the excellent results of this report to the antibiotics alone, but it does suggest a role for antibiotics in high-risk situations.

Before elective cerclage, the clinician should culture the cervix for *Neisseria gonorrhoeae*, group B *Streptococcus*, *Mycoplasma*, *Ureaplasma*, and *Chlamydia*; if culture for any of these is positive, either treatment or prophylaxis is indicated. In addition, an examination of a wet mount of vaginal secretions for evidence of bacterial vaginosis might direct treatment before cerclage placement or prophylaxis during placement. It may be appropriate to employ antibiotic prophylaxis in high-risk situations, such as the placement of a suture under emergent conditions, after 18 weeks, in patients with cervical effacement and dilation.

PROPHYLAXIS FOR BACTERIAL ENDOCARDITIS

Prophylactic antibiotics are indicated for patients at risk of developing bacterial endocarditis following surgical procedures or instrumentation. Those at risk have valvular heart disease with or without a prosthesis, congenital heart disease, mitral valve prolapse, or a history of endocarditis. Those patients with corrected patent ductus arteriosus or atrial septal defect do not require prophylaxis.

Since endocarditis following vaginal delivery is such a rare event, there probably will never be a conclusive prospective study to document the efficacy of prophylactic antibiotics in this situation. However, since bacteremia can occur asymptomatically with vaginal delivery as well as in association with symptomatic infection following vaginal delivery or cesarean section, it is recommended that women at risk undergo antibiotic prophylaxis for either procedure. Although gram-negative organisms are most commonly recovered in these patients, the prophylaxis is directed mainly at the enterococci.

The American Heart Association guidelines for cardiac prophylaxis are summarized in Table 3.

TABLE 3 Guidelines For Prophylaxis Of Bacterial Endocarditis

Aqueous crystalline penicillin 2,000,000 U IM or IV
OR
Ampicillin 1 g IM or IV
PLUS
Gentamicin 1.5 mg/kg IM or IV
OR
Streptomycin 1.0 g IM
The initial dose is given 30 to 60 minutes prior to the procedure (or at the start of labor). Repeat doses are given every 8 hours for two additional doses when gentamicin is used and every 12 hours for two additional doses when streptomycin is used (during labor doses are given every 8 hours or every 12 hours until two doses have been given following delivery).
For patients with penicillin allergy:
Vancomycin 1 g intravenously over 30–60 minutes
PLUS
Streptomycin 1 g IM
The initial dose is given 30 to 60 minutes prior to the procedure (or at the start of labor). Only a single repeat dose is required 12 hours later (or every 12 hours during labor until one dose has been given following delivery).

Data from Kaplan EL, Anthony BF, Bisno A, et al. Prevention of bacterial endocarditis. Circulation 1977; 56:139A–143A.

SUGGESTED READING

Cartwright PS, Pittaway DE, Jones HW, Entman SS. The use of prophylactic antibiotics in obstetrics and gynecology: a review. Obstet Gynecol Surv 1984; 39:537–554.

Duff P. Prophylactic antibiotics for cesarean delivery: a simple cost-effective strategy for prevention of postoperative morbidity. Am J Obstet Gynecol 1987; 157:794–798.

Ledger WL. Antimicrobial agents. In: Infection in the female. Philadelphia: Lea & Febiger, 1986:112.

Swartz WH, Grolle K. The use of prophylactic antibiotics in cesarean section: a review of the literature. J Reprod Med 1981; 26:595–609.

Sweet RL, Gibbs RS. Antibiotic prophylaxis in obstetrics and gynecology. In: Infectious diseases of the female genital tract. Baltimore: Williams & Wilkins, 1985:350.

ACQUIRED IMMUNODEFICIENCY SYNDROME

HOWARD L. MINKOFF, M.D.

The expanding geographic distribution of human immunodeficiency virus (HIV) disease has an ever increasing impact on the practice of obstetricians. In certain endemic areas (Central Africa), up to 25 percent of all parturients are infected. It may be falsely reassuring to assume that seroprevalence rates in Africa reflect a biologically distinct population. It may be more appropriate to think of that area as a sentinel population since certain hospitals in the United States already have seroprevalence rates in maternity wards of 2.5 percent. Since infected women are a reservoir for sexual and perinatal transmission, it is critically important for obstetricians to take the lead in reducing transmission to and from women.

Currently, there is no cure for acquired immunodeficiency syndrome (AIDS), which is the end stage of HIV disease. Therefore this chapter actually concentrates on techniques for counseling and testing women for HIV disease and for taking steps to avoid transmission. AIDS is the small tip of the large iceberg of HIV disease. Thus, rather than dealing with treatment regimens for the many infections that befall AIDS patients, most of this chapter deals with care giving and HIV carriers; techniques for avoidance of nosocomial risks to health providers are included.

HIV DISEASE

For every patient with AIDS, 50 to 300 patients are infected with HIV. AIDS cases are defined as those infected individuals who have a disease at least moderately predictive of a defect in cell-mediated immunity, but who have no other explanation, such as neoplasm malignancy or chemotherapy, for being immunocompromised. Diseases that are indicative of the immunocompromised state include opportunistic infections (*Pneumocystis carinii* pneumonia, cytomegalovirus, and toxoplasmosis) and neoplasias (Kaposi's sarcoma, primary rectal carcinoma, etc.). Patients with symptoms suggestive of AIDS (weight loss, diarrhea, fever, lymphadenopathy) and immunologic alterations, but who lack a conclusive diagnosis of AIDS, are described as having AIDS-related complex (ARC). These definitions were developed before serologic tests for antibody to HIV were available. Accordingly, these definitions are now undergoing modification. Classification systems based on the clinical status of the patient are summarized in Table 1. These symptoms categorize patients as group I if they have acute infection, group II if they are asymptomatic carriers, group III if they have lymphadenopathy, and group IV if they have constitutional symptoms or symptomatic nonHIV disease.

When the disease was first described in 1981, several risk groups were initially identified. These included homosexual males, intravenous drug abusers, hemophiliacs, and Haitians. Beginning in 1985, all blood products were screened for antibody to HIV, so it is reasonable to anticipate that hemophiliacs represent a decreasing percentage of AIDS victims. Haitians have also been deleted as a separate risk group although the Centers for Disease Control (CDC) include "patient from areas where heterosexual spread is felt to play a major role (Central Africa, Haiti)" among those at significant risk. Of particular importance to obstetricians is evidence that heterosexual activity is of increasing epidemiologic significance among women (see next section). By early 1987, there were over 30,000 patients with AIDS, and an estimated 1 to 2 million Americans are believed infected with the HIV virus. Finally, there are projections that, by 1991, there will be more than a quarter of a million Americans with AIDS, including thousands of women and children.

TABLE 1 HIV Disease

Group	*Symptoms*
I	Acute HIV infection
II	Asymptomatic HIV infection
III	Persistent generalized lymphadenopathy
IV	Other disease entities
Subgroup A	Constitutional disease
Subgroup B	Neurologic disease
Subgroup C	Secondary infectious diseases
Category C-1	Specified secondary infectious diseases listed in the CDC
Category C-2	Other specified infectious diseases
Subgroup D	Secondary cancers
Subgroup E	Other conditions

HIV is a retrovirus (RNA virus) with a predilection for cells with receptors for the T peptide. These cells include T4 (helper) lymphocytes, neural tissue, macrophages, monocytes, and perhaps rectal mucosa.

The virus enters a cell where it is acted upon by a reverse transcriptase that leads to the production of deoxyribonucleic acid (DNA); the DNA is incorporated into the cells' genome. Viral replication then ensues, which can lead to infection of more cells. The devastating nature of the disease results from attack on helper cells, which play a key role in coordinating a variety of immune functions, including B-cell activity and induction of killer cells. When the helper cells are inactivated, the host is subject to a variety of diseases, which otherwise would be controlled by the intact immune system.

The virus can be found in lymphocytes, semen, and vaginal fluid. Thus, any sexual act where body fluids are exchanged poses some risk of transmission. Further, recent evidence (in vitro) suggests that the virus can attach to intact rectal mucosa. Anal intercourse represents as clear a risk in transmitting the virus as does vaginal intercourse. Oral intercourse, deep kissing, etc. pose theoretical risks, although the risk of transmission with each of these acts is not precisely known.

The HIV-infected individual frequently has a transient febrile illness several weeks after initial infection. Seroconversion occurs weeks or months later. Ongoing studies are seeking to estimate the probability of a seropositive individual developing clinical illness. According to current estimates, after 7 years as many as 35 percent of infected individuals will have AIDS, and an additional 40 percent will have lesser stigmata of HIV disease. Long-term follow-up studies, beyond 5 years, may reveal that an increasing percentage of individuals develop either infections, neoplasia, or neurologic manifestations of disease. The prognosis for patients diagnosed as having AIDS remains grim. Only a minority of patients are still alive 2 years after substantiation of the diagnosis.

PREVENTING SPREAD TO THE HETEROSEXUAL FEMALE

Since AIDS is not currently curable, the obstetrician's role as a primary care provider to women centers on prevention of spread to his or her patients. Prevention is primarily dependent on an understanding of the heterosexual spread of the disease and the role of "safe sex" practices in reducing the risk of spread. Since the first descriptions of opportunistic infections and Kaposi's sarcoma among previously healthy male homosexuals, AIDS was recognized as a sexually transmitted disease (STD), whereas the ability of the disease to be spread heterosexually has been the subject of more recent inquiry. Several studies have documented that the steady female sexual partner of an infected male can become infected even if she has no other risk factors.

It has been somewhat more difficult to document female-to-male transmission. Male African AIDS patients reported significantly more frequent contact with prostitutes than noninfected controls. However, this may be related to more frequent STDs among those males or treatment with nonsterile needles, which is as likely a vector as the prostitutes. Studies from the US Army, using questionnaires, suggest that many servicemen with AIDS contracted it heterosexually from prostitutes in Germany. However, given the stigma about homosexuality and intravenous drug abuse in the armed forces, the validity of these results has been questioned. However, there are enough anecdotal reports about infection of husbands by wives who have been infected with blood transfusions to indicate that female-to-male transmission can occur, although the facility with which this occurs is unknown. Finally, recent reports on long-term sexual partners of infected patients reveal a seroconversion rate as high as 50 percent in both susceptible males and females. Perhaps the most alarming statistic regarding heterosexual transmission is that the number of women with AIDS who contracted it heterosexually has increased (from 12 to 27 percent) over the last several years. There has been a concomitant increase in awareness by women of these risks, and studies have suggested a modification of lifestyle by many sexually active women. These modifications have not been reflected in surveys of heterosexual males.

The key question for the physician treating sexually active women is what can be done to reduce the risks. The editor of JAMA, Dr. George D. Lundberg, has suggested, "This is a great time to practice sexual monogamy." Of course, monogamy is "no risk" sex only if a woman's partner shares that philosophy and is not himself infected. The history of public health efforts to eradicate sexually transmitted diseases is filled with examples of the failures of programs that are based solely on recommendations for celibacy or monogamy coupled with dire warnings about casual sex. More useful measures involve public education about "safe sex."

It should be understood at the outset that any sexual act that involves an exchange of body fluid cannot be considered absolutely safe. However, some acts clearly involve more risks than others. For example, the virus has only been isolated from the saliva in a small minority of patients infected with HIV disease and then only in small quantities. The risk from kissing, if a patient has no oral cuts or sores, is undoubtedly less than the risk from intercourse. It is generally agreed that rectal intercourse, whether heterosexual or homosexual, is the sexual act that carries the highest risk. Vaginal intercourse also involves the potential for spread. Oral intercourse poses a theoretical risk, but to what degree has not been clearly delineated. Mutual masturbation, however, is an example of safe sex.

An important alternative to solely proscriptive advice is to counsel about and advocate ready access to and routine use of condoms and spermicides as they have demonstrated some transmission-prevention capabilities in the laboratory. On electromicroscopy, the pores in a latex sheath (condom) are not large enough to allow egress of HIV. Of course, as family planning experts can testify, they are not fail safe. If they cannot always prevent conception, they cannot always prevent HIV transmission. Failure may involve inappropriate usage, inconsistent usage, and product defect. Appropriate use includes (1) application of the condom before the penis comes in contact with the external labia, (2) avoidance of petroleum-based lubricants, and (3) the need for the male to withdraw while the penis is still erect and to hold the rim of the condom against the penis so that the condom does not slip off. Despite these shortcomings, seroconversion rates are lower in women whose infected male partners use condoms than among women having unprotected sex with infected males. A final suggestion to heterosexual patients is to "know your partner." Anonymous, casual sex is dangerous. Initial appearances cannot rule out previous sexual contact with intravenous drug abusers or infected sex partners. There is evidence in the medical and lay press that an increased awareness of the risks of heterosexual sex may signal the end of the sexual revolution.

PERINATAL HIV DISEASE AND AIDS

Serosurveys from New York City have indicated that in some hospitals 2.5 to 5 percent of all parturients are infected with HIV. Thus, even using conservative transmission estimates, the frequency with which children in this community are infected with HIV far surpasses the frequency with which they are infected with such other organisms as herpes or rubella. The relatively high seroprevalence in New York City reflects a sentinel population, not a biologically variant population. Thus, in the near future, obstetricians in all communities will have to consider instituting routine, antepartum HIV testing (with confidentiality and consent). The appropriateness of broad scale testing is based upon our current understanding of the significance of infection to the parturient. Consequently, this section focuses on the impact of pregnancy on HIV infection and the impact of the infection on the mother and fetus.

Pregnancy clearly has the potential to modify the progress of HIV disease and vice versa. The pregnant host undergoes immunologic changes that have previously been reported to affect other viral illnesses. In pregnancy, helper to suppressor ratios and lymphocyte functions are altered. Outbreaks of viral illnesses such as influenza have been noted to affect a disproportionate number of pregnant women. For these reasons, it might be assumed that the course of HIV disease would be altered by pregnancy.

Although only a few cases of opportunistic infections associated with AIDS in pregnancy have been reported, their generally poor outcomes would seem to support the theory that the prognosis is worse in pregnancy. The majority of reported patients with opportunistic infections died during their initial hospitalization. However, more careful analyses of the cases reveal that the delay in diagnosis was a major contribution to the poor outcome. In the setting of pregnancy, many nonspecific symptoms such as malaise and nausea may be mistaken for "pregnancy symptoms." Furthermore, until recently, obstetricians and midwives rarely encountered AIDS, and hence, immunocompromise may have been considered as a potential diagnosis relatively late in the course of the illness. These case reports highlight the need for those who care for parturients from risk groups to consider HIV in their differential diagnosis of related illness.

Since patients with AIDS constitute only a small minority of patients infected with HIV, it is appropriate to determine whether pregnancy accelerates the progression from asymptomatic carriage of HIV to clinical illness. A few reports have noted a high rate of progression to clinical illness within several years of the birth of an affected child. However, no reports have included matched controls (nonpregnant, infected women from similar risk groups). These studies have examined women identified as infected because their children developed illness. There is some evidence that seropositive women whose children develop infection are those with more rapidly progressing immunocompromise and hence are at greater risk for progressive disease. The pregnant patient with AIDS would probably only receive treatment for opportunistic infection since most care providers would be hesitant to utilize agents such as AZT in pregnancy because similar drugs, such as methotrexate, have demonstrated teratogenicity.

The most common concern voiced by the pregnant AIDS patient is whether the unborn child is infected. Such potential clearly exists. The majority of cases of pediatric AIDS or ARC cases are the result of perinatal transmission, with the remaining cases attributed to blood transfusion. Three cases have been related to contaminated breast milk. These involved women who seroconverted after being transfused in the postpartum period. Their babies subsequently seroconverted. The remaining cases involve prenatal transmission. Reports of viral isolation in the thymus of preterm infants delivered by cesarean section and description of an "AIDS embryopathy" suggest that transplacental transmission can occur. However, many infants do not have stigmata until several months after birth, and the possibility that infection occasionally occurs during parturition also exists. At this point, no evidence exists that cesarean section is protective for the neonate.

Although descriptions of pediatric AIDS and ARC have been published in great detail, relatively little has been reported about pregnancies among seropositive mothers. Our experience at SUNY Health Science Center at Brooklyn and Kings County Hospital has been that most pregnancies are not subjectively different for seropositive mothers. They rarely report symptoms that can be attributed to immunocompromise. Initially, most mothers were from the CDC's defined risk groups. However, there is recent evidence that HIV is extending beyond the boundaries of previously recognized risk groups and, as such, is behaving like other sexually transmitted diseases. If a physician is to offer counseling and testing to potentially seropositive mothers, one cannot wait until one is actually caring for a symptomatic patient or perhaps an easily recognized risk group member. It is preferable that efforts be directed at heterosexually active women who have engaged in nonmonogamous relations.

Studies designed to accurately determine the rate of transmission from mother to child are currently ongoing in many centers throughout the United States, Africa, and Europe. Earlier studies demonstrated clinical illness in up to 65 percent of children of infected mothers. In those studies, the mothers were initially identified because they had previously given birth to children who developed AIDS. It is possible that they may represent a distinct subgroup whose transmission rate is different from seropositive mothers in general. Other studies have found stigmata of disease in up to one-third of children within several months of birth. The percentage of children followed by prospective studies who have developed illness has ranged from 20 to 50 percent. Although these numbers are not specific, they are useful for counseling.

One potential use of testing, beyond allowing women to make informed decisions about their reproductive options, is to alert pediatricians as to which neonates may be infected. Such information now provides only limited benefit to the pediatrician. For example, although the Centers for Disease Control recommend modification of vaccine schedules for infected children, that recommendation (based on limited data) is only applicable to symptomatic children. This may change if some form of effective, early therapy (i.e., gamma globulins) is shown to modify the course of a child's illness. Currently, the main utility of maternal AIDS testing is to alert pediatricians to the potential significance of coughs, colds, etc. in an HIV-infected child in order to facilitate timely institution of therapy.

Therapy of the pregnant woman with AIDS is directed towards opportunistic infections. Patients with *Pneumocystis carinii* (PCP), the most common infection, are treated with cotrimoxade or pentamidine (as are the nonpregnant) despite the risks of these drugs in pregnancy. The high mortality from PCP obviates use of therapies with lesser effectiveness.

There are no proven immunomodulating co-factors that can modify the rate of progression in the asymptomatic pregnant carrier of HIV. Thus, although it seems logical to recommend avoidance of antigenic stimuli (drugs, sperm) and situations that alter T4:T8 ratios (sleep deprivation, stress), there is no good evidence that actual clinical benefit accrues.

HIV AND THE HEALTH CARE WORKER

Publicity surrounding transfusion-related AIDS has made the lay community increasingly reticent to receive blood and increasingly desirous of using directed donations when transfusion is required. These feelings persist despite universal blood screening for HIV antibodies. Self-exclusion questionnaires also continue to be administered since there is a period of time when a recently infected individual sheds the HIV virus, but does not yet have detectable antibody. It is now estimated that the risk from transfused blood is extremely low (1:30,000 to 1:1,000,000 units). There is, however, no evidence that directed donations (blood from friends, relatives, etc.) hold any greater risk than blood from the general population, so a patient who needs blood, but who wishes to accept only directed donations, should be accommodated. Finally, the safest blood a patient can receive is autologous blood. Patients scheduled for elective surgery can be offered that option, although safety in pregnancy has not yet been documented.

The risk of viral transmission in the hospital has been a concern to health care providers. The experience with hepatitis B virus serves to chasten obstetricians. The risk of transmission of hepatitis B virus after a needle stick ranges from 5 to 30 percent and almost 1 in 5 obstetricians has serologic evidence of a past infection with hepatitis B. This is particularly worrisome since, in a given year, in institutions in highly endemic areas, as many as 14 percent of house officers have been stuck with needles used on AIDS patients. Fortunately, nosocomial infection does not occur with facility. Although there have been a few infections of medical personnel, including three that did not involve needle sticks, the risk appears quite small. There have been tens of thousands of contacts of health care workers with infected blood and secretions. The risk from a needle stick is estimated to be no greater than 0.5 percent and no seroconversions have occurred related to peripartum care. The most cogent advice to health care providers dealing with high-risk patients is to exercise caution. Do not recap needles prior to discarding them; do not attempt to bend or break them; wear gloves at any time contact with body fluids can occur.

There have been no documented cases of patients contracting HIV infections from infected medical personnel. Not surprisingly, there are health care workers from risk groups, and there are seropositives among them. Currently, there are no indications that they cannot continue to perform their normal medical functions.

The appropriate approach to isolation in the hospital has been the subject of several studies. A variety of approaches has been proposed, including universal screening of all patients for serologic status. The current recommendation is to treat all patients in endemic communities with care, rather than to attempt to identify every individual carrier.

ETHICAL AND SOCIAL ISSUES

The dramatic surge in the prevalence of a sexually transmitted, lethal virus has raised a large number of ethical issues. Central among these issues is the appropriate scope of screening and the sanctity of medical confidences. These issues have particular relevance in regard to this disease because of the stigma attached to the diagnosis. There have already been several hundred law suits brought regarding discrimination based on the diagnosis of AIDS or even the presumed diagnosis of AIDS. The factors are in place for the inevitable conflict between the need for confidentiality codified in the Hippocratic oath ("what I may see or hear in the course of treatment in regard to the life of men...I will keep to myself...") and the public's (and health professionals') desire to reduce their own risks by knowing who is infected. The physicians' ethical dichotomy is perhaps most clearly reflected in the Principles of Medical Ethics of the AMA (1957), Section 9: "A physician may not reveal the confidence entrusted to him in the course of medical attendance...unless he is required to do so by law or unless it becomes necessary in order to protect the welfare of the individual or of the community." Although confidentiality clearly serves as the center of gravity for that ethical thesis, the "unless" can confuse the issue if one is dealing with a seropositive individual who refuses to reveal his status to his betrothed, spouse, etc. Although a myriad of potential ethical conflicts have not been resolved, certain facts seem straightforward. The Infectious Disease Society of America and the American College of Physicians have adopted a series of positions. These include the following: 1. AIDS patients should receive competent and humane care "...even at the risk of contracting a patient's disease." 2. Encourage public education about HIV in order to prevent spread of infection and to alleviate discrimination against those who become infected with the virus. 3. Testing for antibody should be used only in situations in which it will be of benefit to public health and will not be discriminatory. 4. Counseling and educational efforts, rather than policies promoting physical restriction and isolation, are appropriate methods for controlling the spread of infection. 5. Beyond mandated reporting requirements, positive results should not be communicated by health professionals to any other party, except the patient whose blood has been tested. 6. Physicians should improve sexual history taking and safe sex counseling.

The rapidly expanding scope of the HIV epidemic is beginning to impact on women. Tens of thousands are already infected and many, if not most, progress to disease. Therefore, it is incumbent upon obstetricians to familiarize themselves with those aspects of the disease that affect women. Obstetricians must immediately involve themselves in efforts directed at disease prevention through counseling of sexually active women and counseling and testing of pregnant women.

SUGGESTED READING

Acquired immunodeficiency syndrome. J Infect Dis 1986; 154:1–7.

CDC. Recommendations for assisting in the prevention of perinatal transmission of HTLV-III/LAV and AIDS. MMWR 1985; 34:721–732.

CDC. Summary: recommendations for preventing transmission of infection with HTLV-III/LAV in the workplace. MMWR 1985; 34:681–695.

Francis D, Chin J. The prevention of acquired immunodeficiency syndrome in the United States. JAMA 1987; 257:1357–1366.

Minkoff HL, Nanda D, Mendez R. Follow-up of mothers of children with AIDS. Obstet Gynecol 1987; 69:288–291.

Minkoff HL, Haynes-deRegt R, Landesman S, et al. Pneumocystis carinii pneumonia associated with acquired immunodeficiency syndrome (AIDS) in pregnancy. Obstet Gynecol 1986; 67:284–287.

Minkoff HL, Nanda D, Mendez R. Pregnancies resulting in children with acquired immunodeficiency syndrome. Obstet Gynecol 1987; 69:285–287.

CHLAMYDIA TRACHOMATIS INFECTION

RICHARD L. SWEET, M.D.

The United States is currently in the midst of an epidemic of sexually transmitted diseases (STDs). The most prevalent of these STD pathogens in the United States is *Chlamydia trachomatis*. It is currently estimated that there are upward of 4 million chlamydial infections annually in the United States. *C. trachomatis* has long been known as the causative agent of trachoma, a disease that is hyperendemic in many developing countries and considered to be the leading preventable cause of blindness in the world. In addition, *Chlamydia* is the pathogen long known to cause inclusion conjunctivitis in the newborn, and lymphogranuloma venereum. More recently chlamydial infections of the genital tract and the consequences of perinatal exposure, both maternal and neonatal, have received considerable attention. It is women who bear the brunt of the *Chlamydia* burden because of their increased risk for adverse reproductive consequences. *C. trachomatis* is a high prevalence agent that is associated with a wide variety of complications. This organism has been associated with acute salpingitis and other long-term consequences such as infertility, ectopic pregnancy, neonatal conjunctivitis, and chlamydial pneumonia of the newborn; an association of chlamydial infection with adverse pregnancy outcome has also been suggested.

C. trachomatis is a unique bacterial organism. It is an obligatory, intracellular bacteria. Thus, it must grow and replicate within a host cell. In addition, *Chlamydia* has a unique growth cycle. The organism exists in two forms: (1) the elementary body, which is the infectious particle and capable of entering uninfected cells, and (2) the initial body, which multiplies by binary fission to produce the inclusions that are identified in properly stained cells. The *Chlamydia* growth cycle takes approximately 48 hours to complete. This slow growth cycle has clinical implications in that slow-growing organisms require long-term therapy. *C. trachomatis* is currently divided into 15 serotypes. In particular, the serotypes D, E, F, G, H, I, J, and K are the sexually transmitted agents that cause inclusion conjunctivitis, newborn pneumonia, urethritis, cervicitis, epididymitis, salpingitis, acute urethral syndrome, and perinatal infections.

Chlamydia is recognized as the major cause of nongonococcal urethritis in men and is the leading cause of acute epididymitis in men under the age of 40. In addition, it is a frequent cause of proctitis in homosexual men. A variety of infections has been associated with *Chlamydia trachomatis* in women. These include mucopurulent endocervicitis, endometritis, salpingitis, and pelvic inflammatory disease. Chlamydial infections have been linked with tubal infertility and ectopic pregnancy. Chlamydial infections of newborns secondary to vertical transmission from infected mothers have been identified; these include newborn conjunctivitis and pneumonia. The role of *Chlamydia trachomatis* in pregnancy is more controversial. There has been some suggestion that *Chlamydia* produces adverse pregnancy outcomes, such as premature rupture of the membranes, preterm delivery, and low birth weight. In addition, several authors have suggested that *Chlamydia* is responsible for postpartum endometritis.

CLINICAL SPECTRUM OF CHLAMYDIAL INFECTION

Endocervicitis

The site within the female genital tract that is most often infected with *C. trachomatis* is the cervix. The organism causes an endocervicitis. However, many asymptomatic infections also occur. The organism is a specific parasite of columnar cells and thus grows only within the transitional zone and the endocervix. The infected cervix may range from a clinically normal appearance to one with an ectropion and mucopurulent endocervical discharge. The entity of mucopurulent cervicitis is a specific one characterized by the presence of mucopus, as demonstrated by the finding with a cotton swab showing yellow or green endocervical discharge, or the presence of polymorphonuclear leukocytes on a Gram's stain, or the presence of ectopy with easy bleeding, erythema, and edema. It is apparent that cervical infection with *C. trachomatis* is a major reservoir for male and neonatal infections associated with this agent. In addition, the cervix is the source of major complications involving the upper genital tract, such as acute salpingitis and its sequelae of tubal infertility and ectopic pregnancy.

Endometritis

Investigations in Seattle have demonstrated that nearly half of the females with mucopurulent cervicitis due to *Chlamydia* have histologic plasma cell endometritis on endometrial biopsy. Moreover, these women have a high incidence of abnormal uterine bleeding, abdominal cramps, and uterine tenderness. The latter findings suggest that many women with chlamydial cervicitis have acute, nonpuerperal endometritis. Of great concern has been the finding by Jones and colleagues at the University of Indiana that in nearly half of the women with asymptomatic chlamydial cervical infection (no abdominal pain, no uterine tenderness, no abnormal bleeding) *Chlamydia trachomatis* is recovered from their endometrial cavity. This suggests that there is a large group of women who already have silent upper genital tract infection with *Chlamydia*. We recently demonstrated that *Chlamydia trachomatis* could be recovered from the endometrial cavity of women with signs and symptoms of acute salpingitis or pelvic inflammatory disease. Moreover, we noted that in these women *Chlamydia* could be recovered, after treatment, from the endometrial cavity despite prompt, clinical response if antimicrobial therapy that did not provide coverage against *Chlamydia trachomatis* was used to treat their pelvic inflammatory disease. Thus the presence of subclinical, persistent chlamydial endometritis among patients with resolving acute pelvic inflammatory disease exists.

Acute Salpingitis

The most serious systemic complication of chlamydial infection in women is acute salpingitis. Without question acute salpingitis is the major medical and economic consequence of the STD epidemic in young women in the United States. The role of *C. trachomatis* as a pathogen in acute pelvic inflammatory disease has received considerable attention. Initially, investigators in Scandinavia had demonstrated the association between *Chlamydia trachomatis* and acute salpingitis. These studies definitely demonstrated that *Chlamydia trachomatis* was an important etiologic agent in this disease. It has been estimated that in Scandinavia between 30 to 70 percent of cases of acute salpingitis are associated with *Chlamydia* as the etiologic agent. Until recently in the United States, evidence has suggested that *Chlamydia*-associated acute salpingitis was much less frequent than what was being reported from Scandinavia. Our own laparoscopy studies initially failed to recover *Chlamydia trachomatis* from the fallopian tubes of women with acute pelvic inflammatory disease. However, recently investigations in San Francisco and Seattle have confirmed a definite role for *Chlamydia trachomatis* as a major etiologic agent in acute salpingitis in the United States, demonstrating that between 25 and 50 percent of such patients will have *Chlamydia trachomatis* recovered from their upper genital tracts. Thus it seems that there is no doubt that *Chlamydia* is a major agent for this devastating disease in the United States.

Of great concern have been the studies that have demonstrated that *Chlamydia trachomatis* is associated with several of the significant sequelae of acute pelvic inflammatory disease. Over 20 reported studies have now confirmed an association between the presence of previous chlamydial infection and infertility due to tubal obstruction. Most distressing in these studies is the fact that over half the women who have infertility caused by tubal obstruction have no history that they had ever been diagnosed or treated for acute pelvic inflammatory disease. Studies by Jones and colleagues at the University of Indiana have suggested that there is a large group of asymptomatic, subclinical, upper genital tract chlamydial infections that may well explain this high incidence of no history of pelvic inflammatory disease but confirmed infertility following chlamydial infection. In a similar vein, recent studies in Scandinavia and the United States have demonstrated a very strong association between ectopic pregnancy and evidence on antibody titers of previous chlamydial infection. Thus the two major sequelae of acute pelvic inflammatory disease have been demonstrated to be associated with previous chlamydial infection in serologic studies. Although this does not definitely prove that *Chlamydia* caused the pelvic inflammatory disease or the infertility and ectopic pregnancies, when so many studies converge on a single theme we must place credence in such findings.

Perinatal Infection

The prevalence of *Chlamydia trachomatis* in pregnancy has been reported to range from 2 to 37 percent; it is estimated that approximately 5 percent of all pregnant women in the United States have chlamydial infections of their cervix. It has been well documented that vertical transmission of *Chlamydia* from the infected, untreated mother to her neonate occurs in approximately 60 percent of cases among infants born vaginally. Prospective studies have demonstrated that somewhere between 20 to 50 percent of infants born to such mothers develop neonatal chlamydial conjunctivitis, and 10 to 20 percent develop pneumonia within the first 2 months of life. The chlamydial conjunctivitis typically appears in the first week of life and is characterized by purulent discharge. The pneumonia manifests by a staccato cough and mild respiratory symptoms. The babies are usually afebrile, but on x-ray examination have a definite interstitial infiltrate. Cost benefit analyses have been performed that clearly demonstrate that it is advantageous to screen pregnant women for *Chlamydia*, identify those who are infected, and treat the chlamydial infection in the pregnant mother in order to prevent the neonatal conjunctivitis and pneumonia. The specifics of this treatment are discussed further on.

More controversial has been the role of *Chlamydia trachomatis* in adverse pregnancy outcome. Initial studies at the University of Washington suggested that patients who had chlamydial cervical infections during their first prenatal visit were significantly more likely to develop late-onset endometritis following vaginal delivery. Subsequent studies performed in a variety of cities failed to confirm this finding. Recently it has again been suggested by investigators in Seattle and Chicago that there is indeed an association between chlamydial infection and postpartum endometritis. Resolution of this controversy will require additional studies.

Of greater concern has been the suggestion that *Chlamydia* may adversely affect pregnancy by being associated with preterm labor, preterm delivery, premature rupture of the membranes, and low birth weight babies. Initial studies from the University of Washington showed a significant association of chlamydial infection with prematurity, low birth weight, and perinatal mortality. Subsequent studies performed in Baltimore, Arizona, and Atlanta failed to confirm such a finding. Recently Harrison, at the University of Arizona, suggested that the subgroup of chlamydial infected mothers who were immunoglobulin M (IgM) positive (which it was felt connoted recent acute chlamydial infection) were at significant risk for preterm labor and low birth weight infants. We at the University of California in San Francisco have confirmed this finding in a much larger study and have shown that those women with cervical *Chlamydia* infection who are IgM positive had a 2.5-fold increased risk of developing preterm labor and delivery or of having premature rupture of the membranes. However, when we controlled for the presence of other sexually transmitted diseases in logistic regression analysis, the significance with chlamydial infections disappeared. Thus we are left with a controversy that is as yet unresolved and one that will require additional future studies.

DIAGNOSIS OF CHLAMYDIAL INFECTIONS

It is clear that a relatively large proportion (somewhere between 50 to 65 percent) of women with chlamydial cervical infections do not have any clinical signs or symptoms of their infection. However, because of the cost of chlamydial culture and the inaccessibility to *Chlamydia* diagnostic tests that have existed in the past, many protocols were established to identify patients at significant risk for chlamydial infection and to intervene with empiric therapy in those patients. Studies in adolescent females suggested that those women who were at high risk for chlamydial infection included the nonwhite, those using oral contraceptives, women with a diagnosis of lower genital tract infection, those who had had onset of sexual activity at an early age, and those who had inflammatory changes on their Papanicolaou smear. In a family planning clinic, Hansfield and colleagues recently demonstrated that those women at significant risk for chlamydial infection were less than 24 years of age, had had a new sexual partner within the previous 2 months, had partners with nongonococcal urethritis, had easy bleeding on swabbing of the cervix, and used either no contraceptives or nonbarrier methods of contraception. However, because of inaccessibility of chlamydial cultures, empiric treatment regimens were proposed. Generally these included patients who were partners of men with nongonococcal urethritis, women with mucopurulent endocervicitis, women with acute urethral syndrome, and women with gonococcal infection. However, studies performed here in San Francisco suggested that only one-third of women with chlamydial infections would fall into one of those risk groups, and that such empiric therapy would miss over two-thirds of cases of chlamydial infection in the United States. In an attempt to come to grips with the epidemic of chlamydial infection, the Centers for Disease Control has recommended that when treating gonorrhea infection, it should be suspected that concomitant chlamydial infection exists, and combination therapy should be used that is effective against both *Neisseria gonorrhoeae* and *Chlamydia trachomatis*.

Current diagnostic capabilities for *Chlamydia trachomatis* infection include cell culture and antigen detection systems. We feel that cytology is an insensitive diagnostic approach to the *Chlamydia* problem. Culture using a cell line for *Chlamydia*, typically cyclohexamide-treated McCoy cells, remains the gold standard of diagnosis. However, this typically takes 48 to 96 hours and often longer in order to obtain the results and requires experience with cell culture lines. There are currently two antigen detection systems available. The first is the fluorescein-labeled monoclonal antibody, and the second is an immunoassay type system. Both systems are very specific and very sensitive in high prevalence populations. However, as the prevalence of the disease drops, the sensitivity begins to drop as well. There are approximately 2 to 3 percent false-positive results with the antigen detection systems, which means that in a low prevalence population of only 2 to 3 percent, there will be a 50 percent false-positive rate. However, the antigen detection systems are readily available to many clinicians in the United States and can be used appropriately in areas where cultures are not available.

TREATMENT OF CHLAMYDIAL INFECTIONS

The current Centers for Disease Control treatment recommendations for *Chlamydia trachomatis* infections of the lower genital tract include (1) tetracycline, 500 mg orally four times a day for 7 days, or (2) doxycycline, 100 mg orally twice a day for 7 days. Alternate regimens include erythromycin base or stearate, 500 mg four times a day for 7 days, or erythromycin ethylsuccinate, 800 mg four times a day for 7 days. An additional regimen would be sulfamethoxazole, 1 g twice a day for 10 days, but this is by far the least frequently used regimen. To date there have been no strains of *Chlamydia trachomatis* demonstrated to have in vitro resistance to tetracyclines. In fact, the overall susceptibility of *Chlamydia* to tetracyclines is so effective that the Centers for Disease Control does not even recommend a test of cure following chlamydial treatment with a tetracycline. The sexual partner(s) of women with chlamydial infection must receive treatment with similar regimens.

Current recommendations for the treatment of acute pelvic inflammatory disease are based on the recognition that this infection is polymicrobic in nature. In general, three major etiologic agents have been elucidated: *N. gonorrhoeae*, *C. trachomatis*, and anaerobic and aerobic bacteria. To provide optimum coverage, the Centers for Disease Control has recommended that combination broad-spectrum therapy be employed in the treatment of acute pelvic inflammatory disease.

In the United States approximately three-fourths of the one million annual cases of acute pelvic inflammatory disease are treated on an ambulatory basis. The recommended outpatient regimens for the treatment of acute pelvic inflammatory disease include a combination of either ceftriaxone, 250 mg intramuscularly, ampicillin, 3.5 g orally, amoxicillin, 3.0 g orally, aqueous procaine penicillin, 4.8 million U intramuscularly, or cefoxitin, 2 g intramuscularly plus doxycycline, 100 mg orally twice daily for 10 to 14 days. Probenecid, 1 g orally, is given concomitantly with ampicillin, amoxicillin, penicillin, or cefoxitin. Currently recommended regimens for treatment of hospitalized patients with acute pelvic inflammatory disease include (1) cefoxitin, 2 g intravenously every 6 hours plus doxycycline, 100 mg intravenously every 12 hours for a minimum of 4 days, followed by doxycycline, 100 mg orally every 12 hours, to complete a 10- to 14-day course of therapy; or (2) clindamycin, 600 mg intravenously every 6 hours plus gentamicin, 2.0 mg per kilogram loading dose and then 1.5 mg per kilogram intravenously every 8 hours for a minimum of 4 days, followed by clindamycin, 450 mg orally every 6 hours to complete a 10- to 14-day course of therapy. In limited prospective studies to date, these doses of clindamycin have resulted in 100 percent eradication of *C. trachomatis* infection in patients with acute pelvic inflammatory disease.

In pregnant women with chlamydial cervical infection, the treatment of choice is erythromycin. Appropriate regimens include (1) erythromycin base, 500 mg four times a day for 7 days, or (2) erythromycin ethylsuccinate, 800 mg three times a day for 7 days. If patients do not tolerate these doses of erythromycin, the daily dose should be decreased by half and the duration of therapy increased to 2 weeks. Preliminary studies have documented the efficacy of erythromycin treatment in eradicating chlamydial infection in pregnant women and preventing vertical transmission of *Chlamydia* to neonates. Schachter and Grossman noted that when the prevalence of *C. trachomatis* cervical infection was greater than 5 percent, the cost-benefit analysis favored screening all pregnant women and treating women positive for *Chlamydia* during pregnancy.

Chlamydial inclusion conjunctivitis is usually treated with tetracycline or erythromycin eye drops. However, because treatment with topical agents does not prevent chlamydial pneumonia, systemic erythromycin therapy is recommended for the treatment of conjunctivitis as well as of pneumonia. The dose is 40 mg per kilogram per day given over a 2-week period of time. Systemic therapy will also eradicate nasopharyngeal colonization and prevent pneumonia secondary to chlamydial infection. To date, no studies exist to answer the question of whether treatment of chlamydial infection in pregnancy enhances a favorable pregnancy outcome. Thus treatment of pregnant women is primarily aimed at prevention of neonatal chlamydial infection and eradication of the reservoir of infection.

Although they are not currently recommended or clinically available, several alternative antichlamydial agents deserve mention. Small, preliminary studies have documented the ability of amoxicillin and ampicillin-like agents such as piperacillin or mezlocillin to eradicate *C. trachomatis*. In particular, in pregnant women amoxicillin has been demonstrated to have a higher rate of eradication of *C. trachomatis* and to be better tolerated than erythromycin therapy.

A great deal of excitement has centered on the potential use of quinolone agents in the treatment of *C. trachomatis*, *N. gonorrhoeae*, and the mixed anaerobic bacteria. Ciprofloxacin, ofloxacin, and perfloxacin have excellent activity against clinical isolates of *C. trachomatis*. The clinical efficacy of these quinolones in eradicating *C. trachomatis* must be determined in clinical trials.

SUGGESTED READING

Schachter J. Chlamydial infections. N Engl J Med 1978; 298:428–435, 490–495, 540–549.

Schachter J, Grossman M, Sweet RL, et al. Prospective study of perinatal transmission of *Chlamydia trachomatis*. JAMA 1986; 255:3374–3377.

Sweet RL, Schachter J, Landers DV. Chlamydial infections in obstetrics and gynecology. Clin Obstet Gynecol 1983; 26:143–164.

Sweet RL, Walker C, Landers DV, Schachter J. *Chlamydia trachomatis* infection and pregnancy outcome. Am J Obstet Gynecol 1987; 156:824–830.

POSTPARTUM INFECTION

RONALD S. GIBBS, M.D.

Puerperal endomyometritis, occurring mainly after cesarean delivery, is one of the most common complications encountered by obstetrician-gynecologists. The etiology is often polymicrobial; involving aerobes, anaerobes, and genital mycoplasmas. *Chlamydia trachomatis* appears to have little role in endometritis after cesarean section but is associated with a late-onset, mild infection after vaginal delivery. Major risk factors for puerperal endometritis are cesarean delivery, abnormal labor (including interrelated factors of prolonged labor, prolonged membrane rupture, multiple examinations, and internal monitoring), and indigent socioeconomic status.

Clinical manifestations of endomyometritis are usually fever (>100 degrees F), tachycardia, lower abdominal pain, uterine and adnexal tenderness, and purulent or foul lochia. These findings typically develop 36 to 48 hours after delivery. However, earlier onset fevers should not be ignored, since those, especially within the first 24 hours after delivery, often are due to infections caused by group B streptococci. In the initial evaluation of a patient with suspected endomyometritis, the differential diagnosis should include acute pyelonephritis, appendicitis, pneumonia, and viral syndrome.

For the vast majority of patients, several simple laboratory tests are sufficient to establish the correct diagnosis. These tests are hematocrit, differential white blood cell count, urine culture, blood culture, and endometrial culture.

It should be noted that the results of the endometrial cultures are more reliable if specimens are obtained with a double-lumen collecting device to protect against contamination by cervical and vaginal microorganisms.

Chest x-ray study should be reserved for women with suspected respiratory infection. Sonography or computed tomographic (CT) scanning is indicated generally when the patient has a persistent fever and a pelvic abscess is suspected.

ANTIBIOTIC THERAPY

Patients with puerperal endomyometritis must be treated with antibiotics that are active against most causative organisms.

Clindamycin Plus Gentamicin

For the past decade, the standard for comparison has been a combination of clindamycin plus gentamicin (Table 1). The combination enjoys wide in vitro activity, with clindamycin providing excellent activity against pelvic anerobes and most aerobic gram-positive organisms. Gentamicin complements the activity of clindamycin by providing excellent activity against aerobic gram-negative rods. Indeed, among commonly encountered genital bacteria, the only one that is resistant to this therapy is the enterococcus (*Streptococcus faecalis*). *Mycoplasma hominis* is susceptible to clindamycin, and *Chlamydia trachomatis* can often be eradicated with high doses of clindamycin. *Ureaplasma urealyticum*, formerly called T-form mycoplasma, is not susceptible to this combination, but this organism does not appear to be of major importance.

Initially, the antibiotics should be administered intravenously. For clindamycin, it had been customary to use 600 mg IV every 6 hours. Gentamicin is given as 1.0 to 1.5 mg per kilogram intravenously every 8 hours. Thus, this dosage scheme resulted in multiple intravenous injections daily. Recently, a new preparation of clindamycin (900-mg vial) has been developed for intravenous dosing every 8 hours. Considering the kinetics of clindamycin, the use of an 8-hour regimen is appropriate. Also, since clindamycin and gentamicin are compatible in intravenous solutions, the number of daily injections may be decreased to three.

When used in the above doses, the overall efficacy of this regimen in most pelvic infections has been 88 to 95 percent. When there has been a good response, we continue intravenous therapy until the patient has been afebrile for 36 to 48 hours. Then we discontinue intravenous therapy and usually discharge the patient from the hospital that day. Formerly, we had continued the patient on oral antibiotics for several days. However, we now believe that oral antibiotics are unnecessary in most patients. We reserve oral therapy for selected patients, such as those with bacteremia or protracted infections.

When a patient does not respond clinically in 48 to 72 hours, she should be reevaluated. Cultures should be checked for resistant organisms, and general and pelvic examinations should be performed to detect a mass, hematoma, abscess, retained placenta, or extensive cellulitis. Also, gentamicin peak and trough levels should be checked at this point, especially if an aerobic gram-negative rod has been isolated. The gentamicin dose should be adjusted to achieve a peak level of 5 to 10 μg per milliliter. If the patient is stable, and no mass is detected, then a resistant organism may be assumed to be the cause of the persistent fever. Most patients respond after the empirical addition of intravenous ampicillin (2 g every 6 hours) or intravenous penicillin G (5×10^6 U every 6 hours) to provide coverage of enterococci. Because a small percentage of anaerobes are resistant to clindamycin, metronidazole can be empirically substituted for clindamycin at this time also. However, I usually just add the penicillin. If the patient is unstable (if abdominal and vital signs deteriorate), then special circumstances, such as myonecrosis or necrotizing fasciitis, must be considered (see further on).

Within an additional 48 hours (after the change in antibiotic), most patients have a satisfactory resolution of their infection. Those who have persistent signs are most likely to have an infected mass. The abdominal incision should be carefully inspected for signs of infection, and if suspect, it should be probed or opened. To rule out a pelvic mass, a repeat examination is in order, followed by a CT scan. I believe that in this circumstance, a CT scan pro-

TABLE 1 Summary of Selected Antibiotic Regimens Used to Treat Pelvic Infection

Antibiotic(s)	*Common Dose Range (IV)*	*Major Resistant Organism*	*Representative Side Effects*	*Reported Cure Rates*
Clindamycin plus gentamicin	600 mg q6h or 900 mg q8h (clindamycin) 1.5 mg/kg q8h (gentamicin)	Enterococci	Diarrhea; nephrotoxicity	>90%
Penicillin or ampicillin plus gentamicin	5×10^6 q6h (penicillin), 2 g IV q4–6h (ampicillin) 1.5 mg/kg q8h (gentamicin)	Selected anaerobes including many *Bacteroides* species	Allergic, nephrotoxicity	65–80%
Cefoxitin (Mefoxin)	1–2 g q6h	Enterococci	Allergic	>90%
Cefotetan (Cefotan)	2 g q12h	Enterococci	Allergic	>90%
Cefoperazone (Cefobid)	2 g q12h	Enterococci, many *B. fragilis*	Allergic	>90%
Cefotaxime (Claforan)	1–2 g q6–8h	Enterococci, many *B. fragilis*	Allergic	>90%
Moxalactam (Moxam)	1–2 g q8–12h	Enterococci	Allergic, bleeding disorders	>90%
Imipenem-cilastatin (Primaxin)	250 mg each q6h	Few	Allergic	>88%
Aztreonam (Azactam)	2 g q8h	Anerobes, gram-positive aerobes	Allergic	>90% when combined with clindamycin
Piperacillin	3 g q4h	*S. aureus*	Allergic	>90%
Ticarcillin/ clavulanate potassium	3 g (ticarcillin) plus 0.1 g clavulanate q 4–6h	Selected strains	Allergic	Not reported
Ampicillin/sulbactam	2 g ampicillin + 1 g sulbactam q6h	Selected strains	Allergic	Not reported

vides a more complete evaluation than sonography. Gallium scans are of limited value in postoperative patients. Based on these studies, surgical intervention may be necessary. An intravenous pyelogram should be ordered if urinary tract obstruction is suspected.

In addition to an infected wound or pelvic mass, another source of persistent fever is septic pelvic thrombophlebitis. This diagnosis may be suggested by CT scan but otherwise is suggested by the following findings: (1) persistent fever despite appropriate antibiotic use, (2) absence of an infected mass, and (3) absence of resistant organisms. Thus, septic pelvic thrombophlebitis is often a diagnosis of exclusion. For this condition, I favor a diagnostic trial of therapeutic doses of intravenous heparin for 48 to 72 hours. If there is a response, then I continue the heparin for 7 to 10 days. I do not continue therapy with oral anticoagulants, but I do continue antibiotic use during the heparin therapy.

It is a rare patient whose fever persists throughout this evaluation and therapy. For patients who are stable, this is the time to consider drug fever, factitial fever, and other sources of fever (e.g., collagen disease, catheter sepsis). However, an occult abscess must still be suspected.

Although clindamycin plus gentamicin has a high cure rate, use of this regimen is not without problems. In 1 to 6 percent of cases, clindamycin therapy is accompanied by diarrhea, severe enough to cause a change in therapy. All patients receiving antibiotics should be asked daily about bowel changes. If the patient develops more than three to five loose bowel movements daily, clindamycin should be discontinued. If anaerobic coverage is still needed, metronidazole (1,000 mg initially, followed by 500 mg intravenously every 6 hours) may be substituted. In most patients, diarrhea will stop promptly (within 24 hours). If diarrhea persists, if it is initially accompanied by blood and mucus, or if the patient is distended or toxic, then it is necessary to evaluate for pseudomembranous colitis. A stool sample should be sent for analysis for *Clostridium difficile* toxin and *C. difficile* culture. Pseudomembranous colitis can also be diagnosed by proctoscopy, but the toxin assay is generally preferred. Clindamycin is rarely accompanied by other adverse effects, but these may include allergic reactions and abnormalities of liver function studies in a small percentage of patients.

Gentamicin may cause oto- or nephrotoxicity, but obstetric patients, in general, are at low risk for these complications. Consequently, we do *not* routinely measure gentamicin levels, but we do measure serum creatinine levels initially and every 2 to 3 days during therapy. We reserve measurement of gentamicin levels for conditions such as (1) prolonged therapy (greater than 7 to 8 days); (2) marked obesity (when determination of proper dose is difficult); (3) poor response to therapy; (4) gram-negative bacteremias; and (5) elevated serum creatinine levels. Indeed, in the last circumstance, it would be wiser, in general, to use an alternative antibiotic.

With gentamicin dosing, the problem is more often not having high enough rather than having too high levels. When puerperal women (with normal serum creatinine values) are given 1.5 mg per kilogram every 8 hours, approximately one-third will have peak levels less than 5μg per milliliter.

Penicillin-Ampicillin Plus Gentamicin

Use of these combinations has been popular in the past, but their limited anaerobic activity has made them less effective than clindamycin plus gentamicin in post-cesarean endometritis. Retrospective studies have reported excellent cure rates with penicillin and gentamicin after vaginal delivery, but I suspect that equivalent results could be achieved with appropriate single drug therapy (see following).

Metronidazole (Flagyl) Plus Gentamicin

Metronidazole has superb activity against obligate anaerobic organisms and has been associated with few side effects when used parenterally. Combining metronidazole with gentamicin provides activity against anaerobes and aerobic gram-negative organisms but leaves little activity against important pathogens (group B streptococci, *Staphylococcus aureus*, and enterococci).

Other Aminoglycosides

In some centers, gentamicin resistance is a problem, leading to use of tobramycin (Nebcin) or amikacin. However, because these resistant organisms are very rarely a problem on an obstetric service, we continue to use gentamicin, since it is effective, safe (when compared to other aminoglycosides), and inexpensive.

Newer Cephalosporins-Cephamycins

Although there are a huge number of these antibiotics, only a few have been evaluated thoroughly for therapy of endometritis or related obstetric-gynecologic infections. The purported advantage of these drugs is broad-spectrum activity with safety and ease of administration. In general, these newer agents have extended gram-negative activity, including activity against anaerobic species. The following discussion is limited to those agents evaluated for therapy in pelvic infections.

Cefoxitin (Mefoxin). Cefoxitin has a very fine spectrum for treating pelvic infections and includes excellent activity against anaerobes, gram-positive aerobes (except enterococci), and the more common gram-negative aerobes. Like all cephalosporins, it is not active against genital mycoplasmas or *Chlamydia*. The initial dose should be 1 to 2 g every 6 hours intravenously. Several trials including gynecologic and obstetric infections have produced cure rates comparable to those obtained with clindamycin plus gentamicin.

If there is a poor response to cefoxitin, the differential diagnosis is similar to that when clindamycin plus gentamicin fails. However, here the resistant organisms may be enterococci, an *Enterobacter* or other resistant gram-negative rods, or, rarely, a resistant anaerobe. Thus, I prefer to stop the cefoxitin and replace it with a penicillin plus clindamycin, plus gentamicin.

Side effects complicating cefoxitin are mainly allergic in type, as with the older cephalosporins. However, antibiotic-associated diarrhea and pseudomembranous colitis also can occur.

Moxalactam (Moxam). Moxalactam also has a very favorable spectrum against anaerobes (similar to cefoxitin) and has greater activity against aerobic gram-negatives. When used as 2 g intravenously every 8 hours, it has produced a high cure rate (equivalent to clindamycin-gentamicin) in several trials of postcesarean endomyometritis. However, moxalactam use in nonobstetric patients has been accompanied by an unusual side effect for a cephalosporin—bleeding disorders. Although these bleeding disorders were nearly all preventable by prophylactic vitamin K administration and although obstetric patients were at very low risk in the first place, moxalactam became a stigmatized antibiotic and is not widely used for pelvic infections.

Cefotetan (Cefotan). Cefotetan is a relatively new antibiotic with a spectrum of activity also similar to cefoxitin. Its major advantage is that it has a longer half-life, making doses of every 12 hours appropriate. Although there have been few published trials of its use in endometritis, the cure rate of cefotetan appears very good, again in comparisons similar to clindamycin plus gentamicin or cefoxitin.

Cefoperazone (Cefobid). Cefoperazone has a somewhat different spectrum from cefoxitin. It is more active against the aerobic gram-negative rods but less active against anaerobes, primarily the *Bacteroides fragilis* group. Approximately 50 percent of *B. fragilis* species are resistant to cefoperazone, but most of the other more common pelvic *Bacteroides* species, including *B. bivius*, are susceptible. Cefoperazone also has a longer half-life than cefoxitin, making it appropriate to use every 12 hours or in some cases, every 8 hours. In two trials, cure rates for cefoperazone have been higher than 90 percent. Adverse effects are few and mainly allergic. Bleeding disorders have been reported in medical oncology patients receiving cefoperazone but not in obstetric-gynecologic patients.

Cefotaxime (Claforan). Cefotaxime has a spectrum similar to that of cefoperazone among pelvic bacteria. Its half-life is shorter, requiring dosing every 6 to 8 hours. A dose of 2 g every 8 hours gave a cure rate higher than 90 percent in a variety of pelvic infections. Adverse effects have been infrequent and mainly allergic.

Imipenem-Cilastatin (Primaxin). Imipenem-cilastatin is a combination of *N*-formimidoyl thienamycin plus cilastatin. The latter improves urinary activity and decreases the renal toxicity of thienamycin. Thienamycin, itself, has extensive in vitro activity, including problem organisms such as enterococci, *Enterobacter* species, and *B. fragilis*. Minimal inhibitory concentrations are usually very low to a wide range of microbes. Thienamycin was chemically unstable, but the addition of the formimidoyl group overcame the problem. Cilastatin is a specific inhibitor of renal dyspeptidase, an enzyme responsible for metabolism of imipenem. Cilastatin, thus, provides prolonged, reversible inhibition of imipenem metabolism, resulting in dramatic increase of urinary activity. Concomitant administration of cilastatin also prevents proximal tubular necrosis, which had been observed in sensitive animals that had received high doses of imipenem alone. Clinical trials with Primaxin have been favorable, although they are not yet extensive. The recommended dose is 250 mg of each drug (imipenem plus cilastatin) intravenously every 6 hours. In one small noncomparative series, the cure rate was 88 percent, a rate previously noted for many other single agents.

Monobactams

Structurally, these antibiotics are similar to cephalosporins but have one ring (thus the name monobactam) rather than the two rings of the cephalosporins and other beta-lactam antibiotics. Aztreonam (Azactam) is an interesting compound with a spectrum of activity limited mainly to the aerobic gram-negative rods. Thus, although aztreonam would be inappropriate for use as initial single-agent therapy of pelvic infections, it offers an alternative to aminoglycosides in combination therapy. In a comparison of gentamicin (1.5 mg per kilogram every 8 hours) versus aztreonam (2 g intravenously every 8 hours), each with clindamycin, in treating postpartum endometritis, the regimens were equivalent and both highly effective. Side effects with aztreonam are infrequent and, as with the cephalosporins, are mainly allergic.

Newer Penicillins

These antibiotics include piperacillin (Piperacil), mezlocillin (Mezlin), and azlocillin (Azlin). They all have a similar spectrum with excellent in vitro activity against most genital pathogens. In comparison to the new cephalosporins, these new penicillins have activity against enterococci but are not active against penicillinase-producing *Staphylococcus aureus* species. Most gram-negative aerobic rods are susceptible, although some strains are resistant. Anaerobic activity is good. These antibiotics are not active against the genital mycoplasmas and possess limited activity against *Chlamydia trachomatis*. High doses are usually administered in the empirical treatment of endomyometritis or other pelvic infections. In one study, reporting a 92 percent cure, piperacillin was used at 3 g every 4 hours. Compared with carbenicillin, an older member of this class, these newer members carry a lower sodium load per daily dose and have less effect on platelets.

Beta-Lactamase Inhibitors Plus Penicillins

These combinations provide a novel approach to combating antimicrobial resistance by combining an older penicillin plus a beta-lactamase inhibitor. Parenteral combinations are ticarcillin plus clavulanic acid (Timentin) and ampicillin plus sulbactam (Unisyn). An orally administered combination is amoxicillin plus clavulanic acid (Augmentin). The minimal inhibitory concentrations of many organisms are lower by fourfold or more to the combination than to the penicillin itself. The resulting combinations have very good in vitro activity against nearly all pelvic pathogens. Trials to date on pelvic infection have been limited, but these novel combinations show great promise.

Interpreting Antibiotic Trials

After reviewing these data on antibiotic efficacy in puerperal endometritis and related pelvic infections, there is little apparent difference between regimens—even though some have a clear in vitro advantage compared with others. Yet, these differences may not translate into in vivo, statistically significant differences for several reasons. First, the sample sizes have often been small (generally 50 or less per treatment group), making it unlikely that a statistically significant difference will be shown, unless absolute cure rates differ by more than 20 percent. Second, organisms resistant to any one antibiotic are usually present in a small percentage of cases. Third, in many infections, especially in endometritis after vaginal delivery, an antibiotic can be curative if it is effective against most but not necessarily all microbes present. Fourth, criteria for success or failure may vary from investigation to investigation, and fifth, with some antibiotics, relative differences in in vitro activity can be overcome by administering a high dose.

SPECIAL COMPLICATIONS

Almost all cases of postpartum pelvic infection are limited to simple endomyometritis, abdominal wound cellulitis or abscess, and simple episiotomy infection. Several rare, life-threatening complications may occur, however. Many of these manifest with characteristic findings that require prompt surgical intervention as well as broad-spectrum, preferably combination antibiotic therapy.

Necrotizing Fasciitis. Nectrotizing fasciitis may involve the abdominal incision or the perineum after episiotomy. The infection spreads along fascial planes. In necrotizing fasciitis of the perineum, infection spreads to the abdominal wall, thigh, or buttock. Findings are variable but usually initially include edema and erythema without clear borders. Later, there is often a progressive, brawny cutaneous edema, with the skin becoming blue or brown. Bullae or frank gangrene may appear. Local anesthesia or hyperesthesia may follow. Associated findings are severe pain, toxicity, hemoconcentration, and hypocalcemia (due to saponification of fatty acids). This infection may involve a variety of organisms, including group A streptococci and anerobes. Broad-spectrum antibiotics plus extensive debridement are essential. At surgery, necrotizing fasciitis may be recognized by separation of the skin from the deep fascia, absence of bleeding along incision lines, and serosanguineous discharge. The dissection should be carried out until all necrotic tissue is excised.

Myonecrosis. Myonecrosis (gas gangrene, anaerobic myonecrosis) may involve the uterus or muscles beneath the deep fascia of the abdominal wall or the perineum. Often, this infection is caused by a myotoxin from *Clostridium perfringens*, but it may occur as a result of necrotizing fasciitis. Onset may be dramatic, with sudden severe pain, toxicity, and shock, often early in the puerperium. For uterine myonecrosis, hysterectomy is indicated, whereas for perineal myonecrosis, extensive debridement is necessary. High-dose, broad-spectrum antibiotics are also indicated.

Progressive Synergistic Bacterial (Meleney's) Gangrene. Meleney's gangrene classically has a central ulcer surrounded by a deep red-purple zone, which in turn is surrounded by an erythematous zone. The central ulcer may be dark gray to black. A combination of synergistically acting organisms is usually responsible, necessitating broad-spectrum antibiotics in addition to sharp debridement. Since this process usually does not involve the deep fascia, fascial removal is often not needed. Serial debriding procedures may be needed, however, to resolve the process.

Pelvic Abscess. Pelvic abscess now is an extremely uncommon complication of delivery. Although it has been reported after vaginal delivery, most pelvic abscesses occur after cesarean delivery. Yet, even then, abscess occurs in far less than 1 percent of cases of postcesarean pelvic infection. By initially using antibiotics with excellent anaerobic activity, we have noted far fewer postcesarean abscesses recently. As noted earlier, pelvic abscess is diagnosed on the basis of a pelvic mass and, at least initially, a poor response to antibiotics. The abscess is best delineated by CT scan, but sonography, plain abdominal films, or a pyelogram may show the abscess as well. After cesarean delivery, pelvic abscess is most likely to be retroperitoneal (behind the bladder flap or at the base of the broad ligament). This may dissect into the cul-de-sac or inguinal region. Another complication is breakdown of the uterine incision (uterine dehiscence). Rupture into the peritoneal cavity is decidedly uncommon.

Treatment of pelvic abscess consists of broad-spectrum combination antibiotics, clearly including a drug of choice for anaerobes (e.g., clindamycin, metronidazole, or cefoxitin), usually with drainage. In patients who are stable, infected pelvic masses may resolve on antibiotic therapy alone, especially if they are small (less than 5 to 6 cm). If the abscess or mass is well delineated on CT scan and fixed, then percutaneous needle aspiration may be possible if no vital structures lie in the needle path. If these approaches are unsuccessful or if the patient is unstable, then exploratory laparotomy is indicated. Here, it is most likely that hysterectomy with pelvic drainage will be necessary.

Septic Shock. Septic shock may complicate a number of these conditions. Although a detailed discussion of treatment of this life-threatening problem is beyond the scope of this chapter, it is important to recognize the importance of vigorous supportive therapy (including hemodynamic monitoring, fluid resuscitation, vasoactive agents, colloid, and perhaps steroids), the need for surgical intervention, and the use of a combination of drugs of choice (such as clindamycin plus gentamicin plus ampicillin).

COST

Although cost of antibiotic therapy is an appropriate concern, there are no good data on *total* comparative costs of therapy. If we assume that two regimens (e.g., a combination versus a single agent) are equally effective, then cost comparisons are pertinent, but indirect as well as direct costs must be considered. The former should include costs of administration; monitoring for adverse effects and serum levels, if indicated; and treating side effects. In general, single-agent therapy has a high direct cost, but total costs may be comparable to the combination of clindamycin plus gentamicin.

RECOMMENDATIONS

For most cases of puerperal infection, a high response rate (>90 percent) can be expected when any of several appropriate antibiotic regimens are used properly. For mild infections, including most cases of endometritis after vaginal delivery, single agent therapy would be appropriate. Antibiotics with more favorable in vitro activities include cefoxitin, cefotetan and piperacillin. Moxalactam has an equivalent spectrum, but is little used because of concern regarding adverse effects, and imipenem-cilastatin might be better reserved for more serious infections. Other antibiotics including cefoperazone and cefotaxime have had good effect, even though their in vitro activity is not so good, especially against *B. fragilis*. Combinations of older penicillins plus a beta-lactamase inhibitor are of interest.

For more serious infections, including most of those after cesarean section, I believe the standard for comparison is clindamycin plus gentamicin, although many alternative regimens may be used.

Patients need careful evaluation in the 10 percent of cases where a prompt response to antibiotics is not obtained. Antibiotic therapy must be modified in an orderly way, and diagnostic studies should be pursued.

SUGGESTED READING

DiZerega G, Yonekura L, Roy S, et al. A comparison of clindamycin-gentamicin and penicillin-gentamicin in the treatment of post-cesarean section endomyometritis. Am J Obstet Gynecol 1979; 134:238–242.

Duff P. Pathophysiology and management of postcesarean endomyometritis. Obstet Gynecol 1986; 67:269–276.

Sweet RL, Gibbs RS. Antimicrobial agents. In: Sweet RL, Gibbs RS, eds. Infectious diseases of the female genital tract. Baltimore: Williams & Wilkins, 1985:314.

GROUP B STREPTOCOCCAL SEPSIS

PHILIP B. MEAD, M.D.

The contribution of the group B streptococcus (GBS) to neonatal morbidity and mortality has long been recognized and was the subject of a National Institutes of Health workshop a decade ago. At that forum, which brought together leading investigators, "emphasis was given...to the definition of priorities leading to programs for the prevention of GBS infection." However, despite 10 years of efforts subsequent to that meeting, no consensus exists for an approach to this problem, and as recently as 1985 the published recommendation of the Centers for Disease Control for dealing with GBS sepsis in "Sexually Transmitted Diseases: Treatment Guidelines" was that "the present state of knowledge about the epidemiology of GBS disease is not sufficient to recommend routine treatment of pregnant women or their sexual partners or routine prophylaxis of the newborn." Without a recommended approach, a wide variety of protocols exist that vary greatly in their scope and impact. The lack of a consensus approach to GBS sepsis stands in sharp contrast to the management of other infectious diseases that command large investments of resources and man hours. The disparate nature of the approaches to perinatal infections is best illustrated by the current management of herpes simplex virus in contrast to that of GBS sepsis.

It is estimated that herpes simplex virus infects only 120 to 1,000 neonates annually in the United States. Seventy percent of these infants die, and many survivors suffer serious sequelae. Current perinatal management involves study of weekly viral cultures in the third trimester and use of cesarean section for viral shedders at term. Although this approach has been noted to be both expensive ($53 million annually, 5,000 unnecessary cesarean sections) and relatively ineffective (75 percent of neonates exposed to asymptomatic shedders are missed by this protocol), it remains the de facto standard of care.

For GBS, on the other hand, it has been estimated that 4,000 to 10,000 newborn infants per year are infected and that the mortality rate for early-onset disease can be as high as 50 percent among premature infants. Hence the number of neonatal deaths from it is several times higher than from herpes simplex virus. Yet, although many antepartum protocols for the prevention of GBS sepsis have been proposed, none has been uniformly adopted because each has problems that have been clearly recognized and that may limit the benefits. Thus the lack of an ideal system has until now precluded the universal institution of any management plan, leaving the broad scope of the problem largely unaddressed.

Clearly there is a need for further research, which has been acknowledged for many years and was the focus of the National Institutes of Health workshop mentioned previously. However, although a protocol should be based on the results of a prospective randomized study, there is need for a standard approach to the prevention of GBS infection until such research is completed. A study seeking to document the effectiveness of a protocol in lowering sepsis rates among preterm infants from 1 percent to 0.5 percent, for example, would have to involve a population base of over 100,000 deliveries (assuming a 9 percent prematurity rate) and hence probably will not be reported in the near future. Therefore, in an attempt to generate a consensus approach that may prevent a proportion of deaths from GBS disease in the interval until a more universal solution is devised (for example, a vaccine), we will summarize current strategies that have been proposed as well as their shortcomings and then offer several protocols for consideration as immediately applicable yet practical solutions to the problem of early-onset GBS neonatal sepsis.

CHARACTERISTICS OF GBS DISEASE

Many characteristics of GBS disease make it particularly insidious and difficult to eradicate. First, since up to 40 percent of pregnant women may be colonized, therapeutic plans directed at all GBS carriers must be very broad-based. Further, there are several types of carriage that can occur during pregnancy. Only 40 percent of colonized patients carry the organisms chronically throughout pregnancy, whereas the rest carry them either intermittently or transiently and may have a different culture status at delivery than they had ante partum. The culture characteristics of the organism also pose potential difficulties. If selective media are used, the percentage of patients who are found to be carriers will be more than double that found with standard media. These additional patients, colonized by low numbers of organisms, may not be at as great a risk of infecting their infants. Colonization rates also vary, depending on the site at which the culture is performed. There is a gradient of colonization, with the highest rates found near the rectum and progressively lower rates found toward the cervix and urethra. Infants may be infected even if the mother is colonized only in the rectum.

Between 40 percent and 70 percent of women who are colonized with GBS will deliver infants who are colonized, and 1 percent of these colonized infants become septic. The mortality from GBS sepsis is closely linked to the gestational age of the neonate, with up to 90 percent of extremely premature infants but less than 5 percent of term infants dying. Compounding management problems is the fact that death frequently occurs despite early institution of appropriate antibiotic therapy. In addition to a higher mortality rate, an increased attack rate has been linked with prematurity. The attack rate among premature infants is seven times that among mature infants. Most neonatal deaths are a result of early-onset disease that has been associated with transmission of GBS from the mother's genital tract, occurring either concomitantly with labor or ruptured membranes or during parturition. Thus high colonization rates, variable patterns and sites of carriage, and the relatively small percentage of colonized mothers being delivered of septic infants have made GBS disease a difficult one to prevent. However, several approaches have been suggested.

PREVIOUSLY EVALUATED MANAGEMENT PROTOCOLS

Maternal Antepartum Protocol. In general, treatment schemes have been directed either at identifying and treating colonized mothers or at identifying and treating colonized infants. One of the first treatment plans proposed that was directed at mothers involved culture studies of all women in the third trimester and treatment of those who were colonized to prevent them from infecting their babies at birth. This approach fails to include patients who are unregistered, a group at increased risk for premature delivery. A second concern is the difficulty of obtaining third trimester (26 to 28 weeks) vaginal cultures from all patients. Speculum examinations are traditionally done at the first antepartum visit—not at 26 weeks—for the vast majority of gravidas. Adding a speculum examination in the third trimester for all patients can cause enormous logistical problems for the private practitioner or busy obstetric clinic. However, the major problem with this approach was the failure of therapeutic courses of antibiotics, administered to the patient and her sexual partner, to eradicate the organism, perhaps because of the decreased effectiveness of penicillins in the lactamase-rich environment of the rectal flora. Eradication could only be achieved if antibiotics were continued until delivery, a duration of therapy that was obviously impractical. Additionally, approximately 10 percent of patients who are not culture-positive at initial testing may become positive by term, whereas one-third of those who are culture-positive at initial testing have spontaneously lost the organism by the time labor commences. Finally, there may be a high rate of false negative cultures if nonselective media are used and inappropriate sites for culturing are chosen (for example, cervix only). Even if this maternal antepartum protocol were to prove effective, concern would still be raised about the number of people requiring treatment (all colonized women and their sexual partners) and the cost and risks (5 percent rate of adverse reactions to penicillin, 0.04 percent anaphylactic reaction rate) of such wide-scale antibiotic therapy.

Maternal Intrapartum Protocol. An alternative suggestion was to identify the patient who is a carrier but then to withhold treatment until labor commences. This bypassed the problem of recolonization after earlier therapy. Further, there is evidence that intrapartum therapy, even if instituted only 2 hours before birth, can reduce or prevent neonatal sepsis. Yow noted no colonization among 34 infants of colonized mothers treated in labor, compared with colonization in eight of 16 infants of untreated colonized mothers. Colonized infants of treated mothers may also have lower inocula of bacteria and a lower likelihood of sepsis. Two additional studies, described herein, have also validated the efficacy of the intrapartum protocol. A problem with this plan is, again, that patients who are culture-negative at initial screening may be positive at term and vice versa. Furthermore, the number of patients who would need treatment and the occurrence of established infections prior to therapy remain problems. However, the greatest objection to this approach involves the ethical and medicolegal issues of withholding treatment (until the onset of labor or premature rupture of the membranes) despite documentation of the presence of a potential pathogen. Although the current literature shows a poor correlation between maternal colonization with GBS and complications such as premature labor or premature rupture of the membranes, it is indeed difficult to explain to some patients that it is presumably safe to withhold therapy until the onset of labor or rupture of membranes but critical to begin therapy at that juncture. This concern is highlighted by the refusal of patients to be included in randomized studies of this approach.

To circumvent those problems that arise because of changes in culture status between initial cultures and labor, rapid identification techniques are being developed. These include slide coagglutination (Phadebact Streptococcus Test, Pharmacia Diagnostics, Piscatawny, NJ), latex particle agglutination (Bactigen GBS system, Wampole Laboratories, Cranbury, NJ, and Directigen Group 3 Streptococcus test kit, Becton Dickinson, Baltimore, MD), and fluorescent antibody techniques. Unfortunately, in the bacterial-rich vaginal environment, most techniques need long incubation periods (5 to 20 hours) to achieve high specificity and sensitivity. This is an even greater problem when processing rectal cultures, yet it is likely that the rectum is the primary reservoir of GBS. Indeed, Boyer has found that infants may be infected even if the mother is colonized only in the rectum. We are unaware of any studies that have evaluated rapid antigen detection methods for identification of rectal colonization with GBS. Current rapid antigen detection systems have not been developed for use by nonlaboratory personnel in the labor unit, although presumably this might be possible. This is an important consideration, since clinical protocols based on rapid antigen detection methods necessitate the availability of the test 24 hours a day, including weekends and holidays. Finally, even if a perfectly sensitive and specific rapid-culturing technique were available and carriers could be treated in labor, there still would be a need to treat up to 40 percent of all parturients.

Another rapid identification technique that has recently been evaluated is the use of a vaginal Gram's stain. This test has the advantage of simplicity and ready availability. It has a high sensitivity, so it might be useful for ruling out the presence of the GBS. However, because of the large number of gram-positive cocci in the vagina, the specificity is low and the predictive value of a positive Gram's stain is only in the range of 33 percent. Moreover, the test has never been evaluated using rectal swabs in addition to vaginal samples.

Neonatal Protocol. A report from the Mount Sinai Hospital gave impetus to consideration of treatment of the neonate instead of the mother. That report noted that when hospital policy was switched from use of silver nitrate to intramuscular penicillin for prevention of gonococcal ophthalmia, a coincident disappearance of early-onset GBS sepsis was noted. This was a retrospective report and covered some time periods (back to 1952) when the pathologic diagnosis of GBS sepsis may not have been uniformly made. Although Lloyd subsequently reported similar findings, his study also used historical controls and the colonization rate in his treatment period was so low that one would not have expected as much morbidity as in the historical control period. Ramamurthy in a prospective controlled trial found no improvement with use of penicillin prophylaxis in newborn infants and noted that large fluctuations over time in colonization rates made studies of GBS disease singularly inappropriate for historical controls. Siegel performed a 2-year prospective study in which infants delivered on alternate weeks received either intramuscular penicillin or ocular topical tetracycline. Although the penicillin group had less GBS sepsis, they had more infections with penicillin-resistant organisms. Finally, evidence that up to two-thirds of infants with GBS sepsis are bacteremic at birth suggests that neonatal therapy may not be the best option.

IMMUNOPROPHYLAXIS

Vaccines have also been considered as a potential answer to the problem of GBS sepsis. Mothers of infants with GBS sepsis are significantly less likely to have high levels of antibody than mothers of noninfected neonates. This fact has fostered the belief that immunoprophylaxis will be the ultimate solution to this dilemma. Although studies in lower animals have been encouraging, only limited success has been noted with passive or active immunization in rhesus monkeys or humans. However, interest persists since effective immunoprophylaxis would not only overcome the limitations of chemoprophylaxis discussed earlier but also because an immunologic approach is more likely to prevent late-onset as well as early-onset infections. Most of the relevant work has been performed with type III group B streptococci, the principal cause of meningitis in both early- and late-onset infections. Baker and Kasper have demonstrated that babies who develop type III GBS infections generally have low titers of maternally acquired type-specific IgG directed against the type III polysaccharide capsular antigen. Not surprisingly, subsequent studies revealed that mothers of uninfected babies had higher titers than mothers of infected newborns, and there was a significant correlation between maternal and cord blood titers.

Baker has developed a native type III-specific polysaccharide vaccine that is immunogenic in women and is associated with a low rate of mild side effects. Similar vaccines have been prepared for types Ia and II. However, up to 40 percent of nonimmune adults receiving type III polysaccharide vaccine fail to have a satisfactory immune response, and nonresponders do not develop specific antibody even with repeated vaccine challenges. It is possible that response to vaccine is genetically determined, and the women who fail to mount an antibody response to their own colonizing streptococci may be the same women who fail to respond to the vaccine. Thus, the highest risk pregnancies would be least likely to benefit from vaccine.

Further studies are clearly required to investigate the potential value of polysaccharide vaccines. However, maternal immunization will never be able to prevent disease in neonates who are born so prematurely that they have not received a significant amount of IgG transplacentally. Perhaps the greatest roadblock to immunoprophylaxis will be currently unsettled liability issues for the manufacturers of vaccines. Given the present negative climate, the pharmaceutical industry has shown little interest in supporting the development and marketing of a GBS vaccine.

PROPOSED PREVENTION STRATEGIES

As previously mentioned, the high rates of carriage of GBS organisms, the frequently intermittent nature of such carriage during pregnancy, its recurrence after appropriate therapy, and the failure of antibiotics in the face of established infection in the neonate have combined to frustrate attempts to safely eradicate neonatal disease. Protocols aimed at all carriers of disease are extremely treatment-inefficient, whereas the more focused protocols that are directed at infected neonates are usually instituted too late to be successful. To be more efficient and more timely, the focus of intervention should remain on the mother yet be narrowed from being on all carriers to high-risk carriers only. After reviewing our own data at the Medical Center Hospital of Vermont, we have suggested that "an alternative approach to these problems would be the identification of risk factors for early-onset disease and treatment of only those...at high risk" (Table 1).

Boyer's Protocol

A major step in the direction of developing a focused maternal intervention protocol is based on the work of Boyer and his colleagues. After performing exhaustive studies on maternal-fetal transmission of GBS, carriage patterns, and the chemotherapeutic impact of intrapartum antibiotics, they proposed a plan based on antepartum screening and intrapartum treatment. Their proposal would result in the treatment of only 4.2 percent of all patients by aiming solely at patients who are both colonized (22.8 percent of their population) and who have risk factors for an increased attack rate (18.3 percent of their population—those with low birth weight, rupture of membranes >18 hours, or intrapartum fever). Pasnick noted GBS morbidity in the same subgroups.

Boyer subsequently validated the efficacy of selective intrapartum prophylaxis both in terms of interruption of mother-to-infant transmission and preventing early-onset neonatal GBS disease. In a randomized controlled trial, he studied the effect of selective intrapartum prophylaxis with ampicillin in 160 high-risk women (prenatal GBS colonization and premature labor, prolonged membrane rupture, or intrapartum fever). In infants born to mothers who received intravenous ampicillin during labor, as com-

TABLE 1 Strategies for Preventing Early-Onset Group B Streptococcal Neonatal Sepsis

Boyer's Protocol

- Vaginal + rectal culture at 26 weeks all gravidas
- If culture positive:
  - Preterm labor OR term delivery with ROM >12 hr: Intrapartum ampicillin plus 4 doses to neonate over 36 hours
  - Term delivery with ROM <12 hr: One dose of penicillin to neonate

Minkoff's Protocol

- Vaginal + rectal culture on admission if:
  - Preterm labor
  - Preterm PROM
- Intrapartum ampicillin if:
  - Cultures positive
  - Cultures pending and labor begins or is not stopped

Individualized Protocol

- Vaginal + rectal cultures beginning at 26 weeks, with attempt to eradicate GBS if isolated, for any patient with history of an infant affected with GBS neonatal sepsis
- Early treatment with parenteral antibiotics for mothers with suspected chorioamnionitis
- Vaginal culture for GBS on admission, with notification of pediatrician if positive, for patients with PROM or preterm labor

ROM = rupture of membranes
PROM = premature rupture of membranes
preterm labor and preterm PROM = <37 weeks gestation
intrapartum ampicillin = 2 gm IV q6h

pared with controls who received no treatment, neonatal colonization with GBS was present in eight of 85 (9 percent) versus 40 of 79 (51 percent; $p<0.001$), and bacteremia occurred in none of 85 versus five of 79 (6 percent; $p=0.024$). The side effects of ampicillin were limited to a single episode of urticaria in a mother who had no history of penicillin allergy.

Boyer asks what proportion of perinatal GBS disease this strategy is likely to prevent (Table 2). In previous prospective studies at his institution, it was shown that 62 percent of cases of early-onset disease occurred in babies whose mothers met their criteria for prophylaxis of prenatal colonization and perinatal risk factors, and that 94 percent of the infants who die from the disease have mothers in this group. Pregnant women who receive only late prenatal care or none at all would not be identified as carriers of GBS and hence would not be candidates. In the United States, such women represent 4 to 9 percent of all deliveries. Thus, selective intrapartum chemoprophylaxis is likely to prevent at least 50 percent of the cases of early-onset GBS disease and 75 percent of the deaths from the disorder.

Although their work represents an impressive body of data in support of intrapartum treatment of high-risk patients, several concerns about the practicality of routine institution of this approach remain.

The first problem with their specific plan is that although it narrows the focus of therapy, it still requires the institution of universal screening, which reduces the chances of its being widely accepted. Costs would be high, since their results are based on screening all patients with both vaginal and rectal cultures and use of selective media. Based on current costs for cultures and therapy, projected to involve 3.6 million births annually, the cost would be $108 million for universal screening and $2.5 million for treatment with ampicillin for 4 percent of all pregnant women. The second problem is that therapy is based on results of screening performed at 26 to 28 weeks. In indigent populations, which have higher prematurity rates and higher attack rates for GBS disease, many patients present in the third trimester or in labor for initial care and do not have culture results available. Also, carriage status may change between the time of culture and that of labor. Boyer found that the overall predictive value of a postive prenatal culture was 67.2 percent, and that 8.5 percent of patients who were initially culture negative became culture-positive by term. Further, the number of patients becoming positive after negative prenatal screens would be substantially higher if rectal cultures were not performed on all prenatal patients. Again, the efforts and costs involved in instituting vaginal and rectal cultures on all patients make adaption of this protocol unlikely. Finally, the ethical problems of withholding therapy in patients with positive antepartum screens have been discussed earlier. Despite these problems, Boyer's work represents an important step toward developing a practical approach to the problem of

TABLE 2 Maximal Proportion of Early-Onset Group B Streptococcal Disease Theoretically Preventable by Various Protocols

Protocol	*Cases Prevented*	*Deaths Prevented*
Boyer	50%	75%
Minkoff	30–50%	40–94%
"Nothing"	<1%	<1%

GBS disease and may constitute a workable policy for certain obstetric services.

Morales and Lim have also validated the efficacy of selective intrapartum prophylaxis in preterm pregnancies with premature rupture of the membranes using a rapid antigen detection system to identify maternal colonization. Although their approach obviates some of the problems inherent in antepartum culturing, it is open to the same criticisms of availability, specificity, and sensitivity presented in the discussion of rapid antigen detection tests.

Minkoff's Protocol

Minkoff has proposed an alternative strategy that would result in an increase in the number of parturients receiving antibiotics in labor while substantially reducing the number of patients needing screening, thereby minimizing the logistic complexities that universal screening entails. Among the groups at high risk for sepsis, Minkoff would focus on preterm infants. Approximately 90 percent of neonatal deaths associated with GBS disease occur in that group. Patients with chorioamnionitis, one of the other risk groups of Boyer, routinely receive antibiotics independent of GBS culture status. Attempting to treat the final risk group delineated by Boyer, all culture-positive term patients with ruptured membranes of more than 18 hours, would reduce the total number of deaths associated with GBS disease only slightly while requiring a tremendous increase in the need to obtain cultures as well as timely results. Further, since sepsis in his study occurred at or beyond 18 hours of rupture, it would be necessary to start therapy earlier in the course of labor to prevent morbidity (he has selected >12 hours of membrane rupture), thus markedly increasing the percentage of patients requiring therapy, since they "might" not deliver until after 18 hours of membrane rupture. The logistic complexities of deciding when to initiate Boyer's protocol based on anticipated duration of membrane rupture in a given patient are obvious to those who have managed a busy delivery floor.

Minkoff suggests that for all patients admitted in preterm labor and/or with preterm premature rupture of membranes (<37-weeks gestation), cultures for GBS should be obtained. If labor is successfully inhibited with tocolysis, antibiotic therapy can be withheld pending culture results. All culture-positive patients should be treated with intravenous ampicillin 2 g every 6 hours for 24 hours, then switched to 500 mg orally every 6 hours for 2 weeks, and then recultured. (Although penicillin G is the most active antimicrobial against GBS, the choice of ampicillin as the prophylactic agent seems appropriate because of its safety, low degree of serum protein binding, rapid penetration into the fetal blood and amniotic fluid during labor, and activity against common obstetric and neonatal pathogens in addition to GBS). Erythromycin is used for the penicillin-allergic patient. If the patient's labor is not successfully inhibited and the culture result is pending, then antibiotic therapy is begun. If a patient being managed conservatively with preterm premature rupture of the membranes goes into labor (assuming tocolysis is not used), antibiotics are given if the culture is pending (2 g intraveneously as soon as possible, then 2 g every 6 hours). Thus therapy and culturing are reserved for the approximately 8.9 percent of the population who deliver prematurely and who account for over 90 percent of GBS-associated deaths. The actual number receiving therapy may be even less, depending on the number of patients whose labor is successfully inhibited while culture results are pending.

Several problems with this protocol can be recognized. A large number of culture-negative patients receive unnecessary antibiotics because of unavailable culture results. At most this number represents approximately 7.4 percent of all patients (prematurity rate 8.9 percent × culture-negative rate 83.3 percent). This is substantially more than the approximately 1.4 percent of patients who would receive unnecessary therapy when all risk groups that are culture-positive at 26 to 28 weeks are treated in labor (18.3 percent of patients at high risk × 32.8 percent of women with positive prenatal cultures whose intrapartum cultures are negative × 22.8 percent overall prevalence of prenatal GBS carriage). This increased need for therapy is balanced against a substantial decrease in the number of patients not receiving needed therapy because although their cultures were positive during delivery, they were negative at initial screening (8.5 percent of risk patients), or because the patient was unregistered and no antepartum culture was obtained.

An additional concern with Minkoff's protocol is the experience of Baker that term infants account for 70 percent of early-onset disease and up to 60 percent of fatal cases. Minkoff's proposal is obviously most applicable for those services where most mortality and serious morbidity from GBS sepsis occurs in preterm infants.

Perhaps the greatest attraction of Minkoff's proposal is its simplicity and ease of implementation.

What proportion of early-onset GBS disease is Minkoff's protocol likely to prevent (see Table 2)? Since this approach is focused on premature delivery, its success is directly related to the proportion of GBS-associated cases and deaths complicating preterm birth. There is variation in the reported series, but most investigators suggest that 30 to 50 percent of cases of GBS sepsis occur in preterm infants, and these account for between 40 to 94 percent of all GBS-related deaths. The corresponding figures from this institution are 50 percent of cases and 83 percent of deaths.

An important question that remains is the safety of waiting for culture results for the preterm patient with ruptured membranes who is being managed conservatively.

Unfortunately, the risk of ascending infection with GBS during the time that culture results are pending is unknown. If rapid screening were available, risks could be minimized, since antibiotics could be instituted within hours of rupture. Without rapid screening it is necessary to consider initiating use of prophylactic antibiotics on admission for patients with premature rupture of membranes. However, the risk-benefit ratio of that approach is difficult to assess pending the results of studies currently under way.

Neither Boyer nor Minkoff directly addresses the question of GBS disease as a cause of preterm labor or premature rupture of membranes. Because attack rates of early-onset GBS disease increase as birth weight decreases, it seems reasonable to postulate an association between maternal colonization and preterm delivery. However, based on a prospective study of 924 parturients with premature labor, premature rupture of the membranes, or intrapartum fever, Boyer failed to find such an association, nor was he able to document significant differences in prevalence of maternal GBS colonization among any of the birth weight categories examined. His findings were consistent with those of Ancona, who found no difference in mean birth weights between infants born to colonized and noncolonized mothers. These results differ from those of Regan, who found a higher proportion of extremely premature infants with gestational ages of less than 32 weeks born to mothers with cervical GBS colonization than to mothers without colonization. Data on overall rates of delivery at less than 36 weeks are not provided in Regan's study, however. Boyer feels that the weight of available evidence favors the conclusion that maternal GBS colonization is not a major determinant of premature delivery. He suggests that the markedly higher attack rates of GBS disease in premature infants are determined by increased host susceptibility or exposure to large inocula in infected amniotic fluid rather than the presence of maternal colonization per se.

As for concern about obscuring the diagnosis of neonatal disease among infants born to antibiotic-treated mothers, Minkoff concurs with Boyer's statement that "when there is a substantial and well-defined risk of intrauterine infection, the potential benefit of intrapartum prophylaxis for the newborn infant more than compensates for increased uncertainty in postnatal diagnosis." Both investigators also agree that although "...the possibility of selecting resistant flora by blanket use of prophylaxis remains a disturbing risk, and additional controlled data documenting safety and efficacy of selected intrapartum chemoprophylaxis in preventing invasive disease will be required before a firm recommendation can be made," it is their clinical opinion that in defined high-risk populations, some therapeutic strategy is warranted while the aforementioned studies are ongoing.

"Do Nothing" Protocol

One of the most perplexing problems related to prevention of early-onset GBS neonatal infection is its widely varying incidence over time. This observation is amply borne out by our own data (Table 3) showing annual incidences from 0.78 to 3.22 cases per 1,000 deliveries. It is evident that, for certain low-incidence years, any protocol may be "looking for a needle in a haystack." Additionally, the proportion of early-onset disease accounted for by term infants varies in the literature from 0 to 60 percent and in our experience from 0 to 67 percent. These wide swings in incidence and gestational age affected make it extremely difficult for individual services to select a GBS prevention strategy that will be continuously cost-effective over time.

TABLE 3 Group B Streptococcal Neonatal Sepsis University of Vermont/Medical Center Hospital 1981–1986

	1981	*1982*	*1983*	*1984*	*1985*	*1986*
No. Births	2299	2363	2395	2416	2484	2561
GBS Sepsis	2	3	6	3	8	2
(Preterm)	(2)	(1)	(3)	(3)	(2)	(1)
(Term)	(0)	(2)	(3)	(0)	(6)	(1)
Cases per 1000 births	0.87	1.27	2.51	1.24	3.22	0.78

Moreover, although the overall number of infants affected with early-onset disease may approach as many as 10,000 in the United States annually, these numbers are small for any given service (0.75 to 3 per 1,000 live births) and vanishingly small for an individual practitioner. Thus, in those areas where early-onset disease is seen at the lower incidence levels cited, some have suggested a policy of individualization. Not really a "do-nothing" approach, this strategy emphasizes antimicrobial therapy for all patients with suspected chorioamnionitis, antenatal culturing with attempts to eradicate GBS in those with a previously infected infant, and selective culturing for GBS on admission to include those with premature rupture of the membranes and preterm labor. Some would argue that not all diseases yield to protocol management and that intelligent individualization is preferable to the use of protocols that have received either less than exhaustive validation or no validation at all (Table 4).

Regardless of which approach is chosen—Boyer's, Minkoff's, "nothing," or something else—several points are worthy of emphasis:

1. If a protocol is instituted, it is imperative that hospitals using it keep a careful record of all neonatal infections and deaths attributable to GBS as well as of any maternal or neonatal side effects associated with

TABLE 4 "Costs" of Three Protocols for the Prevention of Group B Streptococcol Neonatal Sepsis

	Percent of All Gravidas Affected		
	Boyer	*Minkoff*	*"Nothing"*
Antepartum Cultures	100%	0	<1%
Intrapartum Cultures	0	8.9%	15%
Intrapartum Ampicillin	4.2%	8.9%	<1%
Unnecessary Treatment	1.4%	7.4%	0

therapy, so that failures related to parochial resistance patterns, established infection, or other problems are quickly detected.

2. Development of any antepartum or intrapartum protocol should be a joint effort by the obstetrics and pediatric services so that neonatal care can be coordinated most effectively with prenatal data collection and antibiotic administration.
3. Finally, if rapid, sensitive, and specific diagnostic tests for GBS become available in the future, it will be necessary to review approaches to prevention, with the hope of more sharply focusing on the truly high-risk patient.

SUGGESTED READING

Boyer KM, Gadzala CA, Kelly PD, Gotoff SP. Selective intrapartum chemoprophylaxis of neonatal group B streptococcal early-onset disease. III. Interruption of mother-to-infant transmission. J Infect Dis 1983; 148:810–816.

Boyer KM, Gotoff SP. Prevention of early-onset neonatal group B streptococcal disease with selective intrapartum chemoprophylaxis. N Engl J Med 1986; 314:1665–1669.

Howe RS, Voychehovski TH, Uraizee F, Bentsen C, Spear ML, Minkoff H, Mead P, Boyer KM, Gotoff SP. Neonatal group B streptococcal disease. N Engl J Med 1987; 316:1163–1164.

Minkoff H, Mead P. An obstetric approach to the prevention of early-onset group B beta-hemolytic streptococcal sepsis. Am J Obstet Gynecol 1986; 154:973–977.

BACTERIAL VAGINOSIS IN PREGNANCY

DAVID A. ESCHENBACH, M.D.

INFECTION IN PREGNANCY

With a few exceptions, bacterial infections that occur during pregnancy represent no additional threat to the pregnant as compared with the nonpregnant woman. Neonatal bacterial infections represent a constant although small risk to the newborn despite the availability of antibiotics. However, the risk of bacterial infections for the newborn is small, even when the most common neonatal causes of sepsis, group B streptococcal and *Escherichia coli* infections, are considered. The most significant risk of bacteria during pregnancy may occur not from direct maternal and neonatal infections but as an indirect consequence of chorioamnionitis and amniotic fluid infection. It is now becoming apparent that infections at these sites are associated with prematurity.

The cause of premature labor in the vast majority of women remains unknown, and the rate of prematurity has decreased very little over the past 30 years despite preventive methods, including intensive prenatal care, tocolytic therapy, and nutritional supplementation. In contrast, over this same period, the perinatal mortality rate has markedly declined, but 80 percent of this decrease has been due to vastly improved neonatal care that has led to a reduction of mortality in each birth weight interval. The largest amount of perinatal morbidity, perinatal mortality, and costs occur in prematurely born infants, and these factors are greatest for the lowest birth weight infants. It is apparent that only a modest reduction of prematurity would have a major impact on perinatal mortality and the cost of neonatal care.

Infection has been widely studied as a cause of prematurity. Indirect evidence linking infection and prematurity includes similar demographic characteristics for populations with each entity and higher rates of histologic chorioamnionitis and neonatal infection when infants are born prematurely. In addition, there have been a large number of microorganisms associated with prematurity, including *Neisseria gonorrhoeae, Ureaplasma urealyticum,* and, to a lesser extent, *Mycoplasma hominis,* group B streptococci, *Chlamydia trachomatis, Trichomonas vaginalis,* and recently, anaerobic bacteria.

It has been difficult to interpret the significance of these findings because these data represent a large number of diverse organisms, and there has been an insufficient number of patients in each report to study interactions between the organisms. Thus, in some cases, the presence of the organism may not actually be a causative factor of prematurity but rather represent a well-described phenomenon in which the presence of one organism increases the likelihood of another organism. In this scenario, a second organism not sought for in the study could have represented the organism causing prematurity, whereas the first organism was recovered at increased frequency in premature pregnancies only because of its association with the second organism. Recently, more direct evidence of a role for infections in prematurity has been developed linking infection of the amniotic fluid and chorioamnion with premature labor and delivery. Data from amniotic fluid and chorioamnionic infection provide the most convincing evidence of infection in prematurity, but these observations need confirmation. They will be discussed later in the chapter. Despite no definite proof that infection causes prematurity, interest in this possibility remains high because infection is most amenable to treatment.

DEFINITIONS OF TERMS

In 1955, Gardner and Dukes described a new vaginal syndrome that they attributed to a newly described organism, *Haemophilus vaginalis. H. vaginalis* had some but not all the characteristics of other organisms in the *Haemophilus* species, but it also had characteristics of *Corynebacterium* species and at one time was even placed in this genus. It was not until the recent use of DNA homology techniques that it became apparent that the organism was neither a *Haemophilus* nor a *Corynebacterium* species, and a separate species designation was developed. The same organism is now called *Gardnerella vaginalis.* In their classic article, Gardner and Dukes described clinical features associated with the presence of this organism and termed the disease causing vaginal symptoms *Haemophilus vaginalis* vaginitis. Although Gardner and Dukes could isolate the organism only among women who had clinical features of this disease, other investigators began to report the isolation of *G. vaginalis* from a large number of individuals who were believed not to have vaginitis. The designation of who had vaginitis became very confused, compounded by (1) failure of most investigators to apply Gardner and Dukes' specific criteria for the identification of the disease, and (2) failure to appreciate that *G. vaginalis* could be recovered from individuals without the disease. Patients with the clinical criteria proposed by Gardner and Dukes have a readily definable entity that is separable from a normal discharge. This infection can also be accurately distinguished from other causes of vaginitis by distinct signs, and the diagnosis should not be made simply by the absence of *Candida* or *Trichomonas* or both.

G. vaginalis can be isolated from about 95 percent of women with this infection, but it is now evident that the organism is also present in 40 to 50 percent of women who otherwise have no signs or symptoms of vaginitis. Before these points were realized, other terms had been used to define the infection, including nonspecific vaginitis (a total misnomer because it can be very specifically diagnosed), *Gardnerella vaginalis* vaginitis (a term that should not be used because organisms other than *G. vaginalis* are involved and as mentioned, a large proportion of normal women have the organism present), and anaerobic vaginitis or anaerobic vaginosis (also not an accurate description because organisms other than anaerobic bacteria are associated with the disease). Recently, the term bacterial vaginosis has been proposed, "bacterial" represents the finding that a large number of diverse bacteria, including both *G. vaginalis* and anaerobic organisms, are present in the vagina, and vaginosis describes the most distinctive feature of this infection, a fishy amine odor. The term vaginitis would imply the presence of inflammatory cells, and inflammatory cells are typically absent in the vaginal discharge of these women.

CLINICAL FEATURES

Symptoms. Symptoms among women with bacterial vaginosis range from none to a distinctive fishy smelling vaginal odor that typically increases with intercourse. The odor is caused by the presence of amines that are volatized when vaginal fluid is made more basic. Normal vaginal fluid has a pH of less than 4.5. The relative basic seminal fluid (pH 7.2) is able to disassociate the amines from their attachment to proteins, thereby volatilizing the amines to give the distinctive odor. Patients may also complain of an increased vaginal discharge. Symptoms of vulvar pruritus, vulvar irritation, dysuria, a discolored discharge, or lower abdominal discomfort are not features of this disease. Although a proportion of women have symptoms typically associated with this disease, a large proportion of individuals with bacterial vaginosis are asymptomatic or have symptoms associated with other coexisting lower genital tract infections. Patients with bacterial vaginosis commonly have other concomitant lower genital tract infections, and these infections often produce nonspecific genital symptoms not attributable to bacterial vaginosis.

Signs. Women with bacterial vaginosis typically have what is described as a thin, watery, homogeneous discharge. This discharge is distinguished from the normal vaginal discharge, which is thicker and consists of clumps of vaginal epithelial cells providing a floccular appearance. The discharge is often white to gray in appearance. It does not have the yellow or green purulent appearance that is most closely associated with trichomoniasis or cervicitis. Similarly, there is no evidence of vulvar or vaginal inflammation. It should be pointed out that patients with bacterial vaginosis frequently have trichomoniasis or cervicitis, and they thus may have a combination of features associated both with these infections and with bacterial vaginosis.

Risk Factors. The age, demographic characteristics, history of prior genital infections, and history of prior sexual experience suggest that this infection is sexually transmitted. Although sexual transmission is suggested, the evidence is not as clear as with infection caused by a single sexually transmitted organism. Male sexual partners of patients with bacterial vaginosis have a higher rate of *G. vaginalis* isolated from the urethra than control males. However, the presence of *G. vaginalis* does not prove sexual transmission because this organism can be isolated from 15 percent of virgin prepubertal girls. Additionally, male contacts of women with bacterial vaginosis have not been studied for the presence of other organisms in their genital tracts and other data suggest a more complex relationship than exists for other organisms known to be solely sexually transmitted. For example, therapy of male partners with metronidazole has no effect on the long-term recurrence rate of bacterial vaginosis in the female. The male role is further complicated by the possibility that contact with uncircumcised males may be a factor in the development of bacterial vaginosis. Other nonsexual risk factors have been noted. From initial data, it appears that oral contraceptives and barrier methods protect against but IUD's increase the risk of this infection. Intercourse frequency, oral or rectal sexual contact, douching, tampon use, and antibiotics do not seem to be related to bacterial vaginosis.

DIAGNOSIS

Strict objective criteria for the diagnosis of bacterial vaginosis have been formulated and should be applied to establish an accurate diagnosis. The clinical diagnosis of bacterial vaginosis can be made by finding vaginal discharge with (1) a homogeneous appearance, (2) a pH of greater than 4.6, (3) the fishy amine odor upon mixing 10 percent potassium hydroxide with the discharge, and

(4) clue cells (Table 1). As previously mentioned, women with bacterial vaginosis have a thin, watery (homogeneous) appearance to the discharge in contrast to the clumpy, thick appearance of normal vaginal discharge. The pH of normal vaginal discharge ranges from 3.5 to 4.5. Women with a vaginal discharge pH of greater than or equal to 4.6 have either bacterial vaginosis, trichomoniasis, or cervicitis. The presence of the fishy amine odor does not occur in a normal discharge or in vaginal candidiasis. Of course, women with either trichomoniasis or cervicitis together with bacterial vaginosis can have an amine odor caused by coexisting bacterial vaginosis. The so-called clue cell represents a vaginal epithelial cell to which so many bacteria are attached that the cell border appears serrated and is obscured. This definition allows for the very specific determination of a clue cell. Other more subjective criteria can all be misleading. Normal epithelial cells occasionally have enough bacteria on the surface of the epithelial cell that give a hazy or dirty appearance to the cell.

In addition to the clinical criteria for the diagnosis of bacterial vaginosis described earlier, Gram's stain criteria to diagnose bacterial vaginosis have been developed. Women with bacterial vaginosis have (1) an increased number of small gram-negative or gram-variable rods, including a newly described curved rod called *Mobiluncus* and (2) a relative absence of *Lactobacillus* morphotypes (large gram-positive rods) (see Table 1). Women with a normal vaginal discharge have a predominance (usually more than six per high-power field) of *Lactobacillus* morphotypes with only a few (less than five per high-power field) of small rods. Gram's stain features can be accurately used to diagnose both bacterial vaginosis and a normal discharge. Other laboratory criteria using gas-liquid chromatography are not widely available. It deserves emphasis that the disease entity, bacterial vaginosis, must be established by specific clinical or Gram's stain criteria. It is not accurate to make the diagnosis of bacterial vaginosis simply in the absence of trichomonads or *Candida*. It will be further emphasized that the presence or absence of *G. vaginalis* also cannot be used to diagnose bacterial vaginosis.

Role of Cultures for Diagnosis

There are no culture criteria that accurately distinguish patients who have bacterial vaginosis from other patients, and for clinical purposes, cultures have no role in establishing the diagnosis of bacterial vaginosis. With the recent use of selected media, it has become apparent that 40 to 50 percent of all women in the reproductive age range have *G. vaginalis* isolated from the vagina. Although about 95 percent of women with bacterial vaginosis have *Gardnerella vaginalis* isolated from the vagina, the isolation of this organism is too nonspecific to reliably diagnose bacterial vaginosis because of the large number of normal women who also have this organism present. It should also be noted that *G. vaginalis* is recovered from 40 to 50 percent of individuals following successful therapy of bacterial vaginosis, and thus the presence or absence of this organism also cannot be used to determine treatment success. Recovery of other organisms associated with bacterial vaginosis, including anaerobes, is not only difficult but does not accurately establish or exclude the infection.

The bacteriology of this infection is very complex. Perhaps an increased concentration of bacteria rather than an increased prevalence of organisms better characterizes bacterial vaginosis, although both features occur. It has become apparent that there is an increase not only in the prevalence but also a 100- to 1,000-fold increase in the concentration of both *G. vaginalis* and selected anaerobic bacteria, including *Bacteroides bivius, Peptostreptococcus,* and *Mobiluncus* species. In addition, the prevalence and concentration of *Mycoplasma hominis* increase in this milieu. These bacteria combine to produce a very anaerobic vaginal environment with a low Eh that has the features of an intravaginal abscess.

ASSOCIATION WITH PREMATURITY

Bacterial Vaginosis. From 15 to 20 percent of pregnant women have bacterial vaginosis. It has been identified more frequently in women who deliver prematurely or are in premature labor than in control pregnant women at a similar gestational age. An assessment of the relationship between prematurity, selected cervical vaginal flora, and 30 demographic, socioeconomic, and obstetric variables associated with prematurity was recently made. This study included 79 women in premature labor and 455 women who delivered at term. In a univariate analysis, preterm labor of less than 37 weeks occurred among 25 (25 percent) of 102 women with and 54 (13 percent) of the 432 women without bacterial vaginosis ($p = 0.01$). Preterm labor (less than 34 weeks), premature rupture of membranes, birth weight less than 2,500 g, and amniotic fluid infection were also associated with bacterial vaginosis in the univariate analysis (Table 2). Ethanol use and pregnancy-induced hypertension were also associated with premature labor, and a multifactorial analysis was used

TABLE 1 Diagnosis of Bacterial Vaginosis

Clinical Diagnosis	*Gram's Stain Diagnosis*	*Culture Diagnosis*
Homogeneous appearance pH > 4.5	Predominance, usually > 30 of *Gardnerella* morphotypes and other rods per high-power field	At present, cultures have no role in the diagnosis of bacterial vaginosis because no cultures are reliable for diagnosis
Fishy amine odor with addition of 10% potassium hydroxide	< 5 *Lactobacillus* morphotypes per high-power field	
Clue cells		

to adjust ten demographic and obstetric variables associated with prematurity in other reports plus the two outcomes associated with prematurity in the univariate analysis of this study. The presence of *C. trachomatis* was also adjusted in the analysis of bacterial vaginosis, and in a separate analysis, adjustment was made for the presence of bacterial vaginosis when the outcome of women with *C. trachomatis* infection was studied. In all instances adjustments were made for differences in gestational age at the time of study entry. A significant association remained between the presence of bacterial vaginosis and preterm labor of less than 37 weeks (Odds Ratio [OR] 2.0, p = 0.05), and between bacterial vaginosis and premature rupture of membranes (OR 2.0, p = 0.05) in the multifactorial analysis (see Table 2).

In the second study, premature delivery (less than 37 weeks) occurred among 42 percent of 52 women with and 26 percent of 107 women without bacterial vaginosis (p <0.03). In this study, a multifactorial analysis was also used to adjust for educational level and premature rupture of membranes, the two variables that differed between women with and without a premature delivery. A premature delivery was associated with the presence of bacterial vaginosis as determined by Gram's stain (OR 2.3, p <0.03) and with the absence of *Lactobacillus* species (OR 0.2, p <0.02). In both of the studies, *C. trachomatis* infection was also related to prematurity independent of the relationship between bacterial vaginosis and prematurity. In the third study which will be discussed in more detail below, bacterial vaginosis was related to asymptomatic amniotic fluid infection among women in premature labor. Women in premature labor had a 3.8-fold increased risk of bacterial vaginosis compared with control women matched for gestational age at enrollment and selected demographic and obstetric variables (p <0.02). In summary, all three studies have linked bacterial vaginosis with events concerning prematurity. However, a limited number of other organisms were studied in these reports, and all three reports have suffered both from small numbers of subjects and from limited analyses of the interrelationship between prematurity, other organisms, and bacterial vaginosis. Further data are required in which other organisms are simultaneously recovered and then controlled in the analysis.

Amniotic Fluid Infection. Organisms have been recovered from the amniotic fluid obtained by transabdominal amniocentesis among women in premature labor with intact membranes. Approximately 10 percent of women in premature labor have organisms isolated from amniotic fluid (Table 3). Amniotic fluid cultures from women not in labor who undergo amniocentesis (for genetic or prematurity studies) have been sterile. The recovery of organisms from amniotic fluid of women with premature labor and not of women without labor suggests but does not conclusively prove that organisms cause labor. Alternatively, organisms could gain entrance into amniotic fluid as a consequence of labor. Regardless of the timing, once organisms are in amniotic fluid, they are highly associated with premature delivery. Women with bacteria or *Candida* in the amniotic fluid delivered less than 1 day after amniocentesis, compared with women with no organisms in the amniotic fluid who delivered a mean of 25 to 51 days after amniocentesis (Table 4). Patients with genital mycoplasmas isolated from amniotic fluid delivered at the same interval as those with no organisms isolated. The observation that organisms in amniotic fluid are associated with a premature delivery suggests that either the organisms cause the onset of labor or alternatively that contractions at this stage of pregnancy expose placental membranes and the lower uterine segment to the movement of vaginal organisms into amniotic fluid. A wide variety of organisms was recovered, including the isolation of anaerobic bacteria from the amniotic fluid of 57 percent of women in premature labor. A large proportion of the anaerobes that have been recovered from amniotic fluid are those isolated at an increased concentration and prevalence among patients with bacterial vaginosis. It is of interest that neonates generally do not become septic despite exposure to contaminated amniotic fluid, but anaerobic bacteria usually do not cause neonatal sepsis.

Chorioamnionic Infection. There have been a number of recent reports in which organisms have been recovered from between the chorion and amnion of the placenta. A large variety of organisms have been isolated from this space of the membrane. *Ureaplasma urealyticum* was more likely to be isolated from placental membranes of infants admitted to the neonatal intensive care unit (presumably largely related to prematurity) and still-

TABLE 2 Association of Bacterial Vaginosis with Prematurity

Author	*Outcome Variable*	*Univariate* OR*	*Univariate* P	*Multivariate* OR	*Multivariate* P
Gravett	Preterm labor <34 wk	2.2	0.01	1.9	N.S.§
	<37 wk	2.2	<0.01	2.0	<0.05
	Preterm ROM†	2.4	<0.01	2.0	<0.05
	Birth weight <2,500 g	1.7	<0.05	1.5	N.S.
	Amniotic fluid infection	2.1	<0.05	2.7	<0.05
Martius	Preterm ROM	~4	<0.01		
	Delivery <37 wk	~2	<0.05	2.3	0.03
Gravett	Preterm labor	3.8	0.02‡		

* OR = odds ratio.
† ROM = rupture of membranes.
‡ Matched with controls.
§ N.S. = not significant.

TABLE 3 Organisms Recovered from Amniotic Fluid of Women in Premature Labor with Intact Membranes

Author	*Number*	*Positive Amniotic Fluid Culture (%)*
Wallace	25	1 (4%)
Hameed	37	3 (8%)
Garite	59	7 (12%)
Wahbeh	33	4 (12%)
Gravett	54	6 (12%)
Bobitt	31	8 (26%)
Total number of women	239	29 (12%) Mean positive

born infants than infants admitted to the newborn nursery. In this study, organisms other than *U. urealyticum* or *M. hominis* were not associated with prematurity or stillbirth. Although subsequent studies have usually not confirmed a relationship between prematurity and recovery of organisms from the chorion-amnion space, many of these studies were small. A recent study has added evidence that supports a relationship between chorioamnionic infection and prematurity. In this study, women who delivered prematurely had increased recovery of not only *U. urealyticum* but also *G. vaginalis, Bacteroides* species, peptostreptococci species, and *Mobiluncus* species from the chorioamnion compared with those who delivered at term. These four isolates were not only the most common organisms recovered from the chorioamnion but also the organisms found in increased concentration in women with bacterial vaginosis. In fact, vaginal bacterial vaginosis was associated with infection of the chorioamnion and with histologic chorioamnionitis in this study. The presence of both *U. urealyticum* and other bacteria in the chorioamniotic space was independently associated with both premature delivery and histologic chorioamnionitis after multifactorial adjustment for the duration of labor and rupture of membranes. In summary, bacterial vaginosis was associated with infection of the chorioamnion, histologic chorioamnionitis, and prematurity in this study.

Before it can be definitely concluded that bacterial vaginosis causes premature labor, patients with bacterial vaginosis must be treated with an effective antibiotic versus placebo to demonstrate a reduced occurrence of prematurity among antibiotic-treated women. Until these data become available, routine treatment of bacterial vaginosis cannot be advocated during pregnancy. If bacterial vaginosis can be shown to cause prematurity, the importance of this infection will substantially increase several times over its present status as a nuisance problem without serious consequences.

TABLE 4 Delivery Interval (Days) of Women in Premature Labor Stratified for Presence or Absence of Amniotic Fluid Organisms

	Amniotic Fluid Isolation		
Author	*Bacteria or Candida*	*Mycoplasma*	*No Organism*
Bobitt	<1.0	N.D.*	25
Gravett	0.6	35	34
Wahbeh	1.0	N.D.	42
Hameed	<1.0	N.D.	51

* N.D. = Not done.

POSTPARTUM ENDOMETRITIS

The high concentration of virulent organisms in the vagina of women with bacterial vaginosis raises a further possibility that these organisms could cause postpartum endometritis. Vaginal organisms colonize the amniotic fluid compartment during labor and after rupture of the membranes. These organisms contaminate uterine and wound incisions and the abdominal cavity during a cesarean section to produce an infection usually diagnosed as postpartum endometritis.

Recently, a protected endometrial culturing device was used to reduce vaginal-cervical contamination when endometrial cultures were obtained and selective media was used to recover *G. vaginalis.* In this report, both *G. vaginalis* and the same anaerobes associated with bacterial vaginosis were isolated from 20 percent, *G. vaginalis* alone or in combination with other facultative bacteria was isolated from 20 percent and anaerobes associated with bacterial vaginosis were isolated from 20 percent of women with postpartum endometritis. Thus, as many as 60 percent of women with postpartum endometritis had organisms recovered from the endometrial cavity that are associated with bacterial vaginosis. Prospective studies are needed to determine the rate of postpartum endometritis among women with antepartum bacterial vaginosis compared with women without vaginitis.

TREATMENT STRATEGIES DURING PREGNANCY

There is no precedent for routine treatment of bacterial vaginosis during pregnancy at this time. In fact, treatment during pregnancy poses a problem. Metronidazole, the most widely used effective antibiotic in the treatment of nonpregnant women, has a small carcinogenic potential that limits its use during pregnancy, at least the first half of pregnancy. Penicillins can be safely used during pregnancy. However, ampicillin or amoxicillin is clearly not as effective as metronidazole, and in nonpregnant women these two antibiotics have provided modest cure rates of only 35 to 65 percent. Triple sulfa cream may be safe, but in well-controlled studies it is not an effective remedy. Betadine gel is not only ineffective but could produce a fetal goiter in pregnancy.

Two new treatment regimens of bacterial vaginosis offer promise for pregnant women. A new combination antibiotic, Augmentin, contains amoxicillin and clavulanic acid. Clavulanic acid irreversibly binds to beta-lactamase, which otherwise would inactivate amoxicillin. Thus the addition of clavulanic acid increases the activity of amoxicillin. In preliminary trials, Augmentin has been effective in treating bacterial vaginosis. More experience with this drug in pregnancy is necessary to evaluate possible fetal effects, but there are no theoretical risks to using clavulanic acid in pregnancy. Recently, a clindamycin vaginal cream has been used effectively to treat nonpregnant women with bacterial vaginosis. Since clindamycin has no known adverse fetal effects, vaginal clindamycin cream remains an attractive future option for use in pregnancy.

SUGGESTED READING

Amsel R, Totten PA, Spiegel CA, et al. Nonspecific vaginitis: diagnostic criteria and microbiologic and epidemiologic associations. Am J Med 1983; 74:14–22.

Amstey MS, Steadman KT. Symptomatic gonorrhea and pregnancy. J Am Venereal Dis Assoc 1976; 3:14–16.

Blackwell AL, Fox AR, Phillips I, et al. Anaerobic vaginosis (nonspecific vaginitis): clinical microbiological and therapeutic findings. Lancet 1982; ii:1379–1382.

Bobitt JR, Damato JD, Sakatini J. Perinatal complications in group B streptococcal carriers: a longitudinal study of prenatal patients. Am J Obstet Gynecol 1985; 152:711–717.

Bobitt JR, Hayslip CC, Damato JD. Amniotic fluid infection as determined by transabdominal amniocentesis in patients with intact membranes in premature labor. Am J Obstet Gynecol 1981; 140:947–952.

Brand JM, Galask RP. Trimethylamine: the substance mainly responsible for the fishy odor often associated with bacterial vaginosis. Obstet Gynecol 1986; 68:682–685.

Braun P, Lee Y-H, Klein JO, et al. Birth weight and genital mycoplasmas in pregnancy. N Engl J Med 1971; 284:167–171.

Bump RC, Zuspan FP, Buesching WJ, et al. The prevalence, six month persistence, and predictive values of laboratory indicators of bacterial vaginosis (nonspecific vaginitis) in asymptomatic women. Am J Obstet Gynecol 1984; 150:917–924.

Chen KCS, Forsyth PS, Buchanan TM, et al. Amine content of vaginal fluid from untreated patients with nonspecific vaginitis. J Clin Invest 1979; 63:828–835.

Eschenbach DA. Lower genital tract infections. In: Galask RP, Larsen B, eds. Infectious diseases in the female patient. New York: Springer-Verlag 1986:163.

Eschenbach DA, Critchlow CW, Watkins H, et al. A dose duration study of metronidazole for treatment of nonspecific vaginitis. Scand J Infect Dis Suppl 1983; 40:73–80.

Gardner HL, Dukes CD. *Haemophilus vaginalis* vaginitis. Am J Obstet Gynecol 1955; 69:962–976.

Gravett MG, Hummel D, Eschenbach DA, et al. Premature labor associated with subclinical amniotic fluid infection and with bacterial vaginosis. Obstet Gynecol 1986; 67:229–237.

Gravett MG, Nelson HP, DeRouen T, et al. Independent association of bacterial vaginosis and *Chlamydia trachomatis* infection with adverse pregnancy outcome. JAMA 1986; 256:1899–1903.

Greenwood JR, Pickett MJ. Transfer of *Haemophilus vaginalis* to a new genus, *Gardnerella: G. vaginalis* (Gardner and Dukes). Int J Syst Bacteriol 1980; 30:170–178.

Hameed C, Tejani N, Verma UL, et al. Silent chorioamnionitis as a cause of preterm labor refractory to tocolytic therapy. Am J Obstet Gynecol 1984; 149:726–730.

Hammerschlag MR, Albert S, Rosener I, et al. Microbiology of the vagina in children. Normal and potentially pathogenic organisms. Pediatrics 1978; 62:57–62.

Hardy PH, Hardy JB, Well EE, et al. Prevalence of six sexually transmitted disease agents among pregnant inner-city adolescents and pregnancy outcome. Lancet 1984; ii:333–337.

Harrison HR, Alexander ER, Weinstein L, et al. The epidemiology and effects of cervical *C. trachomatis* and mycoplasmal infections in pregnancy. JAMA 1983; 250:1721–1727.

Hillier SL, Martius J, Krohn MA, et al. Case-control study of chorioamnionic infection and chorioamnionitis in prematurity. Vancouver, BC: Abstract of Obstetrics and Gynecologic Infectious Disease Society, 1986:4.

Holmes KK, Chen KCS, Lipinski CM, et al. Vaginal redox potential in bacterial vaginosis (nonspecific vaginitis). J Infect Dis 1985; 152:79–82.

Kaltrieder FD, Kohl S. Epidemiology of preterm birth. Clin Obstet Gynecol 1980; 23:17–31.

Kleinman JC, Kovar MG, Feldman JJ, et al. A comparison of 1960 and 1973–1984 early neonatal mortality in selected states. J Epidemiol 1978; 108:454–460.

Kundsin RB, Driscoll SG. Monson RR, et al. Association of *Ureaplasma urealyticum* in the placenta with perinatal morbidity and mortality. N Engl J Med 1984; 310:941–945.

Leigh J, Garite TJ. Amniocentesis and the management of preterm labor. Obstet Gynecol 1986; 67:500–506.

McCormack WM, Hayes CM, Rosner B, et al. Vaginal colonization with *Corynebacterium vaginale (Haemophilus vaginalis).* J Infect Dis 1977; 136:740–745.

Mengel MB. The effectiveness of single dose metronidazole therapy for patients and their partners with bacterial vaginosis. Masters, Public Heatlh Thesis, University of Washington, May 1986.

Martin DH, Koutsky L. Eschenbach DA, et al. Prematurity and perinatal mortality in pregnancies complicated by maternal *Chlamydia trachomatis* infection. JAMA 1982; 247:1585–1588.

Martius J, Krohn MA, Hillier SL, et al. Relationship of vaginal *Lactobacillus* species, cervical *Chlamydia trachomatis,* and bacterial vaginosis to preterm birth. Obstet Gynecol 1988; 71:89–95.

Naeye R, Kissane JM. Perinatal diseases, a neglected area of the medical sciences. In: Naeye RL, Kissane JM, Kaufman N, eds. Perinatal diseases. International Academy of Pathology. Baltimore: Williams & Wilkins, 1980:1.

National Center for Health Statistics: 1951 and 1977. Vol 1. Natality. Washington DC. U.S. Department of Health, Education and Welfare.

Pheifer TA, Forsyth PS, Durfee MA, et al. Nonspecific vaginitis: Role of *Haemophilus vaginalis* and treatment with metronidazole. N Engl J Med 1978; 298:1429–1434.

Prevedovrakis CN, Strigou-Charalabis E, Kaskarelis DB. Bacterial invasion of amniotic cavity during pregnancy and labor. Obstet Gynecol 1971; 37:459–461.

Regan JA, Chao S, James LS. Premature rupture of membranes, preterm delivery and group B streptococcal colonization of mothers. Am J Obstet Gynecol 1981; 141:184–186.

Rosene K, Eschenback DA, Tompkins LS, et al. Polymicrobial early postpartum endometritis with facultatively anaerobic and anaerobic bacteria, genital mycoplasmas and *Chlamydia trachomatis:* treatment with piperacillin or cefoxitin. J Infect Dis 1986; 153:1028–1037.

Russell P. Inflammatory lesions of the human placenta. I. Clinical significance of acute chorioamnionitis. Am J Diagn Gynecol Obstet 1979; 1:127–137.

Spiegel CA, Amsel R, Eschenback DA, et al. Anaerobic bacteria in nonspecific vaginitis. N Engl J Med 1980; 303:601–607.

Spiegel CA, Amsel R, Holmes KK. Diagnosis of bacterial vaginosis by direct Gram stain of vaginal fluid. J Clin Microbiol 1983; 18:170–177.

Spiegel CA, Roberts M. *Mobiluncus* gen. nov., *Mobiluncus urtisii* subsp. *curtisii* sp. nov., *Mobiluncus curtisii* subsp. *holmesii* subsp. nov., and *Mobiluncus mulieris* sp nov., curved rods from the human vagina. Int J Syst Bacteriol 1984; 34:177–184.

Svensson L, Ingemarsson I, Mardh P-A. Chorioamnionitis and the isolation of microorganisms from the placenta. Obstet Gynecol 1986; 67:403–409.

Totten PA, Amsel R, Hale J, et al. Selective differential human blood bilayer media for isolation of *Gardnerella (Haemophilus) vaginalis*. J Clin Microbiol 1982; 15:141–147.
Vontver LA, Eschenback DA. The role of *Gardnerella vaginalis* in nonspecific vaginitis. Clin Obstet Gynecol 1981; 24:439–460.
Wahbeh CJ, Hill GB, Eden RD, et al. Intra-amniotic bacterial colonization in premature labor. Am J Obstet Gynecol 1984; 148:739–743.
Wallace RL, Herrick CN. Amniocentesis in the evaluation of premature labor. Obstet Gynecol 1981; 57:483–486.
Westrom L, Evaldson G, Holmes KK, et al. Taxonomy of vaginosis; Bacterial vaginosis—a definition. Scand J Urol Nephrol 1984; (Suppl 86):259.
Williams RL, Chen PM. Identifying the source of the recent decline in perinatal mortality rates in California. N Engl J Med 1982; 306:207–211.

SYPHILIS IN PREGNANCY

BRYAN LARSEN, Ph.D.
DAVID CHARLES, M.D., F.A.C.O.G., F.R.C.O.G.

The prevention of congenital syphilis is a major aim in perinatal care provided by the obstetrician. The disease, although devastating to the afflicted individual, is almost entirely preventable because of the availability of effective diagnostic tests and curative antibiotics. Nevertheless, cases of congenital syphilis still occur and may even be on the increase. In 1986, the Centers for Disease Control (CDC) reported that after 8 years of declining rates of congenital syphilis from 1971 to 1978, the number of infants affected began to increase. The number of cases reported more than doubled from 1978 when there were 108 reported cases to 1983 when there were 268 reported cases. In the United States, approximately 0.05 percent of liveborn infants are affected, although the geographic distribution of cases is uneven.

Despite the fact that epidemics of syphilis are not currently moving unabated through the population as in former times, a significant number of adults are affected. During the years when congenital syphilis was on the rise, the rate of primary and secondary syphilis among women increased from 4.7 cases per 100,000 women to 7.6 cases per 100,000 in 1983. As a sequel of an increase in the number of adult cases, there is a proportionate increase in the number of cases of congenital disease. In recent years, between 20,000 and 30,000 new cases of primary and secondary syphilis have been reported annually to the CDC.

Congenital syphilis is not only a consequence of pregnant women acquiring the disease but also is a result of inadequate prenatal care. For example, in 1982, 50 of the 159 reported United States cases of congenital syphilis occurred in Texas, and the majority of these 50 cases occurred in infants born to socially deprived minority groups. Two-thirds of these women had no prenatal care, and those who did received substandard care. In a recent nation-wide survey of 460 cases of congenital syphilis, the CDC reported that the women involved tended to be young; 30 percent were younger than 20 years of age. The majority were Black (52 percent) or Hispanic (36 percent) and made fewer visits for prenatal care than the general population of pregnant women.

Consequently, the prevalence of congenital syphilis reflects the degree to which health services are either unavailable to disadvantaged women or to which these women are unwilling or unable to avail themselves of such services. It is clear that the battle against congenital syphilis must of necessity be waged on two fronts, thus requiring the combined efforts of both public health authorities and the primary care physicians. Whereas some cases of congenital syphilis occur because care is unavailable for high-risk women, a lack of education is undoubtedly also responsible. Rigorous measures must be adopted to educate women regarding the need for medical attention at an early stage of pregnancy and to ensure that medical attention is available for high-risk women. Public health officials, health care providers, and government agencies must all cooperate if these goals are to be achieved.

There is an inherent danger in what may be currently considered an over-reliance on public health authorities in the prevention of congenital syphilis. The tendency to relegate the care for cases of syphilis to public health clinics has diminished the opportunity for medical students to learn about the disease that is commonly referred to as the great imitator. The clinical manifestations of syphilis are often extremely complex in their presentation, thereby emphasizing the necessity of introducing more rigorous sexually transmitted disease teaching for medical students and physicians. The medical graduate must know which tests are available and how to interpret them.

ADULT SYPHILIS

Syphilis is caused by the spirochete *Treponema pallidum*, which is acquired by contact with infectious material from either another person or, in rare instances, via blood products (i.e., needle stick) from a person with the disease. The organism is fastidious, cannot grow saprophytically, and is extremely susceptible to drying and other environmental conditions. As a result, transmission via fomites is virtually impossible. The primary infection is characterized as a painless ulcer. The incubation period is 10 days to 3 months, although most patients develop a primary lesion within 6 weeks. Usually the lesion occurs on the genitalia, but a chancre may be encountered at other sites such as the oropharynx, rectum, or nipple.

In women, a painless intravaginal or cervical primary lesion is not ordinarily noticed by the patient, and the spontaneous healing of such a lesion without therapy may lead to a false sense of security. The Venereal Disease Research

Laboratory (VDRL) test may not become positive for up to 3 months, which may be after the healing of the primary ulcer. Thus, not all patients with primary syphilis have a positive VDRL test. The primary syphilitic lesion should contain spirochetes that are demonstrable on dark-field microscopy. Unfortunately this method is under-utilized, and many laboratories do not have microscopes equipped with dark-field condensers. Confirmation of the non-treponemal test with a specific treponemal test such as the fluorescent treponemal antibody absorption (FTA-ABS) test is essential because of the possibility that a positive VDRL test may be a biological false positive.

If primary syphilis is inadequately treated or not treated, the disease may progress to secondary syphilis 6 weeks to 6 months after the primary exposure. The clinical spectrum of secondary syphilis is broad, potentially including malaise, fever, maculopapular rash, hair loss, condyloma latum, generalized lymphadenopathy, nephritis, hepatitis, meningitis, long-bone periosteitis, and iridocyclitis. The presence of rash on the soles of the feet and the palms should alert the physician to the possibility of secondary syphilis—although neither this nor the other clinical findings is pathognomonic for secondary syphilis. Rather, these findings should arouse suspicion of syphilis and should be followed by appropriate diagnostic measures. As with primary stage, the symptoms of secondary syphilis abate spontaneously as the patient enters a latent phase, which may persist for many years. A recrudescence of the secondary disease may occur at any time in the first 4 years, although the majority of relapses occur within the first year.

CONGENITAL SYPHILIS

The gravid patient who has primary or secondary syphilis may transmit the organism to her offspring in utero as the treponemes have the ability to cross the placenta. The probability that the organism will be transmitted from mother to fetus is nearly 95 percent. It is estimated that there are 1.5 to 1.8 cases of congenital syphilis for every 100 cases of primary and secondary syphilis. In view of these statistics, it is essential to find and treat cases of syphilis occurring in pregnant women.

Formerly, it was believed the fetus was protected from transplacental infection for the first 4 or 5 months by the barrier function of the cytotrophoblast. However, it has been demonstrated that spirochetes can be present in abortuses of 9- and 10-weeks gestation, thus indicating that transplacental infection may occur at any time during pregnancy. In addition to spirochetes in the bloodstreams of the mother and fetus, spirochetes have also been demonstrated in the amniotic fluid of a 30-week pregnancy although it was not clear what pathway led to intra-amniotic infection with the organism. Maternal syphilis results in transplacental infection, which can occur at virtually all stages of pregnancy (although the likelihood of fetal infection is greater in the second and third trimesters).

Demographic studies of cases of congenital syphilis have indicated that young women who belong to ethnic minorities and who receive little or no prenatal care and those with multiple sex partners are at greatest risk for delivering an infant with congenital syphilis. Moreover, there is an uneven geographic distribution of congenital syphilis cases reported in recent years. New York, Texas, and Florida had rates in excess of 10 cases per 100,000 live births. South Carolina, Georgia, Louisiana, New Mexico, Nevada, and California had rates of 4.0 to 9.9 cases per 100,000 live births. These data should not be used to provide a false sense of security to the physician whose patient population does not fit these criteria, but rather to help identify groups that require special attention.

Intrauterine syphilis may result in spontaneous abortion, premature labor, intrauterine growth retardation, stillbirth or neonatal death. A surviving infant who has congenital syphilis may be born with few stigmata or may have multiple systems involved. The CDC indicated that stillbirth in the presence of maternal syphilis occurred in 29 percent of the cases reviewed between 1983 and 1985 and 12 percent of infants were asymptomatic at birth. The stigmata of congenital syphilis may develop early, within the first 2 years of life (early congenital syphilis) or after the first 2 years of life (late congenital syphilis). As summarized in Table 1, the manifestations of early and late congenital syphilis differ, but both reflect multisystem involvement and it should be remembered that not all of these stigmata occur in every patient. As congenital syphilis is a rare occurrence in most practices the clinical presentation may cause some confusion.

Of the myriad of clinical manifestations of early congenital syphilis, the most common are rash on the palms and soles, rhinitis, and hepatosplenomegaly. The bullous vesicular skin eruptions contain spirochetes, which can readily be demonstrated by dark-field microscopy. These vesicles are highly infectious. Other frequent entities noted in patients with congenital luetic infection are periosteitis, which leads to the pseudoparalysis of Parrot, and meningitis.

Physicians must be alerted to the fact that congenital syphilis is a tremendously destructive disease and, despite the diagnostic difficulties, every effort must be made not to miss the diagnosis. It should be emphasized that the VDRL test performed on the cord blood may be a useful diagnostic tool. However, because IgG antibodies cross the placenta, the cord blood is usually positive when the mother's serology is positive. Nevertheless, if the cord blood has a titer significantly higher than the mother's this suggests congenital syphilis. The cord blood titer may be used as a baseline, and a continuous rise of the infant's VDRL titer after birth is indicative of active disease. Although not readily available, specific IgM may be utilized for confirmation of fetal infection.

LABORATORY TESTS FOR SYPHILIS

Of major significance in provision of adequate prenatal care is the use of screening tests even in patients without clinical signs of syphilis. Figure 1 emphasizes the importance of vigorously applying diagnostic methods to patients with symptoms, as well as those without symptoms, in an effort to discover cases of syphilis in pregnancy. The serologic tests for syphilis are not specific and are

TABLE 1 Manifestations of Congenital Syphilis

Early Congenital Syphilis	*Late Congenital Syphilis*
Hepatosplenomegaly	Dental
Generalized lymphadenopathy	Mulberry molars
Pneumonia alba	Hutchinson's teeth
Hematologic	Enamel dystrophy
Anemia	Skeletal
Erythroblastemia	Frontal bossing
Reticulocytosis	Saddle nose
Thrombocytopenia	Saber shin
Disseminated intravascular coagulation	High palatal arch
	Short maxilla
Mucocutaneous	Clavicular and scapular deformities
Rhinitis (snuffles)	
Maculopapular rash	Clutton's joints
Pemphigus (palms and soles)	Ocular
Petichiae	Interstitial keratitis
Jaundice	Uveitis
Renal	Glaucoma
Nephrosis or nephritis	Neurologic
Edema	Eighth nerve deafness
Ascites	Convulsive disorders
Central nervous system	Paresis, paralysis
Hydrocephalus	Mucocutaneous
Meningiovascular syphilis	Rhagades
Delayed mental development	Gummas
Ocular	Palatal perforation
Uveitis	Cardiovascular
Chorioretinitis	Aortitis
Glaucoma	
Gastrointestinal	
Pancreatitis	
Enteritis	
Intrauterine growth retardation	
Placental	
Hypertrophy	
Villitis	
Perivasculitis	
Immature villi	

based on the detection of anticardiolipin antibodies. These include the VDRL test and the rapid plasma reagin (RPR) card test. Such tests are of great value in identifying patients who, despite the absence of symptoms, may require further evaluation and perhaps therapy. Individuals who do not have syphilis may have a false positive serologic test for syphilis, a phenomenon which does not seriously detract from the utility of such tests.

The VDRL test may be performed quantitatively as it provides a useful method for following the course of the disease. A fourfold increase in titer is accepted as evidence of developing infection, and decrease in titer of similar magnitude indicates resolution of acute infection. In a patient who has been adequately treated, the quantitative VDRL titer should eventually approach zero. The VDRL can be utilized in evaluation of the cerebrospinal fluid and should be used in infants exposed to syphilis in utero.

Specific treponemal tests are available, such as the FTA-ABS, which may be used to confirm the presence of disease in VDRL-positive individuals. However, in contrast to the VDRL, which shows decreasing titers in adequately treated patients, the FTA-ABS remains positive after the patient has been treated. It must be emphasized that such specific treponemal tests as the FTA-ABS test are essential because of the possibility that a positive VDRL test may represent a biological false positive.

THERAPY OF THE PREGNANT HOST

The importance of diagnosis cannot be overemphasized because syphilis is a treatable disease. *Treponema pallidum* is exquisitely susceptible to penicillin. The required therapeutic level of penicillin in serum is in excess of 0.03 units per milliliter for 7 to 10 days. The continuing role of penicillin in the therapy of syphilis is universally accepted because it has the potential of curing the disease at any stage in the mother, it crosses the placenta in concentrations which are treponemacidal, has a wide margin of safety in the mother and the fetus, is inexpensive, and can be administered as a single dose.

The CDC guidelines issued in 1985 reaffirm the use of penicillin for syphilis during pregnancy:

> For patients at all stages of pregnancy who are not allergic to penicillin, penicillin should be used in dosage schedules appropriate for the stage of syphilis as recommended for the treatment of nonpregnant patients....For patients at all stages of pregnancy who have documented allergy to penicillin:
>
> 1. If compliance and serologic follow-up can be assured, administer erythromycin in dosage schedules appropriate for the stage of syphilis as recom-

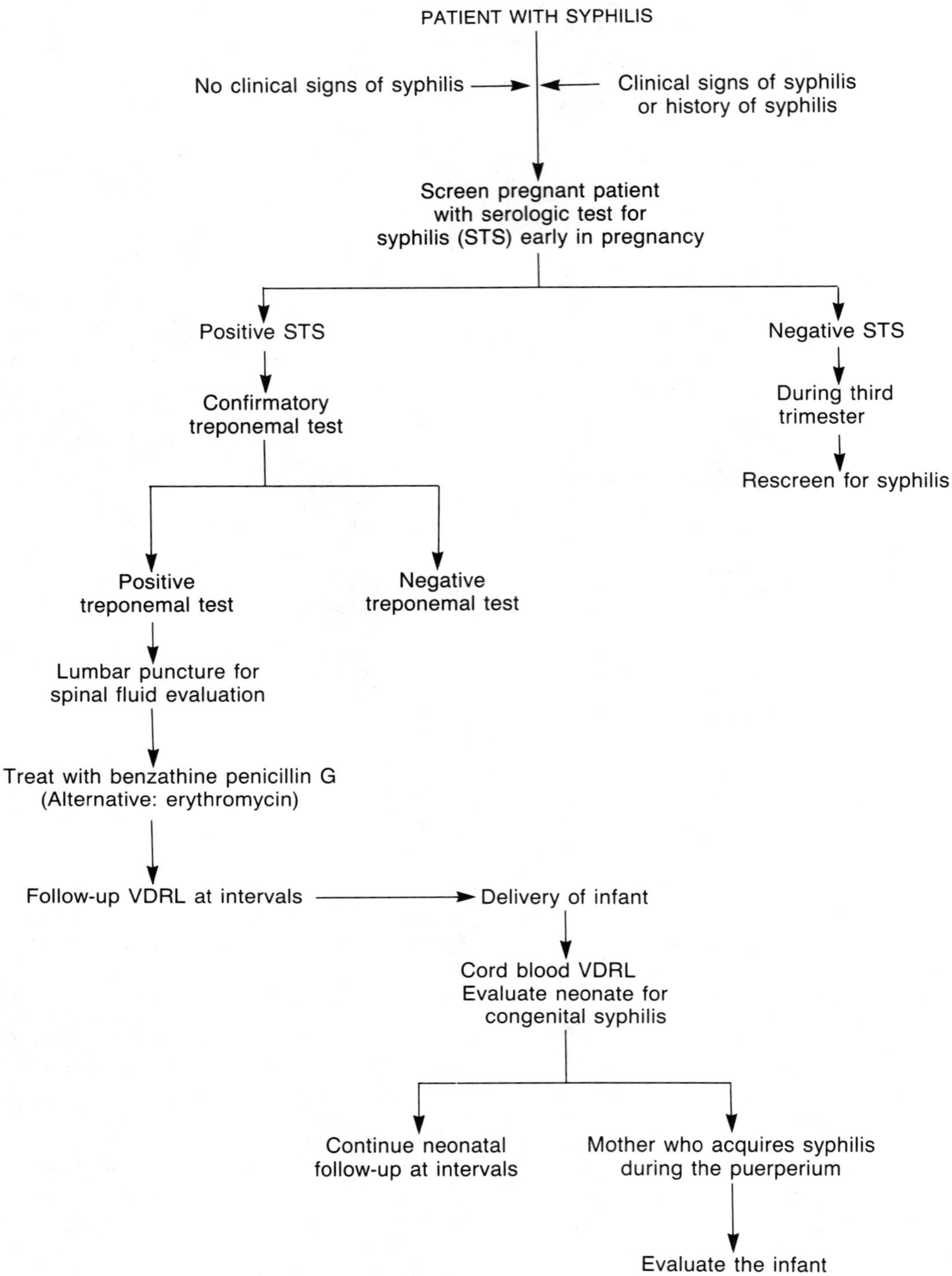

Figure 1 Syphilis in pregnancy.

mended for the treatment of nonpregnant patients. Infants born to mothers treated during pregnancy with erythromycin for early syphilis should be treated with penicillin.

2. If compliance and serologic follow-up cannot be assured, the patient should be hospitalized and treated in consultation with an expert. Tetracycline is not recommended in pregnant women because of potential adverse effects on the fetus.

Consequently, pregnant patients with early syphilis, including primary, secondary, or early latent syphilis of less than 1 year duration, should receive 2.4 mega units of benzathine penicillin G intramuscularly at a single session. The alternative is erythromycin 500 mg orally four times daily for 15 days.

Patients who have syphilis of longer than 1 year duration (except neurosyphilis) should receive 2.4 mega units of benzathine penicillin G intramuscularly once a week for 3 weeks. Pregnant patients may have signs of neurosyphilis more often than is generally appreciated and therefore it should be noted that doses of penicillin G in doses of 6 to 9 mega units administered over 3 to 4 weeks may be necessary to establish treponemacidal activity in the cerebrospinal fluid.

Despite the general usefulness of penicillin, some problems must be acknowledged. Of particular concern is that, in the recent CDC report, among the 81 women who had prenatal care and delivered infants with congenital syphilis, 60 had been treated with benzathine penicillin regimens appropriate to their stage of disease. Other reports also exist, which indicate that treatment failures may occur with penicillin therapy, and although failures with penicillin are not numerous, they do occur often enough to attest to the fact that the recommended penicillin therapy has some deficiencies. Therefore, penicillin is usually but not always effective in preventing congenital syphilis.

It must be acknowledged that the cause of the failure of penicillin to prevent congenital syphilis in all instances is not known and probably relates to a variety of factors. First, the CDC report indicated that more than half of the mothers who delivered infants born with congenital syphilis after appropriate treatment with benzathine penicillin received their therapy in the third trimester. The latter raises the possibility that, in some cases, the duration of fetal exposure to penicillin may have been too short to effect a cure.

A second important fact, which has not been applied by those responsible for recommending therapy, is that the pharmacokinetics of various antibiotics is altered during pregnancy. It is not at all unusual for serum antibiotic concentrations in the pregnant woman to be half the levels furnished by an equivalent dose of the antibiotic levels in the nonpregnant individual. Although it is not known how pregnancy affects levels of penicillin G, other penicillins such as ampicillin and piperacillin are known to achieve significantly lower serum levels in pregnant women than in their nonpregnant counterparts.

A third possible problem in pregnancy associated with the therapy of syphilis is the fact that the treponemes may have invaded the cerebrospinal fluid more often than is commonly recognized. As a result, it is possible that therapy is incorrectly deemed adequate in cases of unrecognized neurosyphilis.

A fourth area of concern is in respect to transplacental penetration of penicillins during pregnancy. Although not all penicillins traverse the placenta with equal facility, it is generally accepted that fetal blood levels equal or exceed maternal blood levels after continuous infusion or after a single dose of long-acting penicillin. However, data are usually acquired by a single measurement on a maternal-fetal pair. It would be useful to have some idea of the area under the concentration-time curve in the fetus, as compared to the mother, which could be helpful in determining the length of time fetal treponemes are exposed to bactericidal levels of drug. Interestingly, it is reported that amniotic fluid levels may reach concentrations 32 times those found in the mother because of intrauterine fetal micturition, but such a contribution would only be present in the latter half of pregnancy. We found that levels of penicillin in the amniotic fluid at 30-weeks gestation were less than 0.5 units per milliliter 20 hours after 2.4 mega units of benzathine penicillin and was not detected 10 days later, even though a further identical dose had been administered 4 days after the first dose. Furthermore, it is known that despite adequate serum levels 24 hours after benzathine penicillin treatment, infants had not attained adequate levels in the cerebrospinal fluid. Moreover, it has been reported that an infant treated in utero, and who received continuous treatment until death at 22 days, had viable treponemes in the aqueous humor. Additional work is required on the pharmacokinetic and pharmacodynamic aspects of penicillins and alternative drugs in the pregnant host, as well as in the neonate.

One further problem of penicillin therapy is the risk of the Jarisch-Herxheimer reaction. Although this phenomenon is well known in the nonpregnant host, it may be manifest in pregnant women by premature labor, occurring soon after the drug is administered, or by intrauterine fetal demise within a month after the Jarisch-Herxheimer reaction occurred. There is currently no way to predict which patients will undergo this reaction, although it may be more pronounced in individuals with secondary syphilis.

The reported failures of penicillin to prevent congenital syphilis suggest that, in the future, it may be necessary to consider the use of more prolonged courses of penicillin therapy or more aggressive follow-up of gravid patients with syphilis or infants born to mothers who have been treated during pregnancy.

Erythromycin therapy, which is utilized as an alternative for penicillin-allergic women, also presents a unique set of problems. During pregnancy, the absorption of erythromycin from the gastrointestinal tract is highly variable. For example, we found that 2 of 10 pregnant women given a 500 mg dose of enteric-coated erythromycin base did not have detectable serum levels 4 hours after drug ingestion. The levels achievable in the cord blood range from 6 to 20 percent of the maternal blood concentration. Consequently, it is necessary to administer a prolonged course of erythromycin. The CDC recommendation is for 500 mg of erythromycin four times daily for 15 days. It is believed that anything less than a 30 g course of drug is unlikely to be efficacious.

A troublesome problem associated with erythromycin therapy is the tendency for the drug to produce gastrointestinal symptoms. Patients may become noncompliant as a result of these untoward effects of the drug. This noncompliance is particularly significant in light of the recognized ineffectiveness of courses of therapy utilizing less than 30 g of drug.

Since there is no therapeutic regimen which is known to be 100 percent effective, it is essential that the physician be vigorous in the follow-up of infected patients. Patients in high risk categories should receive VDRL screening both in early pregnancy and in the third trimester. Those who have been treated for syphilis should receive monthly serologic tests for the duration of the pregnancy. A fourfold decrease in titer within 3 months is considered to be evidence of an appropriate response. Retreatment is warranted if an adequate response is not achieved.

Infants born to mothers who had syphilis during pregnancy must be carefully examined for signs of congenital syphilis and cord blood should be evaluated to establish a baseline VDRL. If the mother was treated with erythromycin during pregnancy, the baby should be treated with penicillin. According to the recommendations of the CDC, infants born to mothers with syphilis should receive repeated evaluation, at 1 month and at 3 month intervals for the subsequent 15 months, and then every 6 months until the VDRL is negative or stabilized at a low level. Evaluation should include cerebrospinal fluid examination. The recommended therapy for all infants with congenital syphilis is penicillin, and therapy should be effective for neurosyphilis. For further details regarding pediatric assessment and therapy the reader should consult the guidelines published by the CDC.

SUGGESTED READING

Anon. 1985 STD treatment guidelines. MMWR CDC Surveill Summ 1985; 34:76s–108s.

Anon. Congenital syphilis—United States 1983–1985. MMWR CDC Surveill Summ 1986; 35:625–628.

Glover DD, Winter CA, Charles D, Larsen B. Diagnostic considerations in intra-amniotic syphilis. Sex Transm Dis 1985; 12:145–149.

Jones JE Jr, Harris RE. Diagnostic evaluation of syphilis during pregnancy. Obstet Gynecol 1979; 54:611–614.

Rathburn KC. Congenital syphilis. Sex Transm Dis 1983; 10:93–99.

Thompson SE III. Treatment of syphilis in pregnancy. Sex Transm Dis 1976; 3:159–167.

YEAST VAGINITIS

DAVID CHARLES, M.D., F.A.C.O.G., F.R.C.O.G.
BRYAN LARSEN, Ph.D.

In recent years, a steady rise in the incidence of vulvovaginal mycoses has been observed. Vaginitis caused by yeast, including *Candida albicans* and to a lesser extent *Candida glabrata*, is a problem having worldwide distribution and affecting countless women. An estimated one-quarter to one-third of vaginitides with a microbial etiology are caused by yeast. Moreover, the discomfort experienced by the patient is only part of the problem. In pregnancy, the disease may occur with increased frequency and with greater severity than in healthy nongravid women and may be especially difficult to treat. Cases of chorioamnionitis due to *Candida* occur more often than is generally appreciated, and intrauterine yeast infection and abortion have been reported. Oral thrush may occur in infants born to women harboring yeast in the vagina.

Because of the importance of deep mycoses in immunocompromised hosts caused by opportunistic pathogens such as *Candida albicans*, considerable research has been conducted in recent years on the host-parasite interaction in yeast infections, and this has led to a better understanding of deep and superficial mycoses. Some advances in therapy have also been achieved, notably, a systemic azole agent has been made available for use in the United States, although it is not approved for use in pregnancy. There have been attempts to shorten the duration of topical therapy for vaginal candidiasis. Such improvements will be welcomed by both patient and physician and should enhance patient compliance.

Vaginal yeast infection is undoubtedly an opportunistic process. The mere presence of yeast in the vagina is not always associated with symptoms. It is well recognized that asymptomatic women (approximately 20 percent) harbor yeast as members of their normal vaginal flora. Whether the development of yeast vaginitis is the result of an increase in the number of viable organisms associated with the vaginal epithelium or the production by the yeast of a particular biologically active substance has not been established. Usually, large numbers of yeast are present in symptomatic women, suggesting that yeast vaginitis may be the result of an increase in the number of organisms present. However, occasionally symptoms may occur despite the presence of relatively few yeast cells. Thus, yeast may produce an end product that causes symptoms, but strains may differ in the quantity they produce.

In addition to the normal vaginal flora, the source of yeast in women with vaginitis may be the flora of the gut. Studies that use sophisticated typing methods indicate a high degree of concordance between vaginal, rectal, and oral isolates. Sexual transmission plays a minor role in vaginal candidiasis. Most cases of male genital yeast infections are the result of transmission from an infected sexual partner. Balanoposthitis can occur as a sequel to or as an antecedent of yeast vaginitis. The latter suggests that in order to prevent reinfection, yeast eradication must be instituted simultaneously in both partners. The presence or absence of a prepuce does not appear to affect the carriage rate of *Candida albicans* on the penis. Studies have shown similar penile carriage rates in circumcised and uncircumcised males. The penis probably becomes transiently colonized after intercourse, and penile cultures may be positive in 5 to 25 percent of male consorts of women with vaginal candidiasis.

The adherence of yeast to the vaginal epithelium is also believed to play an important role in the genesis of vaginitis. For example, *Candida albicans* is more adherent to vaginal epithelial cells than other *Candida* species that are less commonly associated with vaginitis. Adherence is associated with germination; cells with germ tubes or hyphae are better able to attach to epithelial cells than the ungerminated forms. In addition to morphologic considerations, the ability of yeast to produce phospholipases and extracellular proteases is considered to be an attribute of virulence. Therefore, it is appropriate to consider whether conditions occurring within the vagina can enhance these factors.

It is well known that pregnancy may be associated with an increased probability of yeast vaginitis. Specifically, during pregnancy the microenvironment of the vagina is altered in such a way as to promote yeast colonization. The prevalence of yeast colonization among asymptomatic nonpregnant women is approximately 15 percent, and this increases to 30 percent during pregnancy. The prevalence of yeast carriage progressively increases for the duration of pregnancy. With the propensity toward increased rates of colonization comes an increased likelihood of developing symptoms during pregnancy. Moreover, the clinical response to yeast infection is diminished in the pregnant host, and recrudescence of the infection is common. Studies in which volunteers were inoculated with yeast showed pregnant women to be frankly more susceptible to infection than nonpregnant controls.

There are several possible explanations for the enhanced susceptibility of the pregnant patient, but none of them has been established unequivocally as the reason for this phenomenon. The relative pathogenicity of *Candida albicans* is disputed, as it does not always fulfill Koch's postulates. This organism can exist as a saprophyte on mucous membranes, and previous damage to the vagina may be required for vaginitis to develop.

An increase in glycogen production is frequently considered to result in an increase in the potential for symptomatic vaginal candidiasis. Such an increment in glycogen levels occurs in diabetes mellitus and putatively occurs during pregnancy. Most patients who have recurrent infections have no demonstrable carbohydrate intolerance, and this fact implies that recurrent vaginal candidiasis is unlikely to be the only manifestation of occult diabetes mellitus.

Because humoral immunity is of secondary importance in yeast infection compared with cell-mediated immunity, the increased incidence of symptomatic infections in the latter part of pregnancy may be the result of reduced cell-mediated immunity in the presence of normal humoral antibodies rather than increased glycogen production. In the past it has been common to consider the deposition of glycogen and the pH of the vaginal epithelium as exerting control over the vaginal flora. Numerous questions remain about the validity of some of the earlier assumptions regarding this problem. Alterations in glucose metabolism have been cited as responsible for yeast proliferation, although this is probably more relevant to diabetic patients than to nondiabetic pregnant women. Recently, the presence of estrogen receptors in the cytosol of yeast has raised the possibility that the hormones of pregnancy may enhance the growth or pathogenicity of the yeast. This has been established for other deep fungal diseases such as cryptococcosis, and such a supposition appears plausible in the case of vaginal candidiasis. In rats, vaginal colonization can only be achieved by maintaining the animals on estrogen, further emphasizing the hormonal effects on colonization and infection.

Despite the inability to explain why yeast infection and colonization are enhanced during pregnancy, the practical implications are that gravid women who present with yeast infections during pregnancy may have symptoms that are particularly severe and may be difficult to adequately treat, and that they may be subject to recurrent disease. Therefore the physician must be prepared to expend significantly more energy in dealing with such individuals than in treating the average nonpregnant patient with vaginitis.

The initial step in treating vaginitis during pregnancy is to obtain an accurate diagnosis of the type of etiologic agent involved. When a patient presents with a curdy white discharge and plaques adherent to the vaginal walls, especially when accompanied by vulvar irritation, one automatically considers yeast vulvovaginitis. Nevertheless, treatment should not be undertaken solely on the basis of the appearance of the discharge or the clinical symptoms. A specimen of the vaginal discharge should be suspended in a drop of 10 percent potassium hydroxide, and a fishy odor, if present, should be noted. The fishy odor is associated with bacterial vaginosis, and if other appropriate symptoms are present, this condition should be treated differently from yeast vaginitis. The potassium hydroxide preparation should be warmed briefly on a Bunsen burner flame or over an alcohol lamp in order to facilitate the digestion of the epithelial cells. Upon microscopic examination under the high-dry objective (400 ×), the slide from the patient with yeast infection may show budding yeast, pseudomycelia, and possibly hyphae. There may also be an abundance of leukocytes noted in a wet-mount preparation, although some observers find that specimens from the severely affected individual may not exhibit such a feature.

In vaginal infections associated with *Candida glabrata*, no filaments are observed; rather, ovoid spores are seen. *Candida glabrata* accounts for between 5 and 15 percent of all cases of vaginal candidiasis. Utilization of methylene blue or Gram's stain is preferred to a potassium hydroxide preparation for the cytologic diagnosis of such infections.

In cases of bacterial vaginosis or trichomoniasis that

are encountered with some regularity in pregnancy, the wet-mount preparation should reveal either clue cells in the case of bacterial vaginosis or the typical flagellate protozoon forms in cases of trichomoniasis. It is most important not to assume that all cases of vaginitis occurring during pregnancy are due to yeast. Likewise, it is inappropriate to prescribe therapy without examining the patient. If desired, cultural evidence of yeast infection can readily be obtained by the use of Nickerson's medium (Biggy Agar), which is commercially available. *Candida* colonies are typically dark brown in color on this medium and are readily identified.

Several important advances in the treatment of vaginal candidiasis have improved the success rate. One of the earliest successful methods of treatment was the topical application of a 1 percent solution of gentian violet. This was the preferred therapeutic agent from the 1930s, until the introduction of nystatin in 1955. Apart from the staining of clothing associated with the use of gentian violet, some patients had hypersensitivity reactions. *Candida glabrata* is often resistant to other therapeutic modalities but is highly sensitive to this dye. Furthermore, thorough vaginal and cervical painting with a 1 percent aqueous solution of gentian violet brings about rapid and effective symptomatic relief of the infection.

Nystatin represented one of the greatest advances in antifungal therapy in its time and is still available in oral form and as vaginal tablets. Nystatin is a polyene antibiotic that binds to sterols in fungal membranes, thereby causing leakage of intracellular components. It is not absorbed from the vagina and has long been considered the preferred agent for the treatment of *Candida albicans* infections in pregnancy. The oral form is not very well absorbed, and so its use is limited primarily to intraluminal therapy. The drug is rarely associated with hypersensitivity reactions and is usually well tolerated. The 15-day course of therapy generally required is, of course, a drawback, and as stated earlier, some of the newer imidazole agents have obviated the need for such a prolonged course of therapy (Table 1).

It has been demonstrated that nystatin is associated with a higher rate of relapse than the preferred imidazole drugs. However, it should be noted that more information is available about its safety in the pregnant patient than is available for the imidazoles. Because the imidazoles are absorbed from the vagina and little is known about their teratogenic potential in humans, their use during the first trimester of pregnancy is not recommended. In addition, the systemic antifungal, ketoconazole, which is effective against vaginal candidiasis, is not employed during pregnancy.

The imidazoles have a broad antifungal spectrum in vitro, and these compounds are highly efficacious when applied topically against *Candida* species. The imidazole derivatives inhibit the biosynthesis of ergosterol, the major sterol present in membranes of fungi, and thus these drugs affect the integrity and function of the cell membrane of *Candida albicans*.

There is currently considerable effort within the pharmaceutical industry to produce agents that are more efficacious, safer, and easier to administer than compounds already established for the therapy of vaginal candidiasis.

TABLE 1 Summary of Available Antifungals

Agent	*FDA Rating**	*Dosage*	*Comments*
Nystatin	A	1 (100,000 U) tablet intravaginally daily for 2 weeks	Oral form is not well absorbed and is not indicated for vaginitis
Miconazole	B	100-mg intravaginal suppository for 7 days or 200-mg intravaginal suppository for 3 days	Known to be absorbed from the vagina; avoid during first trimester of pregnancy
Econazole	—	—	Not indicated for vaginitis
Butoconazole	C	5 g 2% cream intravaginally nightly for 6 days	—
Ketoconazole	C	—	Not indicated for vaginitis
Clotrimazole	C	100-mg intravaginal tablet daily for 7 days	—
	B	500-mg intravaginal tablet, one dose only	—

* A: Controlled studies show no risk. Adequate, well-controlled studies in pregnant women have failed to demonstrate risk to the fetus.
B: No evidence of risk in humans. Either animal findings show risk but human findings do not, or if no adequate human studies have been done, animal findings are negative.
C: Risk cannot be ruled out. Human studies are lacking, and animal studies are either positive for fetal risk or lacking as well. However, potential benefits may outweigh the potential risk.

Despite the proliferation of different imidazole antifungal agents, the cure rates attributed to them in comparable superficial mycoses are very similar. Thus, clinical and mycologic cure rates for vaginal candidiasis are in the range of 85 to 95 percent after vaginal applications of clotrimazole, miconazole, econazole, or ketoconazole.

Miconazole nitrate is available as a 2 percent vaginal cream or 100-mg suppositories that can be used daily for 7 days for the treatment of vaginal candidiasis. The maximum absorption from the vagina is only about 1 percent. Adverse effects following topical therapy for vaginal yeast infections include pruritus or irritation in about 5 percent of patients, and less frequently headaches or skin rash. Pelvic cramps occur in about 1 of every 500 patients. Miconazole is considered safe for use in pregnancy but should be avoided for the therapy of yeast infections in the first trimester because of the propensity of this compound to produce pelvic cramps in some patients.

When antifungal therapy is instituted in the pregnant patient, several formulations are available. If vaginal tablets or suppositories are prescribed, it may be necessary to also prescribe a cream preparation if the patient has vulvar symptoms. Furthermore, it should be noted that the recommended dosage or duration of therapy may be different for the pregnant patient and the nonpregnant patient because yeast vaginitis has a tendency toward refractoriness in pregnancy.

Ten years ago the duration of most forms of therapy for vulvovaginal yeast infections was at least 10 days. Since then newer compounds have resulted in curtailment of therapy to a few days. Experience has shown that prolonged courses of therapy resulted in poor patient compliance and a high incidence of recurrent infections. The simpler and shorter a course of therapy, the greater the chances are that the patient will comply with the directions of prescribed treatment.

Although the imidazoles are usually the preferred therapy, some physicians advocate the use of boric acid powder. In one double-blind study one group of patients was treated with 600 mg of boric acid powder and the second group with ground tablets (100,000 U) of nystatin daily. The drugs were administered intravaginally in identical gelatin capsules, one capsule per day. The 7- to 10-day cure rate for boric acid was 92 percent compared with 64 percent for nystatin, and the 30-day cure rate was 72 percent for boric acid and 50 percent for nystatin. Serum boron levels were less than 1 μg per milliliter, which was considered to be below the level of toxic effects.

In addition to antimycotic therapy, affected patients must avoid wearing insulating clothing, most specifically nylon underwear and pantyhose, since they are often known to precipitate exacerbations of symptoms in individuals who harbor *Candida albicans* as a vaginal inhabitant. Such clothing decreases ventilation and increases perineal moisture and thereby encourages replication of the yeast. Likewise, deodorant sprays and perfumed toilet paper should be avoided, as they have been known to produce an exacerbation of symptoms.

Women who do not adequately respond to therapy should be reexamined to determine if they still have yeast vaginitis. Other predisposing factors such as diabetes mellitus should also be considered in reassessing the patient. It may be appropriate at this point either to treat the patient's sexual partner with antifungal cream or to recommend the use of condoms until therapy has cleared the symptoms. A repeat culture rather than clinical resolution of symptoms and signs furnishes the best criterion for cure.

SUGGESTED READING

Friedrich E, Derman R, eds. Advances in candida management: a symposium. The Female Patient 1986; Special Edition:5–56.

Hill LVH, Embil JA. Vaginitis: current microbiologic and clinical concepts. Can Med Assoc J 1986; 134:321–331.

Kaufman RH (Guest Editor). Vulvovaginal candidiasis: a symposium. J Reprod Med 1986; 31(Suppl):639–671.

Montes LF, Wilborn WH. Fungus-host relationship in candidiasis. Arch Dermatol 1985; 121:119–124.

Sweet RL (Guest Editor). International symposium on vulvovaginal mycoses. Am J Obstet Gynecol 1985; 152:921–970.

URINARY TRACT INFECTIONS

SUSAN M. COX, M.D.
F. GARY CUNNINGHAM, M.D.

Urinary tract infections are common during pregnancy and may involve both the upper and lower tracts. *Asymptomatic bacteriuria*, or *covert bacteriuria*, defined as actively multiplying bacteria within the urinary tract in a woman without symptoms, complicates 2 to 10 percent of all pregnancies. This prevalence is increased in women of lower socioeconomic status and those with diabetes and is twofold greater in those with sickle cell trait. Symptomatic urinary tract infections, including cystitis and acute pyelonephritis, complicate 1 to 3 percent of all pregnancies. *Acute cystitis* by definition is confined to the bladder, is more common in the second trimester, and probably has a lower recurrence rate following treatment than covert bacteriuria. *Pyelonephritis*, the most common and serious acute medical complication requiring hospitalization during pregnancy, frequently develops from untreated asymptomatic bacteriuria and may be associated with significant maternal and fetal morbidity and mortality. There is inferential evidence that pregnant women with pyelonephritis are more susceptible to the deleterious effects of endotoxemia.

ETIOLOGY

An important tenet in care of urinary tract infections during pregnancy is prevention. Covert bacteriuria usually precedes pregnancy, which does not predispose to acquisition of bacteriuria per se. In fact, less than 1 percent of pregnant women will actually acquire bacteriuria if their initial screening culture is sterile. Pregnancy does, however, predispose to the development of pyelonephritis because of the obstruction and urinary stasis associated with it. Hydroureter and hydronephrosis are caused by mechanical compression of the enlarging uterus as well as smooth muscle relaxation induced by progesterone. Additionally, pregnancy-induced glucosuria and aminoaciduria produce an excellent milieu for bacterial proliferation.

The most frequently identified uropathogens in pregnancy-related urinary tract infections are *Escherichia coli*, *Klebsiella pneumoniae*, *Enterobacter*, and *Proteus mirabilis*. These organisms probably gain access to the urinary tract by ascending infection from the colonized vaginal vestibule or urethral meatus. It is now believed that the initial event necessary for significant colonization of uroepithelium is bacterial adhesion via fimbriae, which are hair-like surface appendages. Most Enterobacteriaceae contain type I fimbriae that adhere to mannose receptors on cell surface glycoproteins. Bacteria then multiply to reach critical concentrations necessary to cause infection. More recently, it has been shown that 10 to 15 percent of *Escherichia coli* have P fimbriae that adhere to α-D-galactopyranosyl-(1$\rightarrow$4)-β-D-galactopyranoside receptors on the uroepithelial cell. This is significant, since almost all nonobstructive pyelonephritis is caused by such P-fimbriated organisms.

ASYMPTOMATIC BACTERIURIA

Diagnosis

Any one of several laboratory techniques is used to screen for asymptomatic urinary tract infections. The Griess test, first described in 1879, is based on bacterial reduction of nitrates normally present in urine. A simple, accurate, colorimetric dipstick is available for the test (Chemstrip LN, Biodynamics); however, false-positive findings are frequent and generally attributed to contaminants. False-negative results may be seen with some pathogens, such as streptococci, which do not produce nitrites. Recently, Lenke and Van Dorsten evaluated the efficacy of nitrite dipsticks in 56 pregnant women at risk for pyelonephritis. Of 146 cultures, 12 percent were positive for uropathogens, but nitrites were present in only 22 percent of these. Thus, the nitrite test proved neither sensitive nor cost-effective.

Bac-T-Screen (Marion Scientific Division), a semiautomated instrument, has recently been employed for prenatal screening. Incubation is not required, and results are available in 3 minutes. Moreover, the test is not affected by antimicrobials. The Bac-T-Screen correctly detected 97 percent of urine specimens with not less than 10^5 colonies per milliliter, 77 percent with not less than 10^4 and less than 10^5 colonies per milliliter, and 28 percent of those with not greater than 10^3 colonies per milliliter. False-negative results were seen predominantly with gram-positive isolates, presumably due to their lower affinity for the safranin dye.

The most accurate simple method to identify urinary tract infection is culture via plate-streaking using a quantitative loop. Demonstration of a single uropathogen in significant numbers, considered by most to be at least 100,000 organisms per milliliter, is diagnostic. False-positive cultures are reduced by prompt processing and careful patient instruction in collection technique.

Bacteriuria may be either urinary or renal in origin. The first test utilized to localize the site of bacteriuria was the bladder washout technique, first reported in 1966. In 1974, an immunofluorescence test was described for detection of *antibody-coated bacteria* of renal origin. This noninvasive technique correlates well with results using the bladder washout technique and ureteral catheterization. Although this technique is simple, reliable, and relatively sensitive, with an overall accuracy rate of about 90 percent, its clinical utility has not been defined.

Treatment

More than 20 years ago, Kass defined asymptomatic bacteriuria as more than 10^5 bacteria per milliliter obtained with two successive midstream urine cultures. However, for clinical purposes, treatment is recommended after a single positive culture. Recent evidence suggests that 10^5 bacteria per milliliter is too restrictive and that fewer organisms may reflect infection rather than just urethral contamination. This has been our experience at Parkland Hospital, as we have seen a substantial number of renal infections follow untreated bacteriuria in patients with 30,000 to 50,000 colonies per milliliter.

It is now well established that eradication of asymptomatic bacteriuria appreciably reduces the risk of acute pyelonephritis and its complications. The choice of initial antimicrobial is empirical, and several drugs have been shown to be safe and efficacious (Table 1). In one study, Whalley and Cunningham reported an overall cure rate of 85 percent—65 percent were initially cured with 14-day drug therapy and an additional 20 percent with treatment of the first relapse. This compared favorably with the 90 percent cure rate obtained with continuous therapy. Thus, the short course is preferred because of decreased cost, equivalent efficacy, diminished toxicity, and patient convenience.

In order to assess the therapeutic response to antimicrobials, it is important to document sterile urine after treatment. Follow-up cultures should be obtained at least once, 1 to 2 weeks after therapy, to detect recurrent infections. Recurrent infections—either relapses or reinfections—should be treated, since one-fourth of these women will develop acute pyelonephritis. *Relapse* is recurrent infection identified shortly after completing a therapeutic course and with the same organism as was identified before treatment. These types of recurrences are best

TABLE 1 Antimicrobial Treatment of Urinary Infections Complicating Pregnancy

Clinical Syndrome	*Drug*	*Dosage*
Asymptomatic bacteriuria	Nitrofurantoin	200 mg PO at bedtime for 10 days
	Ampicillin + probenecid	2 g + 1 g PO
	Sulfisoxazole	2 g PO
Asymptomatic bacteriuria or cystitis	Nitrofurantoin	100 mg four times daily for 10 days
	Ampicillin	500 mg four times daily for 7 days
	Cephalexin	250–500 mg four times daily for 7 days
	Sulfisoxazole	500 mg four times daily for 7 days
Acute pyelonephritis	Ampicillin	2 g IV q6h
	Cephalothin	2 g IV q6h
	Mezlocillin	3 g IV q6h
	Gentamicin	3–5 mg/kg/day in three divided doses

treated based on previous in vitro antimicrobial sensitivities. *Reinfection* is recurrent infection after eradication of the original bacteria. Occasionally, a different organism is identified, but usually *Escherichia coli* is again isolated. Reinfection is frequently limited to the bladder and tends to occur at intervals more remote from the initial infection. In order to detect reinfection, some advocate monthly surveillance cultures for the remainder of gestation. These women should then be given another short course of antimicrobials.

Choice of Antimicrobial

The first antimicrobials utilized to treat bacteriuria were the sulfonamides, which are quite effective and still widely used. They have proven efficacy and safety for use in pregnancy. They are structural analogues and competitive antagonists of para-aminobenzoic acid that block bacterial folic acid synthesis. Side effects include allergic reactions, hemolysis with glucose-6-phosphate dehydrogenase deficiency, and, rarely, blood dyscrasias. Renal damage from deposition of crystalline aggregates (associated with some of the older sulfonamides) is rarely seen with the newer analogues. Sulfonamides compete with bilirubin for albumin binding and increase the likelihood of neonatal kernicterus if given to a woman shortly before delivery.

Nitrofurantoin has also been widely studied and is safe, effective, and inexpensive. Its mechanism of antimicrobial activity is unknown, although it inhibits several bacterial enzymes. The recommended dosage is 50 to 100 mg four times a day for 7 to 14 days. However, we have given 100 mg at bedtime for 10 days with equivalent success. Nitrofurantoin is almost completely absorbed in the upper gastrointestinal tract and, therefore, does not alter the lower gastrointestinal tract flora appreciably. Following administration of 100 mg orally, peak serum concentrations are 2 μg per milliliter and urinary concentraons average 150 μg per milliliter. The most common untoward effects include nausea, vomiting, and diarrhea. Serious side effects are rare but include acute interstitial pneumonitis, cholestatic jaundice, and hepatocellular damage; hemolysis also may occur in women with glucose-6-phosphate dehydrogenase deficiency.

Ampicillin is a Federal Drug Administration (FDA) Category B drug that is well absorbed orally and is given in a dosage of 500 mg four times daily for 7 to 14 days. It is a safe and effective broad-spectrum penicillin whose major site of action is against the bacterial cell wall. It contains a beta-lactam bond that is a structural analogue of D-alanyl-D-alanine, which is a part of muramic acid, a major cell wall component. Ampicillin interferes with alanine transpeptidation, a process that "cements" the cell wall. Beta-lactams also affect penicillin-binding proteins involved in cell division and in maintaining cell shape. Major side effects involve penicillin hypersensitivity, including skin rashes, anaphylaxis, serum sickness, and vaginal candidiasis. Recently, concern has evolved because a number of microorganisms have developed in vitro resistance to the drug based on serum levels. For most urinary tract infections, this does not predict in vivo efficacy, since ampicillin concentration at the site of infection is many fold greater than in serum. For example, following an oral dose of 500 mg, peak serum concentrations are

3 μg per milliliter, whereas urine concentrations are 350 μg per milliliter.

The first generation cephalosporins, especially cephalexin, have proved safe and effective for these urinary tract infections. Most of these, like the penicillins, are in FDA Category B. Their basic structure is a beta-lactam ring to which is fused a dihydrothiazine ring, and their action is inhibition of cell wall synthesis, similar to that of the penicillins. Cephalexin is given four times daily in doses of 250 or 500 mg for 7 to 14 days. Following the 250-mg dose, the peak serum concentration is 9 μg per milliliter, and the urine concentration is 800 μg per milliliter. There is no reported fetal toxicity, and maternal adverse reactions are similar to those seen with penicillin.

Single-Dose Therapy

Several studies have evaluated single-dose therapy for asymptomatic bacteriuria in pregnancy. Williams and Smith used single-dose regimens and reported a 77 percent cure rate with 1 g of streptomycin given intramuscularly. However, Brumfitt and colleagues reported only 44 percent cures with single-dose cephaloridine, 2 g intramuscularly. Harris and colleagues gave a single 2-g oral dose of ampicillin plus 1 g probenecid and cured 71 percent of their pregnant patients with bacteriuria. They also used single-dose nitrofurantoin, 200 mg (73 percent cured), sulfisoxazole, 2 g (75 percent cured), and cephalexin, 2 g plus 1 g probenecid (55 percent cured). Although these reports are promising, the number of women studied is small, and further trials are necessary before single-dose therapy is widely recommended.

CYSTITIS

The diagnosis of acute cystitis is based on urinary frequency, dysuria, urgency, and suprapubic discomfort without systemic symptoms. There is an accompanying microscopic pyuria and bacteriuria and a subsequently positive urine culture. Uncomplicated cystitis responds readily to any of the regimens previously discussed. There are now a number of reports in which single-dose antimicrobials were used successfully for acute cystitis. In pregnancy, kanamycin, 500 mg intramuscularly, amoxicillin, 3 g orally with 1 g probenecid, or trimethoprim (480 mg)-sulfamethoxazole (2.4 g) orally, all have cure rates of nearly 85 percent. These regimens decrease drug cost and toxicity while solving problems with compliance. Moreover, they reduce any significant alterations of vaginal and gastrointestinal flora and are well tolerated. Our reluctance to recommend single-dose therapy comes from our report of more than 500 women hospitalized for antepartum pyelonephritis. Nearly 40 percent of these women had symptoms of lower urinary tract infection, and we are concerned that some women thought initially to have cystitis may indeed have had early pyelonephritis, the treatment for which is certainly not one dose.

PYELONEPHRITIS

About 1 percent of all pregnancies are complicated by pyelonephritis, and most of these women are past midgestation. Clinically these women have fever, chills, flank pain, nausea, and vomiting. Examination discloses fever and costovertebral angle tenderness, and microscopic examination of unspun urine confirms bacteriuria and pyuria with or without leukocyte casts. Quantitative urine cultures yield more than 100,000 colonies per milliliter of a single organism, and blood cultures are positive in 10 to 15 percent of cases. *Escherichia coli*, *Klebsiella pneumoniae*, *Enterobacter*, and *Proteus* are the most commonly isolated organisms. *E. coli* is isolated in 60 to 80 percent of all cases.

Acute pyelonephritis is a potentially catastrophic infection for both mother and fetus. Thus, prompt recognition and treatment are of paramount importance to reduce mortality and morbidity. These women are usually severely dehydrated and unable to tolerate oral medication because of nausea and vomiting; therefore hospitalization is mandatory (Table 2). Careful monitoring is necessary to detect serious life-threatening complications that are common in pregnancy. Close observation with frequent assessment of vital signs is central to their care.

Initial treatment is directed toward restoration of the contracted blood volume. Prompt administration of intravenous crystalloids, either physiologic saline or lactated Ringer's solution, is started along with antimicrobials. Fluids should be given rapidly over the first few hours to ensure adequate urinary output defined as at least 50 ml per hour. A modicum of laboratory evaluation is essential and includes a complete blood count, serum electrolytes and creatinine concentrations, as well as cultures of urine and blood. For the uncomplicated case, further laboratory work is seldom necessary, but for complicated infections that will be discussed below, other considerations are given.

TABLE 2 Management Plan for Women with Antepartum Pyelonephritis

Uncomplicated
Hospitalize
CBC, serum creatinine, electrolytes, urine and blood cultures
Monitor vital signs frequently for at least 24 hours
Monitor urine output
Give intravenous crystalloids to maintain urinary output greater than 30 ml/hr
Give parenteral antimicrobials
Complicated
Chest film if dyspnea or tachypnea is found
Foley catheter if oliguria develops
Imaging studies if significant fever persists after 48 hours
Follow-up
Repeat CBC and serum creatinine at 48 hours
Begin oral antimicrobials after patient is afebrile for 24 hours
Repeat urine culture 1 to 2 weeks after therapy

In the majority of cases, rapid clinical improvement follows intravenous hydration and treatment with antimicrobials. Indeed, 85 percent of the women are asymptomatic and afebrile after 48 hours, and the remainder by 72 to 96 hours. Failure to improve clinically within the first 72 hours suggests underlying obstructive uropathy from anatomic anomalies or more commonly from urolithiasis. Women with delayed response may require radiologic urinary tract visualization to exclude obstruction or renal abscesses.

The choice of antimicrobial therapy is empirical. However, for women who have had a previous urinary tract infection during the pregnancy, in vitro sensitivities should be used to select therapy. For almost two decades, ampicillin has been used successfully for treatment, and we give 2 g intravenously by piggyback infusion every 6 hours until the patient has been afebrile for 24 hours. At this time, oral ampicillin, 500 mg four times daily, is substituted and continued after discharge for a total course of 10 days. This regimen is safe and effective and, as previously reported by Cunningham and colleagues at Charity Hospital in New Orleans, 85 percent of women so treated were afebrile within 48 hours. However, in the past several years, many of the uropathogens that cause community-acquired pyelonephritis have been found to be resistant to ampicillin as determined by in vitro sensitivities. Specifically, in 1986 at Parkland Memorial Hospital, only 17 percent of the *E. coli*, 1 percent of *K. pneumoniae*, and no *Enterobacter* isolated from these women were sensitive to ampicillin in vitro. Therefore, it seems reasonable to prescribe antimicrobials to which bacteria are more sensitive. Unfortunately, there are few studies in which the efficacy of other regimens has been evaluated.

In our hospital, concern for in vitro resistance frequently prompts the addition of an aminoglycoside—gentamicin or tobramycin—to ampicillin therapy. Aminoglycosides are composed of two or more amino sugars connected by a glycoside linkage to a central hexose nucleus. They are bactericidal and inhibit protein synthesis via activity on the 30S and 50S ribosomal subunit. They are active against gram-negative rods and are the mainstay of therapy for patients with serious nosocomial infections, especially with *Pseudomonas aeruginosa*.

We are concerned with the use of aminoglycosides in antepartum pyelonephritis. First, nearly 20 percent of these women have significant renal dysfunction, although transient. Nephrotoxicity as well as the potential for ototoxicity in both mother and fetus are worrisome aspects of such combinations, and serial monitoring of serum creatinine levels is mandatory. In addition, many recommend serial measurements of peak and trough aminoglycoside concentrations, with appropriate alterations in dosage. Second, gram-negative bacteria can develop resistance to the aminoglycosides via either (1) ribosomal alteration, causing inability of the drug to bind to the ribosome, (2) decreased cell permeability, preventing entry of the drug, or (3) development of R factors (plasmids) that govern the production of enzymes that inactivate aminoglycosides. The dose recommended is 3 to 5 mg per kilogram per 24 hours in three divided parenteral doses. Peak levels of gentamicin should be less than 10 μg per milliliter and trough levels less than 2 μg per milliliter. Aminoglycosides are widely distributed in the mother as well as the fetus. Maternal side effects include ototoxicity characterized by tinnitus or a feeling of fullness in the ear, which may be an early sign of potential hearing loss, and nephrotoxicity, which is usually manifested by proteinuria or elevated serum creatinine level.

Given current microbial sensitivities, a number of cephalosporins are reasonable alternatives to ampicillin. These beta-lactam antibiotics are characterized by substituent groups added to 7-amino-cephalosporinic acid. Pharmacologically, they interfere with a terminal step in bacterial wall synthesis and probably increase cell wall breakdown. They are bactericidal against both gram-positive and gram-negative organisms. Most cephalosporins are excreted unchanged by both glomerular filtration and proximal tubular secretion. Therefore, renal dysfunction delays their excretion, and dosage adjustments may be necessary. Bacterial resistance arises from beta-lactamase (cephalosporinase), which disrupts the beta-lactam ring and inactivates the antimicrobial. Maternal toxicity is minimal, and the most worrisome are severe hypersensitivity reactions that include anaphylaxis. Thrombophlebitis at the infusion site is more common than with other antimicrobials and usually can be prevented by slowly injecting a diluted solution or by alternating veins. At least with some cephalosporins, there is synergistic nephrotoxicity when they are given concurrently with aminoglycosides, and therefore caution should be exercised with this combination. As with the penicillins, there are no apparent fetal risks, and there is no evidence of teratogenicity.

We have had considerable experience with cephalothin, 2 g, given by intravenous piggyback infusion every 6 hours. The clinical response is equivalent to that for ampicillin. However, antimicrobial resistance, determined by in vitro microbial sensitivities, has been reported with cephalothin. Additionally, Faro and colleagues have published their experiences with cefuroxime, which was reported to be equally satisfactory.

The extended spectrum ureidopenicillins, mezlocillin and piperacillin, are broad-spectrum semisynthetic penicillinase-resistant penicillins that are classified as FDA Category B. They are bactericidal and interfere with cell wall synthesis. Their in vitro spectrum includes gram-negative and gram-positive organisms and encompasses the common uropathogens. Specifically, at our hospital 78 percent of *E. coli*, 84 percent of *K. pneumoniae*, and 85 percent of *Enterobacter* are sensitive to mezlocillin, while 75 percent of *E. coli*, 84 percent of *K. pneumoniae*, and 81 percent of *Enterobacter* are sensitive to piperacillin. Like other penicillins, excretion of these drugs is primarily by glomerular filtration and tubular secretion. Serum concentrations 2 hours after 2 g given intravenously average 20 μg per milliliter, whereas concentrations of active drug in urine exceed 4,000 μg per milliliter. Low concentrations are found in cord blood, amniotic fluid, and breast milk. Adverse effects include hypersensitivity reactions, gastrointestinal upset, and rarely bleeding disorders and neuromuscular hyperirritability.

During a recent 6-month period, we treated 100 women for antepartum pyelonephritis with mezlocillin, 3 g intravenously every 6 hours, and all were clinically cured by 96 hours. One patient required the addition of an aminoglycoside, and she was subsequently found to have focal segmental pyelonephritis. There were no apparent toxic side effects.

COMPLICATIONS OF PYELONEPHRITIS

Acute antepartum pyelonephritis can be a devastating disease, both to the mother and the fetus. As many as one-fourth of these women with severe infection have evidence of multisystem derangement. Although these complications are more frequent when there is obstruction from urinary calculi, this is certainly not necessary for severe sequelae to occur that include pyonephrosis and perinephric cellulitis or abscesses. In these critically ill women, it should be remembered that complications tend to be multiple.

Urinary Calculi

If a prompt clinical response (defined as stepwise defervescence in 48 to 72 hours) is not forthcoming, then consideration should be given to a search for obstructing lesions of the urinary tract. In most cases, these are the result of urinary calculi, the removal of which will usually be followed by resolution of infection. In some cases, a double-J stent placed by means of cystoscopy relieves the obstruction. Therefore, for the woman who is persistently febrile after 72 hours of appropriate therapy, a plain abdominal x-ray film is recommended. Nearly 90 percent of renal stones are radio-opaque and thus diagnosed by this simple procedure. Certainly, the benefits of finding calculi outweigh any minimal risk for the fetus exposed to radiation. In the event that this examination is nonproductive, a modified intravenous pyelogram is done. A single radiograph is obtained 20 to 30 minutes after contrast injection, and this usually outlines the collecting system sufficiently well to visualize any structural anomalies. Occasionally, a second or third film is needed if there is unilateral urinary tract nonvisualization, which may represent an end-stage obstructed kidney with pyonephrosis. For some, retrograde pyelography is needed to outline the obstruction. In some of these cases, calculi frequently coexist with pyonephrosis, and removal of the infected kidney may be lifesaving.

In a small number of women, bacterial infection spreads beyond the renal capsule and causes perinephric cellulitis. In its earliest stages, a phlegmon is formed, and with intensive antimicrobial therapy, resolution follows in several days. In some, there is suppuration of this space, and surgical drainage of the perinephric abscess becomes necessary. These latter infections are quite serious and emphasize the need for continuing investigation in the woman who does not have the typical prompt response to antimicrobial treatment.

We have employed renal ultrasonography and limited abdominal computed tomography (CT) as well as magnetic resonance imaging to better characterize these lesions. CT is modified by the number of "cuts," since fetal dosimetry with a standard examination may be as high as 5 rads. The use of magnetic resonance imaging appears promising, and although it is probably safe, it is not widely available at this time. Using these methods, other complications have now been identified in some of the nonresponding patients. *Emphysematous pyelonephritis* is characterized by a particularly virulent infection with gas-producing Enterobacteriaceae and results in a gangrenous kidney, for which lifesaving nephrectomy is mandatory. *Acute segmental pyelonephritis*, also called *lobar nephronia*, probably represents a segmental intrarenal phlegmon and may cause a significantly delayed clinical response. In most cases continued antimicrobial therapy is followed by resolution, and surgical intervention is not necessary unless suppuration is documented.

Septicemic Shock

Bacteremia can be demonstrated in as many as 10 to 15 percent of women with severe antepartum pyelonephritis, but fortunately septic shock is rare. Continuing hypotension and diminished perfusion as a consequence of endotoxemia must be differentiated from hypotension caused by dehydration from fever, nausea, and vomiting. Although many women with pyelonephritis have other stigmata of endotoxemia, few have continuing hypotension after fluid resuscitation, and those who do are seriously ill. They generally manifest the full-blown septic shock syndrome, with capillary endothelial damage and severely diminished systemic vascular resistance with low cardiac output. Fortunately, in most cardiac output is restored after intravenous fluid therapy, and vasopressor drugs are rarely required. In general, most of the complications that follow are probably variants of the septic shock syndrome and are endotoxin-mediated.

Renal Dysfunction

In a prospective study of 220 women with antepartum pyelonephritis, one-fourth had seriously diminished glomerular filtration rates defined by creatinine clearances of less than 80 ml per minute corrected for body surface area. This dysfunction is transient, and generally there is return to normal within several days. However, in some women, diminished glomerular filtration persists for several weeks. It is likely that such dysfunction is mediated by the lipopolysaccharide of endotoxin, which is a known nephrotoxin. Management includes close observation with continued intravenous fluid resuscitation, antimicrobials, and serial determination of serum creatinine levels. Attention is given to selection of antimicrobials that do not have substantial nephrotoxicity or to appropriate reduction in dosage of those that do.

Hematologic Changes

There is now abundant evidence that endotoxemia causes hemolysis in these women, and this may result in moderate to severe anemia. Erythrocyte transfusions are seldom indicated; however, they may be necessary in women who have hypoxemia from pulmonary dysfunction, as described below. It is clinically significant that many of these women have worrisome anemia after an episode of pyelonephritis, and it is not unusual for the hematocrit to be as low as 25 ml per deciliter. Unless renal dysfunction persists, either from previous underlying chronic renal disease or from delayed recovery from endotoxin-induced dysfunction, restoration of the hemoglobin mass is usually prompt if there is adequate iron.

Other clinically significant hematologic abnormalities are seldom identified. However, mild aberrations are frequent, and these include thrombocytopenia and minimally elevated fibrinogen-fibrin split products. Rarely endotoxin activates the coagulation cascade to produce disseminated intravascular coagulation. As with any other consumptive coagulopathy, treatment is directed toward eliminating the infection, and unless operative intervention is planned, corrections of the coagulopathy follow treatment and blood component replacement is unnecessary.

Pulmonary Injury

Approximately 1 to 2 percent of women with severe antepartum pyelonephritis develop respiratory insufficiency. Pulmonary injury is also caused by endotoxin, and clinically it is similar to other variants of the so-called *adult respiratory distress syndrome*. Endotoxin results in altered alveolocapillary membrane permeability with subsequent pulmonary edema. Fortunately, in most women, clinical aberrations are transient and usually respond to increased oxygen concentration delivered by face mask.

This complication can be life-threatening, and in addition to monitoring blood pressure, pulse rate, and urinary output, careful attention is given to the respiratory rate and symptoms of dyspnea. Most women with pulmonary injury have clinical manifestations within 48 hours of hospital admission, and it is recommended that tachypnea be investigated by chest x-ray film and arterial blood gas analysis. Prompt recognition with appropriate respiratory therapy, which in a few cases includes intubation and mechanical ventilation, will probably prevent severe hypoxemia, which may cause fetal death, preterm labor, or possibly both.

Pulmonary injury, like other complications discussed here, frequently coexists with other disorders. For example, women with evidence of pulmonary capillary injury frequently have associated hematologic aberrations, renal dysfunction, and other abnormalities when compared with women without respiratory symptoms. These syndromes are more common in women with bacteremia; however, infections caused by *K. pneumoniae* seem more likely to cause them. It is not known whether or not prompt institution of antimicrobials directed against this organism prevents these complications. Unfortunately, we have been unable to identify any risk factors that prospectively identify a woman at risk for these complications. Although in general these women tend to be more seriously ill, most factors indicating severity of illness are only recognized in retrospect or at discovery and thus are not prognostic.

SUGGESTED READING

Bailey RR, Peddie BA, Bishop V. Comparison of single dose with a five-day course of trimethoprim for asymptomatic (covert) bacteriuria of pregnancy. NZ Med J 1986; 99:501–503.

Cunningham FG, Morris GB, Mickal A. Acute pyelonephritis of pregnancy: a clinical review. Obstet Gynecol 1973; 42:112–116.

Gilstrap LC, Cunningham FG, Whalley PJ. Acute pyelonephritis in pregnancy: an anterospective study. Obstet Gynecol 1981; 57:409–413.

Harris RE, Gilstrap LC. Cystitis during pregnancy: a distinct clinical entity. Obstet Gynecol 1981; 57:578–580.

Lenke RR, Van Dorsten JP. The efficacy of the nitrate test and microscopic urinalysis in predicting urine culture results. Am J Obstet Gynecol 1981; 140:427–429.

Roberts JA. Pathophysiology of pyelonephritis. Infect Surg 1986; Nov:633–638.

Whalley PJ, Cunningham FG. Short term vs. continuous antimicrobial therapy for asymptomatic bacteriuria in pregnancy. Obstet Gynecol 1977; 49:262–265.

OBSTETRIC HEMORRHAGES

POSTPARTUM HEMORRHAGE

JAMES A. O'LEARY, M.D.

The occurrence of a postpartum hemorrhage (PPH) is universally recognized as one of the most serious problems in obstetrics. Proper management of the third stage of labor is the obstetrician's greatest responsibility, since more women die from accidents in this stage than in the other two combined. Many cases are unpredictable, and the severity can become torrential in the matter of a few moments.

PPH is not a good term, since hemorrhage is often formidable before the third stage is complete. A better term is third stage hemorrhage. Hemorrhage in the mother has been and always will be a prime cause of mortality in pregnancy. Although the incidence of PPH as a cause of maternal death has improved dramatically, the event can still be catastrophic. The two pitfalls of increased uterine blood flow (500 ml per minute) and increased cardiac output of 20 to 25 percent going to the uterus place the mother at double jeopardy. With cesarean section rates increasing dramatically to as high as 25 to 35 percent, many more mothers are at much greater risk for hemorrhage. In most contemporary studies, hemorrhage accounts for roughly one-third of maternal deaths. Emergency hysterectomy is necessary following roughly 1 percent of cesarean sections and 0.04 to 0.3 percent of all deliveries. The notable trends are the disappearance of uteroplacental apoplexy (Couvelaire's uterus) and simple dehiscence of a uterine scar as indications for performing hysterectomy and the emergence of uterine atony and placenta accreta as the major indications. In two large surveys, uterine atony was the responsible factor in the majority of cases.

In view of the continuing incidence of emergency cesarean hysterectomy and puerperal hysterectomy in the management of PPH, it seems opportune to suggest that the teaching of techniques for the management of this problem be amended. Rather than warning of the risk of last resort hysterectomy and uterine packing, emphasis should be placed on the early use of prostaglandins for the medical management of PPH and surgical techniques such as uterine artery and hypogastric artery ligation.

DEFINITION AND INCIDENCE

The definition of PPH is inadequate. In view of the normal degree of hypervolemia during pregnancy, which increases blood volume by 1,000 to 2,000 ml for the average sized individual, a new definition is in order.

The definition of a 500-ml blood loss or more after completion of the third stage remains firmly entrenched. However, almost half of the women who deliver vaginally and almost all who undergo cesarean section fulfill this criterion. Changes in the hematocrit can be deceiving. A woman can tolerate the loss of 500 to 1,000 ml of blood without significant decrease in her hematocrit. A more realistic definition of PPH is a blood loss of 1,000 ml.

Dramatic changes can occur in the patient's vital signs. Obvious tachycardia and hypotension are signs of significant hypovolemia; however, the reverse can be most misleading. A normal blood pressure, or even hypertension, does not preclude dangerous hypovolemia. The pulse rate can also be misleading. It may be falsely elevated or normal to even slow in the presence of significant hypovolemia. Nonetheless, the rule of a pulse rate over 100 beats per minute and a blood loss greater than 1,000 ml is still most reliable for judging PPH.

Hemorrhage after the first 24 hours is referred to as late postpartum hemorrhage. This bleeding is most often the result of an abnormal involution of the placental site, but it can be caused by retention of some placental fragments, or the development of a placental polyp, or both.

The experience on the author's service is about 3 to 4 percent, of which 10 percent have severe bleeding. Nevertheless PPH ranks as one of our leading causes of maternal death. Severe cases are rare but pose the greatest challenge because they can lead to rapid hypovolemic shock and coagulation disorders.

CONTRIBUTING FACTORS AND PREVENTION

Anticipatory knowledge is a key clinical skill that all obsteticians and midwives must develop. Prevention is based on anticipation, which in turn is based on the identification of risk factors that contribute to the problem.

In order to anticipate the need for possible treatment, all labor floor personnel should be well programmed into instant recognition of those patients who are strong candidates (Table 1) for problems with PPH: (1) the patient whose uterus is markedly distended from polyhydramnios, twins, or a large fetus; (2) the grand multipara; (3) the fatigued woman who has been in labor for many hours with little rest; (4) the patient who is anemic, hypovolemic, or toxemic; (5) the patient whose myometrium is infiltrated with blood, as in Couvelaire's uterus; (6) the patient who has a history of blood dyscrasia or previous PPH; (7) the patient who is a member of the Jehovah's Witnesses group; (8) the patient with amnionitis. The more aggressive management of premature labor with terbutaline, ritodrine, and/or magnesium sulfate can increase the amount of blood loss at the time of delivery.

Prevention must begin in the antepartum period. Anemia should be recognized, investigated, and appropriately treated. Prophylactic oral iron, folate, and vitamins should be administered to all pregnant women.

Patients at high risk of developing postpartum atony must be recognized and their records "flagged". Polyhydramnios and macrosomia should be prevented when possible (for example, through adequate control of diabetes), and patients with premature rupture of membranes should be monitored carefully and delivery carried out as soon as any evidence of chorioamnionitis becomes apparent.

Every patient in labor should be considered a potential candidate for PPH. An intravenous infusion with a large-bore needle must be started at a rate of 150 to 175 ml per hour for adequate hydration. In some instances two infusions should be utilized. Blood should be drawn for hematocrit and hemoglobin readings as well as a coagulation profile in those patients with or at high risk of developing a coagulopathy. A sample of blood must be temporarily stored for every patient in case typing and crossmatching are needed. Two units of blood must be typed and crossmatched for every patient at risk of developing postpartum uterine atony or who has hematocrit below 30 ml per deciliter.

Dysfunctional labor should be avoided by the judicious use of oxytocin and by avoidance of heavy sedation or analgesia. The patient should not be allowed to push until cervical dilatation is complete, so as to avoid edema and laceration of the cervix.

TABLE 1 Major Causes of Uterine Atony

Uterine dysfunction
Mismanagement of the placental stage
Excessive medication, deep general anesthesia
Uterine overdistention
Maternal exhaustion due to prolonged labor
Grand multiparity
Myomas of the uterus
Operative deliveries
Abnormalities during third stage of labor
Cephalopelvic disproportion
Macrosomia
Mg SO_4
Overdistended uterus
Twins
General anesthesia
Tocolytics
Sepsis

The delivery of the infant should be slow and well controlled. Difficult operative deliveries such as midforceps rotations and internal podalic versions should be avoided. An adequate episiotomy must be performed. If low forceps extraction is deemed necessary, it should be correctly applied after complete cervical dilatation and only when adequate anesthesia and patient relaxation are attained.

After delivery of the infant, one should wait until signs of spontaneous separation of the placenta are evident. Gentle traction on the cord is then applied with one hand, while pressure at the junction of the upper and lower uterine segments in a backward-upward direction is exerted with the other. This prevents uterine inversion and minimizes bleeding. Credé's maneuver with or without cord traction before the placenta is detached should be avoided, as it may lead to its incomplete separation. The routine use of oxytocin drip immediately after delivery of the placenta is helpful in minimizing postpartum blood loss.

Careful inspection of the birth canal for lacerations after delivery of the placenta is mandatory. In most instances, I recommend exploring the uterine cavity manually for tears or retained placental fragments. If there is any doubt of the completeness of the placenta and in vaginal deliveries that occur following a previous uterine scar, this procedure becomes a must. It is simple, helpful, and with no undue morbidity if strict aseptic techniques are observed. Digital, not manual, exploration of the uterus can in most instances be accomplished without anesthesia if performed immediately after the expulsion of the placenta and before oxytocics are given.

The conviction that aggressive management of the third stage of labor results in reduced blood loss and therefore lower morbidity prompted us to do frequent early manual removal of the placenta, routine uterine digital exploration, and intravenous administration of methylergonovine maleate and oxytocin.

The advantages of digital exploration of the uterus are considerable, the only possible disadvantage being contamination. It is logical, however, to assume that infection may be the result of trauma, hemorrhage, prolonged rupture of the membranes, anemia, and malnutrition but not of uterine exploration. The occasional finding of a placental cotyledon, membranes, submucous fibroid, uterine malformations, and even an unsuspected uterine rupture is an added dividend of this procedure. Blood loss from episiotomy is less if the uterus is explored and the placenta extracted prior to repair. More often than not manual removal after repair requires a second repair.

Large studies of 3 to 5,000 patients who have had uterine exploration show a lower morbidity in such patients than in those who were not explored.

One of the minimum requirements for all obstetricians should be proficiency in manual removal of the placenta and in digital exploration of the uterus, and appreciation of the normal findings in a postpartum uterus. In our experience, the advantages of routine exploration far outweigh its disadvantages, and we have accepted the procedure as a requirement of good obstetric practice. The techniques of fundus fiddling, cord acrobatics, Credé maneuvers, and multiple halfhearted attempts at placental separation by the introduction of one or two fingers into the uterus are strongly condemned.

The management of PPH is simplified if the uterus has been explored and the vagina and cervix have been carefully inspected for lacerations. Early hemorrhage, then, must be caused by either atony or a clotting defect.

TREATMENT

Proper treatment requires an accurate diagnosis. Most cases of PPH are due to uterine atony (90 percent) with or without a retained placenta, and most of the rest are lacerations or a rare uterine inversion.

If the placenta is retained, a cleavage between it and the uterine wall is created with the fingertips, and it is then shelled out. On occasion it may be removed in pieces. Sometimes it is necessary to apply gauze over the fingers to create a friction curettage. Rarely is a curette necessary. The presence of placenta accreta usually requires a hysterectomy.

The treatment of uterine atony can be divided into mechanical, medical, and surgical, with the first two always being performed simultaneously (Table 2).

Initial external massage of the uterus is frequently successful but sometimes must be combined with simultaneous internal massage. This is then followed by cephalad elevation and compression of the fundus. This places the uterine vessels under tension and closes off the placental site. Uterine rupture must be reconsidered.

Uterine packing is rarely successful but can be attempted. The author has had no experience with packing. The use of uterine and vaginal packs in the control of PPH is now a controversial subject. Whether there is still a place in modern obstetrics for this form of therapy seems very doubtful. However, textbooks advocate the technique and still describe it in detail. The fact that patients have survived this form of treatment may not justify its continued use. Our files contain numerous cases of deaths from hemorrhage in which the uterine pack was used ineffectually. Advocates of the pack would have us believe that it was not properly placed, yet many of these women were attended by obstetricians in leading hospitals. The temporary mental relief afforded the obstetrician by a pack is often purchased only at the expense of additional blood loss. Often the packing not only fails to stop the bleeding but contributes to death by lending a false sense of security as a result of the temporary cessation of blood flow. The filling of a resilient and elastic organ such as the uterus with a pack presents definite mechanical difficulties. The manipulations associated with packing may stimulate temporary contraction of the uterus, only to be followed by subsequent relaxation and hidden bleeding. Control of PPH depends on retraction of uterine muscle fibers, and pack may hinder rather than help that process.

TABLE 2 Therapy for PPH

Mechanical:
Compression
Internal and external massage
Pharmacologic:
Oxytocin
Intramyometrial
Parenteral
Carboprost (Prostin/15M)
Intramuscular/intracervical
Intramyometrial
Intravaginal
Surgical:
Vascular ligation
Hypogastric artery
Ovarian artery
Uterine artery
Hysterectomy
Supracervical
Total
Radiologic:
Hypogastric artery vasopressin (Pitressin) infusion
Selective transarterial embolization

It has been shown that when tightly packed, 10 yards of 3-inch intrauterine gauze packing will absorb 1,000 ml of blood. Much valuable time and even more valuable blood is lost and shock becomes profound, with the result that other and better methods of therapy can no longer be used. Intrauterine packing is more often than not a desperation procedure, poorly done under adverse circumstances. The use of the intrauterine pack should be restricted to those cases of persistent postpartum bleeding in which facilities for laparotomy are not immediately available. However, once the operating room has been prepared, the packing should be removed and laparotomy performed if bleeding continues.

Pneumatic pressure of 20 to 25 mm Hg circumferentially applied to the abdomen and legs by means of a "gravity suit" may be useful in patients with PPH and may be particularly valuable in those requiring transport to specialized facilities.

If uterine atony occurs after the placenta has separated, manual massage of the fundus to promote myometrial contractility, concomitantly with the administration of intravenous oxytocin (20 to 30 U per liter of fluid to run at 5 ml per minute) is sufficient therapy in the majority of cases. Occasionally up to 100 U per liter is required. After the uterus has contracted, continuation of the oxytocin infusion (at a lower rate), with frequent manual stimulation of the uterus for the next 4 to 6 hours, is helpful in maintaining uterine tonicity.

If these preliminary measures are not sufficient to contract the myometrium, the addition of ergotrate (0.2 mg, intravenously), while compressing the uterus between one fist in the anterior fornix of the vagina with the other hand on the patient's abdomen for several minutes, may enhance contractility. We have used up to five doses of 0.2 mg on rare occasions with no adverse side effects. Care should be taken not to push the fundus deeply into the pelvis, as this can result in uterine inversion or broad ligament tears.

Uterotonic agents have potentially serious side effects and must be used cautiously and selectively. Oxytocin should be used in an intravenous drip mixed in a solution containing sodium so as to avoid water intoxication. It should not usually be administered as a quick intravenous bolus, since hypotension, cardiac arrhythmias, and even cardiac arrest may occur. However, direct intravenous injection of oxytocin can be given in serious hemorrhages and can be repeated two or three times. Ergotrate must not be given as a first line of therapy and should be avoided in toxemic patients because of its vasoconstrictive effects.

Manual exploration of the uterus and reinspection of the genital tract for lacerations under general anesthesia become mandatory if uterine atony persists despite the measures described. Placental fragments or a succenturiate lobe of the placenta may have been left behind and should be managed as discussed earlier in this section. A laparotomy then will be necessary, and the choice between surgical repair of the lacerations or a hysterectomy will depend on the extent of the tears, the condition of the patient, and her desire to preserve her reproductive organs. In rare instances, inversion of the uterus may be detected. Repositioning should begin immediately, starting at the edges of the uterus nearest the cervix. An oxytocin drip is maintained after the procedure is over to prevent recurrence. Rarely, surgical repositioning may be necessary. Terbutaline has been used prior to repositioning to relax the uterus.

If no placental fragments or genital tract lacerations are found, the blood coagulation status of the patient should be assessed and medical therapy initiated promptly if it is abnormal.

In most clinical problems, a medical or pharmacologic approach is preferable to an operative or surgical approach. The problems associated with severe PPH from uterine atony can deteriorate very rapidly and lead to maternal mortality. The range of deterioration is often unpredictable, as is the response to routine medical management. In view of these limitations, an early and aggressive approach to uterine atony—15-methyl PGF_{2a} (Prostin/15M)—is logical. The initial dose of 0.25 mg to 0.5 mg is injected into the cervix or myometrium.

Preliminary studies using Prostin/15M in the management of severe PPH due to uterine atony that is unresponsive to a conventional treatment regimen of intravenous oxytocin, intramuscular methylergonovine maleate, and manual uterine compression demonstrated an effective response with no significant side effects. Our personal experience over a 5-year period using the same management protocol supports these preliminary studies. An efficacy rate of 86 percent with an incidence of mild side effects of less than 10 percent has been demonstrated. There were four preeclamptic subjects in this group, and none demonstrated a blood pressure elevation to levels that required additional antihypertensive therapy. Half of the subjects required only one injection into the cervix or uterus. Doses were repeated as frequently as every 10 minutes.

Of those who failed to respond to Prostin/15M therapy, half had chorioamnionitis. This relationship between chorioamnionitis and failure of the prostaglandin analogue to control severe PPH was also noted in preliminary studies. These observations suggest that further studies of the effect of chorioamnionitis on prostaglandin-induced contraction of the uterus may be of importance. Supportive of this concept is an interesting in vitro study that demonstrated that the culture fluid from enteric organisms caused hypomotility of human myometrial strips. Failures can occur in women receiving magnesium sulfate therapy because of interference with the calcium ion.

The use of Prostin/15M is certainly no panacea in the management of PPH. However, there are a number of obvious advantages, all of which merit serious consideration. Every obstetrician should be trained in its performance. Lack of familiarity with the technique leads to a certain degree of anxiety, but once one has acquired some experience with this drug, it becomes evident that the anxiety is unfounded. Such experience is not difficult to obtain. Pharmacologically, there is a sound basis for this end result. However, the half-life requires that the patient continue to receive other oxytocins.

From our personal experience with 32 cases and those reported in the literature, it is evident that the uterotonic property of prostaglandins can be of benefit in the management of severe PPH due to uterine atony. Some authors recommend that myometrial injection of PGF_{2a} should be given at the time of cesarean section; this injection should logically precede arterial ligations and hysterectomy. To obtain maximum benefit from this drug, however, it must be used early during the management of severe uterine atony.

Of the three modalities, E-2 suppositories, PGF_{2a}, and Prostin/15M, the latter is preferred. E-2 suppositories are of the greatest value in delayed PPH and when the hemorrhage is not massive. The effects of Prostin/15M appear to be more predictable than those of PGF_{2a}. The efficacy of intramyometrial versus intramuscular injections is very similar. The former is preferable at the time of cesarean section, whereas intracervical injections can be given at the time of vaginal delivery.

SURGICAL MANAGEMENT

The surgical methods for controlling hemorrhage include bilateral hypogastric artery ligation, bilateral ovarian artery ligation, uterine artery ligation, and hysterectomy.

Uterine Artery Ligation

We believe this to be the first and preferred surgical step in controlling pelvic hemorrhage. It is emphasized that uterine artery ligation will only stop bleeding of uterine origin.

First described by Waters in 1952 and "rediscovered" in 1964, uterine artery ligation has since been somewhat neglected by medical schools and clinicians. This oversight is regrettable, because ligation is a rapid, safe, and effective way to avoid excessive reliance on hysterectomy after noninvasive methods for controlling PPH have failed. Its use can be appropriate for stopping moderate bleeding earlier in pregnancy.

The ascending branches of the uterine arteries are even

less difficult to identify and ligate than those encountered by the general surgeon. The question then arises why a technique of uterine artery occlusion is not employed to control hemorrhage resulting from uterine atony or placental pathology encountered at cesarean section. The only logical explanation appears to be unfounded fear of complications, insecurity regarding the ureters, and, most important, inexperience with the technique.

The technique of bilateral occlusion of the ascending branch of the uterine artery and adjacent veins is very simple and can be rapidly performed. Since during pregnancy 90 percent of uterine blood flow passes through the uterine arteries, with minimal flow from the ovarian, cervical, and vaginal vessels, this step will reduce uterine blood flow and produce uterine ischemia.

The surgeon preferably stands on the left side of the patient and grasps and elevates the uterus with the left hand and holds a large Mayo needle with a No. 1 atraumatic chromic catgut suture with the right hand. To ligate the left uterine artery, he passes the needle into and through the myometrium from anterior to posterior, 2 to 3 cm medial to the uterine vessels, and then brings it forward through the avascular area of the broad ligament lateral to the artery and vein. The ligations are performed a few centimeters below the uterine artery and under direct vision with the index finger identifying the artery.

The right uterine artery is then ligated, the needle being passed from anterior to posterior through the avascular area of the broad ligament and brought anteriorly through the myometrium 2 to 3 cm medial to the artery and vein. After ligation, the musculature assumes a pinkish hue secondary to the ischemia, and increased tone may result. However, the uterus often remains atonic, but bleeding is controlled.

It is not necessary to mobilize the bladder, for the sutures are not placed that low and there is no need to fear ureteral damage because the ureters enter the bladder trigone well below the ligature site. Since the ligation is usually done during the course of a cesarean section, the sutures are placed below the level of the transverse uterine incision beneath the reflected flap of peritoneum. With this technique, the vessels do not require palpation and are not injured. It is important that a substantial amount of myometrium be included in the suture to occlude some of the inferior coronary branches of the uterine artery.

The vessels are not divided; thus only a single ligation is performed on each side. Since recanalization will occur, subsequent menstrual flow and pregnancies are unaffected. In the interim, collateral circulation is sufficient to prevent complications.

No major complications have occurred in any of the patients treated. The development of a late arteriovenous sinus is a potential but unlikely hazard.

Although ligation of the ascending branch of the uterine artery is certainly no panacea in the management of PPH, a number of obvious advantages merit serious consideration. Every obstetrician should be trained in its performance.

Despite two successful reports of transvaginal ligation of the uterine arteries, we believe it is a hazardous and bloody procedure and one that should not be attempted.

In performing uterine artery ligation, we define failure as the need for subsequent hysterectomy, hypogastric artery ligation, or religation of the uterine vessels or placental site. With these criteria, our success rate in over 200 cases of women who had cesarean section was 95 percent. Three of our eight failures occurred in patients who had placenta previa, four in patients who had atony, and one in a patient who had amnionitis and probable myometritis. In retrospect, we probably should not have attempted ligation in the woman who had amnionitis because of the added risk of devascularizing an infected organ.

In three instances, despite failure of the initial ligation, blood loss was controlled sufficiently to allow ligation of the placental site or ovarian vessels and thus to avoid hysterectomy and further hemorrhage. It is notable that two of these three patients had placenta previa.

Two other patients who had atony regained tone after ligation, only to have atony recur as the uterine incision was being closed. In both instances, inspection of the ligature sites revealed slight slippage of the knots. Placing a second ligature stopped the bleeding, this time successfully. Postcesarean lochial flow was somewhat reduced, but subsequent menstrual flow and pregnancies were unaffected. Atony recurred in three other patients after repeat cesarean sections and necessitated repeat ligation.

None of these patients had a major complication. Two had small broad ligament hematomas. In one, surgery had been performed by a resident doing his first ligation. Vein damage caused by multiple needle punctures required salpingo-oophorectomy.

In the second patient, the needle had also torn a broad ligament vein. Further enlargement of the hematoma was prevented by ligating the infundibulopelvic ligament at the injury site. Although this patient had had one ovarian artery and vein and both uterine arteries and veins ligated, her convalescence was uneventful. Moreover, the literature reveals only one instance of complication associated with uterine artery ligation.

All patients were followed up, and no adverse effects were observed. In 11 who subsequently underwent elective repeat cesarean section, no evidence of the previous ligations could be detected. In each case, vessels apparently had recanalized.

Average blood loss for the entire group was 1,000 ml. This amount contrasts with average losses of 2,000 ml seen in an earlier group; for those, we waited longer after other methods had failed before performing ligation. We now recommend proceeding promptly with uterine artery ligation rather than waiting and risking massive hemorrhage and shock.

Other evidence favoring uterine artery ligation comes from animal experiments. In our studies of dogs, we had no postoperative complications after the procedure, and found tissue normal during the second laparotomy. Moreover, others have reported uncomplicated term pregnancies—with no intrauterine growth retardation or preeclampsia—in women after bilateral uterine artery ligation for obstetric-gynecologic hemorrhage. As in our patients, those who underwent repeat cesarean section showed no signs of prior ligation. Either recanalization had occurred in these patients or collateral channels permitted normal uterine growth. Successful use of uterine artery ligation for severe first trimester hemorrhage has also been reported.

Hypogastric Artery Ligation

Hypogastric artery ligation can be a lifesaving technique for both obstetric and gynecologic patients. However, it can be more difficult to perform in the presence of a large, bleeding, boggy, postpartum uterus. In addition, the increased vascularity associated with pregnancy makes the dissection far more difficult. Last, in life-threatening situations the average obstetrician's relative lack of experience with the ligation becomes patently obvious.

Hypogastric artery ligation and internal iliac artery ligation are the same procedure. It is somewhat surprising to find that the method is misunderstood by many surgeons, even though it has proved lifesaving in serious hemorrhage.

The biggest pitfall with hypogastric ligation is waiting too long to perform it.

The second pitfall in treating pelvic hemorrhage is thinking that the vaginal blood supply is derived from the uterine artery or a branch of it. The main blood supply to the uterus is the uterine artery, a branch of the hypogastric (internal iliac). The vagina is supplied by the vaginal artery, another branch of the hypogastric artery. Although uterine artery ligation may stop hemorrhage from the uterus, it will not stop bleeding from the vagina. Ligation of the hypogastric arteries usually stops hemorrhage from both.

Ligation of the hypogastric artery does not cause cessation of blood flow through the uterine artery. Ligation causes the arterial flow to resemble venous bleeding.

In the mid-1960s it was demonstrated that if the uterine artery was transected after the hypogastric arteries had been ligated, blood continued to flow at a rate necessitating ligation of the cut uterine artery. The most dramatic finding was a near elimination of the pulse pressure distal to the ligation, which decreased 77 percent from baseline on the side of the ligation and 85 percent if both hypogastric arteries were ligated but only 14 percent on the side opposite a unilateral ligation.

The effect of hypogastric ligation is to change a pulsating arterial system to one resembling venous flow. When arterial pulsations decrease, blood clots can form distal to the ligations and remain in place rather than be blown off by the pulse pressure.

The ligation may be done on either side or bilaterally, depending on the need. The bowel is walled off and packed as high as possible into the upper abdomen. The anterior superior iliac spine will, from our experience, be at approximately the same level or about a finger's breadth below the bifurcation of the common iliac artery. The peritoneum over the common iliac artery is elevated and cut, exposing 3 or 4 inches of retroperitoneal space. In this area there is a considerable amount of areolar tissue, and the ureter is usually to be found there attached to the posterior peritoneum. The ureter usually crosses the common iliac artery just above its bifurcation. The peritoneum and ureter are usually reflected medially.

The areolar tissue is teased away to expose the common iliac artery. A groove director may be used, or a Mixter's forceps, or a moist sponge to clean away the areolar tissue. The palpation of the common iliac artery, which is recognizable by its bounding pulse, is the first step in anatomic orientation. As one proceeds caudad, the bifurcation (at which the common iliac divides into the external iliac and courses toward the leg) and the hypogastric artery (which dips down and courses toward the pelvis) will be seen.

The hypogastric artery is elevated with a Mixter's forceps, and two braided silk sutures are used to ligate it. Chromic 1–0 catgut or Mersilene may also be used as ligatures. The ligatures are placed one-quarter to one-half inch apart.

After the ligation has been completed, the edges of the peritoneum overlying the vessel are brought together with 3–0 fine chromic catgut in several interrupted sutures. We do not recommend the use of a continuous suture, since it might kink the ureter.

Perhaps the greatest pitfall in ligation of the hypogastric arteries is to wait too long or to wait until the patient's condition becomes irreversible and the possibility of recovery is lost. Allowing hemorrhage to continue without some definitive action to counter it may lead to death of the patient.

Another serious pitfall, which may lead to delay and neglect, is the incorrect belief that a branch of the uterine artery always supplies the vagina and that when the flow in the uterine artery has been stopped, the vaginal hemorrhage will stop as well. Many uteri have been removed to stop vaginal hemorrhage, and many surgeons must have wondered why the hemorrhage continued when the uterus was out and the flow in the uterine artery had been controlled.

Ovarian Artery Ligation

Because bilateral hypogastric artery ligation does not always control hemorrhage, an additional procedure may become necessary; bilateral ovarian artery ligation has been successfully used. Contrary to popular misconceptions, it is not accomplished through ligation of the infundibulopelvic ligation.

The ovarian artery is a branch of the aorta and travels retroperitoneally in the infundibulopelvic ligament. At the fimbriated end of the fallopian tube and the most lateral aspect of the ovary, it enters the mesovarium. From there it courses superior to the ovary, with numerous branches spreading to the fallopian tube. At the point of attachment of the utero-ovarian ligament to the uterus, the ovarian artery anastomoses with the uterine artery, adding to the blood supply of the uterus.

Find an avascular area above the artery in the mesovarium, and under adequate visualization, place a Kelly's or right-angle clamp entirely through the mesovarium. Pass the clamp through this window and place it under the artery. If gentle pressure does not open a second window below the artery, open the clamp and incise the mesovarium, again in an avascular area.

Use two free ligatures on the ovarian artery. There is no need to divide the vessel; in fact, this should be avoided. The absorbable polyglycolic suture, No. 0, is adequate.

The mesovarial defects are repaired with interrupted suture. The ovarian artery is ligated in an area to allow maintenance of adequate blood supply to the ovary and fallopian tube.

Hysterectomy

When is hysterectomy indicated for postpartum hemorrhage? The decision is obviously a difficult one to make. There is a natural reluctance to subject an already anemic and frequently traumatized patient to a major surgical procedure involving the sacrifice of her uterus. Good judgment is necessary, and the decision must be made early. In postpartum hemorrhage, as in placenta previa, the initial hemorrhage is rarely fatal. It is the repeated bleedings that eventually result in death.

We are of the opinion that hysterectomy is not as uneventful as some think but carries with it at least the inherent dangers of any major abdominal operation and probably the equivalent of two operations.

In our experience, complication rates can range from 18 to 50 percent depending on the type of operation performed. Closer analysis reveals that the patients undergoing elective or unintended subtotal hysterectomy have the fewest complications (18 to 20 percent). As anticipated, a higher rate of complications occurs in the indicated groups: subtotal hysterectomy 30 to 33 percent, total hysterectomy 41 to 55 percent. However, a disconcertingly high number of complications accompany the elective total cesarean hysterectomy, 35 to 51 percent.

The bladder is injured in approximately 4 percent of all patients, mostly in women who have had previous cesarean sections.

The morbidity rate following this operation can be significant (21 to 25 percent). The distribution of morbidity is usually a reflection of the type of operation and the indication for surgery. Even the elective total hysterectomy for sterilization carries a significant morbidity rate (31 to 33 percent).

The frequent use of and need for blood transfusion are of grave concern and should not be taken lightly. From 60 to 70 percent of patients require transfusion; the transfusion rate varies according to the indications for surgery.

Under normal circumstances, the vagina cannot be prepared preoperatively. A Foley's catheter is inserted. A vaginal pack is placed against the cervix to aid in its identification and to help keep the operative field clean. It may be necessary at times to close the transverse uterine incision. The standard three-clamp technique usually suffices. In emergency situations the lateral clamps may be left in place until the uterus is removed and then tied. The bladder should be advanced in a stepwise fashion so as not to cause any unnecessary venous bleeding.

Removal of the cervix can be facilitated, on some occasions, by the injection of an oxytocic agent into the cervical area to contract the cervix for definite identification. The insertion of a finger from above through the cervical canal with elevation of the cervix aids greatly in its identification and removal. The presence of the vaginal pack also aids in identification.

The vaginal vault is left open, and a small drain is inserted. Antibiotics are employed for a short course.

It can generally be stated that when things go well at a cesarean hysterectomy the operation is rapid and simple, but when unexpected technical difficulties arise, the procedure may become surgically imprecise and alarming blood loss may occur.

SUGGESTED READING

Clark SL, Phelan JP. Surgical control of hemorrhage. Contemp Ob/Gyn Aug 1984; 70.

Cruikshank SH, Stoelk EM. Surgical control of pelvic hemorrhage; ovarian artery ligation. Am J Obstet Gynecol 1983; 147:6.

Hayashi RH, Costello MS, Noah ML. Management of severe postpartum hemorrhage due to uterine atony using an analogue of prostaglandin F_{2a}. Obstet Gynecol 1981; 58:4.

Keith V, Berger GS. Surgical management of intractable pelvic hemorrhage. In: Sciarra JJ, ed. Gynecology and obstetrics. Vol. 1. Philadelphia: Harper & Row, 1984.

O'Leary JL, O'Leary JA. Uterine artery ligation in the control of intractable postpartum hemorrhage. Am J Obstet Gynecol 1966; 94:920–924.

COAGULOPATHIES IN OBSTETRICS

ROBERTO ROMERO, M.D.
HUNG N. WINN, M.D.

CHANGES IN THE HEMOSTATIC SYSTEM DURING PREGNANCY

During pregnancy, blood vessels become more prominent probably owing to the combination of increased blood volume and vasodilation normally observed during gestation. A specialized regional circulation (the placental vascular bed) develops to ensure adequate supply of maternal blood to the conceptus.

The platelet count tends to decrease with advancing gestational age. This has been attributed to hemodilution and placental trapping. Nevertheless, the platelet count during pregnancy remains within the limits of the normal adult range (150,000 to 350,000 per mm^3). The life span of platelets during pregnancy is similar to that in nonpregnant women.

During pregnancy, there is activation of the coagulation components of the hemostatic system, as evidenced by the increased concentrations of fibrinopeptide A and high molecular weight fibrinogen complexes, as pregnancy progresses. This hypercoagulable state seems to be related to the participation of the hemostatic system in the modeling of the placental bed and spiral arteries in response to maternal preparation for the eventual separation of the placenta.

Fibrin is deposited in the placental bed as pregnancy progresses, and it can be found in the floor of the placenta (Nitabuch's layer), lining the intervillous space, and on the surface of the villi. The spiral arteries undergo important morphologic changes during pregnancy, including the replacement of the elastic lamina and the smooth muscle of the vascular wall by a matrix containing fibrin. Physiological consequences of these changes include: (1) The spiral arteries are transformed into large, distended, nonresponsive vessels known as uteroplacental arteries, which are able to accommodate the increased blood flow to the conceptus as pregnancy progresses. Removal of the elastic lamina also reduces the variation in pressure in the blood flowing to the placenta. (2) Fibrin replacement of the tunica media also facilitates the severance of the terminal part of the spiral arteries at the time of separation of the placenta and their occlusion by the action of the myometrial contractions.

McKay has proposed that normal pregnancy is a state of chronic intravascular coagulation localized to the placental bed. This state would result in a compensatory increase in the synthesis of coagulation factors and a decrease in the platelet count.

The activity of all coagulation factors, except factors XI and XIII, is increased. The decreased level in factor XIII is, however, consistent with the increased deposition of fibrin at the end of pregnancy, since recent evidence suggests that the concentration of factor XIII decreases during the acute phase of thromboembolism.

The activity of coagulation inhibitors has been the subject of contradictory reports, but it does not seem to be substantially altered with pregnancy. The traditional concept has been that fibrinolysis is depressed during pregnancy. Evidence to support that view includes the detection during gestation of the following:

1. Falling levels of plasminogen activator.
2. Decreased fibrinolytic activity of plasma.
3. Decreased fibrinolytic capacity in response to venous occlusion.
4. The presence of an inhibitor of urokinase-induced fibrinolysis.
5. Increased concentration of plasmin inhibitors such as macroglobulin and antiplasmin, with no change in inhibitors of plasminogen activator.

Several investigators, using studies of fibrinogen catabolism, have challenged this concept of fibrinolysis depression during pregnancy. They have proposed that there is an appropriate fibrinolytic response but that the levels of plasminogen activator are depressed because of its sequestration in sites of fibrin deposition.

INDICATIONS FOR HEMOSTATIC TESTING IN THE OBSTETRIC PATIENT

Screening tests are indicated whenever there is a significant risk of hemostatic failure. The most frequent reasons for testing in the obstetric patient are:

1. To evaluate the relative contributions of the different components of the hemostatic system causing excessive spontaneous or surgical hemorrhage.
2. To look for subclinical activation of the hemostatic system in patients with obstetric complications that may be associated with disseminated intravascular coagulation (e.g., preeclampsia, fetal death, abruptio placentae). Detection of significant activation of the hemostatic system could change clinical management in these conditions.
3. For laboratory monitoring of the progress of hemostatic therapy in cases of coagulation failure or of anticoagulation in patients with thromboembolic disease.
4. For antepartum or preoperative hemostatic testing of the patient with a history suggestive of a bleeding diathesis or medical disorder associated with hemostatic problems.

Abnormalities in any of the four components of the hemostatic system may cause an increased bleeding tendency. Screening tests should include evaluation of vascular integrity, platelet number and function, the different pathways of the coagulation cascade, and fibrinolytic activity. Specific tests of hemostatic competence include: (1) tests of vascular integrity, (2) platelet count, (3) bleeding time, (4) prothrombin time, (5) partial thromboplastin time, (6) fibrinogen concentration, and (7) fibrinogen degradation products (FDP).

BLOOD REPLACEMENT THERAPY IN COAGULATION FAILURE

The most common indications for transfusion therapy in the obstetric patient are hypovolemia, anemia, and the need to replace hemostatic components. The optimal use of blood component therapy for hemostatic replacement requires familiarity with the composition of the different available preparations.

Whole Stored Blood

When a unit of blood is drawn, it can be kept as whole blood or separated into its individual components. In general, deterioration of the hemostatic function of whole blood begins 6 hours after collection and this, along with volume considerations, limits the usefulness of stored whole blood for replacement of hemostatic components.

Whole stored blood or the combination of red blood cells and crystalloid solution is appropriate therapy for replacement of volume and oxygen-carrying capacity in the acutely hemorrhaging obstetric patient without a coagulopathy. However, when the amount transfused within a 24-hour period exceeds the patient's circulating blood volume, a bleeding disorder due in part to loss and dilution of platelets and plasma coagulation factors can occur. Because of this possibility, some authors have suggested that during massive transfusions, one-third of the blood administered should be fresh. A more practical alternative is the administration of fresh frozen plasma and/or platelet concentrates.

Fresh Whole Blood

The term fresh blood is generally used to designate blood that has been collected less than 24 hours prior to administration. This preparation has an acceptably minimal loss of hemostatic factors, it is less expensive than blood component therapy, and its use is not associated with the problems of microaggregates of platelets, white blood cells, and fibrin formed during storage of whole blood. The major disadvantages of using fresh blood are the risk of hepatitis, since there may be insufficient time to complete hepatitis screening, and the risk of circulatory overload if fresh blood is administered to replace coagulation factors in a patient who is not actively bleeding. At present, the use of fresh whole blood is being actively discouraged by blood bank services in the United States. Insufficient time for hepatitis screening, limited availability of donors, and more efficient utilization of blood components are the reasons for this policy. The use of fresh blood will probably be limited to those parts of the world where transfusion services are not appropriately developed.

Fresh Frozen Plasma

Fresh frozen plasma is obtained by separation and freezing of the plasma derived during the preparation of red blood cells and platelet concentrates from a unit of whole blood. The plasma must be frozen within 6 hours of donation and stored at temperatures lower than −18 °C. The product is available in 200- to 250-ml bags.

Fresh frozen plasma is devoid of platelets but contains all the other coagulation factors, including factors V and VIII. Its concentration of clotting factors is similar to that found in an equivalent volume of circulating plasma in a normal person. It carries the same risk of hepatitis as a unit of whole blood. The product should be administered to ABO-compatible recipients.

Fresh frozen plasma is a good source of coagulation components and is frequently used to administer these factors, along with volume, to the obstetric patient with hemorrhage and disseminated intravascular coagulation.

Since none of the factors are concentrated, large volumes of fresh frozen plasma are usually needed to achieve hemostatic levels of depleted coagulation components. The risk of circulatory overload is, therefore, the most important limiting factor in the use of fresh frozen plasma for hemostatic replacement. For this reason, most congenital deficiencies of factors are best treated with concentrates of specific factors.

Indications for the use of fresh frozen plasma include:

1. Documented deficiencies of isolated coagulation factors, such as factor XI, for which no concentrate is available.
2. Warfarin (Coumadin) overdose, for which it is unsafe to wait for the time required for correction by administration of parenteral vitamin K.
3. Liver disease complicated by significant bleeding in the presence of a prolonged prothrombin time or partial thromboplastin time.
4. Disseminated intravascular coagulation.

Cryoprecipitate

Cryoprecipitate is the term used to designate the white gelatinous precipitate produced by the thawing of fresh frozen plasma at 1 to 6 °C. A unit of cryoprecipitate has a volume of 15 to 25 ml and is an excellent source of fibrinogen and of factors VIII and XIII.

Once prepared, cryoprecipitate can be stored at −20 °C for up to 1 year. When it is needed for transfusion, cryoprecipitate is thawed at 37 °C. Several units of cryoprecipitate are generally pooled into one bag for ease of administration. Once pooled, cryoprecipitate must be used or discarded within 6 hours because of the danger of bacterial contamination. It is preferable to administer this preparation to ABO-compatible recipients.

The main indication for administering cryoprecipitate in the obstetric patient is the need to replace fibrinogen. Each unit contains about 250 mg of fibrinogen, so that significant amounts of this protein can be delivered in a relatively small volume. Ten units of cryoprecipitate generally increase the circulating fibrinogen in an average-sized person by 50 mg per deciliter. Other uses of cryoprecipitate are for replacement of factors VIII and XIII and in the management of bleeding in von Willebrand's disease. The risk of hepatitis with a unit of cryoprecipitate is the same as with one unit of whole blood.

Platelets

Platelets can be administered in fresh whole blood, platelet-rich plasma, and platelet concentrate. The use of fresh blood and platelet-rich plasma as a source of platelets should be discouraged because a large volume is generally necessary to achieve a platelet hemostatic level, and circulatory overload is likely to occur before such a level is reached.

Platelet-rich plasma is obtained by low-speed centrifugation of a unit of fresh whole blood. Platelets remain in the plasma phase, whereas red blood cells and white blood cells precipitate because of their higher specific gravity. A unit of platelet concentrate is obtained from a unit of platelet-rich plasma by centrifugation at a higher speed to precipitate platelets. Each unit is suspended in 30 to 50 ml of donor plasma, and its platelet content is dependent upon the donor's platelet count and the blood volume from which the platelets were extracted. Platelet concentrates are stored at room temperature (22 °C) for a maximum of 2 to 5 days, depending on the type of bag used. Storage for longer periods of time or at 4 °C results in a shorter platelet life span. In the case of autologous transfusion, cryopreservation of platelets may be necessary to extend the storage period.

The response to platelet concentrate transfusions is

expressed in terms of the increment in platelet count per square meter of body area. This method permits evaluation of the effectiveness of platelet transfusions independently of blood volume and allows comparisons between individuals. One unit of transfused platelets generally raises the platelet count by 5,000 to 10,000 per mm^3 per square meter of body surface. Fever, infection, alloimmunization, and drug-induced platelet antibodies can shorten the life span of transfused platelets. Platelets are contaminated with red blood cells, and Rh sensitization can occur after the administration of platelets from Rh-positive donors to Rh-negative recipients. Therefore, an effort should be made to obtain Rh-negative platelet concentrates for the Rh-negative obstetric patient. If this is not possible, Rh immunoglobulin (50 μg) should be administered to prevent the development of antibodies when platelets from an Rh-positive donor are given to an Rh-negative recipient. Although platelets have ABO antigens, they can be transfused to ABO-incompatible recipients if compatible platelets are not available. Episodes of mild hemolysis can occur if large amounts of group O platelet concentrates (with anti-A and anti-B plasma) are administered to group A or B recipients. Both shortened and normal life spans of nonallogenic platelets with respect to the ABO group have been reported, but this does not seem to be a significant clinical problem.

Indications for the use of platelet transfusions include prophylaxis against and treatment of excessive bleeding caused by thrombocytopenia and platelet dysfunction. The combined use of platelet counts and bleeding times permits assessment of the contribution of platelet abnormalities to hemostatic failure. Platelet concentrate therapy is indicated in the following circumstances:

1. Prophylaxis of bleeding in surgical or antepartum patients with a platelet count below 60,000 per mm^3.
2. Prophylaxis of spontaneous bleeding in patients with platelet counts below 20,000 per mm^3 and prolonged bleeding times.
3. Prophylaxis and treatment of excessive bleeding in patients with known platelet dysfunction.
4. Therapy of excessive bleeding in the patient who has been subjected to massive transfusion therapy and has developed dilutional thrombocytopenia.

Six to ten units of platelet concentrate are usually administered at one time. The optimal dose naturally depends on the cause of the thrombocytopenia, the initial platelet count, the level that needs to be reached, the presence of known platelet dysfunction, and alloimmunization or other factors that increase platelet dysfunction. The common starting dose is 1 U of platelet concentrate per 10 kg of body weight. A platelet count should be obtained 1 hour after the transfusion to determine its effectiveness.

Platelet concentrates are more effective in treating patients with impaired platelet production than in those with increased destruction. A notable example of the latter is the patient with immune thrombocytopenic purpura in whom transfused platelets may be destroyed within hours or minutes.

Occasionally, patients receiving frequent transfusions of platelet concentrates may become refractory to random donor platelets. The underlying mechanism for this phenomenon is the development of alloantibodies to platelet-associated human leukocyte antigens. Under those circumstances, human leukocyte antigen–compatible concentrates can be used if platelet transfusions are necessary. A rare complication associated with the administration of platelets is infection. The etiologic agents are similar to those involved in administration of other blood products and include human immunodeficiency virus, non-A and non-B hepatitis, cytomegalovirus, hepatitis B, and bacterial infections.

Plasma Fractions (Fibrinogen and Factor IX Complexes)

Plasma obtained from whole blood or plasmapheresis can be used as fresh frozen plasma or pooled and fractionated into different components such as fibrinogen, antihemophilic factor (AHF or factor VIII), factor IX complex, gamma globulin, or albumin. Pooling of several units of plasma is performed to allow efficient large-scale preparation of the plasma fractions. However, the act of mixing plasma from many donors increases the risk of hepatitis virus. Heat treatment can inactivate the hepatitis virus. This procedure is used in the preparation of albumin and gamma globulin, rendering these products virtually free of risk of hepatitis. Coagulation fractions, however, cannot be heated; and, therefore, these pooled preparations are associated with a significant risk of hepatitis transmission. For this reason, fibrinogen concentrates are no longer a licensed product in the United States. Cryoprecipitate is the preparation of choice for efficient fibrinogen replacement.

Factor IX complex (Proplex or Konyne) is a stable, dried, purified plasma that contains factors II, VII, IX, and X. It is available in vials whose contents are reconstituted with sterile pyrogen-free water. The concentration of factors II, VII, IX, and X is roughly equivalent to 500 ml of fresh frozen plasma. Factor IX complex is prepared from large pools of plasma and therefore carries a substantial risk of hepatitis. It is preferable to administer fresh frozen plasma to replace the factors contained in the factor IX complex and reserve this complex for those cases in which time and volume considerations prevent therapy with vitamin K and/or fresh frozen plasma. The administration of factor IX complex has been associated with the production of venous thrombosis or disseminated intravascular coagulation in the recipient. These side effects are possibly attributable to the presence of procoagulant activity in most factor IX preparations.

The other plasma fraction with hemostatic value is factor VIII concentrate. This preparation is rarely used in the obstetric patient, except in the occasional instance of a specific factor deficiency or a circulating inhibitor.

DISSEMINATED INTRAVASCULAR COAGULATION

Disseminated intravascular coagulation is a pathological state caused by excessive thrombin activity. It is kinetically and pathologically characterized by increased thrombin generation, increased turnover of platelets and coagulation factors, formation of thrombi in the microcirculation, and secondary activation of the fibrinolytic system. These events are manifested clinically by varying degrees of bleeding and ischemic tissue damage.

Disseminated intravascular coagulation is not a specific disease but rather a sequence of pathological events that can be associated with many different conditions.

Familiarity with the pathophysiology, diagnosis, and management of disseminated intravascular coagulation is important, since this condition is the most frequent cause of acquired coagulopathy in the obstetric patient. Since this book deals primarily with treatment, the reader is urged to consult the various hematology texts for information on pathophysiology and diagnosis. Inappropriate handling of this pathological process can lead to serious and potentially fatal complications.

Management

General Principles

1. Disseminated intravascular coagulation is always secondary to a disease that causes excessive thrombin generation. The most effective treatment is to eliminate the cause of activation of the hemostatic system. This implies therapy of the primary disease and, in obstetrics, frequently indicates the need for delivery.
2. The association of disseminated intravascular coagulation with any obstetric entity (e.g., abruptio placentae, chorioamnionitis) transforms a local disorder into a systemic disease and introduces the risk of multiple organ failure. Therefore, the presence of disseminated intravascular coagulation magnifies the severity of the underlying disease.
3. As a mode of delivery, the vaginal route is preferable to cesarean section or hysterotomy in a patient with a decompensated coagulopathy. The vaginal approach places less stress on the hemostatic mechanism than an abdominal operation, in which there is a significant risk of bleeding from the uterine and abdominal wall incisions. It would be ideal if an episiotomy or any other obstetric operative intervention could be safely avoided during the course of a vaginal delivery.
4. The administration of conduction anesthesia (caudal, epidural, or spinal) is contraindicated in a patient with hemostatic failure because of the increased risk of formation of an epidural hematoma and subsequent neurologic damage.
5. Replacement therapy of the depleted hemostatic components is indicated only in the presence of bleeding or to correct subnormal levels of hemostatic factors prior to surgical intervention or to a vaginal delivery. If the fibrinogen level is above 100 mg per 100 ml and the platelet count is more than 60,000 per mm^3, replacement therapy is not generally required.
6. The rationale for the use of heparin in disseminated intravascular coagulation is to decrease the excessive thrombin generation and activity. This would arrest coagulation factor consumption and fibrin deposition and reduce the risk of consumptive coagulopathy and ischemic damage. Although the most effective treatment for disseminated intravascular coagulation is the elimination of the cause of activation of the hemostatic system, this cannot always be immediately accomplished, particularly when the cause is infection or neoplasia. Heparin has been used with some success under these circumstances to prevent the deleterious consequences of disseminated intravascular coagulation. Heparin therapy, however, is rarely indicated in the obstetric patient because most episodes are self-limited and because detachment of the placenta at delivery or during abruption creates significant vascular disruption and heparin magnifies the potential for life-threatening hemorrhage. Its use should be limited to those cases in which there is an intact intravascular bed and delivery is not anticipated during the period of anticoagulation. Heparin has a high molecular weight and does not cross the placenta; therefore, it is an ideal anticoagulant for obstetric use.

Abruptio Placentae. Abruptio placentae is the most frequent cause of acute decompensated disseminated intravascular coagulation in the obstetric patient. The incidence of abruptio placentae varies from 0.2 to 2.4 percent of all pregnancies, and disseminated intravascular coagulation with fibrinogen concentrations of less than 100 mg per deciliter complicates one-third to one-fourth of the cases. The etiology of abruptio placentae is usually unknown. Risk factors include a history of severe abruptio placentae in a previous pregnancy, high parity, hypertensive disease of the mother, cigarette smoking, and external trauma. The role of other proposed causes, such as polyhydramnios, a short umbilical cord, uterine anomalies, and folate deficiencies, remains obscure and is not likely to be significant.

The initial event is likely to be an ischemic lesion of the decidua, leading to decidual necrosis, vascular disruption, and bleeding. As hemorrhage occurs, laceration and dissection along a decidual plane and placental separation take place. The latter produces more vascular rhexis, arterial hemorrhage, retroplacental accumulation of blood, and further placental separation.

Following delivery, control of uterine bleeding is dependent on myometrial contraction, which constricts the severed vessels at the placental implantation site. This mechanism cannot operate efficiently in abruptio placentae because the uterine cavity remains distended by the presence of the fetus. Since the maternal venous sinuses are opened, thromboplastic material can be infused into the maternal circulation. Bleeding stops following delivery of the fetus and placenta or, less frequently, by self-limitation of the precipitating event.

The clinical manifestations of abruptio placentae depend upon the site of placental implantation, the type and degree of separation, the amount of blood loss, and the presence of disseminated intravascular coagulation. It has been suggested that abruption of posteriorly implanted placentas tends to be less symptomatic than that occurring with anterior placentas. The site of separation also has clinical importance, as it may determine the intensity of blood loss. Central detachments involve disruption of the spiral arteries, and the resulting high-pressure arterial bleeding causes an expanding retroplacental hemorrhage. On the other hand, marginal separations produce bleeding from veins at the edge of the placental disk or from the intervillous space. In either case, the bleeding is not of arterial origin and therefore is less serious than that seen with central separations.

Not all central detachments lead to total separation of the placenta and fetal death. If a hematoma can form before the separation and hemorrhage become extensive, the process may stop and only be detected at the time of delivery as an organized thrombus in an area of infarcted placenta.

It must be remembered that the amount of vaginal bleeding is not a reliable indicator of the degree of placental separation. Significant amounts of blood can be concealed within the uterus until delivery. When fetal death occurs, blood loss commonly amounts to 2,500 ml and may exceed 5,000 ml. Therefore, anemia and hypovolemic shock can be present with little evidence of major vaginal bleeding.

Older studies have reported the maternal mortality rate in abruptio placenta to be 1.0 to 2.8 percent. Maternal complications include anemia, hypovolemic shock, acquired consumptive coagulopathy, renal failure, postpartum hemorrhage, and the sequelae of ischemic damage to distant organs.

The occurrence of disseminated intravascular coagulation seems to be related to the degree of placental separation and retroplacental bleeding. The greater the separation, the higher the likelihood of significant bleeding and acquired coagulopathy.

The fetal mortality rate in abruptio placentae has been reported to be over 50 percent, and a significant number of perinatal deaths occur prior to hospital admission. The fetal complications in this disorder are related to hypoxemia and occasionally to anemia. Hypoxemia results from maternal hypovolemia, anemia, and reduction of the available placental interface for fetal-maternal exchange. When fetal anemia occurs, it is probably caused by bleeding from lacerated villi.

Three main theories have been proposed to explain the fibrinogen depletion and the hemorrhagic diathesis associated with abruptio placentae:

1. Release of tissue thromboplastin into the maternal circulation, with the production of disseminated intravascular coagulation.
2. Intrauterine consumption of fibrinogen and other coagulation factors during the formation of the retroplacental clot.
3. Primary fibrinolysis, with digestion of the circulating fibrinogen.

The first theory seems to provide the most plausible explanation for the occurrence of a coagulopathy in abruptio placentae. The placenta and decidua are rich in thromboplastic material. Disseminated intravascular coagulation has been experimentally induced by injecting placental extracts into animals. It has been postulated that thromboplastic material is introduced through the maternal venous sinuses and that activation of the extrinsic mechanism of blood coagulation results in disseminated intravascular coagulation.

It must be stressed that the bleeding diathesis associated with abruptio placentae is due not only to fibrinogen consumption but also to depletion of other coagulation factors, such as factors V and VIII, and to the anticoagulant effects of fibrin degradation products. The incidence of postpartum hemorrhage has been better correlated with a high level of circulating fibrin degradation products than with the fibrinogen concentration. This underlines the importance of fibrinolysis in the production of clinical manifestations of bleeding in disseminated intravascular coagulation.

The clinical course and laboratory findings of the coagulopathy of abruptio placentae are those of decompensated acute disseminated intravascular coagulation. Fibrinogen and factors V and VIII levels are low, whereas fibrinogen degradation products are elevated. Platelets are either low or normal, and frequently the degree of thrombocytopenia is less than that expected from the hypofibrinogenemia. It has been suggested that a very active fibrinolytic system lyses the clots and avoids excessive traumatic destruction of platelets and red blood cells.

A patient with a placental abruption should be cared for in the labor and delivery unit. Women with extensive placental separations usually present complaining of abdominal pain and vaginal bleeding. The uterus is often tetanically contracted and fetal heart tones may be absent. Initial evaluation includes recording of vital signs, assessment of vaginal bleeding, electronic fetal heart rate monitoring, and drawing blood for baseline studies (hematocrit, platelet count, fibrinogen, prothrombin time, partial thromboplastin time, fibrinogen split products, and clot observation test). A secure intravenous route for administration of blood and fluid should be started by using a 16- or 18-gauge cannula. Because fluid can be administered more rapidly under pressure than by gravity alone, it is ideal to use plastic fluid bags rather than glass bottles. Fluid bags can be compressed by a pressor infusion set to increase the rate of infusion. The infusion should be initiated with a crystalloid solution such as Ringer's lactate. A Foley catheter should be inserted to follow urinary output; 30 ml per hour is indicative of adequate renal perfusion.

Tests that can be performed in the labor floor laboratory include hematocrit, a clot observation test, and a peripheral smear for platelet enumeration. The clot observation test is done by collecting 5 ml of maternal venous blood in a glass tube and inverting it four or five times. An abnormality should be suspected if a clot fails to form in 6 minutes. If the clot forms in less than 6 minutes, the concentration of fibrinogen is likely to be more than 150 mg per deciliter. If a clot is not formed in 30 minutes, the fibrinogen concentration is likely to be less than 100 mg per deciliter. This test is simple and should be performed in every patient suspected of having an abruptio placentae. Rapid clot formation essentially makes the possibility of severe hypofibrinogenemia unlikely, and under these circumstances surgical intervention can be undertaken for fetal indications. If a clot has not formed in 30 minutes, however, a serious disruption of the hemostatis mechanism is likely to exist. In institutions where blood components are immediately available upon request, surgery for fetal distress may be started and replacement therapy begun during the procedure. If a delay in obtaining blood products is anticipated, however, it is best to delay surgery until they are available because of the possibility of maternal exsanguination during the operation. A Wright's stain of a peripheral smear can be used to quickly screen for a platelet deficiency. If less than four platelets per high power field are seen, thrombocytopenia should be strongly suspected.

The management of individual cases of severe abruptio placentae depends on gestational age, fetal status, severity of the abruption, feasibility of vaginal delivery, and the presence of shock and disseminated intravascular coagulation. If the fetus is previable or dead, every effort should be made to accomplish vaginal delivery because this imposes less severe demands on the hemostatic system than hysterotomy or cesarean section. If fetal distress is present in a viable infant, delivery should be accomplished in the most expeditious way. If fetal distress is not present and vaginal delivery is anticipated within 6 to 8 hours, vaginal delivery may be attempted provided the electronic and biochemical means of fetal assessment and anesthesia, blood, and operating room access are continuously available. If these conditions are not present, cesarean section is likely to improve perinatal salvage because fetal distress may suddenly occur.

Induction of labor should begin with amniotomy. The loss of amniotic fluid decreases intrauterine volume and allows more effective hemostasis at the placental site. Oxytocin administration by intravenous infusion should be started immediately following the amniotomy.

If there are signs of circulatory collapse in association with disseminated intravascular coagulation, rapid volume replacement is necessary in order to prevent acute renal failure. Replacement with Ringer's lactate solution is initiated pending availability of blood. When fetal death has occurred, a deficit of at least 1,000 to 2,000 ml of blood can be estimated. A central venous pressure line should be placed to assess the effectiveness of intravascular volume replacement. The average central venous pressure in the third trimester should be 10 cm H_2O, and this value can be used as a guide to follow the progress of fluid replacement.

Packed red cells are indicated if anemia is present. The goal is to maintain the hematocrit at around 30 percent. Each unit of red blood cells can be expected to increase the hemoglobin by 1 to 1.5 g and the hematocrit by 3 points. Fresh frozen plasma can be used as a plasma expander or to replace the hemostatic components consumed in disseminated intravascular coagulation, such as fibrinogen, factor V, factor VIII, and antithrombin III. Cryoprecipitate is the most volume-efficient form of fibrinogen replacement. Its use is indicated when fibrinogen concentrations are below 100 mg per deciliter. Each unit of cryoprecipitate contains approximately 250 mg per bag and raises the fibrinogen concentration by approximately 5 mg per deciliter.

If the fibrinogen level is above 100 mg per deciliter, volume replacement therapy can be given as whole blood, packed red cells and fresh frozen plasma, or packed red cells and crystalloid solutions. The best combination is packed red cells and fresh frozen plasma because it provides more labile coagulation factors than whole blood and avoids crystalloid-induced dilution of circulating coagulation factors.

Heparin therapy has been advocated by some authors to arrest coagulation factor consumption in abruptio placentae. However, in the presence of a disruption of the vascular integrity, it is likely to increase the risk of severe hemorrhage; therefore its use in this setting is not recommended.

Since fibrinolysis in abruptio placentae is a protective mechanism against intravascular coagulation, interfering with its natural course by the use of fibrinolytic inhibitors is potentially dangerous. A recent publication, however, has associated uterine inertia refractory to amniotomy and oxytocin with hyperfibrinolysis and has reported resolution of the hypodynamia after the administration of the fibrinolytic inhibitor Trasylol. Although the explanation for these observations remains speculative, their confirmation could create an indication for fibrinolytic inhibitors in abruptio placentae complicated by refractory uterine inertia.

Occasionally, severe bleeding from the placental site occurs several hours after delivery. Active local fibrinolysis may be responsible for this phenomenon. If a surgical cause for the hemorrhage is excluded and bleeding cannot be controlled by manual or pharmacologic stimulation of the myometrium, aminocaproic acid or other inhibitors of fibrinolysis might be used. This should rarely be necessary, however, and consultation with a hematologist is advised prior to starting a patient on these agents.

Prolonged Retention of a Dead Fetus. The association between prolonged retention of a dead fetus and hemostatic failure has been recognized for many years. The coagulopathy seems to be caused by the slow release of tissue thromboplastin from the fetoplacental unit into the maternal circulation. The resultant activation of the extrinsic pathway of blood coagulation leads to excessive generation of thrombin and disseminated intravascular coagulation. This pathologic process is initially low grade, but the progressively increased and sustained generation of thrombin may eventually transform an early compensated disseminated intravascular coagulation into a decompensated state.

The frequency of disseminated intravascular coagulation associated with fetal demise is related to the length of time the fetus has been retained in the uterine cavity and to the laboratory criteria employed to diagnose disseminated intravascular coagulation. Pritchard studied over 100 patients who had retained a dead fetus for more than 1 week and found that none demonstrated a fibrinogen concentration below 150 mg per deciliter less than 5 weeks after detection of fetal death. When more than 5 weeks had elapsed, one-third of the patients had fibrinogen concentrations below 150 mg per deciliter. The factors responsible for the development of hypofibrinogenemia in some patients and not in others are not known.

Aggressive management of the patient with a fetal death has made prolonged retention of a dead fetus a rare cause of coagulopathy in modern obstetrics. The availability of ultrasonography and of effective means to induce premature labor has virtually eliminated the delay in uterine evacuation due to diagnostic uncertainty or fear of induction failure. All patients with a fetal death should be screened with coagulation studies prior to pregnancy termination because clinical manifestations of disseminated intravascular coagulation are often minimal, and the first sign of hemostatis failure may be a dangerously severe postpartum hemorrhage.

The initial changes in the coagulation profile of a patient with a retained dead fetus are an elevation in the circulating levels of fibrinogen degradation products and a fall in the concentration of fibrinogen. These changes precede the development of abnormalities in the partial thromboplastin time and prothrombin time. The fall in platelet count is less marked than that in fibrinogen levels.

The management of a patient with disseminated intravascular coagulation caused by a retained dead fetus depends on the state of hemostatic compensation and whether or not the patient is in labor. If the disseminated intravascular coagulation is either compensated or overcompensated (elevated fibrinogen degradation products, normal or elevated fibrinogen and platelets), the risk of hemostatic failure is small. The management goal in this setting is to accomplish delivery of the dead infant in order to eliminate the source of thromboplastic material and suppress the excessive generation of thrombin. The duration of pregnancy and the state of cervical ripeness determine whether oxytocin or prostaglandin preparations should be used for induction of labor.

If the patient has decompensated disseminated intravascular coagulation (low fibrinogen or platelets), the management objective should be to decrease the risk of peripartum hemorrhage by restoring hemostatic levels of the consumed coagulation components prior to delivery. This can be accomplished by the administration of heparin if the patient is not in labor or by supplying the consumed factor with blood component therapy if labor is in progress.

When the patient is in labor, potential areas of vascular disruption and injury are likely to develop (e.g., placental implantation site, episiotomy, or lacerations). Under these circumstances, the administration of heparin is contraindicated because it may increase the bleeding tendency by reducing the ability to form clots in areas of vascular injury. Management should be directed at replacing the deficient hemostatic components. Fibrinogen is the most frequently depleted coagulation factor in this setting. Platelet counts and levels of factors V and VIII are frequently within a safe hemostatic range (platelets > 60,000 per mm^3; factor V 10 to 20 percent; and factor VIII 25 to 30 percent). Fibrinogen replacement is best accomplished by administration of cryoprecipitate. Approximately 10 U of this product are necessary to increase the circulatory level of plasma fibrinogen by 50 mg per deciliter. Cryoprecipitate is preferred to fresh frozen plasma because the correction of hypofibrinogenemia with the latter product requires the administration of large volumes of colloids, placing the patient at risk for circulatory overload.

If the patient is not in labor, the administration of heparin can arrest the consumption of coagulation factors, permit restoration of hemostatic competence, and obviate the need for blood replacement therapy. Heparin is best administered by continuous intravenous infusion. This reduces the risk of bleeding that may accompany intermittent bolus administration. A recommended program for heparin therapy is to give an initial bolus of 5,000 U and then start an infusion at 1,000 U per hour. Modification of the maintenance rate may be necessary to avoid bleeding complications and achieve therapeutic goals.

Heparin therapy is monitored with serial fibrinogen levels, platelet counts, and partial thromboplastin times. The objective of therapy is to increase the concentrations of fibrinogen, coagulation factors, and circulating platelets above safe hemostatic levels. A reasonable goal is to achieve a fibrinogen concentration between 200 and 300 mg per deciliter and a platelet count above 60,000 per mm^3. The partial thromboplastin time is performed to assess the risk of excessive coagulation and should not be prolonged for more than 2.5 times the normal range.

Patients should be cautioned to avoid trauma and to report any episode of bleeding during heparin administration. Treatment goals can usually be accomplished in 24 to 48 hours, after which heparin can be stopped. Induction of labor can begin 5 hours after discontinuation of therapy, since heparin's anticoagulant activity is virtually nonexistent 4 hours after the infusion has been stopped.

Another indication for heparin therapy is the management of a multiple gestation complicated by decompensated disseminated intravascular coagulation secondary to the death of one fetus during labor. Heparin therapy should be administered in order to achieve safe levels of hemostatic factors. The anticoagulant should then be stopped and labor induced. If the gestation is preterm, however, significant prolongation of the pregnancy can be achieved by anticoagulation of the mother. This can be accomplished initially with intravenous administration of heparin until the fibrinogen concentration has reverted to acceptable levels and then by subcutaneous therapy. The dose of subcutaneous heparin used for maintenance therapy is 5,000 U every 6 hours. Modification of the treatment plan depends on changes in plasma fibrinogen concentration. Platelet counts should be monitored during heparin therapy because thrombocytopenia can be a side effect of heparin administration. Heparin therapy should be discontinued prior to elective induction when the living twin has been shown to have achieved pulmonary maturity. Total discontinuation of heparin therapy weeks prior to delivery without a recurrence of the coagulopathy was possible in one case.

Pregnancy-Induced Hypertension. Pregnancy-induced hypertension, also known as toxemia of pregnancy, is a common cause of chronic disseminated intravascular coagulation in the pregnant patient.

The mechanism of activation of the hemostatic system in pregnancy-induced hypertension is unknown. Several authors have proposed that such an activation occurs prior to the clinical onset of hypertension and is an integral part of the pathophysiology of the disease. Evidence for excessive thrombin activity is provided by the increased concentrations of fibrinopeptide A and soluble fibrin complexes in preeclamptic patients as compared with normal pregnant women. The kinetic consequences of excessive thrombin generation, namely thrombocytopenia, decreased fibrinogen concentrations and a decreased factor VIII activity/VIII antigen ratio have been well documented in the course of the disease. Thrombi in the microcirculations of the liver, kidney, and placental bed of patients with pregnancy-induced hypertension have been identified and may account for the multiorgan manifestations of the disease.

Elevated levels of fibrinogen degradation products are consistent with secondary activation of the fibrinolytic system. The presence of thrombotic lesions in the microcirculation in pregnancy-induced hypertension, however, may be due to a relative impairment of fibrinolytic activity. Activation of the hemostatic system is important in this disease because a correlation has been demonstrated between the severity of hypertension and proteinuria and the degree of coagulation abnormality.

The most frequent manifestations of disseminated intravascular coagulation in pregnancy-induced hypertension are thrombocytopenia and elevated circulatory levels of fibrin degradation products. Platelet counts of less than 150,000 per mm^3 have been reported in as many as 15 percent of patients with preeclampsia and 30 percent of those with eclampsia. This thrombocytopenia is caused by intravascular consumption of platelets. In preeclamptic women with thrombocytopenia, fibrinogen levels are usually normal or may even be elevated. This may be due to a greater degree of compensation afforded by the liver as compared with the bone marrow. Alternatively, it is possible that platelets participate in the process of initiation of disseminated intravascular coagulation in pregnancy-induced hypertension and, therefore, are consumed to a greater degree than fibrinogen and other coagulation factors.

The typical hemostatic profile of a patient with chronic disseminated intravascular coagulation associated with pregnancy-induced hypertension includes thrombocytopenia; normal prothrombin time, partial thromboplastic time, and thrombin time; normal, low or high fibrinogen levels; elevated fibrinogen degradation products; and microangiopathic hemolytic changes of the red blood cells. Decreased activities of factors XII, XI, IX, and VIII as a result of the activation of the intrinsic pathway have been observed in severe pregnancy-induced hypertension. Bone marrow aspiration typically demonstrates a normal or elevated number of megakaryocytes. Serum levels of lactate dehydrogenase can be elevated, reflecting its release from mechanical destruction of red blood cells. Patients with these laboratory findings frequently present with epigastric pain and elevation of the serum glutamic-oxaloacetic transaminase levels. On occasion the triad of abdominal pain, thrombocytopenia, and liver dysfunction may precede the development of hypertension.

The process of chronic disseminated intravascular coagulation invariably resolves after delivery of the infant. Antepartum resolution of thrombocytopenia and correction of the liver dysfunction have been observed to occur spontaneously or after the administration of antiplatelet agents such as aspirin and dipyridamole. Spontaneous antepartum resolution of the thrombocytopenia does not mean that the process of disseminated intravascular coagulation has resolved. Frequently, elevated levels of fibrinogen degradation products can still be demonstrated despite a normal platelet count. This evidence of fibrinolysis is generally accepted to indicate a state of chronic compensated disseminated intravascular coagulation. The consequences of ongoing compensated disseminated intravascular coagulation have not been established, but worsening of the hypertension and delivery of growth-retarded infants have been observed in patients managed conservatively after resolution of their thrombocytopenia.

Although the thrombocytopenia associated with acute pregnancy-induced hypertension can be severe, antepartum bleeding is rare. Frequently, the nadir platelet count is reached during the first postpartum day, with spontaneous resolution occurring 72 hours after delivery in most cases.

Patients with pregnancy-induced hypertension and thrombocytopenia should be considered to have a severe form of toxemia regardless of the degree of systemic hypertension. These women are at risk of multiple organ ischemic involvement and their fetuses are at risk of intrauterine growth retardation. The mechanism responsible for intrauterine growth retardation has been postulated to be suboptimal placental perfusion and poor fetal-maternal exchange because of platelets and fibrin deposits in the uteroplacental microcirculation.

Delivery of the infant is the treatment of choice for patients with pregnancy-induced hypertension and disseminated intravascular coagulation. Platelet transfusions are not indicated unless the platelet count is less than 50,000 per mm^3, there is severe hypertension or active bleeding, or the patient is being prepared for surgery. A reasonable goal is to raise the platelet count to 50,000 per mm^3 prior to any surgical intervention. Fibrinogen replacement with cryoprecipitate is rarely necessary because serum fibrinogen levels generally exceed 100 mg per deciliter.

The role of heparin and antiplatelet agents in the treatment of disseminated intravascular coagulation associated with toxemia has not been definitely established. Their use in patients with severe hypertension is contraindicated because of the risk of cerebral hemorrhage. On the other hand, they may prove to be useful in prolonging an early gestation in patients with mild hypertension but significant activation of the hemostatic system.

PRESENCE OF CLOTTING INHIBITORS

Circulating Anticoagulants

Circulating anticoagulants are endogenous blood components that inhibit the action of clotting factors. They may be directed against a specific coagulation factor or may interfere with a phase of blood coagulation.

Specific Inhibitors

Specific inhibitors can occur in patients with congenital coagulation defects or in individuals with previously normal hemostasis. Most specific inhibitors are thought to be antibodies. Their appearance has been suggested to be due to an immunologic response of the host to a transfused factor (e.g., factor VIII in hemophilia A), although spontaneous inhibitors have also been reported. Among specific inhibitors, the most frequent one is that directed against factor VIII. The inhibitor generally irreversibly inactivates factor VIII by means of a time- and temperature-dependent reaction. The clinical manifestations of this condition are similar to those of hemophilia A, except for a lower frequency of hemarthroses and a higher prevalence of ecchymosis, muscle bleeding, hematuria, and menorrhagia. The inhibitor may appear at any time during pregnancy, but its most frequent occurrence is in the puerperal period. The hemorrhagic diathesis associated with this circulating anticoagulant may be severe and difficult to treat. The diagnosis is usually made by the presence of a prolonged partial thromboplastin time that is not corrected by the addition of normal plasma; prothrombin time and thrombin time are typically normal. On occasion, demonstration of the inhibitor may require incubation of the mixture of plasmas for 1 hour at 37°C. It is possible to quantitate the activity of the inhibitor, and standardized inhibitor units (Bethesda or Oxford) have been described.

Therapeutic modalities employed in the management of patients with acquired inhibitors to factor VIII include replacement of factor VIII alone (human, porcine, or bovine) or in combination with plasmapheresis, exchange transfusions, corticosteroids, antimetabolites, alkylating agents, and/or Autoplex, an anti-inhibitor coagulation complex. Although the traditional approach to the management of the acute crisis has been administration of factor VIII, encouraging results have been reported recently with Autoplex. This preparation contains activated clotting factors and its postulated mechanism of action is to bypass the site of action of factor VIII in the coagulation cascade. The recommended dose is 76 U per kilogram over 15 to 20 minutes. Therapy can be followed by observing the clinical response and by serial partial thromboplastin times. This preparation is extremely expensive and should not be used without a precise diagnosis. Another promising therapy involves the suppression of autoantibody production by IgG intravenous infusion. The recommended course of treatment includes daily infusions of IgG at a dose of 0.5 g per kilogram body weight for 8 days. Hemostasis with a prolonged concomitant rising serum level of factor VIII and a falling autoantibody titer has been observed. This mode of therapy should be considered when either factor VIII concentrate or plasmapheresis fails to control the recurrent bleeding caused by factor VIII inhibitors. Patients with an acute hemorrhagic diathesis due to a coagulation inhibitor represent serious management problems. They should be treated in conjunction with an expert hematologist and the blood bank service.

The prognosis for patients with factor VIII inhibitor is good provided they survive the acute stage of the disease. Most anticoagulants disappear in months or years after detection. Although most infants born to mothers with circulating anticoagulants have been clinically normal, an inhibitor has been detected in two neonates. The significance of this finding remains speculative. In a recent review of the hemostatic performance in successive pregnancies of 12 patients with a factor VIII inhibitor, nine of whom were found to have uneventful pregnancies and to be in remission at the time of the subsequent delivery. These subjects included two patients with inhibitors present at the onset of their second pregnancies but whose antifactor VIII titers continued to decrease and finally disappeared before the second delivery. Bleeding manifestations persisted in three patients in their subsequent pregnancies and in one of them the disease became worse.

It must be stressed that pregnancy or surgery in a patient with a high titer of a factor VIII inhibitor is a potentially life-threatening condition. It seems wise to follow patients who are known to have this problem with serial inhibitor titers and to advise them to wait until they are in remission to conceive. If the disease is detected during pregnancy or if patients become pregnant before remission is achieved, they should be advised as to their risk and followed with serial inhibitor titers. Consideration should be given to the use of steroids in the event of high or rising inhibitor titers.

Lupus-Type Inhibitors. A lupus-type inhibitor was originally described in patients with systemic lupus erythematosus but now has been observed in association with other conditions and in patients without any demonstrable disease. The presence of this inhibitor may be the first manifestation of systemic lupus erythematosus.

The inhibitor is an immunoglobulin of the IgG or IgM type. Its mechanism of action has not been completely established, but most evidence suggests that it interferes with the reaction in which factor Xa, factor V, and phospholipid form a complex (prothrombinase) that transforms prothrombin into thrombin. It has been proposed that this inhibitor occupies the binding site of the phospholipid molecule, which is generally available for the coagulation factor.

Bleeding is uncommon despite the significant abnormalities in in vitro coagulation. Thrombosis, on the other hand, seems to be a more significant problem in these patients. To explain this paradox, it has been proposed that bleeding does not occur because after saturation of the inhibitor molecule with phospholipid, enough phospholipid is still available to react with the coagulation factors and accomplish effective hemostasis. The mechanism of thrombosis associated with lupus anticoagulant remains unclear, but several hypotheses have been proposed. The anticoagulant, with its antiphospholipid property, may damage both platelets and vascular endothelial cells, resulting in increased thromboxane release and reduced prostacyclin production, respectively. These effects predispose to thrombosis. The presence of the circulating anticoagulant is generally discovered by the detection of a prolonged activated partial thromboplastin time that is not corrected by the addition of normal plasma, or an abnormal kaolin clotting time curve. The kaolin clotting time seems to have a higher sensitivity than the activated partial thromboplastin time. Both tests are not specific for the lupus anticoagulant because they can be abnormal in the presence of other anticoagulants. The presence of the lupus anticoagulant can be confirmed by the platelet neutralization procedure in which the prolonged activated partial thromboplastin time is corrected by the addition of excess platelet phospholipid. The prothrombin time and thrombin time are frequently prolonged. The reasons for the prolongation of the latter are unclear. Thrombocytopenia is occasionally present. Excessive platelet destruction caused by a relative deficiency of prostacyclin or by platelet antibodies could be the mechanism responsible for the low platelet count.

The presence of the lupus anticoagulant is associated with increased fetal loss throughout gestation in addition to recurrent thromboembolic disorders. Extensive atheromatous, thrombotic lesions and infarction in the placenta associated with the anticoagulant have also been reported. These observations are important because they suggest a link between autoimmune mechanisms and reproductive wastage and provide new possibilities for therapeutic interventions. Prednisone and low-dose aspirin have been shown to improve fetal salvage in patients with anticoagulants. The recommended doses of prednisone and aspirin are 20 to 80 mg per day and 80 mg per day, respectively. The dosage of prednisone is adjusted to return the coagulation tests such as activated partial thromboplastin time to normal. At this low dose, aspirin inhibits thromboxane synthesis without much impact on prostacyclin production and appears to be safe for use in pregnancy. Interestingly, successful pregnancies have been observed in patients with anticoagulants who received neither aspirin nor immunosuppressive medications during pregnancy. A well-designed clinical trial is needed to evaluate the impact of corticosteroids and/or aspirin on the pregnancy outcomes of lupus anticoagulant–positive patients.

IMMUNE THROMBOCYTOPENIC PURPURA

Immune thrombocytopenic purpura (ITP)* can be defined as a syndrome characterized by a low platelet count, a normal or increased number of megakaryocytes in the bone marrow, shortened platelet survival time, and the presence of platelet-bound immunoglobulin.

In ITP, shortened platelet life span due to increased platelet destruction is the mechanism of thrombocytopenia. A circulating antibody, which is frequently an IgG, is produced against an unidentified platelet antigen. This antibody coats the platelets, which are then destroyed at an increased rate in the reticuloendothelial system, mainly in the spleen. The severity of the disease correlates with the quantity of platelet-bound IgG and not with serum antiplatelet IgG. The antibody can cross the placenta, coat fetal platelets, and enhance their destruction by the fetal reticuloendothelial system. The antibody may be present in women who are in remission; therefore, their fetuses remain at risk for neonatal thrombocytopenia even though they have normal platelet counts.

ITP is not uncommon during pregnancy, as the disease predominantly affects young women during their reproductive years. The consequences of this disorder are related solely to the thrombocytopenia and to the disruption of the normal hemostatic mechanism that a low platelet count can produce. The ever-present threat of hemorrhage poses special problems for both the mother and her fetus during pregnancy, and the aim of management is to minimize that threat. The risks of antepartum, intrapartum, and postpartum hemorrhage, present in all obstetric patients, are increased in women with ITP, as is the potential for increased surgical bleeding during cesarean section. The main risk to the infant is intracranial hemorrhage secondary to transplacentally acquired thrombocytopenia.

The signs and symptoms of this disease are directly related to the platelet count and are not specific for ITP. Capillary bleeding generally occurs when the platelet count in less than 30,000 per mm^3 and is predominantly dermal or mucosal (e.g., petechiae, ecchymosis, epistaxis, hematuria). Retinal hemorrhages are particularly important to recognize because they are signs of impending intracranial hemorrhage. With the exception of these findings, the physical examination is usually normal. An enlarged spleen suggests that the thrombocytopenia is secondary to another disorder, such as systemic lupus erythematosus, infectious mononucleosis, or a lymphoproliferative disorder.

The clinical course of the disease may be acute (associated with drug reactions or viral infections) or chronic. Chronic ITP usually has an insidious course, with episodes of intermittent exacerbations and remissions.

When the diagnosis of ITP is made in a female of reproductive age, family planning and contraception should be discussed. Since medical therapy and splenectomy during pregnancy are not without risk, patients should be advised to postpone childbearing until a remission of the disease is obtained and steroid or immunosuppressive therapy is not required. Splenectomy may be necessary to achieve this state. Occasionally, however, this goal may not be accomplished, because some patients require medical therapy even following splenectomy. If this is the case, patients who desire to become pregnant should be made aware of the potential risks of steroids or immunosuppressants to the fetus. Patients should also be informed that they may need a cesarean section for fetal indications and that there is an increased risk to both the fetus and the mother with this disease. However, ITP is by no means an absolute contraindication to pregnancy.

Regarding contraception, it is not wise to use intrauterine devices because in addition to the risks of menorrhagia and uterine perforation, there is an increased failure rate of this method in patients taking steroids. There is no specific contraindication to the use of birth control pills in women with ITP.

Once the patient with ITP is pregnant, the management goals are to decrease the risk of antepartum, intrapartum, and postpartum maternal hemorrhage and to prevent intracranial hemorrhage in the neonate. Treatment pro-

* The abbreviation ITP is conventionally used for "idiopathic thrombocytopenic purpura," a term here reserved for a condition similar to immune thrombocytopenic purpura but not involving demonstrable platelet-bound IgG.

grams for patients with ITP during pregnancy largely reflect personal bias, since most of the management recommendations have not been evaluated in well-designed clinical trials.

Management of ITP in Pregnancy

The management of ITP is directed toward preventing platelet underproduction, platelet consumption, and impairment of platelet function. The mainstays of treatment are steroids and splenectomy.

General Measures. Iron, folic acid, and vitamin B_{12} deficiencies impair platelet production. Therefore, identification of a deficiency as well as adequate supplementation of the deficient substances during pregnancy is important. Myelotoxic agents such as alcohol should be avoided. If present, fever and infection should be identified and treated, since they shorten platelet survival. Drugs that impair platelet function or cause thrombocytopenia should be avoided.

Steroid Therapy. Therapy in patients with ITP always begins with steroids. The immediate effects of steroid administration are inhibition of antibody attachment to platelets and suppression of platelet phagocytosis by the reticuloendothelial system. The long-term effect is inhibition of antibody synthesis.

The objective of steroid therapy during pregnancy is not only to increase the platelet count to the level at which spontaneous hemorrhage is unlikely to occur (generally above 20,000 per mm^3) but also to provide an adequate reserve so that hemostatic failure will not occur in the case of an unforeseen maternal hemorrhage. Although the ideal goal is to bring the platelet count to normal levels, this frequently is difficult to achieve or requires the use of prohibitively high doses of steroid therapy. A more reasonable goal is to maintain a platelet count above 50,000 per mm^3, since excessive surgical hemorrhage rarely occurs above this level if platelet function is normal. If platelet dysfunction is identified by a prolonged bleeding time, the goal should be to normalize the bleeding time.

Therapy with steroids usually begins with administration of prednisone at a dose of 0.5 to 1 mg per kilogram per day in divided doses. Because the placental transfer of prednisone is less than that of other glucocorticoids (e.g., betamethasone, dexamethasone), this has been the steroid of choice in the therapy of ITP complicating pregnancy. Some authors have recently suggested the use of corticosteroids that readily cross the placenta with the aim of delivering steroids to the fetus, in whom they might have the same therapeutic effect as in the mother. A short course of steroids prior to delivery has been proposed for this purpose. The effect of this approach in the prevention of neonatal thrombocytopenia has been inconsistent. Some authors have reported a favorable response and others have not. There is a theoretical risk of acute worsening fetal thrombocytopenia with this modality of therapy, since corticosteroids could potentially displace the antibodies from the platelets, resulting in an increase in the unbound antiplatelet IgG antibodies in the maternal circulation.

The effect of steroids on the mother is usually noted within the first 24 to 48 hours but may take as long as 2 to 3 weeks. The therapeutic plan is to give the shortest course of steroids that will bring the platelet count to a safe level. Once the platelet count is above 80,000 per mm^3, the steroids should be continued for 1 week and then tapered slowly. If, on the other hand, the platelet count has not reached 50,000 per mm^3 in 3 weeks, the dose of prednisone should be increased to 1.5 to 2 mg per kilogram per day. If continued steroid therapy is needed, it should consist of the lowest dose that will maintain the platelet count above 50,000 per mm^3. This parameter must be checked during reduction and after termination of steroid therapy because a fall in the platelet count is the earliest indication of relapse in asymptomatic patients. Most pregnant women respond to steroids, and therefore the performance of a splenectomy can be deferred until the postpartum period.

The potential risks of steroid administration during pregnancy are difficult to assess. However, the risk of maternal hemorrhage outweighs the potential hazards of the judicious use of these drugs. Although animal studies have shown an increased incidence of cleft palate, this has not been substantiated by the limited studies done in humans. Other potential complications of steroids that are rarely reported include transient adrenal insufficiency in the neonate, neonatal hypoglycemia, and intrauterine growth retardation.

Estriol production can be decreased if the equivalent of 75 mg of cortisol is administered daily because at this level transplacental steroids can depress the fetal adrenal production of estriol precursors. Prednisone is secreted into the breast milk, but if the dose is less than 30 mg per day, it is unlikely to cause any problems in the breast-fed neonate.

Splenectomy. Removal of the spleen eliminates the major site of platelet destruction and an important site of antibody production. Furthermore, since 40 percent of the platelets are normally sequestered in the spleen, this operation increases the number of platelets available for circulation. Splenectomy is usually performed electively in patients with ITP because it may either eliminate the need for steroids or allow a significant reduction in their dosage. During pregnancy, however, splenectomy is indicated only in those women who have life-threatening hemorrhage and in whom primary therapy with steroids has failed to increase the platelet count and bleeding manifestations continue to occur. The major risks of performing a splenectomy in an obstetric patient are premature labor and the occurrence of a surgical accident when ligating the splenic pedicle. During pregnancy all the blood vessels in the abdomen dramatically increase in size. The technical difficulties of operating on these dilated vessels are compounded by the presence of a gravid uterus, which makes access to the splenic pedicle difficult to attain during the second half of pregnancy. However, the operation can be performed immediately following a cesarean section with few additional complications.

Splenectomy has been reported to produce permanent remission in 60 to 70 percent of patients, temporary remission in 20 percent, and no response in 10 percent. The older literature reports a 9 to 10 percent maternal and a

25 percent perinatal mortality rate when splenectomy was performed during pregnancy. These figures are likely to be different today because of the availability of platelet transfusions and improvements in surgical technique. At present the maternal operative risk of elective splenectomy during pregnancy is probably similar to that for a nonpregnant patient.

Immunosuppressive Therapy. Immunosuppressive agents (vinca alkaloids, cyclophosphamide, and azathioprine) have been used with some success to treat nonpregnant patients whose disease is refractory to steroid therapy and splenectomy. The rationale for their use is to depress the production of antiplatelet antibodies and the host's cellular immunity. Their role in the management of a pregnant patient with ITP has not been established, and concern exists about fetal side effects. There is, however, at least one report in which a woman was successfully treated with cyclophosphamide in the early third trimester without obvious neonatal sequelae.

Immunoglobulin G Infusion. Favorable responses in maternal platelet counts and hemostasis have been reported with the intravenous infusion of immunoglobulin G as a treatment for ITP. Rising platelet counts usually occur within 24 hours. This modality of therapy can be very useful in preparing patients for surgery or delivery and offers an attractive alternative to splenectomy in refractory cases. The dosage varies from 0.3 mg to 0.49 mg per kilogram of body weight given over a 4- to 6-hour period daily for 5 days. This course of treatment can be repeated weekly as needed. No adverse maternal or fetal effects have been reported. Interference with the phagocytosis of the antibody-coated platelets by blocking the macrophage Fc receptors of the reticuloendothelial system has been proposed as a mechanism of action for the infused IgG. Actually, a decrease in the Fc receptor–mediated clearance of autologous IgG–coated erythrocytes following immunoglobulin infusion has been observed. The impact of this modality of therapy on fetal platelet counts remains to be determined because both normal platelet counts and thrombocytopenia have been observed in neonates whose mothers had received immunoglobulin infusion for refractory ITP.

Platelet Transfusions. Platelet transfusions have no place in the maintenance therapy of ITP. Transfused platelets are not only rapidly destroyed but they also become progressively less effective in raising the platelet count because the antigenic load they provide induces the production of antiplatelet antibodies. Platelet transfusions are indicated in the face of life-threatening hemorrhage, to maintain hemostasis during surgery, and in severe preeclampsia because of the added risk of intracranial hemorrhage. A rule of thumb is to transfuse platelets until the bleeding time is normalized in cases of severe preeclampsia and to provide a platelet count above 60,000 per mm^3 and a normal bleeding time prior to surgery. High-dose corticosteroid therapy (prednisone 2 mg per kilogram of body weight or an intravenous preparation of equivalent dose) should be administered with platelet transfusions to prolong platelet survival.

Mode of Delivery. The most serious perinatal problem associated with ITP is fetal thrombocytopenia, which makes the neonate susceptible to hemorrhages and particularly to intracranial bleeding. It is believed that the trauma associated with delivery is a determining factor in the production of intracranial hemorrhage. Since most trauma to the fetal head occurs during its passage through the birth canal, cesarean section has been proposed as the method of choice for delivering these infants. Although this is a logical assumption, it must be noted that the protective effect of cesarean section has not been, and probably will never be, demonstrated in clinical trials. However, adherence to a policy of routine cesarean section as the mode of delivery for patients with ITP exposes the mothers to the risks of defective intra- and postoperative hemostasis. Since 77.5 percent of infants born to thrombocytopenic mothers have no detectable clinical bleeding, a significant number of unnecessary cesarean sections will be performed for putative fetal indications. A more logical approach would be to assess the neonatal risk of thrombocytopenia antenatally. Maternal platelet counts have been proposed to detect those infants at greater risk for thrombocytopenia. However, in one series 27 percent of thrombocytopenic neonates were born to mothers with platelet counts above 100,000 per mm^3. This observation invalidates the maternal platelet count as a reliable predictor of fetal thrombocytopenia.

A platelet count can be determined from the fetal scalp capillary blood obtained at the beginning of spontaneous or induced labor and the result can be used to select the mode of delivery. The technique of scalp platelet count determination has been validated by its good correlation with umbilical cord and heel capillary platelet counts.

The incidence and extent of neonatal bleeding was related to the neonatal platelet count. No bleeding manifestations and only mild cutaneous manifestations occurred in those with counts above 100,000 per ml^3 and 50,000 per ml^3, respectively. Serious bleeding requiring treatment was confined to infants with counts of less than 50,000 per mm^3. These authors have therefore proposed that a platelet count of 50,000 per mm^3 in a scalp sample be used as a cut-off value for selecting the mode of delivery. Cesarean section would be indicated only for those infants with platelet counts below 50,000 per mm^3.

It must be stressed that these recommendations are based upon two retrospective studies and a small prospective study, yet the possibility exists that some infants with platelet counts above 50,000 per mm^3 have had subclinical bleeding. A study including ultrasonographic examination and neurologic follow-up of infants born to mothers with ITP is necessary to assess the prevalence of asymptomatic bleeding and to establish the long-term significance of these findings.

The technique for scalp platelet count is simple but must be mastered before it is used in a patient with ITP. The scalp platelet count should be performed at the beginning of labor or after elective amniotomy in patients with a dilated cervix at term. Ideally, the patient should be in the cesarean section room in the lithotomy position. A plastic cone is placed in the vagina and directly applied to the fetal scalp. A stab wound scalp incision is then created similar to that used for scalp pH capillary collection. A Unopette test 5855 system (Becton-Dickinson) is used to collect the sample. This is a plastic pipet that fills by capillary action to 0.02 ml. This pipet is held in an Allis' clamp to collect the sample. Once the pipet has been filled, it is emptied into a reservoir containing 1.98 ml of diluent and mixed. Platelet count determination is performed by an automated technique or a standard manual hemocytometer method. A critical part of the scalp platelet determination technique is the speed with which the procedure is performed. If the blood is collected slowly, it tends to clot, giving falsely low results. It is wise to confirm the machine results with a smear of capillary blood. Blood collection technique for smear preparation is similar to that previously described. Heparinized tubes should not be used for sample collection because of platelet clumping, which can produce abnormally low results.

Complications with the use of this technique have not yet been reported. Compression of the scalp incision should be maintained until bleeding has stopped completely. The capability of performing an emergency cesarean section is essential when this technique is used, as continued fetal bleeding could become a problem.

It has recently been suggested that the administration of a short course of steroids (10 to 20 mg of prednisone) be given to the mother for 14 days prior to the estimated delivery date with the objective of reducing thrombocytopenia in the fetus. This program has been reported to be effective in increasing neonatal platelet counts. However, severe neonatal thrombocytopenia has been reported in steroid-treated mothers; therefore, even if this therapy has been specifically administered for its transplacental effect, a fetal scalp platelet count should be performed to ensure the adequacy of the infant's platelet count.

The inability to determine the fetal platelet count prior to the onset of labor has been considered a drawback of the fetal scalp sampling technique. Even though the impact of labor and delivery on the thrombocytopenic fetuses, especially those with platelet counts below 50,000 per ml, remains to be determined, it seems desirable not to subject these fetuses to the trauma of labor and/or precipitous delivery. Hobbins and co-workers have proposed the utilization of the percutaneous umbilical cord blood sampling technique to determine fetal platelet counts at term to overcome the above problems. However, further studies need to be done to evaluate the merits of this approach.

THROMBOTIC THROMBOCYTOPENIC PURPURA

Pathophysiology and Laboratory Findings

Thrombotic thrombocytopenic purpura (TTP) is a syndrome characterized clinically by thrombocytopenia, microangiopathic hemolytic anemia, neurologic abnormalities, renal dysfunction, and fever, and pathologically by the presence of intravascular hyaline thrombi consisting of platelets and fibrin.

The pathophysiology of this disease has not been definitively established. Increasing evidence suggests that TTP is a disorder of the mechanism that regulates the blood vessel wall–platelet interaction. The initial event may be an injury to discontinuous segments of the endothelium of small arteries and capillaries. The nature of the insult has not been determined but is likely to be diverse and may involve infectious agents and an immunologic mechanism.

Thrombotic Thrombocytopenic Purpura in Pregnancy

TTP is an uncommon disorder, but it affects women more frequently than men and is seen predominantly in those between the ages of 10 and 40. It is therefore not surprising to see this disorder in association with pregnancy. More than 350 cases have been reported, 30 of which have been associated with pregnancy. Twenty-nine biopsy-proven cases of TTP associated with pregnancy have been reviewed by May, Harbert, and Thornton, who found a 7 percent 2-year maternal survival rate and a perinatal mortality rate of approximately 65 percent. This, however, was prior to the more recent therapeutic approaches to this disease.

When TTP presents in a patient prior to or during the first trimester of pregnancy, the diagnosis is relatively easy to make, and some successful pregnancies after therapy have been reported. When the onset of the disease takes place in the third trimester of pregnancy, the diagnostic problem is more difficult because of the striking similarities between eclampsia and TTP. Both diseases may be manifested by thrombocytopenia, microangiopathic hemolytic anemia, renal dysfunction, fever, and coma and/or seizures.

It is important to differentiate between TTP and eclampsia because the latter responds dramatically to delivery whereas the former requires therapy with infusion of fresh frozen plasma and/or exchange transfusions. It has been suggested recently that gingival biopsies may provide a diagnostic tool to differentiate the two entities. Biopsy specimens of patients with TTP should show microthrombi in small vessels without evidence of vasculitis and peripheral clot lysis, whereas patients with toxemia have been assumed to have no thrombotic lesions. The problem with this approach is that gingival biopsies have been reported to be negative in as many as 40 percent of patients with TTP, and the experience with gingival biopsies in women with toxemia is limited. Furthermore, it is possible that toxemic patients with decompensated disseminated intravascular coagulation have thrombotic fibrin deposits in small vessels similar to those found on light microscopy in cases of TTP. Differentiation between the thrombotic lesions of TTP and disseminated intravascular coagulation currently requires the histochemical identification of plasminogen activator activity. Lesions of disseminated intravascular coagulation have increased fibrinolytic activity, whereas this is absent in TTP lesions. Another useful diagnostic test for TTP based on the detection of the platelet agglutinating factor has been recently developed. This test has sensitivity and false-positive rates of 87 percent and 6.4 percent, respectively. Determination of the plasma levels of the unusually large von Willebrand multimers (vWMs) and the platelet agglutinating factor appears to be promising in the diagnosis and/or follow-up of patients with TTP. The damaged endothelial cells release the unusually large vWMs which act synergistically with a plasma platlet-agglutinating factor to cause the segmental intravascular deposition of platelets and platelet-derived fibrin. The unusually large vWMs are absent from the plasma of normal subjects, are greatly reduced or even absent during the acute episode of TTP, and recur in the recovery or remission periods. In addition, the platelet-agglutinating factor is present in sera of 72 percent of patients with active TTP but absent in patients who have inactive TTP or other thrombocytopenic disorders such as ITP or preeclampsia.

Management of TTP in Pregnancy. Therapy for TTP has been empirical and has involved many different regimens, including steroids, splenectomy, heparin, heparin and urokinase, antiplatelet agents, immunosuppressive agents, hemodialysis, and plasma transfusions. Evaluation of the success of different therapeutic modalities is very difficult because they have frequently been used in combination. Furthermore, it is possible that several disorders with different pathophysiologic mechanisms have been inappropriately labeled as TTP. This, of course, will result in variable responses to different therapeutic modalities.

The management of TTP complicating pregnancy depends on the gestational age at the time of presentation. If a patient presents with the typical TTP pentad in the first or early second trimester, the diagnosis can be established with reasonable certainty because toxemia of pregnancy is unlikely to occur at this gestational age. Therapy should be directed toward inducing a hematologic remission. If the patient presents in the third trimester, however, it is very difficult to distinguish between TTP and eclampsia. Since eclampsia is the more prevalent condition, it should be assumed to be present if clinical and pathologic data are not helpful in differentiating these disorders, and the patient should be delivered. Every effort should be made to accomplish a vaginal delivery, since this imposes less stress on the hemostatic system than a cesarean section. Patient failure to improve following delivery suggests that the correct diagnosis is TTP, and specific therapy for that disease can then be initiated.

Obstetric patients with TTP are best managed in conjunction with the hematology and blood bank services. Therapy should begin with either infusion of fresh frozen plasma or exchange transfusion with fresh frozen plasma or von Willebrand factor-depleted cryosupernatant. The exchange transfusion is preferred over the simple transfusion when heart and/or kidneys are involved because of the potential volume overload associated with the latter. The current rationale for the use of plasma is based on the demonstration that patients with TTP are deficient in a factor that is present in normal plasma and can inhibit platelet aggregation. Plasmapheresis with solutions other than plasma or its cryosupernatant is ineffective. The biochemistry of this factor remains to be determined. The patient's status should be monitored with serial platelet counts, serum creatinine, lactate dehydrogenase, and bilirubin determinations, as well as frequent neurologic examinations. Daily plasma transfusions should be instituted until a spontaneous increase in platelet count to near normal values is obtained and neurologic manifestations have disappeared. The volume of the transfusion should be sufficient to maintain the lactate dehydrogenase concentration below 300 U per milliliter. The initial volume for exchange plasmapheresis has been recommended as 35 to 40 ml per kilogram of body weight. Response rates to plasma exchange transfusions and plasma infusion have been reported to be as high as 82 and 83 percent, respectively. Glucocorticoids alone or in combination with plasma exchange have also been shown to be useful in the management of TTP. In fact, glucocorticoids should be considered as a part of the initial treatment. Antiplatelet agents such as aspirin, dipyridamole, indomethacin, ibuprofen, and prostacyclin fail to prevent the in vitro platelet aggregation induced by plasma from patients with TTP. This observation supports the poor clinical responses to the antiplatelet agents in patients with TTP. Patients who have failed to respond to the initial therapy can be empirically treated with splenectomy or immunosuppressive agents with varying degrees of success. The choice of therapy after initial failure is arbitrary and in most cases reflects the personal experience and preference of the physicians managing the case. The administration of platelet concentrates has been associated with worsening of intravascular thrombus formation. They should only be used in cases of life-threatening hemorrhage and in conjunction with plasma exchange transfusions.

SUGGESTED READING

Brozovic M. Acquired disorders of blood coagulation. In: Bloom AL, Duncan DP, eds. Haemostasis and thrombosis. Edinburgh:Churchill Livingstone, 1981.

Cavanagh D. Clotting disorders in pregnancy. In: Cavanagh D, Woods RE, O'Connor TCF, Knuppel RA, eds. Obstetric emergencies. 3rd ed. Philadelphia:Harper & Row, 1981:7.

Romero R, Duffy TP. Platelet disorders in pregnancy. Clin Perinatol 1980; 7:327–348.

Romero R. Management of acquired hemostatic failure during pregnancy. In: Barkowitz R, ed. Critical care of the obstetric patient. Edinburgh: Churchill Livingstone, 1983:219.

Romero R, Duffy TP, Berkowitz RL, et al. Prolongation of a preterm pregnancy complicated by death of a single twin in utero and disseminated intravascular coagulation. Effects of treatment with heparin. N Engl J Med 1984; 310:772–774.

Wintrobe MM, Lee GR, Boggs DR, et al. Diffuse intravascular coagulation. In: Clinical hematology. 8th ed. Philadelphia:Lea & Febiger, 1981:1213.

Editor's Note: Like all books in the Current Therapy series, this volume is designed to emphasize treatment. Therefore, it behooves the reader to consult the various hematology texts for in-depth discussions of pathophysiology and diagnosis.

ECTOPIC PREGNANCY

DAVID CHARLES, M.D., F.A.C.O.G., F.R.C.O.G.
DOUGLAS D. GLOVER, B.S. Pharm., M.D.

Ectopic pregnancy may be defined as the implantation of a zygote in a location other than the uterine cavity. The fertilized ovum can implant anywhere along its path from the ovary to the uterine cervix; however, the vast majority of cases of eccyesis are located in the oviduct and, in fact, 89 percent of all ectopic pregnancies occur in the distal two-thirds of the tube. The order of frequency of location of ectopic gestation is shown in Table 1.

In 1876, Perry and Lea, in a study of 529 cases, reported a 69 percent mortality rate with eccyesis. Following the introduction of the surgical management of this entity by Tait in 1883, the outcome improved, and by the turn of the century, this pregnancy complication accounted for only 5 percent of maternal deaths. As the maternal mortality related to early pregnancy termination dramatically declined after legalization of abortion, the relative incidence of death due to ectopic gestation assumed greater significance, and it now accounts for 12 percent of the maternal deaths in the United States.

The occurrence of eccyesis has increased tremendously in recent years, probably as a consequence of the increased incidence of pelvic inflammatory disease and the relaxed sexual mores of adolescents and young adults. The incidence varies with the age, race, socioeconomic status, and demography of the population studied. Ectopic pregnancy is more common in older parous women. The prevalence is increased in nonwhites and is inversely proportional to socioeconomic status. Jamaica, followed by Vietnam, the United States, and the countries bordering on the Baltic Sea report the highest incidence, and this is coincident with the prevalence of sexually transmitted disease in these areas of the globe.

The factors predisposing to tubal pregnancy include many mechanical entities relating to the tubes, and it is surmised that anomalies of the fertilized ovum may play a role in the etiology of tubal pregnancy. With regard to the ovum, it has been suggested that the preservation of the zona radiata or the zona pellucida during the time a fertilized ovum is in the tube prevents its implantation in this location and that premature disappearance of the zona radiata favors immediate implantation. Normally by the time the blastocyst has reached the uterus, the zona pellucida has disappeared. Owing to the histolytic faculty of the ectoderm, the developing trophoblast commences to embed in the maternal tissues. If there is some delay, or if the zona pellucida disappears while the ovum traverses the oviduct, eccyesis is liable to occur.

TABLE 1 Sites of Implantation of Ectopic Pregnancy in Order of Frequency

Site of Implantation	*Frequency (%)*
Oviduct	95 (of all ectopic pregnancies)
Ampulla	82 (of tubal pregnancies
Isthumus	13 (of tubal pregnancies)
Fimbria	3 (of tubal pregnancies)
Interstitial	2 (of tubal pregnancies)
Ovary Abdomen Intraligamentous Structures Uterus Cornual Cervical	5% (of all ectopic pregnancies)

Foremost among the conditions that may delay the passage of a fertilized ovum through the tube is preceding inflammatory disease or salpingitis. As a result of the inflammatory process, loss of cilia and epithelium occurs as well as swelling of the mucosa and fusion of the plicae; this causes the tubal lumen to be narrowed and complicated by the presence of polypoidal masses and pseudofollicles. Subsequently, epithelial crypts and diverticula form in the muscularis and result in kinking of the lumen; this further adds to the tubal obstruction. It is thus clear that an inflammatory process is capable of impairing the normal function of the fallopian tube and the transmission of the ovum into the uterine cavity. This occurs either as a result of destruction of the cilia and impairment of motility or because of the formation of mechanical barriers such as crypts and diverticula.

Pelvic inflammatory disease is not the only etiologic factor in the subsequent eventuation of an ectopic pregnancy. Pelvic peritonitis may cause kinking of the tube as well as interfere with its muscular contractions, and thereby result in tubal retention of a fertilized ovum. Likewise, there is no doubt that the inflammatory reaction in the tube can be the result of previous acute appendicitis. After the introduction of the intrauterine device, the incidence of ectopic pregnancy increased, in all probability as the result of a low-grade infection associated with its use attributable to the sexual mores of the individual.

Additional etiologic factors in tubal pregnancy include prior surgery on the fallopian tubes for tubal sterilization and congenital malformations of the tubes, including diverticula and accessory ostia. Transmigration of the ovum from the opposite ovary and low-dose progestational contraceptive agents may also play a role in the etiology of eccyesis.

The number of ectopic gestations nearly tripled in the United States in the 10 years between 1970 and 1980. Antimicrobial agents account for at least part of this increase. Prior to the availability of antibiotics, pelvic inflammatory disease was considered to be the "great sterilizer," and the extent of tubal damage was such that subsequent tubal transport of a zygote was just about impossible. As a result of antibiotic therapy, tubal damage is not as extensive, and consequently nidation in the tube is more frequently encountered in clinical practice. This is particularly true in the woman who acquires postpartum endometritis or a low-grade infection following elective termination of pregnancy when antibiotics are prescribed after completion of the procedure.

Ectopic pregnancy is a disease that affects women during reproductive life and, although it can occur in adolescents, it is characteristically observed in older women; the reported mean age is 28 years. The incidence of eccyesis in women between the ages of 25 and 34 is double that in women between the ages of 15 and 24. Early diagnosis of this clinical entity is based on a high index of suspicion, laparoscopy, specific assays for serum beta-human chorionic gonadotropin (beta-hCG), and ultrasonography. The most common symptoms are the classic triad of pain, amenorrhea, and vaginal bleeding. Pain is experienced by all patients with eccyesis, and it varies from a dull ache to a sudden sharp, lancinating pain in the lower abdominal area that may be associated with syncope and the urge to defecate. The pain may be localized on the side of the abnormal gestation; however, in 25 percent of cases it is on the contralateral side. In the presence of extensive peritoneal inflammation, the pain frequently is diffuse. In about 70 percent of cases the diagnosis is established within 4 days of the onset of pain, and shoulder pain may be present after tubal rupture as the blood migrates cephalad and irritates the diaphragm.

Amenorrhea is a highly variable symptom and may vary from 1 to 12 weeks in duration in ectopic pregnancy. Although some patients report the last menses to have been normal, most experience shorter or lighter flow, which may lead them to suspect that they may be pregnant. Others have periodic bleeding or spotting caused by the inability of the low level of sex steroids to support the decidual reaction of the endometrium. This early bleeding is often painless, in contradistinction to that which occurs with the rupture of the oviduct. Vaginal bleeding is experienced by 80 percent of women with ectopic pregnancies, and it may be heavy in ruptured interstitial or angular pregnancies.

On physical examination, the patient may appear ill, and her facial expression will portray the severity of the pain associated with tubal rupture. The skin may be pale and the blood pressure low in the presence of severe intraperitoneal hemorrhage. On the other hand, the blood pressure and skin color will be normal if the oviduct is unruptured or if the bleeding is minimal. Although abdominal distention may be noted in cases of massive hemorrhage, it is observed infrequently. Most patients exhibit lower abdominal tenderness in response to deep palpation, and the presence of rebound tenderness is usually indicative of a hematoperitoneum.

Pain is elicited on pelvic examination in the majority of patients (Table 2). Although excitation pain on movement of the cervix is usually associated with ectopic pregnancy, only 40 percent of patients have pain on lateral cervical motion. Likewise, not all patients have adnexal tenderness on rectovaginal examination, but when elicited it may limit the patient's ability to cooperate and consequently the clinician will fail to palpate any mass that is present. Attention should be paid to the presence or absence of bulging of the pouch of Douglas, since when it is present it is indicative of blood in the peritoneal cavity.

DIFFERENTIAL DIAGNOSIS

It must be emphasized that ultrasonography is useful as an ancillary aid in the diagnosis of ectopic pregnancy. Clinically, there may be difficulty in differentiating a normal from an ectopic pregnancy, especially when the test for urinary chronic gonadotropin is positive and the findings of culdocentesis are negative. Ultrasonography can play a significant role in establishing a diagnosis. If examination by ultrasound indicates the absence of an intrauterine pregnancy, the physician will rightfully perform laparoscopy, whereas if it demonstrates a normal intrauterine pregnancy, the patient will be spared the hazards of anesthesia and surgery. As shown in Table 3, the uterus may be normal or slightly enlarged in cases of ectopic pregnancy, and the internal echo pattern may consist of weak scattered echoes, strong and weak echoes, or a central linear band of echoes of moderate strength that represents decidual reaction. In eccyesis, evidence of a normal intrauterine pregnancy is absent except in the rare case in which ectopic and intrauterine pregnancies coexist.

On occasion ultrasonographic extrauterine findings may reveal the presence of an intact ectopic gestational sac, but this is uncommon. The sac is usually not seen because of its small size, or it may be obscured by overlying bowel or incorporated in a hemorrhagic mass. When seen, it usually lies adjacent to the uterine fundus. When a gestational sac appears to be located eccentrically in the uterine fundus, it should be ultrasonographically differentiated from a normal intrauterine pregnancy associated with a double uterus, a fundal leiomyoma, or compression by the maternal bladder. Cornual pregnancy may furnish a similar appearance. If an extrauterine mass is identified, it is usually a complex, predominantly cystic mass comprising a mixture of blood clot and products of conception. Occasionally the mass appears cystic but poorly defined. The size and ease by which the mass is discernible vary with the duration of the gestation, the location of the ectopic pregnancy, and the amount of blood in the pelvis. The mass may, however, be seen in the adnexal area, adjacent to the uterine fundus or in the pouch of Douglas.

Ultrasonographic differentiation includes pelvic inflammatory disease, endometriosis, and a benign cystic teratoma of the ovary. When there is rupture of an ectopic sac associated with hemoperitoneum, blood may be seen as a crescentic echo-free area in the cul-de-sac. If bleed-

TABLE 2 Pelvic Findings in Ectopic Pregnancy

Physical Sign	*Patients (%)*
Cervical tenderness	40
Adnexal tenderness	40
Palpable adnexal mass	40

TABLE 3 Uterine Size in Ectopic Pregnancy

Size	*(%) of Pregnancies*
Normal size	70
6–8 weeks size	25
>8 weeks size	5

ing is acute and massive, an ascites-like picture may be demonstrable. A rare type of ectopic gestation is an abdominal pregnancy, and demonstration of fetal or maternal echoes or both outside the uterus is diagnostic. In such cases the placenta is usually mixed with bowel echoes, and there is no well-defined amniotic space or chorionic plate.

In the differential diagnosis, one must always consider threatened or incomplete abortion, an intrauterine pregnancy, or pelvic inflammatory disease. In cases of pelvic inflammatory disease, pain and tenderness are more likely to be bilateral. In cases of acute pelvic inflammatory disease, the findings of an elevated temperature, leukocytosis, and increased sedimentation rate aid in the diagnosis. A tubo-ovarian abscess is usually much larger than any adnexal mass associated with an ectopic pregnancy.

A persistent corpus luteum with intra-abdominal hemorrhage also has to be considered, as it may cause a delay in menstruation followed by persistent light bleeding and symptoms identical to those of eccyesis. The enlarged ovary forms a unilateral mass that may be difficult to distinguish from a tubal gestation. If the corpus luteum bleeds profusely into the peritoneal cavity, differentiation from a ruptured ectopic pregnancy can only be made by laparoscopy or colpotomy.

Torsion of the adnexa must always be considered because this entity may cause acute pain combined with nausea and vomiting and resemble the severe pain of a ruptured ectopic pregnancy. Ectopic pregnancy in the right tube may be mistaken for acute appendicitis, although the history is usually dissimilar. The initial pain in appendicitis is characteristically periumbilical followed by anorexia, nausea, or vomiting and a relocation of the pain to the right lower quadrant. Pain caused by ectopic pregnancy is usually pelvic in origin, and in appendicitis the temperature and white count are more likely to be elevated; the uterus is not tender, nor is cervical motion likely to accentuate the pelvic pain. Unless the patient is coincidentally menstruating, uterine bleeding does not occur with acute appendicitis.

Ectopic pregnancy is indeed a great pelvic masquerader. Novak stated: "It may well be considered the disease of diagnostic surprises." To avoid errors in diagnosis, one should obtain a complete history, perform a thorough examination, and intelligently interpret laboratory data. We firmly believe that all of the diagnostic aids are of importance. In cases of suspected ectopic pregnancy, laparoscopy, ultrasonography, and serum beta-hCG assays should be utilized.

MANAGEMENT

As stated previously, the treatment of eccyesis is well known and necesitates surgery without delay. Blood for typing and crossmatching should be obtained at the time of admission to the hospital, and when necessary a blood transfusion should be instituted to treat and combat shock. The amount of blood administered is governed by the rate and quantity of blood loss and the condition of the patient. In the presence of massive intraperitoneal hemorrhage such as can occur with an acute rupture of a cornual pregnancy, large amounts of blood may be required. Rh negative women can become sensitized by Rh positive blood from an ectopic gestation and should be treated with 300 μg Rh immunoglobulin before leaving the hospital.

The operative procedure carried out should be one to cure the eccyesis. If the patient's condition is good and there is little or no hemorrhage, one may perform any indicated pelvic surgery, and some surgeons include appendectomy. However, if the patient has an appreciable amount of blood loss, only salpingectomy or salpingo-oophorectomy should be performed. The contralateral adnexa should always be inspected to eliminate the rare occurrence of bilateral eccyesis and to ascertain if the oviduct is otherwise normal.

Almost all eccyesis occurs in women of reproductive age, many of whom are interested in future fertility. An ectopic pregnancy causes infertility in a large number of patients, and among those who have failed to conceive, a tubal factor is responsible for the infertility in at least two-thirds. Surgical removal of the affected tube is sometimes essential when rupture of the oviduct has resulted in extensive damage, but ovarian conservation is advisable. The encouraging results of in vitro fertilization mandate that we preserve as much ovarian tissue as possible. The likelihood of obtaining oocytes for in vitro fertilization increases with the greater available areas of ovarian surface. Patients who have had a salpingo-oophorectomy have a least a 50 percent chance of having an intrauterine pregnancy. However, the possibility of a repeat ectopic pregnancy may be as high as one in eight of the patients. The pregnancy rate is higher in women who are under the age of 25 at the time of the initial ectopic gestation, and parity per se does not affect future fertility in these individuals. A past history of pelvic infection in a patient with an ectopic pregnancy appears to have an ominous effect on future fertility. The pregnancy rate in such individuals is poor and, since the inflammation usually affects both tubes, the risk of a second ectopic pregnancy in the contralateral tube is always present.

The standard approach to the patient with a suspected ectopic pregnancy has undergone significant modifications influenced by the use of ultrasonography and beta subunit assays of hCG. Although the incidence of ectopic pregnancy has almost tripled in recent years, evidence is now accumulating that contemporary diagnostic techniques, along with the increased use of laparoscopy, are having a favorable influence on mortality and morbidity rates through enhancement of early diagnosis. Early detection as well as exclusion of ectopic pregnancy permits the physician to be more selective in the choice of surgical candidates as well as more conservative in the choice of surgical procedure.

Prior to the availability of the beta subunit hCG assay, the pregnancy test was insufficiently sensitive to be of any value for the diagnosis of ectopic gestation. Reliable colorometric immunoconcentration assays with sensitivity to 10 mIU per milliliter are now generally utilized to screen patients and thereby permit the physician access to the result in 15 minutes, while the patient is still in the emergency facility. Serum immunoradiometric assay has a sensitivity to as low as 1.5 mIU per milliliter but requires

2 hours of laboratory time and is usually unavailable at night. The accuracy of each of these assays is almost 100 percent and, although they do not identify the site of gestation, a negative result essentially excludes eccyesis.

The quantitative level of hCG, however, may aid the clinician in differentating an ectopic from an intrauterine pregnancy. A gestational sac is recognizable by ultrasonography when the serum level of hCG is in the range of 6,000 to 6,500 mIU per milliliter. Absence of a sac with serum levels in this range should alert the physician to a possible diagnosis of ectopic pregnancy. When the serum hCG is less than 6,000 mIU per milliliter and the patient's condition permits delay, it may prove helpful to repeat the radioimmunoassay in 48 hours. The serum concentration of hCG in normal pregnancy increases in this time span by 66 percent. Pelvic ultrasonography should be repeated when the hCG reaches the critical level of 6,000 to 6,500 mIU per milliliter and, in the absence of an intrauterine sac, diagnostic laparoscopy should be performed. On the other hand, a decline in the hCG levels implies tubal abortion, and surgical measures may not be necessary.

Diagnostic culdocentesis in the emergency room may not only establish the diagnosis of intra-abdominal hemorrhage but may also be the most efficient method of determining the presence of an ectopic gestation. After the insertion of a 15-gauge needle into the cul-de-sac, any fluid that is aspirated should be properly evaluated. Grossly bloody fluid should be allowed to stand and clot. Failure to perceive the formation of a clot is consistent with a diagnosis of eccyesis. Formation of a clot may, however, indicate that the needle inserted into the cul-de-sac has entered a pelvic vessel, in which case the procedure should be repeated. Aspiration of straw-colored peritoneal fluid may denote the presence of an unruptured tubal pregnancy. Culdocentesis remains a useful diagnostic tool and, in some instances, is superior to laparoscopy.

Changes in the treatment of ectopic gestation have accompanied changes in its etiology. There has been some interest in the application of microsurgical techniques for the treatment of patients with ectopic pregnancy. It has been generally accepted that salpingectomy is the safest method of management of a ruptured ectopic pregnancy, especially when much of the tube has been severely damaged or destroyed. Some patients, however, have unruptured tubal pregnancies and, in such cases, a portion of the tube can be preserved. One of the following approaches is usually feasible: linear salpingostomy with removal of the conceptus; resection of the segment of the tube containing the pregnancy to allow for possible subsequent tubal reconstruction; and resection of the segment containing the pregnancy with immediate microsurgical anastomosis. Whichever method is adopted, it is well recognized that conservation of a damaged oviduct increases the risk of a subsequent eccyesis. Whenever possible, one should remove the segment of the tube containing the ectopic pregnancy, leaving the ends of the tube ligated. Such a procedure minimizes the immediate risk of another pregnancy occurring in this tube but allows for subsequent reconstruction if the patient remains infertile and is anxious to have something done. In general, it is considered unwise to attempt reconstruction at the time of the emergency because of the presence of blood and tissue edema, and under such circumstances conditions for accurate surgery are less favorable. In addition, at this time the patient is not in the best condition to understand the problem and furnish informed consent.

The contralateral tube is frequently found to be damaged at the time of surgery for ectopic pregnancy. In our opinion, it is not appropriate at this time to divide adhesions around such tubes in order to perform a limited fimbrioplasy or to do a salpingostomy because of the risk of adding to the existing damage. There is no doubt that in the patients who have contralateral salpingostomy performed during emergency surgery, the majority of the tubes become occluded within a year of the procedure.

Salpingo-oophorectomy has been recommended as a treatment for ectopic pregnancy, stemming from the suggestion made on theoretic grounds that the opposite ovary would ovulate every cycle. In the event that in vitro fertilization is required at a later date, however, unnecessary resection of ovarian tissue would seem unwise, as this may be a factor in reducing the chances of a future successful pregnancy. It is well known that a substantial number of patients seen for infertility are infertile because of pelvic adhesions that have followed relatively minor conservative surgical procedures.

Although salpingectomy is appropriate treatment for a ruptured tubal pregnancy, alternatives present when an unruptured ectopic is discovered. This mandates an early diagnosis based on laparoscopy and supplemented by specific assays for beta subunit hCG and ultrasonography. If the uninvolved oviduct is grossly damaged, conservative surgery is clearly indicated, but even if the opposite tube appears normal at operation, it may not be or remain so. This is well known by those who have followed patients who have had chlamydial salpingitis. Unless tubal patency can be demonstrated, the contralateral tube cannot be assumed to be patent, and indeed adhesions may develop during the postoperative period. Since the majority of ectopic pregnancies are located in the distal and middle thirds of the tube, a conservative approach may be possible when there is no tubal rupture. The incidence of recurrent ectopic pregnancy is higher after expression of the conceptus through the tubal ostium than with other techniques. Although a linear incision along the antimesenteric border through the tubal ostium has been advocated with the incision being left open, others have recommended closure by not extending the incision to the ostium so fimbrial damage can be circumvented. Resection would be more appropriate in the narrow isthmic portion of the tube and, although cornual reimplantation at a later date is recommended, tubocornual anastomosis would seem to be more rational. The decision to delay definitive tubal reanastomosis allows time for edema and hyperemia to resolve and for patency of the involved tube and the contralateral tube to be evaluated. These findings may dictate a different operative approach subsequently, and any associated adnexal disease could be dealt with at that time.

If infertility is a problem after an ectopic pregnancy, hysterosalpingography and laparoscopy should be performed within a year if a pregnancy has not been achieved.

A tubal surgical procedure for infertility in a patient

who subsequently develops an ectopic pregnancy in that tube cannot be considered a success even though the patient became pregnant. Tubal preservation in an ectopic pregnancy has been enthusiastically endorsed by many investigators, but the efficacy of saving a tube previously diseased and repaired in which an ectopic pregnancy subsequently develops must also be given due consideration.

There is great deal to be said for the statement made by Allan Barnes, namely, "you should work as hard as possible to conserve the lady's tube in her first ectopic, just as you would if this was her second ectopic in her only remaining tube."

SUGGESTED READING

DeCherney AH, Boyers SP. Isthmic ectopic pregnancy: segmental resection as the treatment of choice. Fertil Steril 1985; 44:307–312.

Kim DS, Chung SR, Park MI, et al. Comparative review of diagnostic accuracy in tubal pregnancy: a 14-year survey of 1040 cases. Obstet Gynecol 1987; 70:547–554.

Pauerstein CJ, Coxatto HB, Eddy CA, et al. Anatomy and pathology of tubal pregnancy. Obstet Gynecol 1986; 67:301–308.

Romero R, Kadar N, Janty P, et al. Diagnosis of ectopic pregnancy: value of discriminatory human chorionic gonadotropin zone. Obstet Gynecol 1985; 66:357–360.

Smith HO, Toledo AA, Thompson JD. Conservative surgical management of isthmic ectopic pregnancies. Am J Obstet Gynecol 1987; 156:604–610.

MISSED ABORTION

RICHARD L. BERNSTINE, M.D.

The treatment of missed abortion has been significantly altered with the increased effectiveness of ultrasonography in determing the normal progression of pregnancy. By definition, missed abortion refers to embryonic death prior to 20 weeks, with prolonged retention within the uterus. Embryonic death can be diagnosed with ultrasonography within 1 to 2 weeks of its occurrence. Evacuation of uterine contents is performed at that time.

Evacuation of the uterus for missed abortion will be considered in two aspects: dilation of the cervix to provide access to the uterine cavity, and methods to evacuate the contents of the uterus.

Missed abortion is not associated with progressive changes in the cervix. As a result, dilation of the cervix must be produced artificially prior to evacuation of uterine contents. Methods to achieve this goal may be classified according to the agent employed: (1) instrumental (metal dilators), (2) Laminaria (naturally occurring or synthetic [osmotic]), or (3) prostaglandins.

INSTRUMENTAL

Rigid dilators have been the traditional instruments to achieve cervical dilation. Significant forces are exerted on the cervix by these instruments, and forceful dilation may result in persistent structural changes that can be associated with cervical incompetence or premature delivery. The design of the rigid dilator has been modified to reduce injury, but probably the experience of the operator is the most important factor.

When the clinical status of the patient dictates a surgical evacuation of the uterus without delay, dilation of the cervix employing rigid dilators is performed.There are several tapered dilators (e.g., Hanks) that have a more gradual effect on the cervix than the traditional Hegar's dilators. The resultant forces produced by dilation are dissipated in both a longitudinal and a radial direction. The experience of the operator determines the force with which the dilator is used. An experienced operator will accomplish cervical dilation with an axial force of 1 to 3 kg, whereas the less experienced operator may to exert more pressure to achieve the same result. Pressures as high as 700 kPa have been recorded with rigid dilators.

Prior to any surgical procedure, an examination should be performed to determine the size, shape, and position of the uterus. The cervix is exposed with a speculum and infiltrated with local anesthetic (epinephrine 1/200,000). A tenaculum is placed on the anterior lip of the cervix, and the cervical canal is sounded to determine direction and length. Dilation of the cervix is accomplished by rigid dilators, starting with the smallest, which are passed just beyond the internal os. Dilation is continued allowing each dilator to remain in place until it can be easily removed. The process is complete when the size of the dilator inserted is 1 mm less than the estimated length of gestation in menstrual weeks.

Complications may arise from the use of local anesthetic. Severe systemic reaction may occur from intravascular injection of the anesthetic agent and may result in convulsions, cardiopulmonary arrest, or death. Respiratory support with endotracheal intubation and anticonvulsive therapy is required. The occurrence of these complications can be minimized by choice of local anesthetic, by addition of epinephrine to the local anesthetic solution to restrict uptake, and by aspirating prior to injection of the local anesthetic to ensure extravascular position of the needle.

Nonetheless, the use of general rather than local anesthesia increases the risk of the surgical evacuation of the uterus two to three times.

Injury to the cervix is more likely to occur when rigid dilators are used (especially if they are used rapidly), when dilation is accomplished to large diameters with general rather than local anesthesia, with a less experienced physician as surgeon, and in the younger women (17 years or less). The injury may be apparent at the time of surgery, i.e., laceration of the cervix with bleeding, or may involve fractures within the substance of the cervix that may not be recognized at the time of surgery but that may lead to structural alterations and sequelae in the cervix (e.g., cervical incompetence).

The incidence of injuries in the cervix can be decreased with preoperative use of *Laminaria*, vaginal prostaglandin, or synthetic osmotic dilators prior to use of rigid dilators at the time of surgery.

LAMINARIA

For many years, *Laminaria* tents manufactured from naturally occurring algae have been inserted into the cervix to produce dilatation of that structure. More recently, synthetic hydrogels or polymer impregnated with magnesium sulfate has been substituted.

Laminaria are produced in three sizes (3 to 5 mm, 6 to 8 mm, and 8 to 10 mm) for clinical use. Their hygroscopic action results in removal of water from the cervix, causing dissociation of the proteoglycan complexes, softening, and dilatation of the cervix.

The *Laminaria* require a minimum of 4 hours for a significant effect and 8 to 24 hours for maximal effect. The increments of swelling appear to be greater in the early hours after insertion, but they continue for several more hours. The average degree of cervical dilatation was 1.3 cm after a medium-sized *Laminaria* had been in place for 16 hours.

Insertion of the *Laminaria* is accomplished with the patient in the lithotomy position. Following bimanual examination, the cervix is visualized and cleansed with an antiseptic solution. The anterior lip of the cervix is grasped with a tentaculum. The cervical canal is sounded to determine direction, width, and length. The appropriate size *Laminaria* for the dimensions of the canal is grasped at its distal end with a forceps and gently inserted into the cervical canal until it passes just beyond the internal os. A gauze sponge may be placed against the cervix to promote retention of the *Laminaria*. The sponge and *Laminaria* are removed in the operating room at the time of surgery.

In some instances, it may be possible to insert only the small *Laminaria* initially. In 4 to 6 hours, the *Laminaria* may be removed and replaced with the next larger one.

The patient frequently experiences mild menstrual-type cramps following insertion of the *Laminaria*, but usually no treatment is necessary.

Difficulty may be experienced in removal of the *Laminaria* when it extends beyond the internal os. With expansion of this extremity of the *Laminaria*, a larger diameter will be exiting the cervical canal than the width of this structure. It may be necessary to dilate the cervix sufficiently to effect its removal. Care should be exercised during placement of the *Laminaria* to avoid this problem, since injury to the cervix may result.

Infection is a potential problem possibly related to length of time the device is in place.

Rarely, the *Laminaria* may fragment, and a portion may be retained in the cervical canal or uterine cavity. Removal is necessary and usually can be accomplished, although with difficulty. Narrow, grasping forceps are used to detect, ensnare, and remove the fragments.

Pathologic changes following use of *Laminaria* consist of acute and chronic inflammation in the cervical stroma without any associated findings.

When *Laminaria* is used preoperatively, considerably less force is necessary to insert a Hegar's dilator. To achieve 7 mm dilatation with a Hegar's dilator, approximately 4 lb of force are required, but following pretreatment use of *Laminaria*, only 2 lb are required.

SYNTHETIC HYGROSCOPIC DILATORS

The synthetic dilators are composed of a hygroscopic polymer or contain a hygroscopic substance (magnesium sulfate). When the *Laminaria* is inserted into the endocervical canal, it absorbs water from the adjacent cervix, which results in its uniform expansion. In laboratory experiments, there is progressive symmetric enlargement of the hygroscopic dilator over a period of 2 to 4 hours, and usually a single unit will achieve cervical dilatation of up to 10 or 11 mm. The shorter time to achieve satisfactory dilatation associated with the synthetic *Laminaria* allows their use in more instances than the naturally occurring *Laminaria*. If there is no urgency to evacuate the uterus, their use will provide some protection to the cervix during the dilation process. Their use is not indicated except with a uterus of 16 weeks or less in size. If there is a clinically apparent genital tract infection, their use is contraindicated.

The *Laminaria* are sterilized and supplied in three sizes: 4 mm × 50 mm, 4 mm × 65 mm, and 3 mm × 55 mm. They may be impregnated with magnesium sulfate to enhance their action.

Prior to their insertion, a pelvic examination is performed to confirm previous findings. The cervix is visualized and cleansed with an antiseptic solution. The anterior lip of the cervix is grasped with a tenaculum. The *Laminaria* is removed from the sterile package by grasping the looped handle end firmly with forceps. It is inserted into sterile solution (water or antiseptic) to moisten and lubricate it and to initiate the expansion process. The direction of the cervical canal is ascertained and the *Laminaria* is inserted up to its knob or collar. At this point, its distal end will be through the internal os. A few sterile gauze sponges are placed against the cervix to aid in its retention.

The *Laminaria* should not remain in place for longer than 4 hours. It should be removed by grasping the handle (distal to the knob or collar) and withdrawing with steady traction. Avoid twisting the device during removal, since breakage is more likely to occur.

Side effects are uncommon. An allergic reaction to the components of the *Laminaria* is possible but has not been reported. During the first minutes following insertion, uterine contractions may result. They are mild and usually disappear within 10 minutes. No treatment is needed.

A vasovagal reaction may occur with any manipulation of the cervix and has been reported during insertion of *Laminaria* even following the use of paracervical anesthesia. Patients should be carefully observed for syncope or other symptoms. A brief convulsion may occur, but the pulse is slow, recovery rapid, and there is no postictal state. Routine use of atropine or epinephrine in the anesthetic solution can help to prevent the occurrence of this condition.

No elevation of peripheral plasma levels of magnesium occurs following the use of the synthetic *Laminaria* impregnated with magnesium sulfate.

Infection is a potential risk associated with insertion of any intracervical device. None has been associated with use of synthetic *Laminaria*, although the experience is limited.

Therapeutic response is satisfactory based on three- to four-fold increase in cervical canal dilatation.

PROSTAGLANDINS

Prostaglandin E_2 (20 mg) may be used as a vaginal suppository to accomplish cervical softening and dilatation and to initiate uterine contractions that may be sufficient to cause expulsion of the products of conception.

Prostaglandins E_2 and $F_{2\alpha}$ occupy crucial roles in the mechanisms of cervical contractions. They induce the maturational changes of cervical ripening (i.e., activation of collagenase and alteration in relative amounts of the glycosaminoglycans). They have several actions to effect uterine contractility. Primary among these is the movement of calcium from storage in sarcoplasmic reticulum to the cystoplasm and enhancement of myometrial gap junction formation.

The use of a prostaglandin vaginal suppository in clinical practice is straightforward. With the patient in the supine position, a speculum is inserted into the vagina, which is cleansed with a dry sponge. The suppository is then inserted into the posterior formix.

The patient remains in the supine position for at least 20 minutes after the insertion of the suppository. The frequency of dose varies with uterine response and the patient's tolerance to the drug's side effects. One suppository inserted into the vagina the night before uterine evacuation will enhance cervical softening and may produce a degree of dilatation.

Because of the troublesome side effects of the prostaglandins, the need for frequently repeated doses, and incomplete emptying of the uterus, their use is not widespread. More commonly, prostaglandin is used in the more advanced instances of missed abortion.

Side effects of prostaglandins include nausea, vomiting, diarrhea, hyperthermia, and hypotension. One of these will occur in approximately 60 to 70 percent of patients. Within 1 hour of insertion of the suppository, most patients will experience nausea or vomiting or have loose stools. A minority (10 percent) will have temperature elevations; and a few of these latter patients may have a minor degree of hypotension. An intravenous infusion containing 20 mg of prochlorperazine (Compazine) in 1,000 ml 5 percent dextrose in lactated Ringer's solution will reduce the incidence of the side effects. Uterine rupture has been reported but is a remote complication.

Therapeutic response is satisfactory, with the development of cervical softening and possibly a small degree of cervical dilatation.

EVACUATION OF THE UTERUS

Evacuation of the uterus may be accomplished by surgical means through the cervix, by mechanical scraping of the uterus, or by vacuum aspiration, or by a combination of these methods.

Medical methods of evacuation of the uterus include systemic and local administration of certain oxytocic drugs.

Dilation and Curettage

Pelvic examination at the time of surgery is essential to confirm the size and position of the uterus. Local anesthesia may be administered into the cervix, or paracervical block may be performed. The anterior lip of the cervix is stabilized with a tenaculum.

If *Laminaria* is present in the cervical canal, it should be removed.

Dilation of the cervix is accomplished as previously described. The final dilation should be adequate to allow a curet to readily pass through the internal os of the cervix without causing injury to that structure.

Traction is made downward on the tenaculum to straighten the cervicouterine angle. Any tissue present in the cervical canal should be removed. The uterine cavity is sounded to determine its depth. If further dilation of the cervix is necessary, it should be performed at this time.

An ovum forceps is introduced into the uterine cavity to detect tissue masses that can be removed. A curet (usually a smooth one) is introduced into the uterus to the fundus. The cavity is curetted in a systematic manner. An attempt to ascertain the implantation site should be made. The curet may be removed with each stroke to make this determination. No pressure should be applied to the curet as it passes the internal os of the cervix in order to avoid damage to this structure. Once the yield of tissue decreases significantly, the surgical procedure is complete. Bleeding should be minimal at this time.

A sharp curet may be employed to gently complete the procedure. A grating sensation indicates that the procedure has gone beyond the extent required, and the surgery should be stopped.

The distinction between a complete surgical procedure and one in which retained products of conception are present in the uterus can be confirmed by ultrasonography. The performance of a real time ultrasound examination while the patient is on the operating table will provide an immediate answer. A discrete midline echo confirms the completeness of the procedure.

Other complications of the procedure include injury to the cervix (previously discussed), uterine perforation, persistent bleeding or hemorrhage, pelvic infection, and late formation of uterine synechia.

Perforation of the uterus can occur when an instrument is passed through the cervix into the uterine cavity. It occurs most frequently with passage of the uterine sound. Accurate determination of uterine orientation in the anteroposterior and lateral diameters of the pelvis reduces the possibility of perforation. Downward traction of the anterior cervical lip via the attached tenaculum is important, since it will straighten the cervicouterine angle and reduce perforations at that site.

Perforation should be diagnosed when there is a sudden decrease in resistance to an instrument or passage of an instrument or passing of an instrument occurs to a greater depth than that indicated by initial sounding. Recovery of obvious extrauterine tissue confirms the diagnosis of perforation.

Perforation should be suspected if abdominal pain develops when the patient is under local anesthesia. Depending on the site of perforation, the pain may be lateral or in the midline of the lower abdomen.

Perforation of the lateral wall of the uterus may not be suspected because of the confining structure of the broad ligament. Delayed unexplained shock may be the presenting finding.

Diagnosis of a uterine perforation is usually obvious at the time of surgery. With a lateral perforation, pelvic examination may detect the development of the hematoma. Confirmation, if required, can be obtained by sonogram.

Management depends on the magnitude and site of injury to the uterus, the patient's general status, the removal of extrauterine tissue (ie., fat) from the uterus, and the need to continue with the curettage.

Usually the injury to the uterus is small, secondary to the uterine sound, and careful clinical observation is indicated. If curettage has not been initiated and there is no bleeding, the surgery can be delayed until a later date. If there is bleeding or the need to proceed is apparent, curettage should be performed under direct visualization of the uterus via laparoscopy. The physician observing through the laparoscope can direct the physician performing the curettage away from the perforation site and avoid any further injury.

A laparotomy is indicated if tissue foreign to the uterus has been removed, if the patient is in shock, if the urine is bloody, or if there has been previous extensive abdominal surgery.

Careful observation for 24 hours is necessary to confirm clinical stability.

If the perforation is in the midline of the fundus and no other confounding factors are present (e.g., shock or the need to complete surgery), then the best course to follow is clinical observation and performance of the dilation and curettage (D&C) at a later date.

If there is a lateral hematoma, follow-up with serial sonograms and hematocrit and hemoglobin readings may be performed. It may be elected to perform laparoscopy to visualize the broad ligament areas and to determine the extent and any progression of a hematoma.

Persistent uterine bleeding following completion of D&C indicates incomplete evacuation of the products of conception. Real time ultrasonography will readily demonstrate the absence of a midline uterine echo and the presence of mottled echoes, indicating clots and tissue. Procrastination with oxytocics is not indicated as definitive treatment. A repeat D&C under real time ultrasonographic guidance is necessary.

Other sites of bleeding, especially the cervix, should be excluded.

Pelvic infection may coexist with missed abortion as a separate disease process or may result from extension of infection from uterine contents to parametria. The latter possibility is less likely than the former. The presence of uterine infection as evidenced by uterine tenderness, foul cervical discharge, fever, and leukocytosis warrants antibiotic coverage followed by D&C. Cultures of cervical smears should be obtained for organisms associated with sexually transmitted diseases.

Uterine synechiae and associated hypomenorrhea and infertility (Asherman's syndrome) are most frequently related to curettage of a gravid or recently gravid uterus. The clinical syndrome suggesting this condition can be confirmed by hysterogram and hysteroscopy.

A satisfactory clinical response occurs with complete evacuation of uterine contents in the absence of immediate or delayed complications.

VACUUM CURETTAGE

Whether the traditional D&C or vacuum curettage is used in the treatment of missed abortion is usually a matter of physician preference or availability of instrumentation. Evacuation of the larger uterus (i.e., second trimester) is probably more easily performed via vacuum. Blood loss also should be less with this method. Frequently, after completion of vacuum curettage, the physician will confirm findings by going over the area with a curet.

The traditional curettage with a metal curet depends on the mechanical action of the instrument to disrupt and evacuate uterine contents. Vacuum curettage depends on the suction created at the tip of the curet to dislodge the products of conception.

The preparation of the patient for vacuum curettage is similar to that described for conventional D&C. Examination should be performed to confirm previous findings. The cervix is exposed and the anterior lip of the cervix is grasped with a tentaculum, and downward traction is performed to straighten the cervicouterine angle. If *Laminaria* has been used, it is removed and the uterus is sounded and further dilation of the cervix is performed as necessary. The suction curet is introduced beyond the internal os and the procedure initiated.

The tip of the suction curet should be beyond the internal os prior to induction of the negative pressure. Each time the curet is removed from or inserted into the uterine cavity there should not be any negative pressure in the system. Failure to observe this rule may result in injury to the internal os. Negative pressure within the system is controlled by occluding the aperture in the proximal part of the curet. The curet is slowly rotated within the uterine cavity to ensure that all fragments are dislodged. Their passage can be observed within the transparent suction tubing. The procedure is completed when the tissue yield within the tubing is greatly reduced and a foamy serosanguineous fluid appears.

It should be emphasized that the plastic curet used in vacuum curettage is not intended to "scrape" tissue from the uterine walls.

Side effects and complications are as described under conventional D&C.

Following the surgical procedure, there should be minimal vaginal bleeding, which should quickly change to a brownish discharge. Mild lower abdominal cramps may be present for a short period of time.

Prostaglandins

The use of a vaginal suppository of prostaglandin E_2 (20 mg) in the second trimester of pregnancy frequently results in the expulsion of the fetus and less frequently in the expulsion of the placenta. Its use is discussed under "Prostaglandins" when used to dilate the cervix.

Oxytocin

The sensitivity of the uterus to oxytocin in the first half of pregnancy is minimal and variable. Prior to 20 weeks of pregnancy, response to oxytocin is frequently absent. If the cervix has dilated spontaneously or from use of another drug (e.g., prostaglandin), the effect of oxytocin to evacuate the uterus may be increased.

The woman whose gestation approaches 20 weeks is more likely to respond to oxytocin infusion than she who is earlier in her pregnancy. The oxytocin concentration of the intravenous solution can exceed that used with a living fetus. The drug should be prepared in an electrolyte solution to avoid the possibility of water intoxication. The time from administration of oxytocin to when effective contractions ensue may be prolonged, and the patient should be prepared for this possibility.

Oxytocin acts to regulate Ca^{++} concentration in the cytoplasm and sacroplasmic reticulum.

Side effects of oxytocin administration at this period of gestation are minimal, but occasional reports have appeared of uterine rupture in women of high parity or when it is used in combination with prostaglandins.

Incomplete expulsion of the products of conception from the uterus may occur. Water intoxication may result from high concentration of oxytocin, rapidly administered in an electrolyte-free solution. Transient hypotension may result from rapid administration of oxytocin.

Generally, a satisfactory response to oxytocin should occur early in its use, or an alternative method of emptying the uterus should be employed.

Treatment of unsensitized Rh-negative mothers with anti-Rh immunoglobulin is required. In most instances, there is not sufficient time to perform the usual immunologic studies prior to the departure of the patient. It is recommended that the unsensitized Rh-negative patient receive immunoglobin prior to discharge.

SUGGESTED READING

Bernstine RL. Surgical aspects of spontaneous abortion. In: Iffy L, Charles D, eds. Operative perinatology. New York: Macmillan, 1984:302.

Freiman SM, Wulff GJL. Management of uterine perforation following elective abortion. Obstet Gynecol. 1977; 50:647–650.

Hulka JF, Leffer HT, Angone A, et al. A new electronic force monitor to measure factors influencing cervical dilation for vacuum curettage. Am J Obstet Gynecol 1974; 120:166–173.

Nicolaides KH, Welch CC, Koullapis EN, Filshie GM. Cervical dilatation by Malicel—studies on the mechanism of action. Br J Obstet Gynaecol 1983; 90:1060–1064.

SPONTANEOUS ABORTION

DAVID CHARLES, M.D., F.A.C.O.G., F.R.C.O.G.
DOUGLAS D. GLOVER, B.S. Pharm., M.D.

The loss of any pregnancy in the first 20 weeks of gestation or prior to the time the fetus attains a weight of 500 g is defined as abortion. Expulsion of the products of conception during the first 12 weeks is termed early abortion, whereas pregnancy failure during the next 8 weeks is referred to as late abortion. The incidence of spontaneous abortion is usually stated to be 10 to 15 percent of all pregnancies. However, this does not take into account those losses that occur soon after implantation and before it is recognized that the woman is pregnant. The true incidence of spontaneous abortion is unknown and, in the majority of cases, the cause cannot be determined.

Of all cases of pregnancy loss, those that occur in the early weeks of gestation are least well understood. It is generally accepted that the majority of early abortuses have chromosomal abnormalities, the more common of which are trisomy and x-monosomy. On the other hand, late abortions are frequently associated with defects of placentation or fetal anomalies. Adding to the confusion is the probability that at least some abortions thought to be spontaneous are, in fact, the result of pregnancy intervention. In support of this concept are data that show that since the legalization of abortion the number of hospital admissions for incomplete abortion has steadily declined and inversely correlates with the rise of induced abortions. Those women who have had one or two previous abortions have a slightly increased risk of another abortion, although there are no data to substantiate this observation. Likewise, there is no unanimity pertaining to the increased risk of spontaneous abortion following voluntary termination of pregnancy.

ETIOLOGY

Infection is an infrequent cause of abortion. The low incidence of abortion caused by microbial infection attests to the efficacy of the maternal host defense mechanisms present in the vagina, uterine cervix, and amniotic fluid. Morbidity related to intrauterine bacterial infection is considerably less than that caused by viruses in the first trimester of pregnancy. In contrast to viral infections, which involve transplacental passage of the pathogen during the viremic phase of the infection, bacterial infections are predominantly vertical infections. *Treponema pallidum* and *Listeria monocytogenes* are, however, organisms that gain entrance to the fetus by placental transmission. Once thought to pose no risk to the conceptus before midpregnancy, the treponeme in recent years has been demonstrated in the tissue of embryos examined after voluntary termination of pregnancy. The association of *T. pallidum* with spontaneous abortion, however, has not yet been fully established. On the other hand, *L. monocytogenes* causes a febrile illness that resembles influenza. In addition to fever and general malaise, the patient may experience cephalagia, pharyngitis, myalgia, loss of appetite, and chills associated with bacteremia. The illness is sufficiently mild that it may be ignored by the woman or, if medical care is sought, considered not to be serious by the physician. For these reasons, listeriosis is rarely diagnosed prior to death of the intrauterine passenger. Fetal demise most commonly occurs in late pregnancy. The clinician should be aware of the fact that listeriosis may mimic pyelonephritis. Consideration should always be given to this diagnosis when the pregnant woman presents with an illness suggestive of renal infection that cannot be confirmed by microscopic urinalysis. It is a fact that the organism has been isolated from ejaculates of men whose wives have had recurrent abortions. Organisms of the same serotype have also been isolated from cervical cultures in these cases. How frequently *L. monocytogenes* is the cause of early abortion is unknown, but it is well established that this organism has a predilection for the fetoplacental unit.

Although viral infections may cause death of the embryo, most commonly the morbidity associated with viral disease results in anatomic defects caused by maternal infection during organogenesis. Such is the case with rubella, which has been recognized as a cause of congenital defects as well as abortion for more than 4 decades. Of equal importance from the public health point of view is the herpes group of viruses. A primary Herpesvirus hominis infection in early pregnancy may result in abortion in at least one-third of the patients.

Uterine anomalies, principally those that decrease the volume of the uterine cavity or reduce the area available for implantation, may lead to second trimester abortion. Leiomyomas of the uterine corpus may also cause pregnancy wastage if they are submucosal in location and significantly distort the uterine cavity. The trend in recent years to have small families and delay childbearing has resulted in this factor being a more frequent cause of abortion. Likewise, retroposition of the uterus can cause early second trimester abortion if incarceration occurs.

DIAGNOSIS

Vaginal bleeding in the first trimester of pregnancy suggests threatened abortion, which may progress to inevitable abortion. Ultrasonic evaluation of such a patient may aid the clinician to distinguish between those pregnancies with impending pregnancy wastage and those that may be salvaged. When confronted with first trimester bleeding, the physician should evaluate:

1. the location, appearance, and volume of the gestational sac;
2. the presence of fetal echoes, the crown-rump length, and detection of fetal life by time-motion mode, real-time imaging, or both;
3. the location, size, and appearance of the placenta.

When evidence of progressive fetal development is demonstrable by ultrasonography, the prognosis is favorable, since over 80 percent of pregnancies in which early bleeding occurs progress normally thereafter. A number of abnormalities may be detected on ultrasonographic evaluation in threatened abortion. Some anomalies have a characteristic appearance on ultrasonography and thereby allow for a definitive diagnosis from the initial evaluation, whereas others may require further assessment before confirmation is feasible.

The diagnosis of blighted ovum is made by demonstrating an intrauterine gestational sac with volume in excess of 2.5 cm without fetal echoes. The wall of the gestational sac may appear to be thin, broken, fragmented, or accoustically invisible because of poor development, degeneration, or necrosis.

An ultrasonographic diagnosis of complete abortion is made by demonstrating an empty uterus, which may reveal a thin central echo. On the other hand, if there is an enlarged uterus with a central clump of echoes, one has to consider a possible diagnosis of missed abortion or molar pregnancy.

An abortion is said to be complete when the products of conception are expelled in their entirety. In the first trimester the gestational sac is frequently expelled intact, whereas in the second trimester the ecbolic process is analogous to parturition at term. When amniorrhexis precedes expulsion of the fetus, which in turn is followed by the placenta and membranes in the process of abortion, dilation and effacement of the cervix occur prior to the expulsion of the products of conception. When the abortion is complete, the uterus rapidly involutes, and blood loss is minimal.

The term incomplete abortion indicates retention in the uterus of a portion of the conceptus. More specifically, this implies a remnant of the chorion frondosum with a portion of the decidua containing chorionic villi or fragments of placental tissue. In the initial trimester of pregnancy before the decidua capsularis and decidua vera fuse, it frequently happens that the conceptus with the capsularis is expelled, and the decidua vera remains in the uterus. On rare occasions, the decidua vera may be expelled and the gestational sac retained. Later in pregnancy, portions of the placenta or even the entire placenta may fail to be expelled from the uterus. In instances in which only a small portion of tissue is left behind, some time may elapse before this is recognized. Sooner or later there will be bleeding or evidence of infection, as exemplified by an offensive discharge, slight fever, or pelvic pain.

If the patient with an incomplete or inevitable abortion is found to be Rh negative, after the evacuation of the uterus the unsensitized patient should be given a full dose of 300 μg of Rh-immune globulin.

The differential diagnosis of any abortion includes threatened abortion, in which the cervix is closed and bleeding is minimal; inevitable abortion, in which the cervix is dilated or the amniotic sac is ruptured; and complete abortion, in which the uterus is empty. If the abortion is complete, bleeding is minimal, and there is no evidence of infection, curettage is not required. In such cases ultrasonographic confirmation of the diagnosis is desirable. Ergotamine tartrate or methylergonovine maleate, 0.2 mg orally three times a day for 2 or 3 days, is sometimes prescribed to stimulate uterine contractions, but in the majority of cases oxytocic agents are not required.

MANAGEMENT OF INCOMPLETE OR INEVITABLE ABORTION

Once partial extrusion of the products of conception has occurred or bleeding becomes excessive, prompt evacuation of the uterus is indicated in order to minimize both blood loss and the risk of infection. Hospitalization is not required, since vacuum curettage can be performed in any well-equipped emergency care facility. More and more of these procedures are being conducted on an outpatient basis. Prior to curettage, the patient should be instructed to empty her bladder. Intravenous hydration is then initiated by infusion of 1,000 ml of 5 percent dextrose in Ringer's lactate, to which has been added 10 units of oxytocin. The latter agent helps to reduce blood loss by stimulating the uterine contractions while evacuation of the products of conception is being performed. Systemic analgesics, such as meperidine, or tranquilizing agents, such as diazepam, may be administered to reduce any discomfort to the patient. After determining the uterine size, shape, and position by bimanual examination, a sterile speculum is inserted in the vagina in order to visualize the cervix. The upper vagina and cervix are cleansed with an antiseptic solution such as povidone-iodine and the anterior lip of the cervix is grasped with a nontraumatic instrument, such as an Allis clamp, and any retained products of conception present in the lower uterine segment or cervical canal are removed with sponge forceps. In the absence of infection, a paracervical block with 1 percent lidocaine is highly efficacious for relief of pain.

Since the cervix is already dilated by prior passage of the conceptus, an 8- or 10-mm suction cannula can usually be inserted easily into the cervical canal. Aspiration is then accomplished with suction, which should not exceed 170 cm mercury. The cannula is gently rotated until no further blood or tissue can be removed from the uterine cavity. All tissue is submitted to the laboratory for histologic examination. To confirm that the uterus is empty, the cavity may be explored with an ovum forceps or curette. On completion of the procedure, 0.2 mg methylergonovine maleate may be administered in order to stimulate uterine contraction and minimize any blood loss.

In the absence of complications, the patient may be sent home following observation for 2 to 4 hours. Continuation of oxytocic therapy is usually unnecessary unless the uterus is atonic and bleeding persists. Likewise, a mild analgesic, such as a combination of acetaminophen with codeine, may be indicated for short-term use; however, when needed, 650 mg of acetaminophen usually suffices. Each patient should be encouraged to take supplemental iron to replenish any blood loss. If the bleeding has been profuse, a blood transfusion may be necessary.

The patient should be advised to contact the physician if she has profuse bleeding, pelvic pain, or a temperature above 100.4° F. She may rapidly resume her usual activities, but coitus and douching should not be allowed for at least 2 weeks. Menstruation may resume in 4 to 6 weeks, but in 10 percent of women it is delayed for as long as 10 weeks. Patients should be reassured that spontaneous abortion is common and that 10 to 15 percent of all pregnancies terminate in this manner. If a patient has an abortion associated with chromosomal abnormalities, she should be referred for genetic counseling if she has any concern pertaining to her reproductive potential.

Because of the anatomic arrangement of the spiral arteries, hemorrhage from the uterus is automatically occluded by uterine contractility. Myometrial contractions are ineffective if any tissue is retained in the uterine cavity. The remedy is curettage with a large curette, although exploration of the uterine cavity with polyp forceps may recover a tissue fragment that is interfering with uterine contractility. Occasionally the procedure may be accompanied by brisk bright red bleeding, and in such cases the physician must be alert to the possibility that perforation of the wall of the uterus by the curette has occurred and that the bleeding may be coming directly from the uterine artery or one of its branches. In such instances, laparotomy is mandatory if the blood loss is severe.

Hospitalization may be preferable for the anxious individual who requires general anesthesia for curettage, but it is essential for any patient with profuse bleeding, hypovolemia, intrauterine infection, molar pregnancy, or associated medical problems.

Bleeding can be severe in cases of abortion, and hypovolemic shock may ensue. The latter is by far the most common variety of shock observed in the obstetric patient. The causes of hypovolemic shock range from ectopic pregnancy, which must always be considered if there is shock in early gestation, bleeding from the placental site, or, in later pregnancy, uterine rupture, atony, or inversion.

Ectopic pregnancy with tubal rupture is associated with abdominal pain, intra-abdominal hemorrhage, a rapid, thready pulse, and hypotension. These patients have marked pallor, slight perspiration, and respiratory excursions that are shallow and rapid. In such cases measures must be instituted immediately to replace blood loss; hypovolemic shock requires blood replacement as soon as possible.

The possibility that one is dealing with a hydatidiform mole or choriocarcinoma instead of an inevitable abortion must always be included in the differential diagnosis of any form of vaginal bleeding in the first half of the pregnancy. Although the history may suggest gestational trophoblastic disease, this is not always so, and at times it is difficult to distinguish between this clinical entity and a threatened or incomplete abortion. Curettage and examination of any retained products generally substantiate the diagnosis. An exception is the rare case of choriocarcinoma that is entirely in the myometrium without any involvement of the endometrium. An immunologic pregnancy test may be of great value, but the quantitative determination of serum beta-human chorionic gonadotropin by radioimmunoassay is of inestimable value in formulating a diagnosis. Normally the serum pregnancy test becomes negative 1 week after an abortion or term pregnancy and from 6 to 12 weeks after evacuation of a molar pregnancy. If the test becomes positive after being negative, it implies the presence of another pregnancy or choriocarcinoma. One must remember that with choriocarcinoma the reaction may be only weakly positive and may in fact be negative. It is probable that variations in the reaction depend on the degree of anaplasia in the Langhans' cells, and the more anaplastic cells may produce a weaker reaction. A weak reaction may, therefore, indicate a highly malignant growth, and when the tumor is deep in the myometrium, the curettings may not be diagnostic.

Spontaneous abortion is one of the more common problems that confronts the physician in an obstetric practice. In the majority of cases there is no doubt as to the diagnosis, and the management is straightforward. It must, however, always be remembered that the potential for disaster is high if due attention is not paid to all aspects of the care of patients with this entity.

SUGGESTED READING

Heinonen OP. Spontaneous abortion, stillbirths and birth defects in epidemiological search for risk factors. Dev Toxicol Environ Sci 1986; 12:63–76.

Miller WA, Erbe RW. Medical genetics. In: Kistner RW, ed. Gynecology: principles and practice. 4th ed. Chicago: Year Book, 1986:657.

Rock JA, Zacur HA. The clinical management of repeated early pregnancy wastage. In: Wallach EE, Kempers RD, eds. Modern trends in infertility and conception control. Chicago: Year Book, 1985.

PLACENTA PREVIA

JAMES G. PULLANO, M.D., M.B.A.
LESLIE IFFY, M.D., F.R.C.S.(C)

DEFINITION AND CLASSIFICATION

Etymologically, the term placenta previa means obstruction of the birth canal by the placenta. In the clinical sense, it refers to the situation in which the cervix is covered, wholly or in part, by the placenta. The inevitable end result is bleeding during pregnancy, especially in the third trimester.

The overall incidence of placenta previa is approximately 1 in 250 births. This, however, varies considerably from as high as 1 in 20 births in grand multiparas to as low as 1 in 1,500 births in nulliparas. In some parts of the world, a marked increase in the rate of placenta previa has been observed during the past decades. The rate rose quite dramatically following the introduction of liberal abortion laws in Hungary where, by the mid-1960s, the majority of pregnancies were terminated utilizing the dilation and evacuation method of induced abortion. A comparable increase was observed in the rate of occurrence of abruption of the placenta. (Fig. 1).

Placenta previa is usually classified according to the degree of involvement of the cervix. When the internal os is covered completely, the term used is total or complete placenta previa. When only a part of the internal cervical os is covered by the placenta, the previa is partial. In the case in which the placental edge just reaches the cervical os, it is referred to as marginal previa. Lateral or low-lying placenta previa denotes implantation on the lower segment in the absence of extension to the internal cervical os. This classification derives from the distinct possibility of severe hemorrhage from the site of a low-lying placenta during labor.

NATURAL HISTORY

Before the days of cesarean section and blood transfusion, the rate of maternal deaths ranged from between 25 and 50 percent and all but a few fetuses in women with placenta previa perished. This outcome resulted from massive bleeding with detachment and delivery of the placenta before the birth of the fetus. The treatment of this disorder before the 1900s followed Braxton-Hicks' ill-fated concept of "internal podalic version" performed at 4 cm cervical

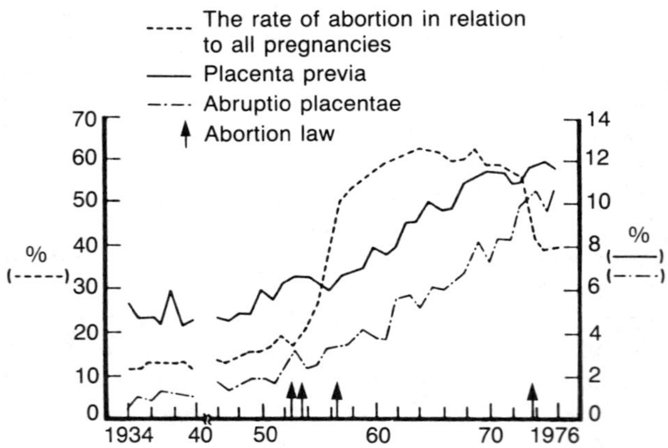

Figure 1 Relationship between the rates of artificially induced abortion, placenta previa, and abruptio placentae in Hungary between 1932 and 1976.

dilatation for the purpose of achieving tamponade of the placenta by pressure from the breech, accomplished by traction on the fetal leg.

ETIOLOGY

It has been suggested that placenta previa is caused by defective vascularization of the endometrium, causing the blastocyst, with limited choice of implantation sites, to implant near the internal cervical os. Patients whose uterine endometrium tends to be defective include grand multiparas, patients with a previous cesarean section, those with induced abortions, and women in the high reproductive age group.

An extension of the above concept is the "menstrual flux theory" that attributes low implantation to delayed ovulation and defect of the corpus luteum. Failure to suppress the next period leads to bleeding and displacement of the unimplanted or poorly embedded ovum by the "menstrual" flow to an ectopic site, such as the lower segment of the uterus. This phenomenon may cause markedly erroneous interpretations of the length of the gestational period and the expected date of confinement.

It has been postulated that large placentas impose increased risk of low implantation (e.g., fetal erythroblastosis and multiple pregnancy).

Once placenta previa has occurred, the risk of recurrence in the next pregnancy is between 4 and 8 percent. Similarly increased is the risk of other reproductive abnormalities, such as ectopic pregnancy, congenital defects, early abortion, placenta accreta, and hydatidiform mole.

SIGNS AND SYMPTOMS

Sudden onset of painless bleeding in the second or third trimester is the usual clinical presentation. The bleeding may produce uterine contractions on rare occasion.

The hemorrhage is usually painless. In general, the greater the degree of the previa, the earlier the bleeding is noted. In about one-third of the cases bleeding manifests before the 30th week, in another one-third between the 30th and 36th weeks, and in the remaining one-third after the 36th week. Apparently, the bleeding is secondary to the formation of the lower uterine segment, with consequent detachment of a portion of the placenta.

The occurrence of congenital defects is increased about three-fold in those cases of placenta previa that extend to 20 weeks or more. Although the rate of previa in the general population is about 1 in 250 births, about 10 percent of first trimester spontaneous abortions are associated with low implantation. Thus, the majority of instances of placenta previa result in early reproductive wastage. This fact implies that the actual frequency of low implantation is approximately three-fold higher than the generally quoted data would indicate.

DIAGNOSIS

In modern obstetrics the diagnostic method used to determine the presence of placenta previa is ultrasonography. With increasing use of this modality in early pregnancy, the diagnosis often precedes the occurrence of painless vaginal bleeding, the classic first sign of low placental implantation. The far less accurate radiologic methods rely on the presence of radioactive isotopes in the hypertrophic uterine vasculature at the implantation site.

An apparent placenta previa, sonographically diagnosed as such in the second trimester, is frequently found to be nonexistent at term. This is because of overdistention of the bladder at the time of the initial examination, which may cause approximation of the anterior and posterior walls. As a result, the placenta may appear to be closer to the internal os than it really is. New techniques, such as fetal elevation in an attempt to facilitate visualization of the internal os, and perhaps the use of magnetic resonance imaging, may improve the chances of accurate early diagnosis in the future.

When placenta previa is confirmed in the third trimester, the chances of hemorrhage at delivery are considerable. For this reason, when previa is noted on an early ultrasonographic examination, reconfirmation of the diagnosis at 36 weeks at the latest is necessary in order to permit advance planning of appropriate management.

Because of the increased incidence of congenital malformations in placenta previa, careful sonographic evaluation of the fetal central nervous, cardiovascular, respiratory, and gastrointestinal systems is warranted. Vaginal examination under double set-up was used in the past to diagnose placenta previa. Its use in current practice is restricted to instances when ultrasonography is unavailable or the results are inconclusive.

When vaginal bleeding is the presenting sign in the second or third trimester, the differential diagnosis includes abruptio placentae, vasa previa, cervical erosion, trauma, hemorrhagic diatheses, endometrial polyps, vaginal infection, and carcinoma of the cervix.

No vaginal examination is permitted in a bleeding gravida beyond the 20th week of gestation until a sonogram has ruled out placenta previa.

MANAGEMENT

The nature of hemorrhage, whether obstetric, surgical, gynecologic, or medical, should be determined and classified, and the patient should be properly treated without delay. The total amount of unreplaced blood loss is directly related to perinatal mortality.

Bed rest in the hospital for at least 72 hours should be offered to any patient who experiences vaginal bleeding when the diagnosis of placenta previa is confirmed by sonogram. The course of action after this period of time depends on an analysis of all the factors involved. The first episode of bleeding in placenta previa rarely, if ever, is fatal for the mother or the fetus. Subsequent episodes of bleeding tend to be of greater severity, however, than the preceding ones. Regretfully, the number of bleeding episodes, and their frequency, are not predictably related to the degree of previa. Since the subsequent bleeding may be fatal, and because the amount of bleeding seldom decreases from one episode to another, it is necessary to hospitalize all patients with placenta previa who have bled two or more times or had a severe hemorrhage even once until delivery. A significant hemorrhage may be defined as one producing a drop in hemoglobin of 1 g or more, excluding the expected decrease from intravenous fluid administration. The rationale is that if the first bleeding was severe, the patient may not be able to tolerate the second episode. If a patient is to be allowed to return home after a moderate first bleeding episode, she must be under continuous surveillance by family members or friends, and ready means of communication with and transportation to the hospital must be available. Otherwise, she must remain hospitalized until delivery. The conditions in the home environment should be reviewed before allowing the patient to leave the institution. If she has children to look after, her ability to rest at home will be impaired. In this case bed rest in the hospital should be advised. The patient herself should understand that the bed rest is essential. Sexual activity is not permitted until after delivery. The time of the gravida at home should be spent in much the same way as in the hospital.

Naturally, a prolonged hospital stay is costly. The average time between the initial bleeding and the delivery ranges between 2 and 6 weeks. However, the costs of intensive neonatal care are even higher. Since studies have shown that in-hospital management permits extension of the gestational period and is conducive, therefore, to the birth of a mature fetus, the actual costs for both mother and infant are probably decreased if the patient is hospitalized after the initial bleeding.

When a gravida presents with bleeding, an attempt at assessing the amount of blood loss must be made. The usual methods include vital signs, urine output, blood indices, and visual estimation of the blood loss. A period of 3 to 4 hours is often needed before significant changes are noted in the hematocrit level after an acute bleeding episode. Complete equilibration requires 48 hours. Unfortunately, the infusion of intravenous fluids can distort the values, and visual estimation of the blood loss is often inaccurate.

Tachycardia usually is present and is proportional to the blood loss. Tachypnea is a relatively early sign of mild volume loss and can be marked at a time when all other parameters are still normal. Orthostatic blood pressure changes, frequently referred to as "tilting", are a common finding and helpful in assessing the degree of hypovolemia. Tilting can be elicited when approximately 25 to 35 percent of the blood volume has been lost.

Evidence of mild peripheral vasoconstriction can be elicited by squeezing the hypothenar area of the hand for 1 to 2 seconds. The normal return to a pink color in 1 to 2 seconds is the expected finding in the absence of significant blood loss.

Narrowing of the pulse pressure is frequently found in cases of mild to moderate degree of blood loss. Blood perfusion of the brain and heart continues at the expense of nonvital body organs, including the uterus and the adrenals. The latter results in sympathetic-adrenal stimulation, which causes a rise in the diastolic blood pressure. With mild to moderate volume deficits, the systolic pressure is maintained.

The concentration of the urine increases in mild to moderate blood loss. Rapid decrease in renal blood flow tends to shift the circulation from the outer renal cortex to the juxtamedullary portion. There are fewer glomeruli and longer loops of Henle in this region, leading to increased reabsorption of water and sodium. The urine, therefore, becomes more concentrated with a reduced level of sodium and a higher degree of osmolarity.

As a guide to treatment, the following yardstick should be used to classify hemorrhage from placenta previa.

Class I—Blood loss is usually under 1 L, representing less than 15 percent of blood volume. These patients rarely exhibit signs or symptoms of volume deficit.

Class II—Blood loss totals 1 to 1.75 L, representing 20 to 25 percent of blood volume. These patients show physical signs.

Class III—Blood loss totals 1.75 to 2.5 L, representing approximately 25 to 35 percent of blood volume. These patients show overt hypotension.

Class IV—Blood loss totals 2.5 L or greater, representing more than 35 percent of the blood volume. These patients are in profound shock and frequently have no discernible blood pressure.

Because of both vasoconstriction and transcapillary refill (e.g., fluid shifts from the interstitial space into the intravascular space), Class I patients rarely exhibit signs or symptoms of volume deficit. These patients, as well as those with more serious blood loss, should receive intravenous fluids as soon as the classification of hemorrhage is completed. The rate of replacement should be based on the approximation of blood lost using the methods mentioned above. Rates of 2 to 3 L per hour are not uncommon in severe cases.

Patients showing signs of Class IV blood loss should be managed according to the principles of management of hypovolemic shock.

After the patient is stabilized, delivery by cesarean section is indicated in most instances.

BLOOD REPLACEMENT

Some champion the use of whole blood when replacing blood loss caused by acute hemorrhage. This is probably reasonable when a replacement of 2 L or more is needed. Most blood banks, however, suggest the use of packed red blood cells even when the volume being replaced exceeds 2 L. Because packed cells have only small amounts of white blood cells and isohemaglutinins (anti-A and anti-B), the incidence of nonhemolytic transfusion reactions is reduced. Packed cells should be administered with normal saline, since Ringer's lactated or dextrose solution can cause the blood to clot or the red cells to lyse.

For every 4 to 5 units of packed red blood cells administered, one unit each of platelets and fresh frozen plasma should be provided. Each unit carries the transfusion risk of a single unit of blood.

The hemoglobin and hematocrit values are of use to direct the further care of the patient. In a normal pregnancy, a hematocrit less than 34 ml per deciliter is indicative of anemia. When transfusion is needed to restore the volume loss in placenta previa, the goal is to achieve a hematocrit of 35 ml per deciliter. Although this may well remain the goal, realistic compromises may need to be made on account of the decreasing availability of blood and the increasing risks of hepatitis, acquired immunodeficiency syndrome (AIDS), and other infections. Thus, since the benefits of blood replacement can reasonably be weighed against the risks of blood-borne diseases, a hematocrit of 30 ml per deciliter is probably a more realistic goal than mentioned earlier.

Fully crossmatched blood is needed at the time the patient presents and the need for transfusion is confirmed. After this period, however, a "type and screen" is more cost-effective. Blood typing and an indirect Coombs' test should be performed on admission and after each series of transfusions. When atypical antibodies are discovered, the patient should be fully crossmatched while in the hospital at 48-hour intervals.

FETAL EVALUATION

Once bleeding has occurred, fetal evaluation should become a part of the standard management. After the 30th to 32nd week of gestation, in case of bleeding a nonstress test is recommended, followed by a biophysical profile in case of suspected fetal jeopardy. The contraction stress test is contraindicated.

THE TIMING OF DELIVERY

Delivery is often necessitated by the inability to control the bleeding. When possible, it is desirable to wait for fetal maturity before effecting delivery. This usually is achieved by the 36th completed week of gestation. The determination of the length of the gestational period must be made on the basis of sonographic data, preferably obtained in early gestation and confirmed on two occasions at least 4 weeks apart. This approach is advisable because of frequent discrepancy between calculated and actual gestation lengths. In case of doubt, prior to elective abdominal delivery an amniocentesis should be performed. In those few cases in which the diagnosis of placenta previa is not accompanied by bleeding (10 percent), elective delivery by the 38th week at the latest is probably advisable.

Cesarean section, either electively or on an emergency basis, is the accepted mode of delivery. The perinatal mortality rate in placenta previa patients does not exceed 2 to 3 percent when a cesarean section is performed at 36 weeks' pregnancy. Using the same criteria, in the case of vaginal delivery the perinatal mortality rate can approach 40 percent.

The incidence of abnormal fetal presentations is increased with placenta previa. This fact further underlines the importance of surgical delivery.

The type of uterine incision is a controversial issue. A cesarean section at or around 28 weeks usually demands a vertical incision, since the transverse diameter of the lower uterine segment is usually small. A shoulder presentation also necessitates a vertical incision. When the vertex is presenting at an advanced gestational age, a transverse incision in the lower uterine segment may be utilized. Much has been written about the necessity for avoiding the placenta when making the uterine incision. This undoubtedly is preferable and will result in reduced total blood loss. However, it is obvious that cutting through the placenta using a transverse incision entails less risk of maternal morbidity than does the use of a vertical incision.

The location of the placenta should be determined by ultrasonography before the operation. The site of the implantation will influence the decision concerning the type of incision needed. An abdominal breech delivery frequently requires extra time. The choice of the incision in such a case varies, therefore, with the type of the breech presentation, the location of the placenta, the size of the uterus, and the preference of the surgeon.

Surgical delivery in case of placenta previa frequently results in excessive blood loss. Therefore, two units of crossmatched packed cells should be present in the operating room and two more units should be immediately available in the blood bank. Some consider it advisable to prepare one unit of low titer O Rh-negative blood for the infant, especially if cutting through the placenta is contemplated. Even if the placenta is avoided on opening the uterus, the bleeding can be a problem after delivery, particularly when the implantation site is posterior, because of the limited contractile ability of the lower uterine segment. Hemostasis by suturing is often unsuccessful in this area. Recently, the injection of prostaglandin F2α (Prostin–0.25 mg) directly into the myometrium has been advocated as a useful measure for the control of bleeding.

Vaginal delivery is no longer considered an option even in moderate degrees of placenta previa, except in cases of fetal demise, prematurity incompatible with life, or a major fetal malformation. Even in these cases, however, cesarean section is often needed to minimize the risk of maternal morbidity and mortality.

Fetal morbidity and mortality rates can be reduced by adequate blood replacement, operative rather than vaginal delivery, and proper timing of the performance of cesarean section. The standards of care regarding the first two objectives have developed over the last five decades and today represent an accepted practice.

Neonatal intensive care has contributed significantly to the reduction of the perinatal mortality rate. Naturally, increased gestational age at delivery greatly enhances fetal survival. There is no general agreement, however, as to how to accomplish this. A large array of terms, such as expectant, conservative, traditional, and aggressive conservative have all been used to describe the same idea. A controversial concept of expectancy is the use of tocolysis to delay delivery and the utilization of steroids to enhance fetal lung maturity.

The theory underlying the use of tocolysis in placenta previa is not without merit. Stated simply, cervical dilatation and effacement in the presence of placenta previa lead to hemorrhage, necessitating delivery. Tocolytics are medications used to stop uterine contractions and their administration therefore should halt the cervical changes conducive to hemorrhage. Regretfully, the use of tocolytic agents is often associated with hypotension. Some, such as ritodrine and terbutaline, cause peripheral vasodilation and are contraindicated, therefore, in the face of active bleeding. Some studies, however, seem to favor their use in cases of placenta previa. Their limits of safety in these studies are often vaguely defined. Other side effects include maternal tachycardia (which makes the evaluation of volume status difficult) and inhibition of calcium production (which may cause myometrial relaxation). Thus, if severe bleeding after the administration of beta-mimetic agents makes an emergency cesarean section necessary, reduced myometrial contractility may increase the likelihood of severe intraoperative and postoperative bleeding. This being the case, the clinical use of tocolytic agents does not seem to be justifiable at this time.

Some favor the use of magnesium sulfate over beta-mimetic agents for the expectant management of placenta previa. This preference is based on its known depressant effect on myometrial contractility, with fewer cardiovascular effects. This drug is more familiar to most obstetricians, having been in use for years for the treatment of preeclampsia. The myometrial relaxation seems to be readily reversed by oxytocin and is, therefore, less likely to cause intra- or postoperative bleeding as compared with the beta-mimetics. Initial infusion rates as high as 3 g per hour are often necessary for adequate effect.

Since keeping the cervix closed should theoretically reduce the bleeding from placenta previa, some advocate the use of cervical cerclage. This reasoning, however, has one essential flaw: Although a suture could well stop dilation, the effacement still may proceed, resulting in torrential bleeding. In addition, cerclage in the third trimester is far from risk-free. If the suture is placed at the level of the internal os (as it should be), then the risk of rupture of the membranes is considerable. Suturing the cervix at any time during pregnancy is conducive to heavy bleeding, especially during the third trimester. This being the case, it seems logical to avoid the use of this procedure in placenta previa.

The use of steroid hormones for the purpose of enhancing fetal lung maturation in placenta previa is contraindicated when terbutaline or ritodrine is being used for tocolysis, since these drugs can cause pulmonary edema. Steroids can, however, be used in conjunction with magnesium sulfate, another drug with tocolytic potential. Steroids are also known to slow the ability of the body to combat infection. In addition, wound healing may be impaired as a result. Since the likelihood of operative delivery approaches 100 percent, in cases of placenta previa the use of steroids appears risky.

Some feel that a low-lying or lateral placenta previa may permit vaginal delivery if the site of the placenta, determined ultrasonically, is far from the cervix. In the absence of accurate criteria for predicting the amount of bleeding in such a clinical situation, we do not recommend this approach.

The following management plan is derived from the above considerations:

1. Diagnose, classify, and treat blood loss as explained above. Stabilize the patient as soon as practical.
2. If stabilization is not possible, proceed to cesarean section.
3. Once stabilization has been accomplished, proceed to ultrasound examination.
4. If placenta previa is confirmed and the evidence indicates a fetal gestational age of 36 weeks or more, proceed to cesarean section as soon as possible. (At cesarean section, have hysterectomy instruments at hand).
5. If the gestational age is less than 36 weeks, try expectant management.
6. After 72 hours of in-hospital observation, outpatient management may be considered if only one incident of minimal bleeding has occurred. Subsequent hemorrhage, or heavy initial bleeding, necessitates hospital management until delivery.
7. Amniocentesis at the calculated 36th week may be used if the length of the gestational period is uncertain.
8. Avoid the use of double set-up, vaginal delivery and/or steroids.

PLACENTA PREVIA ACCRETA

Placenta accreta, increta, and percreta represent trophoblastic invasion up to, into, or through the myometrium, respectively. There is absence of the decidua basalis and incomplete development of the fibrinoid layer. In various reports, the incidence in association with placenta previa varies from 1 to 15 percent. The thin, poorly formed decidua of the lower uterine segment offers little resistance to placental invasion. Attempts at removal of the placenta result in profuse bleeding. Attempts to induce myometrial contractions by uterine massage or through the use of oxytocic agents are usually futile because of the limited contractile ability of the lower uterine segment.

The therapeutic plan chosen in these situations will produce successful results more frequently if the condition is anticipated. This potential complication should be considered in any case of placenta previa, especially when there is a previously scarred uterus. Since cesarean section is the method of delivery advised in almost all cases of placenta previa, the problem can be quickly identified.

The aggressiveness of the management will depend on the amount or rapidity of the blood loss as well as on the reproductive desires of the patient. When the latter is not an overwhelming consideration, removal of the uterus, without any procrastination, is the management method of choice.

All blood should be replaced as it is lost. Frequently, all conservative methods fail, resulting in the need for surgical control of the bleeding. If future pregnancy is desired and the bleeding is not alarming, ligation of both uterine arteries should be attempted. If this is done properly, the results are often dramatic. Care should be taken to avoid including the ureter in the ligation. The proximity of the ureter to the uterine artery, as well as the large amount of blood in the surgical field, can lead to injury of the ureter that may be unrecognized by the surgeon. A postoperative intravenous pyelogram should be done if a uterine artery ligation is performed under difficult circumstances.

Another logical step in achieving hemostasis is hypogastric artery ligation. However, the vessels in this region are dilated significantly during pregnancy, thus increasing the risk of hemorrhage. Nonetheless, when this procedure is performed by an experienced surgeon, the effect can be very satisfying. The hypogastric artery should be ligated in two places but without transection.

When one of the methods fails to produce the desired hemostasis, hysterectomy needs to be performed. In actual fact, hysterectomy is the first line of defense in all those instances in which the hemorrhage deriving from placenta previa accreta is life-threatening.

Since a supracervical hysterectomy can be performed rapidly and will control the blood loss, it is often preferable to total hysterectomy.

VASA PREVIA

Vasa previa refers to vessels traversing the membranes outside the area of the placenta and crossing that of the internal cervical os. It exists in conjunction with velamentous insertion of the umbilical cord and abnormal placentation (e.g., placenta succenturiata, bilobate placenta).

Vasa previa is a rare complication, occurring in about 1 in 3,000 childbirths. When the vessel ruptures, the likelihood of perinatal fetal loss due to exsanguination is between 50 and 75 percent.

PLACENTA PREVIA SUCCENTURIATA

This condition exists when one or more small accessory lobes develop at a distance from the periphery of the main placenta and become implanted over the internal cervical os. The ultrasound examination may only demonstrate the main placenta, well away from the cervix, giving the erroneous impression that no previa is present. If diagnosed, this condition requires the same treatment as described for placenta previa. Care should be taken at cesarean section to ensure that the placenta is completely removed.

Intrauterine Growth Retardation

To a moderate extent, placenta previa predisposes the fetus to intrauterine growth retardation. A good deal of confusion probably results from frequent miscalculation of the gestational period on account of postconception bleeding. Therefore, the ultrasonographic examination should invariably include careful assessment of the age and growth rates of the fetus to permit appropriate choice with regard to the time of the delivery.

Congenital Anomalies

The most common coincidental congenital anomalies with placenta previa are those of the central nervous, cardiovascular, respiratory, and gastrointestinal systems. This fact necessitates that a level II sonogram be done for any pregnancy complicated by placenta previa, with special attention to these organs and systems.

Rh Sensitization

Antepartum bleeding, secondary to placenta previa, can cause a fetal-maternal transfusion and sensitization of an Rh-negative mother. Unless it is known that the father is Rh negative, testing by the acid elution technique of Kleihauer and Betke is probably indicated. This is true despite the recent suggestion that this test is unreliable because the mother is capable of producing fetal cells. Using this method, the fetal red blood cells stain with eosin and appear pink, whereas the adult red blood cells do not stain and appear empty (ghost cells). If fetomaternal hemorrhage is detected, the appropriate dose of immune globulin is given, sufficient in amount to turn an indirect Coombs' test positive within 48 hours. The same investigation may be advisable when a cesarean section is performed for placenta previa, another risk factor for severe fetomaternal hemorrhage.

SUGGESTED READING

Creasy RK, Resnik R. Maternal fetal medicine: principles and practice. Philadelphia: WB Saunders, 1984:539.

Danforth DN. Obstetrics and gynecology. 4th ed. Philadelphia: Harper & Row, 1982:443.

Gabbe SG, Niebyl JR, Simpson JL, eds. Obstetrics: normal and problem pregnancies. New York: Churchill Livingstone, 1986:494.

Iffy L, Kaminetzky HA, eds. Principles and practice of obstetrics and perinatology: New York: John Wiley & Sons, 1981:1105.

Pauerstein CJ. Clinical obstetrics. New York: John Wiley & Sons, 1987:336.

Pritchard JA, MacDonald PC, Gant NF. Williams obstetrics. 17th ed. Norwalk, CT: Appleton-Century-Crofts, 1985:407.

ABRUPTIO PLACENTAE

DAVID CHARLES, M.D., F.A.C.O.G., F.R.C.O.G.
DOUGLAS D. GLOVER, B.S. Pharm., M.D.

Abruptio placentae has been defined as premature separation of a normally implanted placenta, a descriptive definition that attempts to distinguish it from another complication of late pregnancy associated with hemorrhage, namely, placenta previa. The connotation of abruptio placentae signifies the rendering asunder of the placenta, with implication as to the suddenness of the event. Another less frequently used expression, ablatio placentae, makes reference to the carrying away of the placenta from its site of attachment. Likewise, the term accidental hemorrhage, which was used in the United Kingdom, refers to the bleeding that occurs as a sequel to placental abruption. Such varied nomenclature merely serves to highlight the deficits in our knowledge of the etiology of this potentially catastrophic complication of pregnancy.

Approximately 4 percent of pregnancies are complicated by hemorrhage in the third trimester. Of these, 20 percent of the cases are due to placenta previa, 30 percent are the result of abruption, and the remaining etiology cannot always be delineated. The incidence of placental abruption has been variously reported to be 0.5 to 3.79 per 1,000 births. However, the true incidence is undoubtedly higher, since many cases go unrecognized because of a concealed hemorrhage sufficiently small to allow the pregnancy to continue. Abruptio placentae is important in that it accounts for about 25 percent of the perinatal mortality rate, and the fetal death rate following complete abruption has been reported to be as high as 87 percent. Although the cause of abruptio placentae is unknown, the majority of cases are associated with certain risk factors that are listed in Table 1. Of these, hypertension is the predominant etiologic factor, whether it is the result of chronic hypertensive vascular disease or pregnancy-induced hypertension.

The pathophysiology of abruption in association with hypertension is not fully understood. Nicotine is known to diminish uteroplacental perfusion in smokers and may lead to ischemic changes in the decidua basalis. Likewise, chronic hypertension causes ischemia in the placental bed. Prostaglandin production and release from the site of tissue necrosis may likewise play a role in the pathogenesis of abruptio placentae. The chronology of events leading to abruption is most likely similar in women who smoke, those with chronic hypertension, and individuals with pregnancy-induced hypertension.

It has been shown that an association exists between placental abruption and intrauterine growth retardation. It is also considered that impaired fetal nutrition may indeed precede placental separation. Pregnant women who smoke are prone to have infants who are small for gestational age, and abruption is prevalent among such individuals. Women with abruptio placentae have reduced blood levels of vitamin A, beta-carotene, and vitamin E, which is in accord with the concept of defective nutrition.

It has been generally accepted that a decrease in uterine volume may contribute to placental abruption. Reduction in uterine volume is a normal event during the process of parturition. After expulsion of the fetus, the uterus contracts, resulting in a sudden diminution in uterine size and a smaller surface area for attachment of the placenta. Consequently, the placenta buckles and allows a retroplacental hemorrhage to occur, thereby delineating a plane of cleavage. There is presumptive evidence that implies a similar sequence of events resulting in premature separation of the placenta after delivery of the first twin in multiple pregnancy, rupture of the membranes in the presence of polyhydramnios, or as a terminal event in the third stage of labor.

TABLE 1 Risk Factors Associated with Abruptio Placentae

Hypertension
Chronic hypertensive cardiovascular disease
Pregnancy-induced hypertension
Smoking
Previous abruptio placentae
Multiparity
Multiple pregnancy
Trauma

Prolonged preterm premature rupture of the membranes has been reported to increase the risk of abruptio placentae to threefold that noted in association with intact membranes. Furthermore, prolonged preterm premature rupture of the membranes is the most commonly associated complication of pregnancy in those women who later have placental abruption. Most likely the mechanism of placental separation in these cases is similar to that of abruption in late labor. The clinician should be cognizant of the higher risk of abruptio placentae in women who have prolonged preterm premature rupture of the fetal membranes.

Some authors believe that placental abruption can be of either arterial or venous origin. Situated around the periphery of the placenta is a series of discontinuous vascular lakes known as the marginal sinus, which is part of the placental venous drainage system. Hemorrhage from this vascular network may cause separation of the membranes from the decidua and lead to ischemia of the amnion and chorion. The ischemia may result in tissue necrosis, activation of the prostaglandin cascade, amniorrhexis, and preterm labor.

Aspirin was once used with impunity throughout pregnancy. However, ingestion of this substance in the third trimester is now discouraged because of concern related to the hemorrhagic consequences of salicylates. An infrequent complication of bleeding following administration of salicylates is abruptio placentae. A favorite over-the-counter liquid preparation for the treatment of traveler's diarrhea is Pepto-Bismol. Some physicians recommend this product for prophylaxis when a patient is planning to travel to Central America. The active ingredient of Pepto-Bismol is bismuth subsalicylate. The dose recommended on the label is one or two tablespoons every 30 minutes for a maximum of eight doses per day. Ingestion of the higher dose of this antidiarrheal liquid will deliver a 2,105-mg salicylate load that is the equivalent of 2,736 mg of aspirin, equal to eight standard tablets. This amount of salicylate taken daily for several days can place the gravid woman at risk for a bleeding diathesis and certainly should be avoided.

Although the pharmacokinetics of bismuth subsalicylate has not been studied in the pregnant woman, it has been investigated in healthy adult males. Absorption of the bismuth salt appears to be complete, as 95 percent of a single oral dose is recovered from the urine in 24 hours. The plasma half-life for a single dose is 2.8 hours, but the nonlinear kinetics of salicylate elimination with a multiple dose regimen causes the half-life to increase to 7 hours after the fifth dose. Furthermore, accumulation of salicylate in the plasma occurs with any multiple-dose regimen, and this increases the risk to the patient who is receiving long-term prophylaxis for traveler's diarrhea.

Over 3 decades ago, Page and associates devised a grading classification for abruptio placentae to assist the clinician in the evaluation of the patient with placental abruption and aid in formulating the prognosis. Grading was based on the presence or absence of vaginal bleeding, hypotension, coagulopathy, and fetal stress. Grade 0 was usually only recognized when the placenta was examined on completion of the third stage of labor. Grade 1 abruption was the mildest clinical variety and was, in most cases, due to marginal sinus rupture. Grades 2 and 3 were of a more severe nature and required prompt intervention. Over the years, numerous studies have utilized the Page classification to equate the severity of the abruption with the method of management and obstetric outcome. To date, it is still unclear if premature separation is a progressive process preceded by multiple accidents leading to small areas of separation that eventually coalesce or is a single acute event. If one accepts that it is a progressive process, it is essential that delivery of the fetus be expedited.

MANAGEMENT

In the treatment of abruptio placentae, one must consider the following complications that can occur:

1. Renal failure. This may be manifest by the presence of transient oliguria or anuria accompanied by renal tubular or cortical necrosis. In the majority of instances, renal failure is reversible.
2. Pituitary necrosis. This possibility must always be kept in mind in any patient who suffers severe hemorrhagic shock.
3. Coagulation failure. This is encountered in about 25 percent of all cases of placental abruption.
4. Postpartum hemorrhage. It is well known that an antepartum hemorrhage predisposes to postpartum hemorrhage. The incidence of this complication in patients with abruption of the placenta is at least doubled. When placental separation is associated with coagulation failure, its occurrence is seven to eight times that in the general obstetric population because of postpartum uterine atony and an increase in serum fibrinogen degradation products. It is possible that a causal relationship exists between the increase in fibrinogen degradation products and uterine atony.

In all instances the patient with abruptio placentae must be admitted to the hospital. When initially seen, the patient may be in a state of shock. Her general condition must be reviewed, and after evaluation the patient should be placed in the left lateral position so as to prevent any aggravation of the hypotension caused by the weight of the gravid uterus on the inferior vena cava. A blood sample must be obtained for hematologic investigation, specifically evaluation of any coagulation defect and an active fibrinolytic state. In all but the mildest cases, blood transfusion is essential and at least four units are required initially. These patients have a severe degree of hypovolemia, and their natural response to this is one of vasoconstriction. Vasoconstrictive drugs are neither indicated nor necessary, and the first effort should be directed toward restoring the effective circulating blood volume. Hypovolemia can be demonstrated by a low central venous pressure and reduced urinary output. The hematocrit and hemoglobin determinations are less reliable parameters and, as a rule, in the more severe cases a central venous pressure line not only provides a route for massive blood transfusion but is a guide to the amount of blood required. The patient should be transfused until the central venous pressure rises above 4 cm of mercury and adequate amounts of urine are excreted. Blood pressure recordings are not a good indicator of hypovolemia in patients at term, since such individuals can tolerate a large volume of blood loss without exhibiting significant hypotension.

It is essential to evaluate the patient for the presence or absence of any disseminated intravascular coagulopathy (DIC). Placental abruption is the most frequent cause of coagulation failure in the majority of obstetric units. Premature separation of the placenta can occur in apparently healthy women with no clinical warning or in conjunction with pregnancy-induced hypertension. As previously stated, it is possible that clinically silent placental infarcts may predispose to the placental separation and cause alteration of the hemostatic system. There is a broad spectrum in the severity of the hemostatic failure in this entity that appears to be directly related to the degree of placental separation and concealed hemorrhage. In the majority of patients with small degrees of abruption, there is a minor degree of failure of the hemostatic process, and fetal demise is unlikely. On the other hand, when the uterus is tense and tender and no fetal heart sounds are audible, there is a massive retroplacental clot, and in such instances the severity of the coagulopathy is obvious.

Hemostatic failure may be suspected if there is persistent oozing at the site of venipunctures or bleeding from mucous membranes. Simple rapid screening tests should be instituted to confirm the presence of DIC. The blood is frequently incoagulable if the plasma fibrinogen level falls below 100 per deciliter and approximately 25 percent of such patients will develop postpartum hemorrhage. Each unit of blood for replacement delivers 500 mg of fibrinogen, which increases the circulating plasma fibrinogen concentration by 12.5 mg per deciliter. Four units of blood, therefore, can raise the fibrinogen level from 50 mg to 100 mg per deciliter. A fibrinogen level of 100 mg is adequate for reducing the risk of hemorrhage, and further transfusions should be withheld in order to reduce the risk of post-transfusion hepatitis. In the presence of DIC, in addition to a low fibrinogen level, there will be thrombocytopenia and a prolonged prothrombin time as well as elevated fibrinogen degradation products. The therapeutic goal is to maintain the circulating blood volume by correcting the hypovolemic state. This not only prevents renal shutdown but averts further hemostatic failure.

As soon as the patient's general condition begins to improve, no time should be lost in inducing labor by artificial rupture of the fetal membranes. If fetal heart sounds are audible and the pregnancy is of adequate maturity, cesarean section is the most expeditious way of terminating the pregnancy. In most instances, however, labor rapidly supervenes following induction, especially if the patient is parous. It is often difficult to ascertain with certainty when labor has commenced because of the extreme pain suffered by the patient, and frequently vaginal examination must be performed to assess progress. The appearance of blood at the vulva in renewed amounts signifies that the uterus has commenced to contract; otherwise the blood would have remained concealed. There is no evidence to indicate that oxytocic agents aggravate thromboplastin release from the uterus, and in the presence of fetal demise oxytocin infusion following amniotomy is the procedure of choice. The judicious use of oxytocin in cases in which the cervix does not dilate within a short period of time can be extremely beneficial. In the management of abruptio placentae, there is no place for masterly inactivity.

Following emptying of the uterus, myometrial contractions greatly reduce bleeding from the placental site and spontaneous correction of the hemostatic defect usually occurs. If postpartum hemorrhage does occur (not an infrequent complication), it is essential that uterine contractions be sustained with the use of oxytocin, and in the absence of hypertension ergonovine can be prescribed. In instances in which the abruption is small and the fetus is still alive, prompt cesarean section may save the baby if vaginal delivery is neither feasible nor imminent. Fresh frozen plasma, banked red cells, and platelet concentrates should be available to correct any potential severe coagulation defect of the maternal circulation. In rare instances in which vaginal delivery cannot be promptly accomplished and hemorrhage continued, cesarean section may be indicated even in the presence of a dead fetus. In such circumstances, normal hemostasis should be restored by the administration of fresh frozen plasma and platelet concentrates as well as red cells prior to abdominal delivery. Despite extravasation of blood throughout the uterine muscle, myometrial function is not impaired and good contraction will follow emptying of the uterus. Regional anesthesia can cause expansion of the vascular bed of the lower extremities and add to the problem of uncorrected hypovolemia. Additionally, in the presence of hemostatic failure, there is the hazard of bleeding into the epidural space. For surgery in cases of abruptio placentae, general anesthesia is preferred.

In recent years heparin has been used to treat DIC regardless of the etiology. There is, however, no objective evidence that its use in abruptio placentae decreases morbidity and mortality. Although anecdotal reports continue to support its use, large prospective studies have demonstrated that good results can be achieved without the use of heparin. This agent, in the presence of already defective hemostasis with a large bleeding placental bed, may prolong bleeding and cause a massive local or generalized hemorrhage.

Treatment with antifibrinolytic agents can result in occlusion of small vessels with fibrin in such vital organs as the kidney or brain and therefore is contraindicated.

It is important to remember that the unsensitized Rh-negative patient should be given RhoGAM if she has abruptio placentae. About 30 percent of women who deliver vaginally experience transfusion with fetal erythrocytes after manual removal of the placenta. This figure increases to over 50 percent in those who have a cesarean section. A standard dose of Rh-negative immune globulin contains 300 μg of anti-D, which is sufficient to prevent immunization by 15 ml of Rh-positive red blood cells, the equivalent of 30 ml of whole blood. It is essential that the standard dose of RhoGAM be administered. The very fact that the patient received RhoGAM at the 28th week of gestation does not suffice in the case of severe abruption.

The acute defibrination syndrome associated with abruptio placentae may be acute and life-threatening. DIC is a pathologic disorder resulting from intravascular activation of the hemostatic system in response to injury. Such activation of coagulation leads to production of thrombin and proteolytic enzymes that cause the formation of intravascular fibrin, platelet deposition, and secondary activation of the fibrinolytic system. The major clinical problem in DIC is hemorrhage, since intravascular consumption of the coagulation factors results in depletion of fibrinogen and platelets as well as the production of fibrinogen degradation products, which act as anticoagulants. DIC may be acute and overwhelming, and in such cases total defibrination takes place in association with profuse bleeding and shock. The physician must always be alert to the fact that DIC is a pathologic response to an underlying disorder, and the diagnosis and correct management of the latter will restore normal hemostasis.

The hemostatic mechanism represents a dynamic process in which the platelets and coagulation system, which promote hemostasis, are balanced by the repair of the proteolytic mechanism of the fibrinolytic enzyme system. The main hemostatic abnormalities caused by DIC are enumerated in Table 2.

It is probable that many, if not most, cases of DIC are induced by the entry of tissue thromboplastins into the circulation. This is perhaps most frequently seen in obstetric accidents such as abruptio placentae, which leads to the liberation of placental thromboplastic substances.

The most important principle in the treatment of DIC is to remove, if possible, the precipitating cause. If this cannot be achieved, it is unlikely that successful resolution of DIC will occur. In the obstetric patient with abruptio placentae, delivery of the fetus usually produces a rapid return to normal hemostasis. In the presence of uncontrolled bleeding if the precipitating cause cannot be removed rapidly, replacement therapy is indicated. Adequate whole blood may be needed to counteract possible exsanguination. Fresh frozen plasma is useful, since it provides a plasma expander and replaces clotting factors. If cryoprecipitate is available, it is a useful adjunct, since each pack contains approximately 100 to 150 units of factor VIII. Initially 10 bags of cryoprecipitate should be used, following which the fibrinogen level is reassessed and whole blood clot inspection performed. It could be argued that providing replacement coagulation factors adds fuel to the fire, but in practice this does not seem to occur, and hemostasis is not achieved without replacement therapy in many instances. Antithrombin III replacement therapy has been suggested to correct antithrombin III deficiency caused by its consumption. At present, there are no controlled studies to confirm the efficacy of such therapy, although anecdotal reports have suggested that it may be useful. The use of heparin remains controversial, although less credence has been given to the early enthusiastic reports that it was highly beneficial. These communica-

TABLE 2 Mechanisms of Hemostatic Alterations in Disseminated Intravascular Coagulation

Hemostatic Alterations	*Mechanism*
Coagulation factors	
Reduced or absent fibrinogen	Conversion to fibrin
Reduction in factors V and VIII	Activation and destruction by thrombin
Reduction in factor XIII	Activation and then possible consumption during fibrin cross-linking
Reduction in antithrombin III	Formation of complex with thrombin
Reduction in prekallikrein and factor XII	Consumption
Activation products	
Increased fibrinogen degradation products	Proteolytic degradation of fibrin by plasmin
Increased fibrinopeptide A	Generated from fibrinogen by thrombin
Fibrinolytic system	
Reduced plasminogen	Consumption converted to plasmin
Platelets	
Thrombocytopenia	Aggregated in microcirculation
Defects of platelet aggregation and adhesiveness	High levels of fibrinogen degradation products affect platelet aggregation
Activated platelets	
Platelet factors III and IV	Both released from platelets by contact with thrombin or subendothelium

tions date back more than a decade, during which time there have been no convincing controlled clinical trials to show that heparin is efficacious in the therapy of DIC. Perhaps antiplatelet agents will be more extensively utilized in the future. There have been some encouraging preliminary reports of the use of prostacyclin for DIC, and this agent could well play an important role in the future in the therapy of coagulation defects associated with abruptio placentae.

SUGGESTED READING

Abdella TN, Sibai BM, Hayes JM Jr, et al. Relationships of hypertensive disease to abruptio placentae. Obstet Gynecol 1984; 63:365–370.

Cardwell MS. Ultrasound diagnosis of abruptio placentae with fetomaternal hemorrhage. Am J Obstet Gynecol 1987; 157:358–359.

Sher G, Statland BE. Abruptio placentae with coagulopathy: a rational basis for management. Clin Obstet Gynecol 1985; 28:15–23.

LABOR AND DELIVERY

PREMATURE RUPTURE OF THE MEMBRANES

JAY D. IAMS, M.D.

Prematurely ruptured membranes (PROM), defined as amniorrhexis prior to the onset of labor at any gestational age, must be one of the most widely debated topics in obstetrics. This is true for several reasons: the etiology is obscure, the complications are many, and the treatment strategies are multiple and diverse. PROM is a significant cause of neonatal and maternal morbidity at any gestational age, but especially in the preterm gestation. Although PROM occurs in approximately 10 percent of all pregnancies, it precedes 25 to 45 percent of preterm births and has a 20 to 25 percent recurrence risk in preterm gestations. The proper management of PROM requires great care in diagnosis, determination of gestational age, and assessment of fetal and maternal risks.

DIAGNOSIS

Every obstetrician knows the rudiments of confirming the diagnosis of PROM using nitrazine and ferning of pooled vaginal fluid; the diagnostic and therapeutic processes begin, however, with the history, a technique sometimes forgotten in this technologic age. A woman who complains of perineal wetness must be examined in order to distinguish PROM from involuntary loss of urine or vaginitis. This examination is not possible via the telephone. During this initial examination, data are collected that later assist the obstetrician in formulating a management plan: vaginal culture for group B *Streptococcus*, cervical culture for gonorrhea, and vaginal pooled fluid for phosphatidyl glycerol (PG) determination. The color of the fluid is noted, looking for meconium or blood. The cervix is inspected to look for cord prolapse and to assess visually the dilation and effacement.

ASSESSMENT OF GESTATIONAL AGE

Once the diagnosis is secure, the next and most important step is assessment, or reassessment if the woman has received adequate prenatal care, of gestational age. The sequelae of amniorrhexis—including the onset of labor, development of intrauterine infection, and increased compression of the fetus, placenta, and umbilical cord—all have variable significance, depending on the gestational age at the time of rupture. All traditional dating criteria should be reviewed and supplemented by an extensive ultrasound examination, ideally performed in the labor and delivery area. Because the biparietal diameter of the fetus may not be an accurate means of determining gestational age in fetuses exposed to chronic oligohydramnios from any cause, the cephalic index (biparietal diameter/occipitofrontal diameter [BPD/OFD]) should always be recorded in scans done on patients with PROM. Length of the femur and humerus, orbital diameter, and head circumference may be used if the cephalic index is low (less than 0.72) The sonogram should also confirm a subjective disease in the volume of fluid; if this finding is absent, attention to the criteria used for the diagnosis of PROM should be reviewed. The sonographer should note the fetal presentation and look for the umbilical cord in the supracervical area. The remaining volume of fluid should be assessed, since there is a direct relationship between remaining fluid volume and perinatal outcome. Infants born after total fluid loss not surprisingly have been reported to suffer an increased frequency of cord problems and perinatal morbidity.

MANAGEMENT OF PREGNANCIES OF LESS THAN 37 WEEKS

The next step is collection of data to allow an individualized assessment of the relative risk of intrauterine versus extrauterine life for those pregnancies less than 37 weeks and for those in which an accurate gestational age cannot be established (because of no prenatal care, maternal obesity, decreased amniotic fluid, or a poor technical quality scan). The obstetrician may find it useful to proceed by answering a series of questions, as follows.

Is There Reason to Believe the Infant is Safer in the Nursery, Regardless of Its Pulmonary Maturity?

Infection. Evidence of intrauterine infection should be diligently sought; maternal temperature, pulse, and white and differential blood cell counts should be measured. Testing for maternal C-reactive protein has been championed by some, but we have not found it useful in preterm PROM. Maternal fever greater than or equal to 101° F and leukocytosis (20,000 or more white blood cells per cubic millimeter) without an obvious extrauterine cause yield a presumptive diagnosis of amnionitis, and the diagnostic evaluation need proceed no further in these patients. Delivery is in the best interests of both mother and fetus in almost every instance. If the diagnosis of amnionitis is equivocal, then amniocentesis and serial observation of maternal temperature, pulse, leukocyte count, and fetal heart rate may resolve the issue.

Fetal Distress. Evidence of fetal distress should also be sought. Some authors report protocols in which patients with preterm PROM are watched with 12 to 24 hours of continuous electronic fetal heart rate monitoring before being moved from the labor-delivery suite. We have not used monitoring for more than 6 to 8 hours unless decelerations (or labor) were evident in that initial period of assessment, and we have been happy with that approach.

The biophysical profile has also been suggested as a method of early detection of intrauterine infection and distress in pregnancies complicated by preterm PROM. The technique is time-consuming, however, and has not yet been shown to alter outcome in a prospective study of sufficient size to have statistical validity.

Is the Infant Better Off in the Nursery Because of Documented Pulmonary Maturity?

As described earlier, the initial examination should always include analysis of vaginal pool fluid for PG when possible. The presence of PG indicates that the risk of infection probably exceeds the risk of prematurity. When vaginally pooled fluid is insufficient or not available, amniocentesis should be attempted whenever possible. Amniotic fluid obtained via transabdominal amniocentesis can be sent for analysis of lecithin-sphingomyelin ratio, aerobic and anaerobic culture, and Gram's stain as well as PG analysis. It therefore is an extremely useful procedure in the initial evaluation of the preterm PROM patient, providing information on the risks for the fetus of both intrauterine and extrauterine life. If the amniotic fluid analysis produces evidence of pulmonary maturity or of unexpected bacterial colonization, delivery is usually indicated.

This initial evaluation should require no more than 6 to 8 hours and will ensure selection of a group of patients for whom delivery is safer for the fetus: those with documented pulmonary maturity, intrauterine infection, or fetal distress. Mode of delivery is determined by traditional obstetric criteria.

For those who remain, the risks of delivery and prematurity are assumed to be greater than the risks of continuing the pregnancy: infection, cord prolapse, compressed intrauterine environment, and placental abruption. In these women, the next question is:

Can the Risks of Preterm Delivery Be Avoided or Decreased in Order to Avoid the Ongoing Risk of Infection?

Steroids have been evaluated extensively in this situation in a number of trials, as shown in Table 1.

Seven of the ten prospective random trials did not reveal any reduction in respiratory distress syndrome, and five suggested increased risk of neonatal or maternal infection or both. The conclusion to be drawn from these studies is that any neonatal benefit from the use of steroids must be of extremely small magnitude and may be gained at the cost of an increased risk of infection. Steroids do not appear to be the answer once hoped for in the management of preterm PROM.

Can the Risks of Continuing the Pregnancy, i.e., Infection, Be Reduced or Eliminated?

There have been no studies demonstrating improved neonatal outcomes in women with preterm PROM treated prophylactically with antibiotics, but this has not been extensively studied in recent years. Women with preterm PROM found to carry the group B *Streptococcus* or gonorrhea should, however, be treated immediately with intravenous antibiotics, e.g., ampicillin, in order to eradicate these organisms from the vagina before labor occurs. The duration of treatment is not a settled issue. It is clear that intravenous treatment should be initiated as soon as a report of a positive group B *Streptococcus* culture is received, should be continued until a negative vaginal group B *Streptococcus* culture is obtained, and should be reinstituted at the onset of labor. For the majority of women who labor and deliver within 72 hours of rupture, this means they will be given intravenous ampicillin from the time of admission through delivery. For those in whom labor does not occur soon after rupture, it may be possible to obtain a negative group B *Streptococcus* culture. Should these patients then be continued on prophylactic

TABLE 1 Effect of Corticosteroids on Respiratory Distress Syndrome in Preterm Labor (Randomized Controlled Studies Only)

	No. of Patients		
Author	*Steroids*	*Control*	*Effect on Respiratory Distress Syndrome*
Block	43	26	No difference
Taeusch	17	24	*No difference
Papageorgiou	17	19	Decreased
Young	38	37	Decreased
Garite	80	80	*No difference
Collaborative	153	135	No difference
Iams	38	35	*No difference
Nelson	22	46	*No difference
Simpson	112	105	*No difference
Morales	121	124	Decreased

* Studies also suggesting an increased incidence of maternal and/or neonatal infection in the group using steroids. From Garite T, Druzin ML. Management of the patient with preterm premature rupture of the membranes. Intervention 1987; Summer:10.

antibiotics? Those who say "no" cite fear of infection with resistant organisms and claim that reinstitution of intravenous antibiotics at the onset of labor is adequate to prevent neonatal sepsis. Those favoring continuous antibiotic treatment of women with preterm PROM who have been colonized with group B *Streptococcus* argue that since the gastrointestinal tract is the reservoir for these bacteria, recolonization of the vagina is likely to occur promptly after discontinuation of antibiotics. This, in fact, has been observed in clinical trials, making a strong argument for continuing oral or intravenous antibiotics through delivery in women colonized by group B *Streptococcus* with preterm PROM who are managed conservatively.

Can the Risk of Preterm Labor Be Eliminated or Reduced?

Research trials of the generally accepted treatment modality of hospital bed rest are lacking; nevertheless, bed rest with only minimal bathroom privileges is certainly a logical and safe means of minimizing further fluid leakage and avoiding cord prolapse. Recent studies have evaluated prophylactic tocolysis in women with preterm PROM and have found no evidence of benefit when tocolysis was initiated at the first sign of uterine activity. A protocol using prophylactic beta-mimetics and sedatives immediately after hospital admission, without waiting for the onset of contractions, yielded only a modest (3 days) increase in the mean interval from rupture to delivery compared with results in a control group treated with bed rest alone.

The management plan thus far has selected a group of patients who have no evidence of fetal pulmonary maturity, who have no evidence of infection or distress, who have not developed labor, and who have neither received steroids nor tocolytics. Some, usually 25 to 40 percent of preterm PROM patients, have a positive culture for group B *Streptococcus* and therefore would be receiving antibiotic therapy. The next series of questions is aimed at reassessing on a frequent basis the selective risk of delivery versus continued observation.

What Methods Should Be Used to Detect Amnionitis?

The traditional indicators of intrauterine infection (leukocyte count, differential count, temperature, maternal and fetal pulses, and serial manual palpation of the uterus) have never been totally satisfactory individually but together have provided a basis for infection surveillance in these patients. Recent literature has championed increased use of repeated amniotic fluid analysis in detecting intrauterine infection. A Gram's stained smear of fluid is examined for the presence of bacteria, which appears to be more predictive of intrauterine infection than the presence of leukocytes. There are several problems with this approach. Rates of success of obtaining fluid in this setting vary widely from one institution to another, from 5 to 50 percent of patients who are candidates for the procedure. It is therefore not applicable to all. The predictive value and interobserver variability of the Gram's stain findings remain somewhat uncertain as well. Most important, it has not yet been demonstrated that perinatal mortality is improved by more aggressive use of amniocentesis in PROM patients. Still, the direct examination and culture of amniotic fluid are rational methods that honor the traditions of infectious disease. It is particularly reassuring to find a benign smear and negative culture of fluid obtained from a patient in whom traditional indicators of infection were conflicting or equivocal.

Another technique recently applied to amniotic fluid analysis is the leukocyte esterase reagent strip, which indicates white blood cells' phagocytic response to bacteria. This technique has not been widely studied but may prove to be a rapid method of identifying or excluding intra-amniotic infection within minutes of obtaining fluid. The presence of maternal C-reactive protein, a nonspecific acute phase response to inflammation, has also been correlated with the development of amnionitis in PROM but appears to be no more reliable than other traditional indicators of infection such as the leukocyte and differential counts. Initial enthusiasm for this test has now waned.

Although not yet established, frequent, even daily, use of the nonstress test and the fetal biophysical profile have been proposed, as potentially sensitive and specific indicators of fetal compromise caused by sepsis and/or cord compression or both. These tests have not been studied in prospective trials of PROM patients. Retrospectively collected data have indicated a correlation of biophysical profile score and neonatal sepsis, but no difference in perinatal mortality was seen. Biophysical profile testing is time-consuming and expensive. Whether it contributes to a decline in perinatal mortality in conservatively managed PROM patients awaits the results of a prospective random trial.

Besides Infection, What Other Risks Are Present in Conservatively Managed Preterm PROM?

There are several additional hazards to the conservative management of preterm PROM that must be kept in mind. Cord prolapse, placental abruption, fetal physical compression deformity, and pulmonary hypoplasia have all been reported with increased frequency. Beyond bed rest and patient and staff awareness of these problems, little can be done to prevent them.

The patient should be educated fully and repeatedly about the uncertainties of management for preterm PROM. It is not possible to predict each complication in time to prevent it or to treat each complication successfully. Some infants develop sepsis despite the best management, and some suffer respiratory distress syndrome because of preterm delivery prompted by false-positive signs and symptoms of amnionitis. The patient, her family, and the nursing staff must be aware that each day following amniorrhexis requires reassessment of the relative merits of delivery versus continuing the pregnancy.

Should Women with Preterm PROM Be Referred to a Tertiary Perinatal Center?

The answer to this question depends principally upon neonatal facilities in each hospital. Since most (80 percent) of women with preterm PROM labor and deliver within a week of rupture, it is logical to transfer women with preterm PROM below 32 to 34 weeks to a tertiary center capable of continuous ventilation of the preterm infant. Improved survival rates have been reported with maternal rather than neonatal transport of infants below 32- and especially below 30-weeks gestation. Those women who neither labor spontaneously nor become infected can then be reverse transferred to a level I or II facility at 34 to 36 weeks, depending on local custom and facilities.

How Should Labor Be Managed in Preterm PROM?

Women in labor (spontaneous and induced) following preterm PROM are at risk for cord compression, and continuous electronic fetal heart rate monitoring is required. A cord compression pattern that fails to respond to the customary maneuvers of position change and administration of oxygen may be treated with saline amniofusion. In this procedure, sterile normal saline solution in boluses of 250 to 500 ml is infused into the intrauterine pressure catheter to relieve compression of the umbilical cord and may allow labor to continue safely for the fetus.

Medical induction of labor in women with preterm PROM for either pulmonary maturity or suspected infection has a reported failure rate of 50 percent or more in some series. Cesarean section in these cases is rarely done for cephalopelvic disproportion and infrequently done for fetal distress. Most cesarean sections are the result of failure to progress, lack of progress, or failed induction. In such instances, oxytocin has been administered for several hours without producing uterine activity or cervical change. This is a common problem unrelated to a specific region of the country, patient class, or ethnic group. The only common denominator appears to be medical induction of labor in the woman with preterm PROM. This risk of failed induction must be considered whenever a patient with PROM has labour induced.

How Should PROM Be Managed in the Patient with a Previable Gestation?

When PROM occurs before 26 weeks, the prognosis is poor but not as grim as traditionally thought. In a review of 53 such cases managed expectantly, 13 neonates survived. This was accomplished without serious long-term maternal complications. Prolonged preterm PROM carries an increased risk of pulmonary hypoplasia, fetal compression deformity and placental abruption, as well as the usual risks of infection. The patient with PROM before 24-weeks gestation may reject expectant management and request immediate delivery rather than undergo an emotionally difficult and prolonged period of bed rest with only a 25 percent chance of a surviving infant. Prostaglandin gel or suppositories may be used to accomplish that goal.

When conservative management is elected in an effort to salvage the pregnancy, the patient must be made to understand the relatively low probability of success. Bed rest in the Trendelenburg position, prophylactic subcutaneous heparin, aggressive treatment of group B *Streptococcus* colonization, and meticulous attention to bowel function and perineal hygiene are useful in prolonging pregnancy in this difficult situation.

PROM in the second trimester should prompt a careful examination of the cervix after delivery for evidence of cervical incompetence. The etiology of PROM remains uncertain but it probably involves infection. The reader is referred to the chapter on *Incompetent Cervix*.

PREGNANCIES BEYOND 37 - WEEKS GESTATION

The initial evaluation of PROM at term is no different than in the preterm gestation. The diagnosis must be confirmed and the gestational age assessed. Since there is presumed to be no advantage to the fetus by continuing the pregnancy, traditional obstetric teaching has favored induction of labor for women with PROM after 36 weeks who do not labor spontaneously within a few hours of amniorrhexis. This has been done in recognition of the fact that there is an association of the span of time from amniorrhexis to delivery with the incidence of neonatal sepsis. However, the incidence of sepsis in term newborns born to women with PROM appears to be lower than is commonly thought and in recent studies ranges from 0 to 3.5 percent. Sepsis in infants born to women with amnionitis is also less common than expected and ranges from 1 to 13 percent. This, in conjunction with an incidence of cesarean section for failed induction that approaches 50 percent, has prompted a reassessment of the management of PROM at term. Management of PROM at term may also be described by posing a series of questions. Unlike preterm PROM, in which continuation of intrauterine life is the goal if possible, management of PROM at term proceeds from the opposite assumption: The infant, if delivered, should do well. Why shouldn't labor occur promptly?

The first question then is:

Are There Risks to the Fetus or Mother If Labor Is Induced Now?

If the cervix is unripe, labor may not be easily induced. The risk to the mother and fetus of amnionitis and newborn sepsis is increased by a long difficult labor, sometimes complicated also by cord compression and often culminating in cesarean section. Assessment of cervical status requires a pelvic examination, however, which may carry perineal and vaginal bacteria toward the amniotic sac, thus increasing the risk of infection. A single, *sterile*, digital examination has not been found in one series to alter the rate of amnionitis. If, as is usually the case, the cervix is found to be ripe, then induction of labor should be carried out promptly. If an unripe cervix is encountered, then additional questions should be posed.

Are There Additional Risks of PROM in this Patient?

Does she have a history of genital herpes simplex or of group B streptococcal colonization? If so, then prompt delivery is indicated. In those with a history of herpes simplex virus, a careful inspection of the vulva and vagina and detailed inquiry regarding prodromal symptoms should be carried out. Any suspicious lesions or prodromal symptoms should lead to cesarean birth. When vaginal delivery is indicated with a history of herpes simplex virus, we avoid the use of the spiral electrode for fetal heart rate measurement in order to minimize the chances of fetal scalp inoculation of the virus.

Women with PROM who undergo induction despite an unfavorable cervix are candidates for a long latent phase and therefore are at increased risk for group B streptococcal neonatal sepsis if they happen to be carriers. Therefore, when labor is induced in a PROM patient with an unripe cervix, a vaginal group B *Streptococcus* culture should be obtained and intravenous ampicillin begun at a dose of 1 g intravenously every 4 hours throughout labor. This precaution for women with PROM at term is advisable only for those who are expected to have a long latent phase because of an unripe cervix.

Is there meconium-stained amniotic fluid or other evidence on fetal heart rate monitoring of possible fetal compromise? Women with PROM at term with meconium or fetal heart rate abnormality should be delivered promptly regardless of the status of the cervix.

Is there an unstable fetal lie that might allow a cord prolapse? Continuing observation would not be advisable in this situation.

In the relatively few remaining patients whose cervices are quite unripe and who have no special risk of continuing the pregnancy, it appears to be safe to await the onset of spontaneous labor for as long as 3 to 4 days. The safety of this approach has been reported in series from both sides of the Atlantic and may allow an opportunity to avoid cesarean delivery for failed induction. Still, it seems safest to induce those at term in whom there is a reasonable chance of successful induction.

SUGGESTED READING

Crenshaw C. Preterm premature rupture of the membranes. Symp Clin Obstet Gynecol 1986; 29(4):735–862.
Garite TJ. Premature rupture of the membranes. The enigma of the obstetrician. Am J Obstet Gynecol 1985; 151:1001–1005.
Kitzmiller JL. Preterm premature rupture of the membranes. In: Fuchs F, Stubblefield PG, eds. Preterm birth: causes, prevention and management. New York: Macmillan, 1984:298.
Taylor J, Garite TJ. Premature rupture of membranes before fetal viability. Obstet Gynecol 1984; 64:615–620.

CESAREAN SECTION

EDGAR O. HORGER III, M.D.

Trends in obstetric management have led to a cesarean section rate in the United States of approximately 22 percent. This rate has quadrupled from the 5.5 percent rate reported in 1970 and currently exceeds that reported by other industrialized countries throughout North America, Europe, and the Pacific. Some have argued that the increase in frequency of cesarean section is unimportant because it results in improved perinatal outcomes. However, the high operative rate unquestionably places a greater financial burden on health care resources and leads to increased maternal morbidity and mortality. In many cases, perinatal morbidity also is increased.

REASONS FOR RISING CESAREAN SECTION RATE

Medical and sociologic factors have combined to increase the rate of cesarean section. The risk of surgical mortality has decreased markedly, allowing more operative deliveries with less risk of maternal death. Obstetric management has placed greater emphasis on infant quality and has recognized damage caused by birth trauma and asphyxia. The fear of malpractice allegation has made cesarean delivery a form of defensive medicine. The obstetric patient is commonly older and plans fewer pregnancies. More third-party payment of obstetric and neonatal expenses reduce the need for short hospital confinement. Cesarean sections command higher physician fees than vaginal deliveries. Finally, the accepted indications for cesarean section have broadened greatly. Efforts to curb the rising cesarean birth rate require careful consideration of the indications for cesarean section. Four categories of indication are particularly signficant: dystocia, breech presentation, fetal distress, and repeat cesarean delivery.

Dystocia

The diagnosis of dystocia may be the largest contributor to the increasing cesarean rate. It must be emphasized that the causes of dystocia are multiple, and not all require cesarean delivery. Dystocia may result from inadequate uterine forces, fetal malpresentation, pelvic obstruction, true fetopelvic disproportion, or inappropriate analgesia or anesthesia. In the absence of fetal distress, a diagnosis of dystocia demands an explanation of its cause prior to cesarean section or other efforts at delivery.

Failure to progress is a descriptive term with little value in labor management. More specific assessment of dysfunctional labor may lead to the diagnosis of prolonged latent phase, protracted dilation or descent, or arrested dilation or descent. Prolonged latent phase presents no increased risk to either mother or fetus and does not justify cesarean delivery. Appropriate management may include patient rest and hydration, ambulation, and/or oxytocin. Disorders of the active phase of labor may result from inadequate contractions or some fetopelvic disproportion and may lead to increased perinatal morbidity and mortality. Complete assessment requires internal uterine pressure monitoring and graphic recording of cervical dilation and fetal descent. Findings may suggest management through ambulation, oxytocin, or cesarean section. (For a more complete review, see the chapter on *Dysfunctional Labor.*)

Breech Presentation

Although the incidence of breech presentation in the obstetric population remains constant, there has been a remarkable move in obstetric management to deliver these infants by cesarean section. This change is due to the greater frequency of intrapartum and neonatal complications associated with vaginal delivery of the breech presentation. Retrospective studies have confirmed increased risks of umbilical cord prolapse, head entrapment, and perinatal asphyxia. In addition, those breech presentations delivered vaginally have more intraventricular hemorrhage and neurologic abnormality than those delivered abdominally. However, such retrospective studies may be misleading. In many cases, the choice of vaginal or cesarean delivery may have been based on circumstances additional or peripheral to the fetal presentation. Other retrospective reviews extended over a long time period during which a shift toward more cesarean deliveries was taking place. Those infants born in more recent years—and likely by cesarean section—may have benefited more from advances in neonatal care than from cesarean delivery per se. In other cases, gross underestimation of fetal weight may have led to a laissez faire approach to labor management, thereby preselecting poor outcomes for vaginal breech births.

There is general agreement that the very low birth weight breech infant should be delivered by cesarean section. However, there is considerable disagreement regarding the breech presentation when fetal weight exceeds 1,500 g. Vaginal delivery is appropriate provided the fetal weight falls between 2,500 and 3,800 g, the fetus is in the frank breech presentation, there is no hyperextension of the fetal head, the maternal pelvis is of normal achitecture and dimensions, and the physician is experienced in breech birth. Controversy remains when the fetal weight lies between 1,500 and 2,500 g. Assuming the presence of the other factors mentioned previously, vaginal delivery of these smaller infants should not lead to poor outcomes. Macrosomic fetuses in breech presentation should be delivered by cesarean section.

External version of the breech presentation also should play a role in decreasing the cesarean section rate. In experienced hands, external version is successful in approximately 70 percent of cases, and nearly 90 percent of these infants deliver vaginally (see the chapter on *Breech Presentation*).

Fetal Distress

The increasing diagnosis of fetal distress as an indication for cesarean section bears a close temporal relation to the introduction of electronic fetal monitoring. Although some of these diagnoses may result from earlier and better recognition of fetal jeopardy, misinterpretation of fetal heart rate (FHR) patterns commonly leads to the overdiagnosis of fetal distress. Good FHR patterns are 99 percent accurate in predicting good perinatal outcomes, but poor patterns are only 50 percent accurate in predicting poor outcomes. Fetal scalp pH monitoring offers much greater reliability in the diagnosis of fetal distress and asphyxia. Scalp pH monitoring should be used to clarify confusing FHR patterns, such as those showing late decelerations but good short-term variability or loss of variability but no decelerations. In the preterm fetus, acidosis occurs more rapidly and with less ominous FHR patterns. In all cases of apparent fetal distress, intervention by cesarean delivery must be made before severe asphyxia leads to irreversible sequelae, even though this approach may result in some cesarean sections that retrospectively may appear unnecessary.

Vaginal Birth After Cesarean

Craigin's 1916 advice of "once a section, always a section" has been proven repeatedly to be inappropriate. At least 60 to 70 percent of all patients with previous cesarean section can be offered trial of labor in subsequent pregnancies, and roughly 75 percent of these are able to deliver vaginally. Prerequisites for allowing such trial of labor must include the immediate availability of a physician capable of evaluating labor and performing cesarean section, institutional capability to perform cesarean section within 30 minutes of the first recognition of its need, availability of continuous electronic fetal monitoring and full-time blood banking services, and a physician-patient discussion of trial of labor and decision for its use prior to the onset of labor.

Contraindications to Vaginal Birth After Cesarean. Contraindications to trial of labor include previous classical cesarean scar, more than a single previous cesarean section, multiple pregnancy, and fetal macrosomia. However, many anecdotal reports have confirmed safe vaginal delivery despite the presence of such contraindications, and some individual judgment seems appropriate. There is a much greater risk of uterine rupture during labor with a classical scar, and the frequency of perinatal deaths associated with such uterine ruptures reaches nearly 100 percent. On the other hand, vertical scars in the lower uterine segment do not contraindicate trial of labor. Uterine scar type should be determined prior to labor. However, since the classical cesarean section rate is only about 5 percent, many authorities allow trial of labor when the uterine scar type is unknown. There are only limited data regarding trial of labor after two or more previous cesarean sections. Repeat cesarean delivery of these patients seems appropriate. Multiple pregnancy leads to uterine overdistention, causing attenuation of the uterine scar and rendering it more susceptible to rupture during labor. In addition, manipulation of the second twin during delivery may have some effect on the integrity of the scar. Lastly, the increased frequencies of low birth weight infants and abnormal presentations associated with multiple pregnancy suggest that these pregnancies should not be allowed trial of labor following previous cesarean section. Retrospective reviews of trial of labor with unanticipated fetal macrosomia have shown no greater risk than that encountered with delivery of large infants from unscarred uteri.

Uterine Rupture. Uterine rupture is the potential complication most feared in patients allowed to labor after previous cesarean section, and avoidance of this complication is the major rationale for repeat cesarean section. However, multiple reports of vaginal birth after previous cesarean have shown the incidence of uterine rupture to be only 0.7 percent. Maternal death from ruptured cesarean section scar has not been reported in more than 25 years, and perinatal mortality due to ruptured uterus occurs in 0.93 per 1,000 trials of labor. The risk of rupture during labor is greater following classical cesarean section. Postcesarean febrile morbidity does not influence the risk of uterine rupture during subsequent trial of labor. Although the use of oxytocin after previous cesarean does not of itself pose additional hazard, the likelihood of successful vaginal delivery is decreased and the risk of uterine rupture is increased in patients who require oxytocin treatment of abnormal labor. Uterine scar separation, or dehiscence, is found incidentally in about 2 percent of patients undergoing trial of labor. The incidence of dehiscence following successful vaginal delivery is comparable to that found at elective repeat cesarean section prior to labor. Repair of these asymptomatic defects is unnecessary.

Fetal distress necessitating emergency cesarean section occurs in less than 1 percent of laboring patients with previous cesarean section scars. This rate is comparable to that reported during labor in patients without uterine scars. In addition, fetal distress is the primary indication for approximately 5 percent of cesarean sections done in patients who had planned trial of labor and vaginal delivery, whereas 5 to 12 percent of all primary cesarean sections are done for fetal distress. Fetal distress appears to present no greater problem in patients with previous cesarean section than in those with unscarred uteri.

Perinatal and maternal mortality rates are not increased by trial of labor after previous cesarean section. Elective repeat cesarean section does carry a perinatal loss rate slightly higher than that of vaginal delivery following normal labor at full-term gestation. This increased perinatal loss results primarily from unexpected prematurity, which can be eliminated by awaiting spontaneous labor or by appropriate use of ultrasonography and amniocentesis. No maternal deaths have been reported in a very large trial of labor series.

Acceptance of Trial of Labor. Although 60 to 70 percent of obstetric patients with previous cesarean section scars fulfill the criteria for trial of labor, less than 25 percent of them ultimately undergo trial of labor. Hospitals with fewer than 500 deliveries per year report much less frequent use of trial of labor than hospitals with more than 2,000 deliveries annually. Although some correction of the escalating cesarean section rate can be achieved by trial of labor and avoidance of the self-perpetuating contribution of repeat cesarean section, the lack of acceptance of this philosophy may be blamed on both physician and patient attitudes. The data do show trial of labor to be safe if practiced according to appropriate guidelines. Although some hospitals claim to have inadequate facilities and staff, any hospital that can perform emergency primary cesarean section for other reasons should be able to handle trial of labor. There may remain some reluctance of the physician to abandon the convenience of scheduled repeat cesarean section. Pregnant women with previous uterine scars have been found to base their choices of delivery mode on social motives and previous experiences rather than statistical information about medical risks. Further educational efforts must be directed toward both professional and consumer groups.

REPEAT CESAREAN SECTION

Repeat cesarean section is used for delivery of more than 75 percent of pregnancies in women who previously underwent cesarean section. Premature birth is an unfortunate and unnecessary complication of many elective repeat cesarean sections. Up to 15 percent of intensive care nursery admissions result from elective repeat cesarean delivery of premature infants. Alternatives for prevention of such iatrogenic prematurity include repeating cesarean section only after spontaneous onset of labor and delay of scheduled repeat cesarean section until fetal lung maturity has been confirmed by amniotic fluid studies. Awaiting spontaneous labor for performance of cesarean section does carry additional hazards of anesthesia and major surgery on unprepared patients. In addition, although the risk of labor with a lower segment scar is quite small, this approach offers little reassurance when the previous scar is classical or unknown. Amniotic fluid assessment of fetal pulmonary maturity requires amniocentesis, an invasive procedure that is not entirely without risk. Major fetal trauma or fetal death due to hemorrhage has been reported in up to 1 percent of amniocenteses. Other complications of the procedure include infection, premature rupture of membranes, and premature onset of labor. Although ultrasound guidance has increased the safety of amniocentesis, some risk remains. Consequently, performance of routine amniocentesis prior to every elective repeat cesarean section must be questioned.

The incidence of neonatal respiratory distress syndrome (RDS) varies conversely with gestational age at delivery. In the absence of asphyxia, the incidence of RDS is minimal after 38 weeks' gestation, although development of pulmonary maturity may be delayed in some conditions, such as erythroblastosis fetalis or maternal diabetes mellitus. To avoid RDS, elective repeat cesarean sections should be delayed until completion of the 38th week of pregnancy.

Confirmation that pregnancy has achieved 38 weeks' gestation commonly presents some difficulty. The date of the last menstrual period is the most accurate determinant of gestational age available from history and physical examinations. However, in at least one-fourth of pregnancies, the last menstrual period cannot be recalled. Estimation of uterine size by bimanual examination in the first trimester should be predictive of gestational age to within 2 weeks. Urinary immunologic pregnancy tests rarely become positive before 6 weeks' gestation, and Doppler detection of fetal cardiac activity rarely is possible before 10 weeks. Other clinical parameters, such as uterine growth, first detected fetal movements, and first fetoscope detection of fetal heart tones, are more variable but can provide useful information in determining gestational age and predicting estimated date of confinement.

The wide availability of obstetric ultrasound and documentation of its accuracy in determining gestational age have made it the parameter used most commonly in scheduling elective repeat cesarean sections. Ultrasonographic measurements during the second trimester of pregnancy are of greater statistical reliability in predicting estimated date of confinement than either the last menstrual period or early uterine size. However, toward the end of the second trimester, when more variation in fetal size is encountered and the weekly growth increment is decreasing, ultrasonography loses some reliability as an indicator of gestational age.

Elective repeat cesarean section should be scheduled only after completion of the 38th week of pregnancy. Documentation of this gestational age should be based on the date of last menstrual period, which has been confirmed by certain clinical landmarks: (1) pelvic examination before 10 weeks, (2) positive urine immunologic pregnancy test before 6 weeks, and (3) fetal heart tones heard by fetoscope by 18 weeks. Ultrasound findings also must confirm the date of last menstrual period and may include crown-rump length before 13 weeks or second-trimester measurements. Repeat cesarean section may be scheduled if the last menstrual period is confirmed by at least one clinical landmark and one ultrasonographic study. In the absence of an acceptable menstrual history, two clinical landmarks and one ultrasonographic study must confirm 38 weeks' gestation. In all other cases, amniocentesis and appropriate amniotic fluid phospholipid studies must be used to confirm fetal pulmonary maturity before elective repeat cesarean section is performed.

Maternal Risk

The risk of maternal mortality with cesarean section is at least double and perhaps as much as 11 times greater than that noted with vaginal delivery. Much of the increased mortality rate is related in part to the indication for cesarean section, such as maternal hemorrhage with placenta previa or dehydration and infection following secondary arrest of labor. Maternal deaths generally accompany eight to ten of every 10,000 cesarean sections. The causes of death are similar to those found with other abdominal surgery and include hemorrhage, sepsis, pulmonary embolism, and anesthetic complications.

Infection. The frequency of postpartum complications is much greater following cesarean section than after vaginal delivery, and infection is found quite commonly. Puerperal endometritis occurs 7 to 20 times more often after cesarean section. The incidence of postoperative endometritis varies between 5 and 40 percent and is dependent on many risk factors. Although the most significant factor in postcesarean infections is duration of ruptured membranes, other risk factors include prolonged labor, obesity, anemia, operator inexperience, and socioeconomic deprivation. The use of internal fetal monitoring probably does not contribute to the increased rate of infection, and the role of the number of vaginal examinations during labor is uncertain.

There is a much greater risk of infection following primary cesarean than after repeat cesarean section. The use of prophylactic antibiotics reduces the incidence of postoperative infection by 50 percent in primary cesarean sections, but its value following repeat cesarean sections is less certain. Ampicillin or a first-generation cephalosporin should be given intravenously immediately after clamping of the umbilical cord and continued in a short course of no more than three doses.

Although endometritis is the infection that most commonly complicates postcesarean recovery, infections in the urinary tract and operative wound each occur in 1 to 9 percent of cases.

Blood Transfusion. Blood transfusion may be the second most common complication of cesarean section and has been needed in 2.8 to 7.3 percent of these operations. Although the risks of blood transfusion formerly were measured in terms of cost, blood group isoimmunization, and tranfusion reaction, transmission of infection is now of more concern. Approximately 7 percent of patients receiving blood from volunteer donors develop posttransfusion hepatitis. Although more than 90 percent of these cases are non-A, non-B hepatitis, histologic cirrhosis and serious hepatic impairment ultimately develop in 0.1 percent of transfused patients. All volunteer blood donors are screened for human immunodeficiency virus. However, a lag of 8 to 12 weeks remains between viral infection and positive human immunodeficiency virus testing. The Centers for Disease Control estimates that the chance for contracting acquired immunodeficiency syndrome through a single screened blood transfusion is one per 1,000,000.

Storage of autologous blood for possible later transfusion is gaining popularity and has been endorsed prior to elective surgery by the Committee on Hospital Transfusion Practice of the American Association of Blood Banks and the Council on Scientific Affairs of the American Medical Association. A healthy, nonanemic individual can donate up to one unit per week, and this blood can be stored for 6 weeks. However, autologous blood storage during pregnancy has not gained popularity.

A screen and hold procedure prior to cesarean section seems most appropriate. A blood specimen should be obtained to determine the patient's ABO group, Rh factor, and antibody status. If no antibodies are found, the laboratory should assure the availability of a reasonable quantity of type-specific blood. If intraoperative transfusion becomes necessary, the laboratory should be able to supply blood within minutes. The antibody screen will prove to be positive in 0.7 to 3.5 percent of obstetric patients, and the presence of antibodies requires a complete crossmatch of blood. Complete crossmatch prior to cesarean section also is appropriate in the presence of preoperative anemia, active bleeding, placenta previa, coagulation disorder, or any condition that predisposes to uterine atony.

Perinatal Risk

The risk of perinatal mortality associated with cesarean section relates primarily to gestational age at delivery and indication for cesarean section. Iatrogenic prematurity with elective repeat cesarean section can be avoided by awaiting spontaneous labor at term or by scheduling surgery only after confirmation of completion of 38 weeks' gestation or assurance of fetal lung maturity by amniotic fluid studies. Nonetheless, perinatal morbidity secondary to mild, transient respiratory difficulty does occur more frequently after cesarean section than after vaginal delivery, particularly if the birth weight is below 2,500 g and general anesthesia has been used. The presence of labor before cesarean section has little or no effect on this increased incidence of neonatal respiratory morbidity.

Assessment of the indications for cesarean section independent of gestational age suggests that those infants born after labor dystocia or fetal distress have the greatest need for neonatal resuscitation and the highest incidence of perinatal morbidity. Elective repeat cesarean sections and those done because of breech presentation are more commonly followed by little or no perinatal morbidity.

NEW INDICATIONS FOR CESAREAN SECTION

Efforts to slow the rising incidence of cesarean section are contraindicated by the addition of new indications for operative delivery.

Macrosomia

Cesarean section is performed not uncommonly for suspected fetal macrosomia, both prior to and during labor, independent of intrapartum evidence of fetopelvic disproportion. This policy stems from the likelihood of shoulder dystocia in diabetic pregnancies in which fetal weight is over 4,000 g. Infants of diabetic mothers have different body conformation with larger chest and shoulder dimensions, and it is generally accepted that those exceeding 4,000 g should be delivered by cesarean section. However, the degree of macrosomia that justifies cesarean delivery in the nondiabetic pregnancy is less well defined. Cesarean section does seem appropriate for estimated fetal weight of 4,500 g with no engagement of the presenting part. Engagement of the fetal head deep in the maternal pelvis prior to labor warrants a trial of labor even with an estimated fetal weight of 4,200 to 4,300 g. In addition, the errors inherent in estimation of fetal weight must not be overlooked.

Multiple Gestation

Pregnancies with three or more fetuses large enough to consider viable should be delivered by cesarean section. Abnormal presentation occurs frequently in multiple gestation pregnancies and leads to increased risk of umbilical cord prolapse. Placental separation may follow delivery of one or more infants and lead to asphyxia of undelivered fetuses. However, the presence of twins per se does not indicate a need for cesarean section, especially if both fetuses are in vertex presentation. Nonetheless, labor in twin pregnancy often involves low birth weight infants, and abnormal presentation of one or both fetuses is found in 55 percent of cases. Although there is an increasing tendency to deliver by cesarean section if either twin is in breech presentation, the data fail to show improved outcome from cesarean delivery. Vaginal delivery from frank breech presentation is appropriate if fetal weights are at least 1,500 g and labor progresses without difficulty. The feasibility of external version of the second twin from breech to cephalic presentation after vaginal delivery of twin A has been documented. In addition, prompt cesarean section may be used for twin B after vaginal delivery of twin A if any difficulty is encountered or anticipated in the second vaginal birth.

Very Low Birth Weight

Some reports have suggested improved outcomes by cesarean delivery of all very low birth weight (less than 1,500 g) infants. There is general agreement that the outcome for very low birth weight infants in breech presentation is better after cesarean delivery than after vaginal delivery. However, cesarean delivery of the very low birth weight infant in vertex presentation offers no significant reduction in perinatal morbidity or mortality.

Genital Herpes

Patients with active lesions of genital herpes should be delivered by cesarean section. Although both transplacental and ascending herpetic infections of the fetus can occur, the vast majority of neonatal infections result from inoculation by genital lesions during birth. The risk of infection for an infant born vaginally to a mother with primary genital herpes is about 50 percent, and the risk with active recurrent genital herpes is about 5 percent. Neonatal infection carries a 60 percent mortality rate, and one-half of survivors have neurologic or ocular sequelae.

The presence of genital lesions suspicious for herpes at labor onset or rupture of membranes warrants cesarean delivery, regardless of the duration of ruptured membranes.

Pregnant women with a history of genital herpes ideally should have weekly viral cultures from the cervix and labia beginning at 36 weeks' gestation. Some individualization is necessary in pregnancies at increased risk for premature delivery. If cultures are negative within 1 week of delivery and no new lesions are noted, vaginal delivery is appropriate. There is no justification for cesarean section in women with a history of genital herpes but no active disease and in whom a culture was negative within the preceding week. Furthermore, most authorities argue that there is no justification for cesarean section when no active lesions are present, even if no cultures have been done.

Nongenital herpetic lesions generally do not require cesarean delivery. These lesions can be covered to prevent neonatal contact during delivery.

Immune Thrombocytopenic Purpura

Most pregnancies complicated by immune thrombocytopenic purpura are delivered by cesarean section because of the fear of fetal thrombocytopenia and its attendant risk of intracranial hemorrhage resulting from head trauma during vaginal delivery. However, a large number of these cesarean sections ultimately prove to have been unnecessary. Although transplacental transfer of antiplatelet antibodies may lead to thrombocytopenic infants, most neonatal thrombocytopenia is mild and self-limited. Neonatal platelet counts of 50,000 per mm^3 or greater are not associated with serious bleeding problems, but counts below 50,000 per mm^3 carry significant risk.

Appropriate management of the pregnancy with ITP includes measurement of the fetal platelet count. Fetal blood may be obtained by ultrasonically directed percutaneous umbilical blood sampling prior to labor or scalp blood sampling early in labor. If the count is less than 50,000 per mm^3, cesarean delivery is recommended. If the count exceeds 50,000 per mm^3, vaginal delivery should be anticipated.

Elective Cesarean Section

Prophylactic cesarean section has been suggested for the pregnancy that fails to enter spontaneous labor at full-term gestation. Although quantitative estimates of morbidity, mortality, and cost associated with both cesarean section and vaginal delivery remain uncertain, such elective cesarean sections are unwarranted.

SUGGESTED READING

Danforth DN. Cesarean section. JAMA 1985; 253:811–818.

Flamm BL. Vaginal birth after cesarean section: controversies old and new. Clin Obstet Gynecol 1985; 28:735–744.

Philipson EH, Rosen MG. Trends in the frequency of cesarean births. Clin Obstet Gynecol 1985; 28:691–696.

Read JA. The scheduling of repeat cesarean section operations: prospective management protocol experience. Am J Obstet Gynecol 1985; 151:557–563.

Shiono PH, Fielden JG, McNellis D, et al. Recent trends in cesarean birth and trial of labor rates in the United States. JAMA 1987; 257:494–497.

TOCOLYTIC AGENTS

EROL AMON, M.D.
ROY H. PETRIE, M.D., Sc.D.

CLINICAL PERSPECTIVE

A tocolytic agent is one that can inhibit uterine activity by inducing uterine smooth muscle relaxation. These drugs are used primarily for the inhibition of preterm labor. They are additionally used for obstetric procedures, e.g., external cephalic version and invasive fetal therapy, and they are an important adjunct in the management of obstetric emergencies such as spontaneous or iatrogenic hyperstimulation of uterine smooth muscle with resultant fetal distress.

Historically, a host of agents have been utilized in the management of preterm labor. These include progesterone and its analogues, sedatives, intravenous ethanol, diazoxide, and aminophylline. The drugs commonly in use are the beta-sympathomimetic agents such as ritodrine and terbutaline, intravenous magnesium sulfate and its oral analogues, nonsteroidal anti-inflammatory agents such as indomethacin and aspirin, and intramuscular progesterone. The pharmacologic approach to the inhibition of preterm labor is fundamentally limited by our understanding of the factors that initiate labor. The mechanisms for the initiation and continuation of preterm labor have not yet been clearly elucidated. Research activities have focused primarily on the smooth muscle of the myometrium, with specific attention to the gap junctions between muscle cells, the cellular organization of contractile elements within the smooth muscle cells, beta 1 and 2 receptors, oxytocin receptors, and prostaglandin receptors. The biochemical mechanisms studied include enzymatic phosphorylation and dephosphorylation of myosin light chains, cellular calcium transport, cellular levels of cyclic adenosine monophosphate, and mechanisms involving stimulation and inhibition of adenyl cyclase.

CURRENTLY USED AGENTS

The agent hydroxyprogesterone caproate (Delalutin), a potent progesterone analogue is primarily used as a prophylactic agent because a relative decrease in progesterone to estrogen levels appears to allow for a permissive effect on the onset of labor. Delalutin has its primary use as a prophylactic agent in patients with histories of previous preterm deliveries or previous spontaneous abortion or both. It has also been used in patients with twins and in those with a history of incompetent cervix. The results in these patients have been variable and are considered controversial. Surgical procedures during pregnancy are associated with an increased risk of preterm pregnancy. In these situations the use of Delalutin may be effective. The side effects and possible teratogenic risks of the drug also must be considered. The possibility of hypercalcemia and cholestatic jaundice in the mother exists, although their occurrence is very uncommon. Little is known about the fetal effects, but there is a significant data base and clinical experience that tend to argue against Delalutin as a significant teratogenic agent in the short term. Long-term effects of early prenatal exposure to this agent are virtually unknown. It is likely that we will have to wait for several more years and then to study the relationship of injection of the drug to vaginal and cervical lesions, as was done in women who had been prenatally exposed to diethystilbestrol (DES). We do believe that if one is inclined to use Delalutin, it appears that it can be safely used as a form of prophylaxis in the second and third trimesters of pregnancy.

Magnesium sulfate, in addition to its widespread use in the management of preeclampsia and eclampsia, has been effectively used for the inhibition of uterine activity. Clinical experience with magnesium sulfate as a tocolytic agent has revealed its efficacy primarily in well-selected patients with intact or ruptured fetal membranes, the absence of chorioamnionitis, and cervical dilatation of less than or equal to 1.0 cm. The magnesium cation plays a major role in neuromuscular transmission and contractility of smooth, skeletal, and cardiac muscles. The clinically observed hyporeflexia and hypotonia are due primarily to inhibition of acetylcholine release at the neuromuscular junction. The mechanism of action on smooth and cardiac muscle is less well understood. There appears to be competition with intracellular calcium. This effect may ultimately lead to uterine relaxation. Side effects of this medication include a peripheral vasodilatation seen in most patients. The toxic effects of magnesium sulfate have been clearly demonstrated in patients receiving this medication in toxic doses for management of preeclampsia and eclampsia. These include loss of peripheral reflexes, respiratory arrest, and cardiac arrest. Since magnesium sulfate, like most inorganic ions, is almost 100 percent excreted via the kidneys, knowledge of the patient's creatinine clearance or renal function allows one to safely individualize therapy with this agent. Clinically significant effects of neonatal hypermagnesemia have seldom been demonstrated and should not be of major clinical concern. Most nurseries acquainted with hypermagnesemia in preterm neonates have seldom reported any clinically significant problem associated with intrapartum maternal therapy. Magnesium sulfate is the safest and currently the second most commonly used class of tocolytic agents in the United States.

Beta-sympathomimetic agents are the most widely used tocolytic agents in the world and in the United States. Currently, the most popular drug in this regard is ritodrine. In 1980, it was approved by the Food and Drug Administration (FDA) with a labeled indication for use in the management of preterm labor in well-selected patients. The second most popular beta-sympathomimetic agent in clinical use in the United States is terbutaline, with an unlabeled tocolytic indication. Their molecular resemblence to epinephrine and norepinephrine is striking. These betamimetic agents may be dangerous because of their significant cardiovascular, metabolic, and fluid retention properties. Serious cardiovascular complications have been reported. These include maternal pulmonary edema, myocardial ischemia, cardiac arrhythmia, cerebral vasospasm, and maternal death. The decreases in renal blood flow and glomerular filtration rate in association with avid sodium and water retention predispose the patient to pulmonary edema. Serious metabolic abnormalities that have been reported include lactic acidosis and diabetic ketoacidosis. More common and less significant complications in healthy patients include hyperglycemia and hypokalemia. The absolute medical contraindications to the use of these drugs include New York Heart Association Class II heart disease or greater, active hyperthyroidism, uncontrolled diabetes mellitus, and severe hypertension. Neonatologists have reported the onset of hypoglycemia if the infant is delivered very soon after the mother has been exposed to high doses of beta-sympathomimetic therapy.

Indomethacin and other nonsteroidal anti-inflammatory agents have been shown to be highly effective in inhibiting uterine activity by blocking prostaglandin synthesis—in particular, the inhibition of the cyclooxygenase enzyme. However, there has been considerable concern about a variety of potential adverse neonatal effects, which has limited the use of these agents in the United States. The concerns primarily relate to premature closure of the fetal ductus arteriosus with resultant pulmonary hypertension, heart failure, and fetal death. Additional potential adverse effects include a syndrome of persistent pulmonary hypertension of the newborn, a drop in the glomerular filtration rate, potential hemorrhagic complications probably secondary to inhibition of platelet aggregation and adhesiveness, gastrointestinal complications, and fetal and neonatal central nervous system complications. These potential side effects have most often been cited in isolated uncontrolled case reports, in association with hypoxia, acidosis, and sepsis, and when the agent has been used in pregnancies beyond 34-weeks gestation. It is known that the syndrome of neonatal pulmonary hypertension does occur in the absence of antiprostaglandin administration. There is a growing international data base of uncontrolled trials suggesting that indomethacin and other nonsteroidal anti-inflammatory agents not only are effective but have only minimal human fetal and neonatal side effects. Until further data are available, it is recommended that their use be limited to very preterm gestations and that they be administered only for short courses of less than a few days.

Currently the only drug with a labeled indicated tocolytic use by the FDA is ritodrine. It is important to note that the FDA does not and cannot regulate the practice of medicine but can and does regulate the pharmacologically approved indications for labeling purposes of a variety of drugs. Magnesium sulfate, which is standard prophylactic therapy in severe preeclampsia, has never been approved for such use by the FDA. The FDA recognizes that drugs may be used legitimately when supported by the literature for unlabeled indications. The use of magnesium and other beta-sympathomimetic agents for tocolysis falls into the category of unlabeled indication. We therefore believe in and practice the concept that clinical judgment and patient concern, and not an eye to the FDA or the legal profession, should be the prime driving forces behind medical decisions in difficult clinical situations.

CLINICAL USE

The prime use of tocolytic agents is for the management of preterm or threatened preterm labor. Unfortunately, despite the widespread and increasing use of tocolytic agents during the past 3 decades, the incidence of low birth weight and very low birth weight infants does not appear to have changed appreciably. Fortunately, there has been a decrease in birth weight-specific neonatal mortality as a result of improvements in perinatal care. It is well known that not all preterm labor patients are eligible for tocolysis. Accordingly, tocolytic agents have only limited potential in reducing neonatal mortality. Among normally developed newborns, preterm birth, which is largely nonpreventable (more than 70 percent of cases), represents the single most important cause of neonatal mortality and morbidity. Opinions vary widely about the usefulness of tocolytic agents in the treatment of preterm labor. This difference of opinion relfects not only regional traditional teaching practices but also the quality of scientific evidence available on which to base rational clinical practice. The main problems with these scientific endeavors are related to the following: (1) the inherent placebo effect of any therapy is at least 50 percent effective; (2) most controlled trials have used small sample sizes; (3) there have been major problems in research design related to the diagnosis of actual preterm labor; and (4) the inclusion and exclusion of patients in and out of a study based on differing criteria.

THREATENED AND ACTUAL PRETERM LABOR

Threatened preterm labor is a phenomenon in which there are "frequent" uterine contractions with at least one contraction every 10 minutes, but there is no noted associated cervical change. The diagnosis of actual preterm labor requires the documentation of cervical change.

In order to optimize the efficacy of tocolytic agents for the management of preterm or threatened preterm labor as well as to protect the mother and fetus from serious side effects, a careful individualized evaluation of the status of each pregnancy should be performed. Etiologic factors associated with preterm labor should be sought. A deliberate search is performed for infection, pulmonary maturity, abruptio placentae, a bleeding placenta previa, severe congenital anomalies, intrauterine growth retardation, and rupture of the amniotic membranes. A decreased response to tocolysis occurs with these conditions. A lethal congenital anomaly, frank chorioamnionitis, and significant vaginal bleeding are absolute obstetric contraindications to tocolysis. The presence of pulmonary maturity as a contraindication is a controversial issue, since there are those who feel that the hazards of nonrespiratory problems associated with prematurity outweigh the risks of complications caused by tocolysis. Although tocolysis has been used in patients with the clinical suspicion of a low-grade intrauterine infection, most clinicians feel that this and frank chorioamnionitis represent an absolute contraindication to its use. It should be noted that intra-amniotic infection can be manifested as preterm labor alone; the presence of maternal fever is not necessary for this diagnosis. What is required is amniocentesis followed by a Gram's stain and cultures. In fact, we and others have found culture-proven cases of *Listeria monocytogenes* from the amniotic fluid of patients with preterm labor but without fever. In addition to the identification of pulmonary maturity or intra-amniotic infection and/or colonization by the use of amniocentesis, bloody amniotic fluid that does not subsequently clear can be identified. This finding may be associated with abruptio placentae. In some of these cases, no evidence is found of external vaginal bleeding or uterine tenderness, nor is there ultrasonic evidence of abruptio placentae. Amniocentesis may be efficiently and objectively used to decide whether or not to administer tocolytic agents, steroids, or antibiotics in patients with both intact and ruptured membranes.

If tocolytic agents are utilized in all patients with threatened preterm labor, at least 50 percent will be treated unnecessarily and be subject to significant complications. In these cases our drug regimen of choice is either intravenous magnesium sulfate or subcutaneous terbutaline. This is because both drugs cause minimal untoward effects on the mother and the fetus. These drugs are generally available, their cost is low, there is significant clinical experience with their use, there is general availability of laboratory monitoring of plasma concentration of magnesium during its use, and there is a pharmacologic safety factor to counteract the toxic effects of magnesium in the use of the calcium ion. Furthermore, the effects of hypermagnesemia on the newborn are minor, particularly when personnel involved are thoroughly familiar with the action of this cation on the mother and newborn.

We administer a loading dose of 6 g of magnesium sulfate intravenously as a 10 percent solution over 20 to 30 minutes. Subsequently an infusion rate is continued at 2 g per hour, and the dose is titrated against uterine activity and serial blood levels. If these patients are well selected, one can expect an efficacy rate of higher than 90 percent. After uterine contractility has decreased in frequency to less than one contraction in every 10 minutes, the infusion is continued for another 6 to 24 hours and the patient is placed on magnesium therapy per mouth in the form of either the oxide, gluconate, peroxide, or aspartate salt. If these are not available, the practitioner may place the patient on an oral beta-sympathomimetic agent such as ritodrine or terbutaline. Another option is the use of no oral prophylactic therapy, since it has never been conclusively proved that subsequent oral prophylaxis with any class of agents is effective. Magnesium levels should be less than 8 mEq per liter during intravenous therapy. The urine output should be adequate. Oral therapy may be continued until the patient has reached 36- to 37-weeks gestation.

We administer subcutaneous terbutaline according to the following protocol. First absolute and relative contraindications to this beta-sympathomimetic agent are deliberately searched for. If it is deemed safe to use this agent and the patient is in threatened preterm labor, 0.25 mg is administered subcutaneously and repeated every 20 to 30 minutes for up to three doses as long as the maternal pulse does not rise above 120 beats per minute and uterine activity remains unabated. If this treatment significantly diminishes uterine activity, then the patient is placed on oral terbutaline in a dosage of 2.5 to 5 mg every 4 to 6 hours. If uterine activity remains unabated after three doses of subcutaneous terbutaline and the maternal cardiac status does not contraindicate continued use, the patient is placed on intravenous terbutaline therapy. One should note that this situation is an unusual occurrence in the presence of threatened preterm labor.

Some authorities feel one can safely await evidence of cervical change by the same examiner before tocolytic therapy is instituted despite the widely held belief that earlier treatment is more effective. This belief does not seem to hold true, however, if the cervix is long and closed versus being 1 cm dilated and 50 percent effaced. Efficacy appears to be diminished when cervical dilatation is greater than or equal to 2 cm or effacement greater than 50 percent. In the situation of actual preterm labor, i.e., with documented cervical change by the same examiner, if there are no contraindications one may use intravenous ritodrine therapy as described in the package insert of the *Physicians' Desk Reference* or intravenous terbutaline. Even though cervical change may have been demonstrated, it is still our preference to utilize intravenous magnesium sulfate or subcutaneous terbutaline, since they appear to be much safer and to be just as effective.

There are times when one or the other drug is not effective. If the clinical situation does not contraindicate continued use, then combination dual agent therapy with magnesium sulfate and a beta-sympathomimetic may be used. In any situation in which therapy with these agents is undertaken, a careful watch of maternal fluid status is required. An intravenous fluid rate of no greater than 70 ml per hour of a solution of no greater than 0.45 percent saline is recommended to aid in the prevention of pulmonary edema. Special concern regarding this complication is emphasized in patients with multiple gestation, polyhydramnios, decreased creatinine clearance, and maternal anemia and tachycardia prior to treatment. Note that parenteral tocolytic agents commonly cause a hemodilution manifested in a drop in maternal hematocrit values. In most of these situations blood transfusions ordinarily should be avoided. The use of a beta-sympathomimetic agent with fluid restriction is associated with ketonuria due to caloric reduction lipolysis. This is a side effect of treatment and should not be treated reflexively by increasing the rate of intravenous fluids. It is unclear whether this acute form of ketonuria requires treatment. However, if this ketosis is treated, the caloric quality of fluid or oral intake should be increased. In healthy patients a plasma glucose level of less than 200 mg per deciliter or hypokalemia of greater than 2.0 mEq per liter does not ordinarily require treatment, and these acute metabolic effects will resolve spontaneously. A pregnant woman on continued terbutaline therapy should be screened for drug-induced glucose intolerance and treated appropriately.

The rupture of fetal membranes concomitant with preterm labor is a common occurrence. The use of tocolysis in these instances is widely debated. It is our opinion that a tocolytic agent may be used only in selected cases in which there is a demonstrated absence of infection and/or colonization, an absence of pulmonary maturity, and no signs of fetal distress. Employment of amniocentesis is pivital in this form of management. The use of steroids to accelerate pulmonary maturity when there are ruptured fetal membranes is controversial. If there are no absolute contraindications and uterine activity can be safely inhibited with tocolysis, then one may employ a short course of tocolytic therapy in order to gain 24 to 48 hours for the use of steroids to induce pulmonary maturation. If a patient presents in advanced preterm labor (i.e., greater than 4 cm cervical dilatation) without contraindications to a delay in delivery, then the use of a short intensive course of tocolytic agents for 24 to 48 hours may be indicated if one believes in the usefulness of steroid therapy.

PRETERM LABOR PROPHYLAXIS

Tocolysis has been advocated by many clinicians as well as investigators for prophylaxis. Indications have included patients at high risk for preterm delivery with a history of preterm birth, the presence of multiple gestation, maternal surgery such as cervical cerclage, appendectomy, or ovarian cystectomy during pregnancy, or placental abnormalities such as a placenta previa. There appears to be no strong evidence that prophylactic treatment is of any benefit. In fact, prophylaxis may desensitize and down-regulate the hormonal receptors to such a degree that if actual therapy is needed, the agents may then prove *less* effective. Despite the lack of proof and the potential for side effects, the use of prophylaxis in these cases is recommended by some investigators. Most clinicians will use a short course of parenteral prophylactic tocolysis in the perioperative period of surgery. The use of tocolysis in a patient with bleeding placenta previa is controversial. Some will use it in order to arrest uterine activity and thereby diminish bleeding. Others feel this form of therapy is contraindicated.

OBSTETRIC PROCEDURES

With regard to intrauterine manipulation, a bolus administration of beta-sympathomimetic agent or intravenous magnesium sulfate is quite useful. Antepartum external cephalic version as well as intrapartum external version are certainly more successful in patients in whom the uterus is well relaxed. Fetal therapy such as placement of bladder shunts and intravascular or intraperitoneal transfusions is aided by the use of uterine relaxation. Contractions occurring during chorionic villus sampling can be ameliorated with the use of tocolytic agents, thereby aiding proper catheter placement. Acute tocolysis also can be useful at the time of cesarean section. It is not uncommon for the uterus to contract tightly around the head of a premature breech presentation at the time of cesarean section or to contract around the second twin after delivery of the first at cesarean section. In these instances, a bolus of a tocolytic agent may be useful. Furthermore, by inducing uterine relaxation acute tocolysis can assist the operator in the performance of a low transverse cervical incision rather than a vertical or classic incision. One may inject 0.125 to 0.250 mg of terbutaline or 2 to 3 mg of ritodrine intravenously slowly within 30 seconds to 1 minute or 4 to 6 g of a 10 percent solution of magnesium sulfate over 15 to 20 minutes to attain acute uterine relaxation. With this method we have safely performed intra-abdominal external cephalic version at the time of cesarean section in order to deliver the fetus as a vertex and through a low transverse incision. Careful selection of these patients is mandatory. At the time of vaginal delivery, an internal version can be dramatically assisted by the use of uterine relaxation without having to put the patient to sleep. Likewise, external version for a second malpresenting twin is facilitated by the use of tocolysis. It has been reported that uterine inversion can be successfully treated with the aid of tocolytic therapy. A postpartum constriction ring can form at the junction of the lower and upper uterine segments and can be a major cause of retained placenta. The need for general anesthesia can be obviated by the use of a bolus of tocolytic agent. We have managed a few such patients successfully and none unsuccessfully.

OBSTETRIC EMERGENCIES

With regard to the management of labor, the use of tocolysis can be of benefit in the acute assessment of the pregnancy. In these cases it is of utmost importance to watch closely for contraindications to these drugs prior to their use. If there is fetal distress secondary to a cord prolapse, tocolysis may be an important temporizing procedure as preparation for cesarean section is being made. Likewise if there is an occult prolapse, as manifested by severe variable decelerations, uterine relaxation may be obtained through tocolysis as preparations for cesarean section are made. If there are excess spontaneous contractions of uterine activity induced by oxytocin or prostaglandin, they may be effectively diminished with tocolytic therapy. Fetal hypoxia of any cause is generally made worse when there are associated uterine contractions. The frequency and intensity of uterine contractions may be reduced with a tocolytic agent for intrauterine resuscitation. Subsequently additional labor or cesarean section may be warranted.

MATERNAL TRANSPORT

The final indication for tocolytic therapy is with maternal transport to a tertiary level perinatal center. During maternal transport, a dose of 0.25 mg of subcutaneous terbutaline is safe and may be effective if the patient has no absolute medical contraindication. Intravenous magnesium sulfate or intravenous beta-sympathomimetic therapy should be used with caution in these situations. An intravenous pump and personnel experienced in its use are prerequisites to the use of these intravenous drugs. Another alternative to subcutaneous terbutaline is use of intramuscular magnesium for maternal transport.

SUGGESTED READING

Beard RW, Sharp F, eds. Preterm labor and its consequences. London: Proceedings of the Thirteenth Study Group of the Royal College of Obstetricians and Gynaecologists, 1985.

Fuchs F, Stubblefield PG, eds. Preterm birth—causes, prevention and management. New York: Macmillan, 1984.

Hollander DI, Nagey DA, Pupkin MJ. Magnesium sulfate and ritodrine hydrochloride. A randomized comparison. Am J Obstet Gynecol 1987; 156:631–637.

Petrie R. Tocolysis using magnesium sulfate. Semin Perinatol 1981; 5:266–273.

PREMATURE LABOR

J. PATRICK LAVERY, M.D.

The birth of a premature infant is associated with increased hardship, expense, and potentially compromised quality of life. Despite monumental strides in increasing survival rates and improving well-being over the last decade, preterm birth still accounts for 65 to 75 percent of all perinatal deaths occurring in the United States. To achieve improvement in this aspect of perinatal mortality, a thorough appreciation of labor and the factors that lead to preterm birth is critical in order for techniques of prevention to be employed. This chapter reviews the physiology of labor, the clinical aspects and associations of preterm birth, and the components of preterm birth prevention programs now being implemented throughout the United States. Specific labor inhibition techniques and uterine tocolysis are addressed in other chapters.

DEFINITION

The first World Health Assembly in 1948 defined an immature infant as one with a birth weight less than 5.5 lb (2,500 g). In records in which weights were not specified, a gestational age of less than 37 weeks was considered the equivalent. This set of definitions was adopted by the World Health Organization. This definition was reaffirmed in 1950, but limitations were appreciated, particularly in the case of the low birth weight baby who was affected by intrauterine growth retardation. Finally, in 1961, the World Health Organization Expert Committee on Maternal and Child Health recommended that the word "premature" be reserved for infants of less than 37-weeks gestational age and that the "low birth weight" infants be classified as either the *low* birth weight infant (37 weeks or longer, birth weight 2,400 g or less) or the *premature low* birth weight infant (37 weeks or less, birth weight 2,500 g or less).

This classification is useful in delineating populations suffering from intrauterine growth retardation versus pure prematurity, but some ambiguities still persist. Approximately one-third of all infants weighing less than 2,500 g suffer from intrauterine growth retardation due to maternal, placental, or primary fetal factors that interfered with normal development. This distinction is critical in terms of prognosis. The outcome, both in terms of survival and morbidity, is determined by the particular etiology of the low birth weight.

The overall preterm birth rate varies depending upon factors such as institution, population group, level of care, and socioeconomic status. In the United States, the preterm birth rate is between 5 and 10 percent. Despite all efforts to date, this rate in the United States has not declined more than 1 percent in the last 12 to 15 years. We have seen a dramatic reduction in perinatal mortality, but this improvement has been the result primarily of advances in newborn care rather than in obstetric intervention.

PERINATAL MORTALITY

Since perinatal survival prospects are in large part related to successful neonatal management, awareness of the prognosis for perinatal survival at given gestational ages is necessary to make appropriate obstetric management decisions. Knowledge of survival rates in one's own hospital or referral center is critical to such deliberations. Table 1 lists general survival rates for preterm infants born in tertiary care centers by gestational age. These figures were derived from data generated in the mid-1980s. Not only have mortality rates decreased, but long-term morbidity (including neurologic sequelae) due to prematurity is only in the 15 to 20 percent range at present. This complication rate is much lower than that reported in the 1960s and 1970s, demonstrating the effectiveness of concerted efforts toward achieving good perinatal outcome. Uncertain or mistaken estimates of gestational age or erroneous presumptions of nonsurvivability may lead to obstetric decisions that can jeopardize an optimal prognosis. Decisions of crucial significance are, of course, those related to technique of delivery, location of delivery, or availability of neonatal resources.

TABLE 1 Perinatal Survival for Premature Infants Born in Tertiary Care Centers; Data from 1985

24–26 weeks	0–25%
26–28 weeks	50–75%
28–30 weeks	75–88%
30–32 weeks	88–95%
32–34 weeks	95–98%
34–36 weeks	>98%
>36 weeks	>99%

Early establishment and clinical appreciation of true gestational age are essential for achieving optimal outcome. Not only is perinatal outcome improved with accurate gestational dating, but other pitfalls of management can be avoided. Clinicians tend to underestimate the survival rates of premature infants, particularly in the 26- to 30-week range. This is perhaps due to the rapid development of new technology in this area of neonatology. An appreciation of therapeutic modalities such as extracorporeal membrane oxygenation, for instance, is not always evident in areas remote from metropolitan tertiary centers. Secondly, estimates of gestational age and weight may be in error, particularly if early care was not obtained or ultrasonography not performed before 16 weeks, the time frame of greatest reliability for gestational age calculation (Table 2).

The most common causes of mortality in preterm but appropriately grown (AGA) infants are related to extreme immaturity, respiratory distress, intraventricular hemorrhage, and infections. Congenital malformations and other factors are also involved but have a less prominent role. The small for gestational age infant (SGA), stunted by the environment, who is born preterm faces the greatest survival risks from extreme prematurity, infection, and necrotizing enterocolitis, followed by other conditions, particularly congenital malformations. The SGA infant, however, who is born functionally mature and who does not suffer from acute asphyxia or a traumatic delivery has an excellent developmental prognosis. Although he is apt to lag behind his AGA peers in growth, this will not impair his cognitive development. Problems such as chronic infection or a genetic abnormality, of course, will render the prognosis somewhat more guarded for the growth-retarded infant than for the AGA neonate. Because of the association of SGA infants and malformations, it is imperative to perform an ultrasound evaluation of any fetus who presents in premature labor. The information obtained can be an important aid to management decisions. Further, in cases of inhibited preterm labor in which a congenital malformation is identified that has an association with chromosomal abnormalities (e.g., omphalocele or ventricular septal defect), consideration should be given to the performance of an amniocentesis or cordocentesis for karyotyping.

TABLE 2 Reliability of Ultrasonography in Assessing Gestational Age

Gestational sac	± 1 week
Crown rump	± 1 week
Biparietal diameter <20 weeks	± 1 week
Biparietal diameter 24–30 weeks	± 2 weeks
Biparietal diameter >30 weeks	± 3 weeks
Abdominal circumference	24–30 weeks ± 2 weeks
	>30 weeks ± 3 weeks
Femur length	24–30 weeks ± 2 weeks
	30–42 weeks ± 3 weeks

PHYSIOLOGY OF LABOR

The onset of parturition is the result of a complex interplay of fetal and maternal factors. It is well studied in the sheep, in which the fetus initiates the sequence of labor through its pituitary-adrenal axis. An elevation in cortisol, at least in this species, is the most important factor influencing steroidogenesis in the placenta. This steroid surge initiates the biochemical process leading to the increased production of prostaglandins, particularly from precursors stored in the chorion and amnion, and concomitantly changes the sensitivity of the uterine musculature to make it more responsive to uterotonic stimuli such as oxytocin.

In the human, the fetal pituitary-adrenal axis is less important, and attempts to correlate the animal model have been thwarted because decreases in peripheral progesterone toward term have not been consistently appreciated. In human studies related to endocrine changes with term and preterm labor, steroid measurements have failed to predict its onset. Other factors of fetal origin may play critical roles in labor initiation.

Despite the identification of myriad hormonal factors involved in the onset of labor, approximately only one-third of patients clinically presenting in preterm labor can be considered to have idiopathic premature labor and thus be possibly suspect for abnormal endocrine events. Other definable and sometimes preventable factors exist that can predispose a gravida to the early onset of labor.

Based on studies of sheep and associated investigations in humans, the onset of labor suggests that the initiating mechanism comes from a fetal stimulus. In sheep this change in the hormonal environment in the fetal-placental unit leading to labor occurs over a 10-day period (gestation), whereas in humans similar events occur over a 5- to 6-week period (Fig. 1).

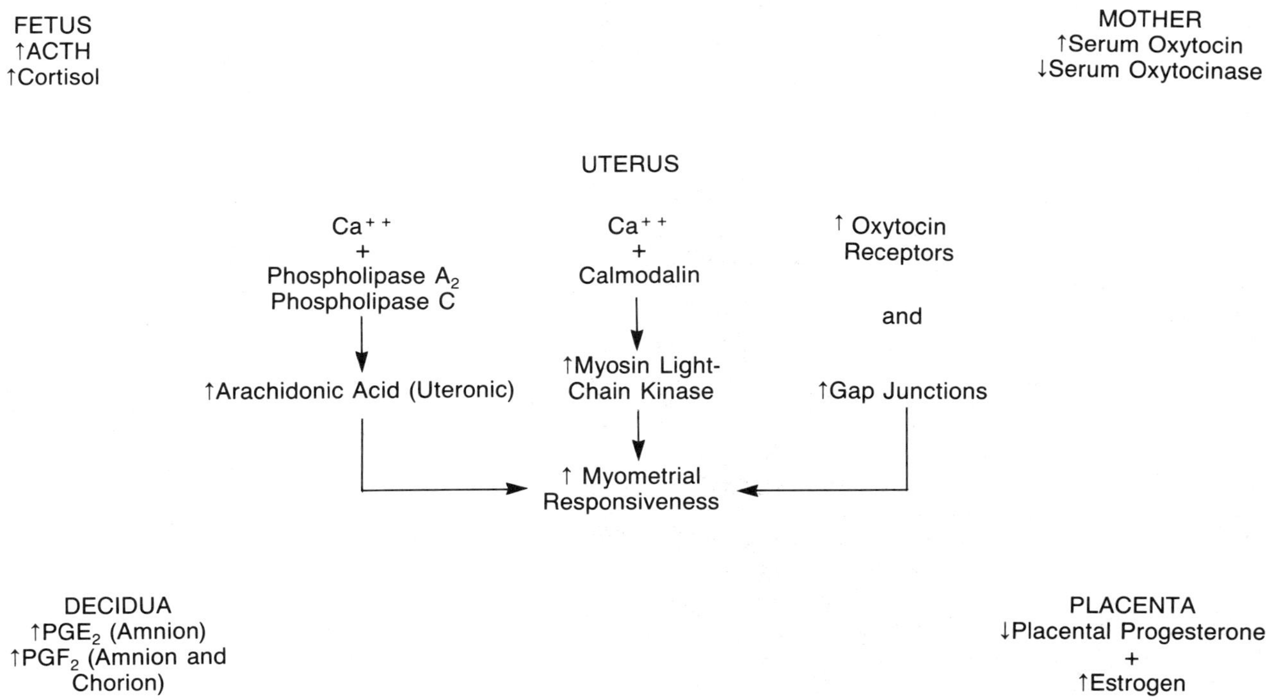

Figure 1 Biochemical factors occurring in the initiation of labor.

As term approaches in the human, the uterus becomes more sensitive to endogenous as well as exogenous oxytocin. As the number of receptors to this octapeptide increases, uterine contractions are more frequent and ultimately more intense. Uterine activity, i.e., measurable contractions, takes place in the uterus from the second trimester. Usually this contractile activity is without consequence and hardly appreciated by the pregnant woman. As term approaches, the frequency and intensity of these contractions increase. As long as contractions occur less frequently than six per hour, cervical changes are unlikely. An increasing estriol to progesterone ratio appears to occur toward term as well as in some cases of preterm labor. Relatively higher estriol levels are found and increased progesterone metabolism occurs most likely secondary to adrenal steroid stimulation, with the result that the uterus is more sensitive to the effects of oxytocin. An increase in uterine gap junctions (anatomic structures important in the synchronization of uterine contractions) and in the number of myometrial oxytocin receptors has been found in a majority of women in term labor and in some during preterm labor. The uterus, which has been stabilized by a high progesterone environment, now is becoming more sensitive to external uterotonic factors (oxytocin), is more capable of synchronous and efficient contractile activity (more gap junctions), and is in an environment with a higher concentration of primary uterotonic agents (prostaglandins). These prostaglandin metabolites have also been found to be elevated in amniotic fluid in the presence of preterm and term labor. Whether this is in response to a primary stimulus or the sequential result of uterine activity is unclear.

Observations made by several investigators raise the issue of multiple causation for preterm birth, an interplay of varied factors not restricted to maternal or fetal origin alone. Thus it follows that the approach to preventing prematurity must also be multifactorial and interdisciplinary. In the clinical setting, different therapeutic regimens have evolved. Attempts at intervention may take the form of trying to block specific steps in the endocrine cascade such as the use of (1) ritodrine to inhibit cyclic adenosine monophosphate and decrease light-chain myosin kinase activity, (2) magnesium sulfate to inhibit free Ca^{++} and thus decrease myometrial activity, (3) alcohol to decrease oxytocin output, or (4) prostaglandin antagonists to decrease prostaglandin production.

However, since only a minority of preterm births actually occur because of pure premature labor, such approaches at tocolysis will not solve the problem of premature birth. Based on several studies, we now know that approximately one-third of preterm births occur because of premature membrane rupture (see the chapter *Planned Prenatal Care: Key to the Future*); one-third because of medical exigencies, either fetal or maternal (e.g., diabetes, hypertension, third trimester hemorrhage); and only one-third because of a prematurely triggered labor process itself. Even though there naturally is some crossover between these three categories, this separation by causality places the prematurity problem into a clinically appropriate and useful perspective.

There are many classifications of risk factors associated with prematurity. Table 3 offers one such categorization that should be reviewed in any obstetric patient to classify her potential risk of preterm birth. Aspects of each category will be reviewed. Their relative significance will of course vary in differing clinical settings.

Maternal factors include the demographic risks of age (<17 or >35 years), low socioeconomic status, unmarried status, low level of education, race (particularly black), short stature, low prepregnancy weight (<50 kg), poor obstetric history, and multiple abortions (particularly if induced and especially if second trimester losses). Relative progesterone deficiency usually associated with habitual abortion is also a possible factor suggested by subsequent preterm birth after initial first trimester therapy. Maternal medical disorders such as diabetes, acute or chronic hypertension, and systemic diseases of a renal or collagen vascular nature would also be included. Their better management should allow for an extension of the pregnancy and the avoidance of preterm birth. In general, the more severe the condition, the more likely the occurrence of preterm birth, either from spontaneous labor or from medical necessity. Events such as first trimester bleeding, previous pregnancies with preterm births, or closely spaced (<1 year) pregnancies also would be factors. Indeed, the occurrence of a preterm birth is the single most significant historical risk factor related to subsequent preterm birth. Other areas of investigation include psychological stress and occupational fatigue. These areas are difficult to quantitate, but associations have been made correlating extremes of such situations with preterm birth.

Fetal factors would include multiple gestation, congenital anomalies, and genetic disorders placing the infant at high risk such as osteogenesis imperfecta. Genetic problems such as trisomy 13 and 18 are associated with the birth of an infant suffering from growth retardation and, not infrequently, preterm delivery. With multiple gestation, decreased physical activity with bed rest beginning at 26 weeks has shown some association with extended pregnancy. Prophylactic oral tocolytics and cervical cerclage have not met with any success.

Placental factors such as placenta previa and abruption often lead to preterm delivery because of associated maternal hemorrhage. First trimester bleeding is likewise associated with early delivery. Although as many as 40 percent of all pregnancies have some early bleeding, the majority continue and do not end in abortion. However, the risk of preterm birth in this population is nearly twice that of normal gravidas, and the occurrence of growth retardation is likewise increased. Early identification of placentas covering the cervix should be followed up by ultrasonography at 30 to 34 weeks. It is only then that the diagnosis of a previa can truly be made. Anatomic abnormalities such as circumvallate placenta and marginal and velamentous placental insertions are also seen with greater frequency in preterm births. Unfortunately, such anatomic variations (occurring in about 1 percent each of all pregnancies) are not predictable and cannot be consistently diagnosed antenatally.

Uterocervical factors include uterine abnormalities, both congenital (such as a uterus didelphys) and acquired (such as leiomyomas). Cervical incompetence must be

TABLE 3 Factors Associated with Preterm Birth

Maternal Factors	Age (<17 or >35)
	Socioeconomic status
	Marital status
	Short stature
	Low prepregnancy weight
	First trimester bleeding
	Stress
	Poor obstetric history
	Race
	Low level education
	Insufficient corpus luteum
	Medical diseases
	Previous preterm birth
	Work
Fetal Factors	Multiple gestation
	Congenital anomalies
	Genetic disorders
Placental Factors	Placenta previa
	Abruptio placentae
	First trimester bleeding
	Circumvallate placenta
	Marginal cord insertion
Uterocervical Factors	Uterine malformations
	Cervical incompetence
	Leiomyomata uteri
Infectious Factors	Urinary tract infections
	Cervicitis vaginitis
	Premature membrane rupture
	Phospholipase release by local organisms
Environmental Factors	Height above sea level
	Stress
	Substance abuse
	Strenuous physical activity
Nutritional Factors	Poor pregnancy weight
	Closely spaced pregnancies
	Weight loss efforts
	Significant malnutrition
	Fad diets
Iatrogenic Factors	Inappropriate inductions/repeat cesarean sections
	Misjudged gestational age

considered: it may be congenital, as associated with diethylstilbestrol exposure; traumatic, as after multiple dilation and curettage procedures or induced abortions, especially second trimester terminations; or functional, as associated with increased second and early third trimester uterine activity (see chapter *Fetal Heart Rate Monitoring*). After the delivery of a preterm infant, particularly a spontaneous second trimester loss, a hysterosalpingogram might be warranted as well as hysteroscopy. Uterine septae are recognizable on ultrasound examination and may afford the clinician insight into subsequent pregnancy management. Early cervical dilation of the internal os has been identified by ultrasonography, and this diagnostic technique can be employed to assist in the management of patients at such risk (Fig. 2).

Infectious conditions have long been associated with preterm birth, the most notable association being with urinary tract infections and pyelonephritis (see chapter *Urinary Tract Infection*). Classically the presence of organisms in the urinary tract, most commonly *Escherichia coli*, has

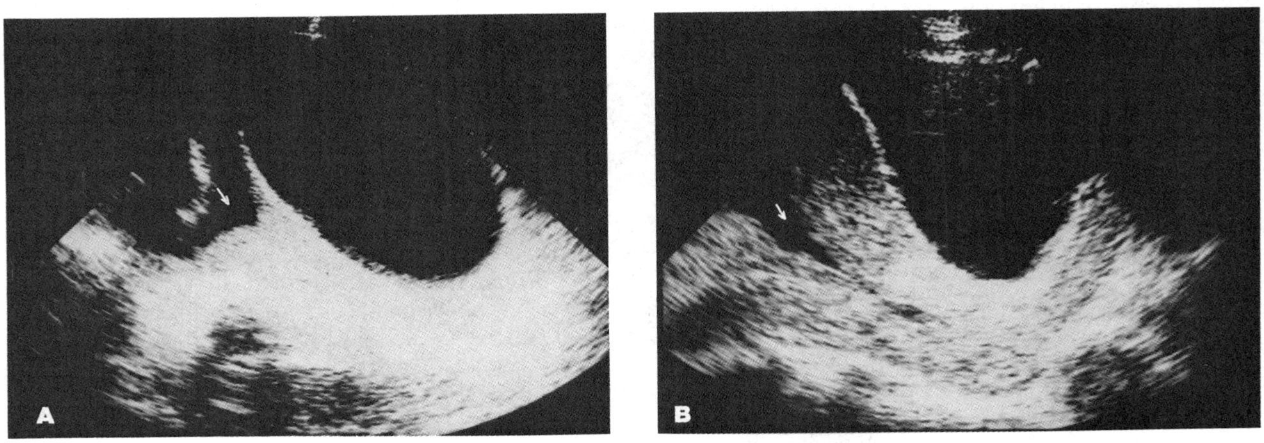

Figure 2 Sonographic view of lower uterine segment and cervix. *A*, Internal os closed (arrow); *B*, internal os open (arrow).

been associated with preterm labor whether the condition was symptomatic or not. The high frequency of asymptomatic urinary tract infection (5 to 10 percent) makes this a possible diagnosis that should be ruled out in all cases of preterm labor. A greater concern is now developing in regard to cervicovaginal infection, as some pathogens have been found capable of initiating the prostaglandin cascade and leading to increased uterine activity (see chapter *Bacterial Vaginosis in Pregnancy).* Cervical infection may likewise have an association with premature membrane rupture. Localized weakness of the membranes due to any cause may contribute to preterm birth, particularly after the 28th week when the membranes are under greater stress.

The exact role of infection, vaginal or systemic, in stimulating preterm labor is not clear, but implications and clinical associations are strong. The presence of several pathogenic organisms has been associated with preterm labor. These would include group B streptococci, herpes simplex primary infections, *Chlamydia trachomatis, Mycoplasma* spp. and, in some studies, *Neisseria gonorrhoeae*. Several organisms are capable of releasing phospholipase A_2 (Table 4), an enzyme critical in the prostaglandin cascade to producing uterine contractions.

In older studies employing antibiotic prophylaxis for urinary tract infections (specifically with tetracycline, which is now contraindicated in pregnancy) and more recent work with erythromycin, lower rates of preterm birth have occurred in the treated populations when drug administration occurred early in the third trimester. The basis for the impact of such success remains speculative.

Premature rupture of the membranes precedes approximately one-third of all preterm births. The exact etiology of premature rupture is unclear, but most of the literature suggests localized factors in the membranes as predisposing to this event. An inflammatory process or one of localized uterine activity could theoretically predispose the membranes to rupture. Thus multiple organisms, if capable of penetrating the endocervical canal, would have two possible mechanisms of promoting preterm delivery, namely, local irritation and membrane weakness as well as biochemical stimulation of uterine activity.

Environmental factors leading to preterm birth include those related to birth location above sea level (more premature infants are being born at altitudes of more than 5,000 feet above sea level); work habits; social habits such as smoking and alcohol consumption and other substance abuse; and stress—both physical and psychosocial. It is difficult to quantitate these risk factors, but some data on athletes in training have suggested that when pulse rates become excessive (>120 to 140 beats per minute), uterine blood flow is compromised and the fetus may suffer. Decreased blood flow, either from decreased cardiac output or from endogenous vasoconstriction, may also lead to increased uterine irritability.

Nutritional factors such as poor diet leading to anemia, poor fetal growth, inadequate plasma volume expansion, and inappropriate food substitutes (e.g., alcohol and drugs) both directly and indirectly contribute to preterm birth (see chapter *Nutrition in Pregnancy).* Low prepregnancy weight (i.e., less than 50 kg) is not infrequently associated with low birth weight babies, particularly when related to inadequate dietary intake. Fad diets and weight loss during pregnancy may pose problems for fetal development. Appropriate supplementation is of valuė, as is counseling against closely spaced pregnancies that create a greater nutritional drain.

Finally, iatrogenic factors can play a role in preterm birth. Scheduled cesarean sections or inductions have led to prematurity complications in as many as 15 percent of elective births. Liberal use of ultrasound examination for early pregnancy dating when performed before 20 weeks is best for most accurate assessment of gestational age. Later in pregnancy, with amniocentesis to determine pulmonary maturity (lecithin-sphingomyelin ratio >2 and presence of phosphatidylglycerol), unexpected preterm birth should not occur (see chapter *Respiratory Diseases*). The Food and Drug Administration's prohibition of the use of oxytocin for "elective" induction has contributed to the reduction of this cause of preterm birth.

Although it is important to have a thorough understanding of risk factors associated with preterm birth, one must remember that only two-thirds of all preterm births have any such associated factors. Therefore the clinician must be ever alert to the signs and symptoms of preterm birth even in low-risk patients.

TABLE 4 Organisms Associated with Phospholipase A_2 Activity

*High**	*Some*
Bacteroides fragilis	*Streptococcus faecalis*
Peptostreptococcus	*Escherichia coli*
Fusobacterium	*Staphylococcus epidermidis*
Streptococcus viridans	Pneumococcus
	Streptococcus groups A and B
	Lactobacillus
	Mycoplasma hominis

* Higher production of phospholipase A_2 activity than seen in membranes.

DIAGNOSIS OF PRETERM LABOR

The diagnosis of preterm labor is often difficult. Uterine activity increases progressively after 14-weeks gestational age, and women's appreciation of uterine activity varies. Subtle symptoms of preterm labor (Table 5), including low backache, especially if rhythmic, menstrual cramps, pelvic pressure, and change in character of vaginal discharge, are all nonspecific. However, close attention to and questions regarding possible changes in the character of these symptoms must be sought.

The difficulty of establishing the diagnosis of preterm labor is reflected in studies with tocolytic agents in which success in control and placebo populations may reach 40 to 60 percent. More objective criteria for preterm labor would include:

1. appreciable cervical change noted by a single examiner,
2. cervical dilatation of 2 cm or greater prior to term,

TABLE 5 Preterm Labor Symptoms

Mild menstrual cramps
Pelvic pressure
Low backache or change in symptoms
Increased vaginal discharge, particularly if blood-stained or mucoid
Rhythmic contractions of more than six per hour

3. cervical effacement of 80 percent or greater prior to term,
4. uterine contractions (palpable or detected by monitor) of four or more every 20 minutes.

If any or several of these findings are present, the diagnosis can be made and appropriate treatment initiated. In all cases, causative factors should be sought (e.g., urinary tract infections) and appropriately treated.

A new clinical association has been detected by close observation of fetuses on ultrasonography. Fetal breathing movements, i.e., the presence of sustained diaphragmatic movements for 20 seconds or more, constitute active breathing. In cases of intact membranes without chorioamnionitis, the absence of fetal breathing has been correlated with continued preterm labor and delivery. In some studies the presence of fetal breathing was associated with 85 percent success in labor inhibition, suggesting some other etiology for the uterine contractions.

In cases of continued preterm labor and intact membranes that are unresponsive to tocolytic therapy over a prolonged period (>24 hours), consideration should be given to amniocentesis to assess for possible chorioamnionitis (white blood cell count, Gram's stain, presence of bacteria on unspun specimen, and culture). Maturity studies (lecithin-sphingomyelin ratio, phosphatidylglycerol) should also be performed on the fluid taken.

PRETERM DELIVERY PREVENTION

The acute management of preterm labor is covered in the chapter *Tocolytic Agents*. The use of tocolytic therapy, while efficacious in a majority of candidates, is applicable in only a minority of all patients who deliver premature infants. For that reason primary efforts at preterm labor prevention have concentrated on population risk assessment and patient education. Early symptoms of preterm labor are not specific and require sensitive questioning and thorough patient education.

Early detection programs have been initiated around the United States and are meeting with varying degrees of success. In addition to patient education, increased frequency of visits for at-risk populations is warranted. Nearly two-thirds of all preterm births will occur in high-risk groups. However, since the corollary of this is the fact that the other third of all preterm births occur among the low-risk population, all patients must be educated in prematurity prevention, perhaps at a lesser degree of intensity.

Frequent and in some cases weekly cervical examinations without penetration into the endocervical canal form a critical component of many preterm labor prevention programs. Early cervical dilatation, i.e., 1 to 2 cm at less than 32 weeks, has been associated with a nearly threefold higher rate of preterm birth than is found in comparable patients in whom no dilatation has taken place. The use of tocographic techniques, either in hospital settings, in clinic facilities, or by home monitoring (Term Guard), has been recommended to promote early detection of uterine activity.

The application of such intense programs (Table 6) has met with success in general obstetric populations and particularly in the largest such program in Haguenau, France. However, reservation has been voiced about its potential success in extremely high-risk low socioeconomic populations where the extreme indigent status of the population is a significant factor. Indeed, in groups such as these, basic needs of nutrition, reading ability, desire for or interest in obtaining any type of care, and other nonmedical factors are of greater significance. Populations receiving no prenatal care have higher prematurity rates than those receiving such care in the same socioeconomic strata. The delivery of such care must be an essential first step before the details of an elaborate prevention program can be implemented.

However, as has been demonstrated by Papiernik in France over an 11-year period, a prematurity prevention program was able to decrease the rate of preterm birth from 5.4 to 3.7 percent, even when standardized for the patients' social class distribution. Thus diligent effort may prove worthwhile, although the time expended will be considerable and by necessity the process will have to be ongoing.

DELIVERY OF THE PRETERM INFANT

In those cases in which attempts at prevention and therapy for preterm labor have failed and delivery is inevitable, efforts must be made to accomplish the delivery in a tertiary care center or one prepared for the stabilization of a preterm infant. Data suggest that among infants in the 27- to 32-week range (800 to 1,500 g), the perinatal survival may be improved from 10 to 20 percent by delivery in the appropriate setting. This necessitates active as-

TABLE 6 Essential Aspects of Preterm Prevention Program

Educate patient and staff on signs of preterm labor.
Have patient report on signs and symptoms of preterm labor, including pelvic symptoms and uterine activity.
Perform cervical evaluation by trained individuals at periodic (weekly after 20 weeks—high risk; single screening exam 28 to 32 weeks—low risk) intervals.
Use external tocography aggressively for suspected preterm labor.
Provide appropriate and accessible channels of communication for patient.
Use tocolytic therapy aggressively within margins of safety with suspected preterm labor.

sessment and maternal transport programs to complement efforts at preterm labor prevention. Such transport programs will ultimately be cost-effective by decreasing complications and morbidity that would otherwise be incurred by deliveries in inappropriate facilities.

The technique for delivery of the preterm infant has been discussed at great length. Certain principles seem to remain valid. Most critical is the maintenance of a well-oxygenated, nondistressed infant. Close fetal monitoring is a necessity. In the 26- to 32-week range, routine use of cesarean section is not necessary, nor will it invariably prevent intracranial hemorrhage. A well-oxygenated, nontraumatic delivery is most critical for successful outcome. Because the infant's head circumference is greater than that of the abdomen until 32 to 34 weeks, the use of cesarean section has been utilized more frequently in breech presentations. However, even in this circumstance, the literature occasionally provides conflicting opinions.

The documented fact of reduced perinatal mortality and the trend toward greater utilization of cesarean section require more detailed analysis before a causal relationship can be demonstrated.

SUGGESTED READING

Beard RW, Sharp F, eds. Preterm labour and its consequences. Proceedings, 13th Study Group, Royal College of Obstetricians and Gynaecologists. London: 1985.

Committee to Study the Prevention of Low Birthweight. Preventing low birthweight. Washington DC: National Academy Press, 1985.

Creasy RK, Resnik R, eds. Maternal-fetal medicine. Principles and practice. Philadelphia: WB Saunders, 1984.

Vidyasagar D, ed. The tiny baby. Clin Perinatol 1986; 13:2.

POSTDATE PREGNANCY

WILLIAM N. SPELLACY, M.D.

The first description of postdate pregnancy has been attributed to the 1902 article by Ballantyne who described not only its occurrence but its risks. In the 1950s, the syndrome was widely discussed in the literature from Western Europe where this diagnosis was a frequent reason for the induction of labor. A few American papers cited the significance of the problem in those years, but most obstetricians did not consider it a serious or frequent perinatal event. During the past twenty years, perinatology has changed significantly. Regionalization of obstetric care became recognized as a preferred method for the management of high-risk pregnancies and some physicians took fellowships in Maternal Fetal Medicine to become subspecialists in order to manage those referred complicated cases. Following this change, in the late 1960s, the general obstetrician began to recognize women with problem pregnancies early in gestation and to refer them to perinatal centers for their obstetric care. In addition, advances in science provided new ways to manage some diseases and many of former significance (such as Rh sensitization) were virtually eliminated from practice. Others, such as diabetes mellitus, became treatable with excellent outcomes. As a result of these changes, the American obstetrician began to manage a more normal population of pregnant women. Suddenly, one of the new complications that was being frequently seen in that type of practice was the gestation that went post date. The definition of the postdate pregnancy is one reaching 42 or more weeks and its frequency has been reported to range between 3 and 12 percent. This chapter will describe: 1) The accurate dating of gestation that is essential to making the diagnosis; 2) causes of postdate gestations; 3) maternal complications; 4) infant complications accompanying these pregnancies; and 5) a management plan to provide optional outcomes.

DATING THE PREGNANCY

One of the most important aspects of early prenatal care is to determine accurately the length of gestation and the expected date of confinement (EDC). In general, the accuracy of this process depends upon two things, namely seeing the pregnant woman early in her gestation and having several dating methods that all agree. Most calculations begin with the use of the last menstrual period (LMP). It is important to ask specifically for the date of the *first* day of the last normal menses as the woman may not know that this is what is important and may provide the last day, thereby introducing an automatic error for the calculated EDC of 2 to 7 days. Using Naegele's rule, the last menstrual date minus 3 months plus 7 days gives a reasonable estimate for the EDC. Studies have been done to determine the mean duration of gestation. Kortenoever reviewed 7,054 pregnancies in Holland in which the last menses was known and considered normal and found the mean duration was 282 days. In another study of 5,596 singleton gestations that exceeded 28-weeks duration (where the last menses was known), Nakano found the mean duration to be 278.5 days. Thus a 280-day mean duration from last menses seems fairly reliable. The calculations make the assumption that ovulation occurs about midcycle or on the fourteenth day of a 28-day cycle. Since the follicular phase is the variable portion of the cycle, if ovulation is delayed and the follicular phase is prolonged, then this method of calculating the EDC is in error. In one study by Saito and associates, there were 15.5 percent pregnancies that reached 42 weeks by the LMP definition, yet when a review of recorded basal body temperature records was done in the same women to determine the precise time of ovulation, no pregnancies exceeded 285 days from ovulation to delivery.

There are also many clinical parameters that are useful in dating gestations. The size of the uterus on pelvic examination in early pregnancy is helpful. As the uterus grows into the abdomen, the fundal height measurements from the symphysis are also useful. The uterus reaches the umbilicus at about 17-weeks gestation and the fundal height is approximately 20 cm at 20-weeks gestation. Jimenez and co-workers found that the mother's perception of first fetal movements was not different for primigravida and multigravida and that this occurred on the average at 17-weeks gestation, with a range of 12 to 21 weeks. In addition, fetal heart tones could first be heard with a stethoscope at a mean time of 17 weeks, with a range of 14 to 19 weeks. Thus, it is important to see patients frequently during these critical early weeks if there is uncertainty about the pregnancy duration, in order that several clinical parameters can be recorded as precisely as possible.

A number of laboratory studies can also help to date a gestation. Measurements of serum placental hormones such as human chorionic gonadotropin (hCG) or human placental lactogen (hPL) have proven to be good indices of gestational age. The accuracy of dating with early pregnancy hCG measurements has been found to be accurate to $\pm$ 3.2 days between 29 and 60 days of gestation. Pregnancy-specific proteins such as SP_1 can also be used as duration markers, but accuracy is not significantly better than with hPL.

The use of ultrasonography to determine gestational age is now well accepted and is probably the most widely used laboratory method today. In the early gestational weeks (from 5 to 10), the gestational sac diameter can be measured—this has a standard error of $\pm$ 0.64 for predicting the weeks. There is a 2-week window of time between 11 and 12 weeks of pregnancy when ultrasound dating is difficult. However, after the twelfth week until the twentieth week, the fetal head biparietal diameter is accurate for dating and has a prediction error of only 6.3 days. Other fetal bone studies such as femur length can also be used. O'Brien and co-workers found an accuracy of $\pm$ 6.7 days between weeks 12 and 23 when dating with this method. Chervenak and associates found ultrasound crown-rump measurements the most accurate and superior to the use of serum hCG in early pregnancy. In general, the accuracy of ultrasound dating decreases as the pregnancy advances since there is more variation in fetal size with age and therefore reliability can only be certain if the examinations are done before the third trimester. Women with uncertain menstrual or clinical dates in early gestation need ultrasound studies to help set the EDC. Women who reach the thirtieth week in pregnancy should not have their EDC changed by further testing as it would not be more accurate and could make the obstetrician miss a postdate problem.

CAUSES OF POSTDATE GESTATIONS

The most frequent cause of this problem is inaccurate pregnancy dating due to a failure to know the time of ovulation. This is a double problem. First, it causes a large number of normal pregnancies to be labeled "postdate"; therefore, the use of more intensive management programs occur, thus resulting in more expensive tests and possibly more operative intervention with induction of labor and/or cesarean section. Thus the costs for patients and the work effort for the health care providers is unnecessarily increased. Second a false "postdate" label puts many normal gestations into the high-risk classification and their obvious normal outcome dilutes the importance of the syndrome and lulls the obstetricians into believing that this is rarely a serious complication. Obvious causes of this problem are irregular menstrual cycles with delayed ovulations, and inaccuracy in recalling last menstrual dates, and not having early prenatal care when dating of pregnancy is most accurate. Another contributor is the discontinuation of oral contraceptives, which delays ovulation by 2 or more weeks in the first spontaneous cycles.

Less common contributors have been unusual problems like anencephaly of the fetus or sulfatase deficiency in the placenta. While the anencephalic infant can deliver early as well as late, the pregnancy with sulfatase deficiency, which is an X-linked problem, routinely delivers the male in the postdate period. Normal ripening of the cervix as term approaches is closely associated with increased blood levels of dehydroepiandrosterone sulfate (DHEA-S). Thus DHEA-S plays a key role in preparing the cervix for labor.

Finally, most of the true postdate gestations are of unknown cause. It is accepted today that prostaglandins produced in the uterus have a pivotal role in initiating labor. It is also common for the gravida with postdate gestation to have an "unripe" cervix. Many recent studies have shown that the cervix can be rapidly changed by the local application of prostaglandin gels. These data suggest that an important etiology may be cervical disease, either as a deficiency in prostaglandin production or as a refractoriness of the cervix to respond to endogenous prostaglandins. Further research in this area should be rewarding in terms of a better understanding of the etiology of the condition, in addition to more effective therapy.

COMPLICATIONS

Maternal

There are several problems posed for the woman who goes past her EDC by 2 or more weeks; these include the following: (1) emotional stress, (2) inconvenience and cost, and (3) birth trauma. The emotional strain of apprehension, expectation, and anxiety occurs because of failure to start labor "on time." Since the mother has focused on a due date for many months, to reach that date and then to continue with no signs of labor leaves her frustrated and concerned. The second problem relates to the medical intervention in terms of assessments and attempted delivery. The many additional tests and doctor visits plus the attempts at labor induction and/or cesarean section further the anxiety, cause inconvenience, and increase the cost of the pregnancy. Sometimes these aggressive undertakings also result in additional complications. The final potential hazard is the physical trauma that can be experienced when delivering a large macrosomic infant. Vaginal and cervical lacerations complicate the immediate delivery, as well as potentially creating long-term problems such as cervical incompetence, pelvic relaxation, and urinary stress incontinence. Although all of the maternal complications are important, none are life threatening for the woman.

Infant

The complications for the infant in a postdate gestation are much more serious than those for its mother and are as follows: (1) oligohydramnios with cord accidents, (2) macrosomia and birth trauma, (3) meconium passage and aspiration, and (4) placental insufficiency and perinatal hypoxia—death. Oligohydramnios can result in acute cord compression. Normally amniotic fluid increases in pregnancy until about the 37th week of gestation. There is a gradual decrease after that time. The mean volume at 37 weeks is 1,000 ml and by 40 weeks it has fallen to 800 ml. This decrease continues past term and at the 42nd week it has reached 250 ml. Maternal diseases like hypertension can produce an even lower volume. Cord compressions with oligohydramnios are frequently not predictable, although variable fetal heart rate decelerations on continuous monitoring and the disappearance of amniotic fluid with smaller measurable pockets on real time ultrasonography scanning are clues to the occurrence of this problem.

Macrosomia, or birth weights greater than 4,500 g, results from continued growth over an extra 2 or more weeks. The possibility of this increases even further if the woman is obese or has diabetes mellitus. The consequences of macrosomia can be obstructed labor or, more importantly, shoulder dystocia during delivery, which can lead, on occasion, to permanent nerve injury to the arm. Prediction of the macrosomic infant is often possible by ultrasonographic assessment of fetal weight. These estimates generally are best done with fetal liver-abdominal circumference scans, but they have an error of about 10 percent. In these cases, it is important to determine fetal weight by ultrasonography before attempting a vaginal delivery.

A third and important problem is meconium aspiration. The fetus rarely passes meconium between the 16th and 32nd weeks of gestation, then it progressively increases the frequency of meconium passage as it gets older. The frequency of meconium passage in postdate gestations ranges from 25 to 30 percent compared to a frequency of about 10 percent at term. The associated complicating problem is that as the amount of amniotic fluid decreases post date, the passed meconium is less likely to be well diluted and this results in a thicker meconium being available for aspiration by the fetus. The thicker the meconium, the more likely it is to obstruct small airway passages if it is carried deep into the lung structure. If the fetus develops hypoxia during labor, it gasps, thereby pulling the meconium deep into the respiratory tract. Neonatal respiratory distress, pneumonia, atelectasis, and pneumothorax can result.

The final problem for the infant is placental insufficiency. The placenta's peak functions also occur at about 37-weeks gestation, after which there is a gradual reduction. If the infant continues to grow, then the placenta-infant ratio decreases, and the reserve for transfer and support may reach a point where intrauterine existence is compromised. In order to survive in the compromised intrauterine environment, the fetus must decrease its energy requirements. It can do this in two ways: first, the fetus may decrease its growth rate and may also lose its deposited fat and glycogen. It then shows signs of fetal growth retardation and dysmaturity. Secondly, as a further means for the fetus to adjust to the poor intrauterine environment and to decrease its energy requirements, the fetus can stop moving. Although it can also demonstrate hypoxia at rest, this is most often apparent when there are uterine contractions, especially if they are strong enough to dilate the cervix as in true labor. These infants often demonstrate late-type fetal heart rate decelerations, bradycardia, and acidosis during early labor. This compromised placental reserve could reach the point where fetal death occurs. Thus the postdate pregnancy can present with a spectrum of infant problems including poor fetal growth, dysmaturity, meconium passage, decreased fetal movement, loss of amniotic fluid, nonreactive fetal heart rates, late-type fetal heart rate decelerations with uterine contractions, hypoxia, acidosis, low Apgar scores, central nervous system damage, and death.

Management

Since the complications of postdate pregnancies significantly rise after 42-weeks gestation, the women must be identified at 41 weeks so that they can be managed appropriately from the 42nd week on. There are four principal concepts in management, namely: (1) The fetus is mature and should have few neonatal problems; (2) Terminating the pregnancy will end the problem; (3) The in utero environment must be monitored for the risks of oligohydramnios and placental insufficiency if termination is not done; and (4) During delivery, problems of shoulder dystocia, meconium aspiration, acidosis, and hypoxia must be avoided. The specific plan for management is as follows:

Weekly Vaginal Examinations

The patient must have weekly vaginal examinations in order to assess the condition of the cervix. When the cervix reaches a dilatation and effacement whereby the induction of labor will be easy and probably successful, then she should be admitted into the hospital for that procedure. This is usually easily and safely accomplished if the cervix is 3 or more cm. If the vertex is at zero station, induction can be started by amniotomy and occasionally oxytocin infusion is also needed. The success of locally applied prostaglandin gels in changing the cervix from unfavorable to favorable is encouraging for future practice.

Weekly Real-Time Ultrasound Scans

One of the physiologic changes that accompany the maturation of the pregnancy is the gradual reduction of the amniotic fluid volume. The gradual and continued loss of amniotic fluid creates the ominous oligohydramnios environment whereby fetal compression of the umbilical cord becomes a serious risk. Since cord compression is not usually predictable, occurs abruptly, and can result in sudden fetal death, it must be a major concern to the obstetrician. Many studies have demonstrated a significant increase in perinatal mortality with oligohydramnios. The uterus should thus be scanned with real-time ultrasonography on a weekly basis in order to assess the amniotic fluid volume. One useful way is to measure the diameters of the visible fluid pockets, and if the largest of these is less than 2 cm in diameter, the fluid volume is severely reduced. The ultrasonographic diagnosis of oligohydramnios should be an indication to proceed to delivery. If induction of labor is attempted, then continuous electronic monitoring of the fetal heart rate must be done to watch for signs of cord compression in the form of variable decelerations. Some investigators have attempted to treat this problem during labor with amnion infusions of saline with some success, but it is not universally done at this time.

Weekly Fetal-Placental Function Tests

As the pregnancy progresses, there is a gradual decrease in the functional surface area for transfer across the placenta. There continues to be a gradual growth of the fetus giving a decrease in the fetal/placental reserve. At some point this will be below the limit of adequacy for normal intrauterine existence. This change is a slow one and as a result most placental/fetal function tests become abnormal days before fetal death, and thus they provide a long enough lead time and are clinically useful. There are many tests that can be applied to these pregnancies in order to assess this risk. The tests that have been extensively studied include the following:

Antepartum Fetal Heart Rate (FHR) Monitoring. Both the nonstress test (NST) and the contraction stress test (CST) have been utilized in many studies to assess fetal health in postdate pregnancies, and they both seem to provide similar valid assessments in these gestations. Since oligohydramnios and cord compression are also potential risks, these FHR strips should be carefully reviewed for evidence of subtle variable decelerations as they may be predictive of that problem and have been associated with a significant increase in perinatal mortality. These FHR and ultrasonographic studies have been combined into a "biophysical profile" assessment, which also includes evaluations of fetal tone and breathing, but there are little data in randomized controlled studies to suggest that improved perinatal outcomes result from such complicated monitoring compared to FHR and ultrasonographic amniotic fluid volume studies alone.

Estriol (E_3). The amount of estriol in the maternal blood and urine is dependent upon the size of the placenta and fetus and their functional state. As the placenta decreases its function for a given gestational age, there is a gradual decrease in estriol production, and many studies have demonstrated that this decrease is a useful biochemical marker of fetal-placental compromise in postdate gestation. Most laboratories today utilize plasma-free estriol as the test since the assay systems are easy to perform and it eliminates the problems of 24-hour urine collection.

Human Placental Lactogen. Serum hPL is a useful marker of the functional mass of the placenta, and it decreases as the placental functional mass decreases. Accordingly, it has been utilized as an adjunct marker for placental reserve. Studies with postdate gestations have shown some predictability of intrauterine compromise by the test, but not enough to be able to utilize it as the only assessment of the intrauterine environment.

The fetus in postdate pregnancies is clearly mature and therefore if delivered healthy and not having congenital anomalies, it will do well in the nursery and survive. Thus if there is any test that begins to show increased risk in utero, it must be acted upon immediately by proceeding to delivery. The use of these tests is shown in Figure 1.

Delivery

Once the decision has been made to deliver the patient or once she spontaneously begins labor, then there are several significant problems that need to be guarded against.

Labor Dysfunction—Shoulder Dystocia. This problem is significantly increased in the pregnancy where the fetus has reached macrosomic size. Because this is a risk in the postdate woman, the fetus must be screened with ultrasonography in order to estimate fetal weight. If the estimate reaches 5,000 g an elective cesarean section should be considered since there is a 10 percent error in the estimate, which makes the likelihood of the fetus truly being 4,500 g or more very good.

Meconium Aspiration. The passage of meconium is frequent in the postdate pregnancy with usual incidences in excess of 25 percent. If the pregnancy also has oligohydramnios, then the meconium remains thick. Fetal hypoxia may result in increased fetal gasping, thus pulling the meconium deeper into the respiratory tract. Fetal distress with meconium is especially dangerous for the infant. The major problems concern the neonate's respiration. Despite modern therapy, there will be more respiratory distress, pneumothorax, and death. There has been an attempt to reduce these problems by aspirating the respiratory tract with a DeLee suction before the chest is delivered and then to immediately intubate the neonate and suction below the vocal cords if they are meconium stained. Studies have shown that even this aggressive approach will not prevent all of the serious neonatal problems. Meconium aspiration still remains as a very serious complication of pregnancy.

Fetal Distress. The postdate fetus is in double jeopardy for distress in labor because of the associated oligohydramnios with umbilical cord compression accidents and because of possible placental insufficiency. When these infants are in labor they must be continuously and carefully assessed. This is best done with continuous electronic FHR monitoring. The information derived from FHR monitoring is better with internal monitoring, which should be done as soon as obstetrically feasible. If there are ominous signs of potential fetal hypoxia in late labor,

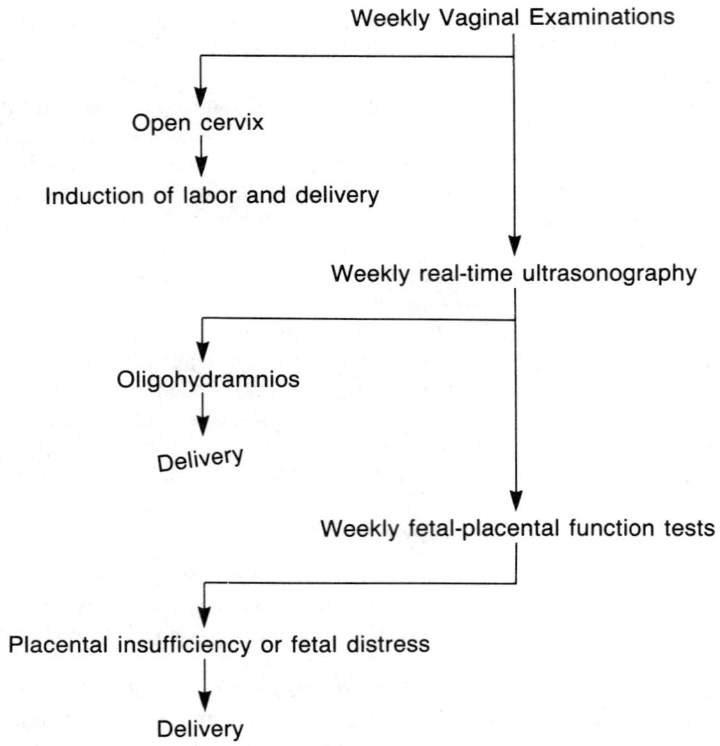

Figure 1 Management of postdate pregnancies.

such as loss of variability or subtle late decelerations, then a fetal scalp blood sample may be useful in selecting out the hypoxic-acidocic fetus for immediate delivery. This test can reduce the number of unnecessary cesarean sections done for heart rate changes alone. There must be the possibility of doing a rapid emergency cesarean section if fetal distress develops, and this means a decision—delivery time of less than 30 minutes and hopefully closer to 15 minutes. During the preparation time for an emergency cesarean section for fetal distress, there should be an attempt to resuscitate the fetus. This is best carried out by administering oxygen to the mother, moving her to the left side, elevating the presenting fetal part, and stopping uterine activity with a tocolytic drug, such as 0.25 mg of terbutaline given subcutaneously. If the FHR returns to normal the cesarean delivery should be delayed for at least twenty minutes to allow the fetus to recover and to restore its acid-base balance. Intrauterine resuscitation is preferred to extrauterine resuscitation because the need to establish lung function is not a critical step in the process.

In conclusion, for the practicing general obstetrician the postdate pregnancy represents a common and potentially serious high-risk pregnancy complication. The problem of postdate pregnancy is compounded by inaccurate pregnancy dating. The use of biochemical-biophysical assessments of gestational age is useful in the first half of pregnancy when menstrual data are unreliable. The cause of true postdate (42+ week) pregnancies is usually not known. The maternal complications include anxiety, apprehension, increased expense, and possible traumatic birth of a large infant. The infant complications include oligohydramnios with acute cord compression, meconium passage and aspiration, macrosomia and labor abnormalities or shoulder dystocia, and placental insufficiency with dysmaturity, hypoxia, acidosis, and death. Management requires weekly vaginal examinations, real-time ultrasonographic assessment of amniotic fluid volume, and fetal-placental function tests, such as fetal heart rate (NST-CST) monitoring and/or estriol measurements. Delivery should be done if the cervix is favorable, the amniotic fluid is lost, or fetal distress occurs. Continuous assessment of the fetus during labor is critical since many are so compromised they are not able to deliver safely via the vagina. Before vaginal delivery is attempted, the fetal weight should be estimated by ultrasonographic studies to avoid shoulder dystocia with the macrosomic infant.

SUGGESTED READING

Bastida A, Manning F, Harman C, Lange I, Morrison I. Ultrasound evaluation of amniotic fluid: outcome of pregnancies with severe oligohydramnios. Am J Obstet Gynecol 1986; 154:895–899.
Clifford SH. Postmaturity with placental dysfunction—clinical syndrome pathologic findings. J Ped 1954; 44:1–13.
Jimenez JM, Tyson JE, Reisch JS. Clinical measures of gestational age in normal pregnancies. Obstet Gynecol 1983; 61:438–443.
Knox GE, Huddelston JF, Flowers CE Jr, Eubanks A, Sutliff G. Management of prolonged pregnancy: results of a prospective randomized trial. Am J Obstet Gynecol 1979; 134:376–384.

DYSFUNCTIONAL LABOR

EMANUEL A. FRIEDMAN, M.D., Sc.D.

Essential to proper therapy of the patient experiencing aberrant labor progress is clearly focused diagnosis of her condition. The management of dysfunctional labor has been facilitated in recent decades by the recognition that it is now possible to use objective clinical criteria for diagnosing the several specific types of disorders encountered in practice. Despite a paucity of understanding of the pathophysiology of the human gravid uterus and why it sometimes fails to function adequately to empty its contents effectively at or near term, there is general acceptance of the concept that experiential data can be assessed to optimize results for the gravida and her fetus for purposes of guiding therapeutic programs. By these means, those who attend women in labor are now more knowledgeable about and better able to deal with potentially critical labor problems than in the past.

DIAGNOSIS

The diagnosis of dysfunctional labor is readily accomplished by simple graphic portrayal of the patterns of advancing cervical dilation and of fetal descent (station of the fetal presenting part estimated in centimeters cephalad or caudad to the reference plane of the ischial spines) plotted against the time elapsed from the onset of regular uterine contractions as perceived by the gravida. In all normal cases, dilation proceeds along an S-shaped pathway. Its initial arm is the latent phase, during which there is little progress. The active phase, characterized by rapid and linear dilation, follows with little alteration in uterine contractility. Prior to full cervical dilation and retraction, the pattern appears to slow in the deceleration phase that precedes the onset of the second stage of labor. Simultaneously, the descent pattern evolves its characteristic hyperbolic shape. Little descent is ordinarily seen until the active phase of dilation is in progress; active descent, which is most rapid after the deceleration phase begins, generally continues without interruption until the leading edge of the fetus reaches the perineum.

Three types of dysfunctional labor can be readily differentiated by tracing the labor graph, namely, prolonged latent phase, protraction disorders (two variants are recognized), and arrest disorders (of which there are four known). The latent phase seldom exceeds 20 hours in nulliparas (14 hours in multiparas), so that a patient who fails to show active dilation after this duration of time has elapsed from the onset of labor can be diagnosed as having prolonged latent phase. Similarly, the maximum slope of the active phase is normally at least 1.2 cm dilation per hour in nulliparas (1.5 cm per hour in multiparas). Those whose rate of active dilation is less than these limits have protracted dilation. If fetal descent in late labor does not exceed the critical rate of 1.0 cm per hour in nulliparas (2.0 cm per hour in multiparas), diagnose protracted descent. Once active dilation or descent has begun, it should continue apace. If dilation halts in the active phase for 2 hours or more, consider secondary arrest of dilation. If the station, once descent has begun, does not advance over a period of 1 hour, arrest of descent exists. Prolongation of the deceleration phase is an abnormality in which this segment of the pattern continues beyond the normal duration of 3 hours in nulliparas (1 hour in multiparas). Failure of descent is an abnormality characterized by active fetal descent not occurring as expected at the end of the first stage and in the second stage of labor.

It is important to be able to distinguish these several kinds of labor aberrations. Unless one can recognize the specific disorder as it develops in a given patient, one cannot ensure that the appropriate program of evaluation and management will be undertaken. The recommendations for therapy that follow have been found to be effective when applied to the care of parturients affected by the specific type of labor problem under consideration. A regimen applicable to one kind of disorder, however, is not equivalently beneficial for another. It follows, therefore, that proper identification of the abnormality must precede any form of treatment.

PROLONGED LATENT PHASE

The latent phase may be abnormally prolonged for a number of reasons, none of which is necessarily serious or threatening to the mother or fetus. Not uncommonly, for example, the ineffectual uterine contractions may merely represent false labor. It is often indistinguishable in every characteristic from the early phase of true labor, except by hindsight; when the contractions stop in due course, the diagnosis becomes patently clear. Alternatively, the latent phase is often prolonged inadvertently by analgesic or anesthetic agents administered to the laboring patient for relief of discomfort. Because the myometrial contractile elements are not yet fully coordinated in the latent phase of labor, the efficiency of the uterus as an integrated muscular organ is easily inhibited by such agents. Assessment should principally address these factors. Be especially alert for medical or obstetric problems that warrant aggressive intervention. This becomes important for weighing the therapeutic options available for managing a patient with prolonged latent phase and for choosing among them. If one recognizes that the disorder of prolonged latent phase is basically innocuous in the sense that, if managed well, it offers no special hazard to either mother or fetus, one will not be tempted to intervene aggressively and inappropriately. Prolonged latent phase can be treated with equal efficacy by either therapeutic rest or uterotonic stimulation. With few exceptions, we prefer to institute a program aimed at providing an interval during which the patient can sleep and recuperate from her already long, tedious, and unproductive efforts. Carefully explain the benign nature of the problem to allay growing anxieties. Use the time to advantage to replenish fluid losses and correct electrolyte imbalance. Morphine sulfate is given subcutaneously or intramuscularly in a dose of 15 mg to the woman of average weight. Consider adjusting the dose upward to 20 mg for a large patient or down to 10 mg for a small one. Although we have had no personal experience with other medications, some have used barbiturates or ataractics instead to good effect. Reassess after 20 minutes to determine the impact of the drug on the patient. Watch for respiratory depression. If uterine contractions have subsided, allow the patient to sleep undisturbed unless periodic reevaluation or continuous monitoring is indicated by prevailing risk status. Persistent contractions suggest the possibility that the labor may already have progressed into the active phase. Verify by ascertaining whether there has been any measurable change in cervical dilatation. If none is observed (and respiratory function has not been depressed), consider giving one additional injection of 10 mg morphine sulfate to halt the contractions and ensure adequate uterine rest. It is not at all clear why this approach is so effective, but when patients treated in this manner awaken after 6 to 10 hours, nearly all will promptly resume effective uterine contractions, advancing rapidly in the active phase of labor, and progressing uneventfully to delivery.

Most of the remaining patients, about 10 percent overall, are out of labor when they awaken. For them, the treatment has demonstrated that the antecedent event was merely an episode of false labor. There is no need for further care (other than continuing routine ambulatory prenatal care) until they reenter labor at a later date. Only a few (about one in 20 overall) awaken and resume their former ineffectual pattern of uterine contractions without active phase progression. It is clear that these women have been helped physically and emotionally by the rest provided them, but they will soon be discouraged and tired again unless they see some real progress. To accomplish this, oxytocin can be given by carefully titrated infusion to augment myometrial activity, provided there is no counterbalancing contraindication against its use.

As previously mentioned, patients with prolonged latent phase are just as effectively treated with uterotonic stimulation as by therapeutic rest. Amniotomy has not been shown to have any consistent value in these cases for correcting this specific labor disorder. The preferential choice of narcotic agents over oxytocin is based on several compelling considerations. Many of them are in false labor, but they cannot be identified prospectively as such. Using oxytocin thus constitutes an attempt to induce labor for this subgroup. It not only subjects them to all the potential hazards of labor induction in general but it magnifies those risks based on the suboptimal condition of the patient as regards hydration, acid-base balance, energy state, anxiety level, and the condition of the cervix. The cervical condition is especially important as an index of the likelihood that the induction will be successful. Too often, the attempt will fail if it is undertaken in a gravida with unprepared soft tissues, compounding the problem and then ostensibly justifying a cesarean section that might readily have been averted by a more conservative approach. These gravidas benefit greatly by being given the opportunity to rest and recover from an already overly long period of "labor." Moreover, the rest regimen appears to be especially useful as a therapeutic trial for differentiating true labor from false. Oxytocin as a first-line therapy for prolonged latent phase, therefore, is called for only in those few cases in which any delay, even for a few hours of rest, would be considered inappropriate.

The outlook for patients with prolonged latent phase is quite good. The labor aberration itself appears to be entirely harmless. Affected patients, if permitted to progress into the active phase and beyond, generally do very well. The frequency of other labor problems is no greater among them than among gravidas with a normal latent phase pattern. Those few who do develop a protraction or arrest disorder (see below) can be expected to respond to appropriate management in the same way as any other gravida without any enhancement of outcome risk for mother or fetus. Those whose labor course in the active phase and the second stage follows a normal pattern have an especially good prognosis for uncomplicated vaginal delivery of an uncompromised infant. In view of this good outlook for patients with prolonged latent phase, the abnormal labor pattern can never be considered an ample justification by itself for cesarean section.

PROTRACTION DISORDERS

In contrast to the inoffensive nature of the prolonged latent phase pattern, both protraction and arrest disorders have much more serious potential impact in relation to operative delivery and adverse fetal results. This appears to be related principally to their common association with cephalopelvic disproportion, fetal malposition, and fetal compromise. About one-third of gravidas who are diagnosed as having either protracted dilation or protracted descent (conditions often appearing sequentially in the same labor) show objective evidence of obstructed labor. As soon as the diagnosis is made, therefore, one should carefully evaluate the cephalopelvic relationship. This is generally facilitated in advanced labor because the cervix is partially dilated and the fetal presenting part is well down into the pelvis. Digital examination can easily assess the degree of molding and deformation of the fetal head, particularly noting asynclitism, malposition, and overlapping of the cranial plates. In addition to assessing the pelvic shape, architecture, and capacity, the examination should address the spatial relation between head and pelvis. This is best achieved by palpation through the course of a contraction, perhaps with additional caudad force applied to the uterus by an assistant to impress the head more strongly in the pelvis. This is the Müller-Hillis manuever that we find useful as an objective means for evaluating for cephalopelvic disproportion. If the fetus fits tightly with no apparent space between it and the pelvic bones and does not advance at all when forced downward in this way, disproportion is very likely to exist. Contrariwise, palpable descent clearly rules out insurmountable disproportion, at least at the fetal station in which the examination was done.

Finding documentable bony dystocia in a patient with a protraction disorder warrants cesarean section. This avoids the kinds of problems that can be anticipated to result from a long course of labor and a difficult delivery in these cases, including ascending infection and fetal damage from hypoxia or intracranial hemorrhage. If there is ample room for descent to occur safely, the labor should be allowed to continue without interference. Careful continuous electronic fetal heart rate monitoring is essential. Oxytocin stimulation has not been shown to be at all effective in speeding up the abnormal process. In fact, use of oxytocin may actually prove deleterious, because although it does not appear capable of augmenting the rates of dilation and descent, it does enhance myometrial contractility. It may thereby intermittently diminish uterine and placental blood flow and thus reduce fetal oxygenation. A fetus with little or no reserve can be made overtly hypoxic as a consequence. It is not yet known why patients with these desultory types of labor patterns are refractory to uterotonic stimulation or why there is this apparent dissociation between the uterine contractions and the work they are intended to accomplish.

Gravidas permitted to continue in labor with a protraction disorder need a great deal of support by personnel and family because progress is so slow and cannot be prodded to move more quickly. Reassure them repeatedly to allay fears. Maintain assiduous surveillance, observing for evidence of developing amnionitis, fetal distress, and arrest of labor. Ensure proper maintenance of adequate fluid and electrolyte status. Provide for their comfort, but recognize that the dysfunctional labor reflects myometrial function that is readily inhibited to become even less efficient by narcotic analgesic agents (despite a contractile pattern that may outwardly appear to be quite good). This means minimizing the dosage and frequency of administration of such agents and perhaps relying more on tranquilizers or nonpharmacologic measures. Amniotomy is often necessary for application of a fetal scalp electrode for monitoring purposes, especially if the tracing obtained from the external abdominal transducer is not entirely satisfactory. However, rupturing the membranes does expose the patient to two added risks. Uterine infection may develop during the course of the long labor still to come and, inexplicably, the labor may thereby be further complicated by a superimposed arrest disorder. Because fetal monitoring is such an important component of management, however, these risks must perforce by considered acceptable on balance.

If the patient with a protraction disorder is allowed to labor and no complication develops, she can be expected to progress along her prescribed slow, dilatory pathway to full cervical dilatation and ultimately to bring the fetal presenting part down to the perineum. Spontaneous vaginal delivery is entirely feasible under these circumstances and is the preferred delivery mode for these cases. However, to accomplish this requires one to revoke the concept that the second stage of labor must be limited in duration to a specific time interval, such as 2 hours. Not uncommonly, it takes several hours to effect normal delivery with protracted descent, and this is acceptable provided neither mother nor fetus is compromised. Be sure there is no disproportion and the fetal status remains good. Avoid the temptation to deliver by forceps because of the potential trauma such instrumentation is likely to cause in these cases, even when employed in a skillful fashion and under ideal conditions.

ARREST DISORDERS

The very common association of arrest disorders with cephalopelvic disproportion, seen in about one-half of affected patients, makes it essential to evaluate the cephalopelvic relations with care in every case before undertaking any form of therapy. Just as for gravidas who develop a protraction disorder in advanced labor, these relations are readily assessed by a skillful pelvic examination invoking the principles of the Müller-Hillis maneuver (see above). Other factors that have been related to and perhaps causative of arrest disorders, such as fetal malposition and heavy analgesia or conduction anesthesia superimposed on a protraction disorder, are of far less clinical significance in regard to their fetal effects. Nonetheless, if remediable conditions are disclosed, measures may be taken to counter the inhibitory influences, for example, by allowing the anesthetic level to fall or the analgesia to abate. Even when such items are found, however, it is still important to be sure there is no concurrent disproportion. To assume arrest of dilation or descent is due to peridural anesthesia without first ruling out the much more serious problem of disproportion risks delay in diagnosis and exposes the gravida and her fetus to possible aggravation of its hazards.

Documentation of cephalopelvic disproportion in a patient presenting with one or more of the arrest disorders is sufficient grounds to justify cesarean section without any further trial of labor. Although this may seem unduly aggressive and constraining, the recommendation is based on the empirical observation that few, if any, patients affected by the combination of adverse factors can deliver vaginally with safety. The rate of delivery trauma is high among those few who are delivered by this route, and the frequency of fetal death and damage is unacceptable. Nearly all come to cesarean section regardless of the efforts made to attempt to achieve vaginal delivery. Nonetheless, some authorities now recommend uterotonic stimulation for these cases without regard for the cephalopelvic relations in the form of a trial of augmented labor to assess the functional capacity of the pelvis to accommodate the fetus. Careful continuous fetal monitoring is essential under these conditions, watching for evidence of fetal distress. The end point for a trial of oxytocin stimulation in the presence of possible cephalopelvic disproportion does not seem entirely logical. Although currently available monitoring techniques properly flag hypoxic events, they do not appear capable of recognizing harmful changes in intracranial stresses or shearing forces before damage occurs so that appropriate interventive action can be undertaken for prevention. In the absence of objective clinical evidence to verify the safety of this practice, therefore, it cannot be fully condoned.

By contrast, if one can rule out a bone impediment by demonstrating ample compensatory space between the fetal head and the maternal pelvis, oxytocin infusion is clearly in order. It is given by cautious titration to enhance myometrial function while monitoring that function and the fetal status most carefully. Augmentation of uterine contractility is usually very effective in yielding progressive dilation and descent in these cases irrespective of the apparent cause of the arrest pattern. Moreover, this seems to apply regardless of the type of contractile pattern existing before the stimulation was begun, even if the contractions were clinically indistinguishable from those of strong, normal labor. Of considerable importance is the kind of response one obtains insofar as the resulting dilation or descent is concerned. Using the prearrest slope as a reference (that is, the maximum rate of change achieved in the active phase or the second stage before the labor arrested), one can assess whether postarrest progression in response to uterine stimulation by oxytocin is appropriate. This serves as a useful index of prognosis. If the postarrest response slope is the same as or greater than the prearrest slope of the curve, one can usually anticipate uneventful vaginal delivery without serious fetal complication. Contrastingly, if the postarrest rate of change is of lesser magnitude (or if one cannot accomplish any additional dilation or descent by oxytocin stimulation), it is unlikely that a safe vaginal delivery will occur. Under these latter circumstances, it is imperative to reevaluate the cephalopelvic relations to ensure that an obstruction to labor has not been overlooked. Cesarean section will probably be required in such cases in the best interests of mother and fetus.

The outlook for vaginal delivery in patients with an arrest disorder thus depends primarily on the presence or absence of cephalopelvic disproportion. If disproportion is present and detected early in the course of an arrested labor, prognosis for the infant delivered by cesarean section is good. Similarly, an arrest disorder occurring in a patient with ample pelvic capacity should ultimately result in the vaginal delivery of an uncompromised neonate. Outcome results are not necessarily so optimistic, however, for cases in which dystocic problems exist but are undetected or revealed late, perhaps as a product of a failed trial of uterotonic stimulation or a prolonged delay in the recognition of the arrest pattern. In the era before fetal monitoring was widely available, fetuses delivered after an arrest disorder did not fare well as a rule. Introduction of meaningful surveillance of the fetal status, coupled with appreciation of the significance of the postarrest slope as a means for flagging previously undetected pelvic impediments, has improved the results considerably. This change substantiates the value of these measures and supports a firm recommendation that they should be used in all arrested labor patients who are permitted to continue in labor after the aberration has been verified.

SUGGESTED READING

Friedman EA. Physiology of labor. In: Cohen WR, Friedman EA, eds. Management of labor. Baltimore: University Park Press, 1983:1.

Friedman EA. Effects of labor and delivery procedures on the fetus. In: Cohen WR, Friedman EA, eds. Management of labor. Baltimore: University Park Press, 1983:307.

Friedman EA. Aberrant labor problems. In: Labor: clinical evaluation and management. 2nd ed. New York: Appleton-Century-Crofts, 1978:45.

Friedman EA. Hydramnios. In: Labor: clinical evaluation and management. 2nd ed. New York: Appleton-Century-Crofts, 1978:279.

Friedman EA. Prolonged latent phase. In: Friedman EA, Acker DB, Sachs BP, eds. Obstetrical decision making. 2nd ed. Toronto: BC Decker, 1987:236.

PROSTAGLANDINS

LUIS SANCHEZ-RAMOS, M.D.

Prostaglandins are lipids formed from polyunsaturated fatty acids released from phospholipids in the plasma membrane of cells. Membrane phospholipids such as phosphatidylcholine and phosphatidylinositol provide the precursors to the prostaglandins. Phospholipase A_2 hydrolyzes phosphatidylinositol with the release of arachidonic acid, which serves as the precursor for prostaglandin E_2 (PGE_2) and prostaglandin F_2 alpha (PGF_{2a}). These compounds are the principal prostaglandins in humans and are of the greatest significance biologically.

Both PGE_2 and PGF_{2a} have a marked oxytocic effect on the pregnant uterus. In addition, it has been found that PGF_{2a} contracts nonpregnant uterine muscle. Both of these compounds exert distinct effects on target organs (Table 1).

Twenty years ago PGF_{2a} was used intravenously for the induction of labor. This was the first clinical application of prostaglandins in obstetrics and provided the stimulus for further extensive research. Since then, prostaglandins have been used successfully in several clinical situations (Table 2).

TABLE 1 Effects of Prostaglandins on Target Organs

Actions	*PGE_2*	*PGF_{2a}*
Myometrium	Contractions	Contractions
Gastrointestinal smooth muscle	Increased motility	Increased motility
Blood vessels	Vasodilation (hypotension)	Vasoconstriction (hypertension)
Hypothalamus	Pyrexia	None
Respiratory	Bronchodilation	Bronchoconstriction

TABLE 2 Indications for the Use of Prostaglandins

PGE_2:
- Termination of pregnancy from the 12th through the 20th gestational weeks
- Evacuation of the uterine contents in the management of missed abortion or intrauterine fetal death up to 28 weeks of gestational age
- Management of nonmetastatic gestational trophoblastic disease
- Cervical ripening prior to induction or abortion
- Induction of labor

PGF_{2a}:
- Termination of pregnancy between the 16th and 20th weeks of gestation
- Induction of labor
- Post partum hemorrhage

CERVICAL RIPENING

A considerable amount of data suggest that prostaglandins soften and ripen the cervix, rendering it more favorable for induction and thereby affecting the duration of labor, the incidence of maternal and fetal complications, and the need for cesarean section.

The cervix that is unfavorable for induction of labor is associated with elevated levels of chondroitin sulfate, dermatan sulfate, collagen, and decreased concentrations of hyaluronic acid. The collagen that is coated by dermatan and chondroitin sulfate is held as a rigid, strictive structure. Synthesis of hyaluronic acid is stimulated by the process of cervical ripening, thereby increasing the water content of the cervix, leading to swelling and "ripening."

PGE_2 at low doses and suspended in a viscous gel has been shown to improve the state of the cervix, reduce the length of labor, and decrease the incidence of cesarean section, especially that due to failure of induction. PGE_2 and PGF_{2a} inhibit the adenosine triphosphate–dependent sequestration of calcium in sarcoplasmic reticulum and thereby act to increase the concentration of cytosolic Ca^{++}, a process that leads to activation of myosin light-chain kinase, phosphorylation of myosin, and, thereby, the interaction of phosphorylated myosin and actin. PGE_2 and PGF_{2a} cause the rapid appearance of myometrial gap junctions. Comparisons have been made between extra-amniotic prostaglandin E_2 gel and other methods utilizing PGE_2, i.e., oral, intravenous, and intravaginal PGE_2. All forms and methods have resulted in an improvement in cervical status, but the response appears to be greater in those patients who receive extra-amniotic prostaglandin gel.

Many different protocols have been described using PGE_2 extra-amniotic jelly for cervical ripening. The methods have varied with the number of applications, dosage of PGE_2, and preparation of the gel. Currently there are a number of studies comparing intracervical versus vaginal application. However, none of the preparations has received Federal Drug Administration (FDA) approval for use in cervical ripening. Since the extra-amniotic application of PGE_2 gel is a reasonable use of an approved drug, the gel should be used only under institutional protocol to include continuous electronic fetal monitoring. Permission should be requested of the institutional review board of the hospital and results reviewed by peer review and quality assurance committees.

We have noted, as have others, that a significant number of patients (30 to 40 percent) do not achieve cervical ripening after one application of PGE_2 gel. Currently we are assessing the cervical condition every 6 hours and utilizing multiple dose administration of the gel. Our protocol follows.

After the Bishop's score is determined and informed consent is obtained from the patient, she is transferred to the labor and delivery suite. Electronic external fetal monitoring is applied, and 2 mg of PGE_2 mixed in hydroxyethyl cellulose gel is administered into the cervical canal via a soft plastic catheter. After the catheter is removed, the patient is observed for a 6- to 8-hour period. Detailed assessment of contractions and electronic monitoring of maternal and fetal health parameters are used throughout the observation period. The cervix is reevaluated, and if it is found to be unfavorable for induction (Bishop's score <4), a second dose of gel is given and a second 6- to 8-hour observation period initiated. The same procedure is performed at the end of the second observation period. Subsequent labor induction with continuous intravenous oxytocin is started if the patient is not in labor after the third dose or after obtaining a favorable Bishop's score. Amniotomy is performed as soon as possible, and oxytocin is continued until delivery. Approximately 80 percent of patients undergoing cervical ripening with PGE_2 gel experience uterine contractions and 30 to 40 percent actually go into labor. For this reason, patients undergoing cervical ripening with PGE_2 gel must be under close observation with continuous electronic fetal monitoring, especially when applying the gel to high-risk patients (e.g., those with uteroplacental insufficiency).

The following are contraindications for cervical ripening with PGE_2 gel:

1. previous uterine scan,
2. placenta previa,
3. abruptio placentae,
4. asthma,
5. sickle cell disease, and
6. fetal distress.

Most patients tolerate the gel without adverse reactions. An occasional patient may experience mild nausea, vomiting, and diarrhea.

INDUCTION OF LABOR

Prostaglandins, especially PGE_2 and PGF_{2a}, are effective agents for the induction of labor. The intravenous route was initially utilized, but other modes (i.e., intravaginal, buccal, and oral) have become more promising.

The intravenous infusion of prostaglandins has been shown by many investigators to be a successful method of labor induction. Prostaglandin infusions have no advantage over oxytocin in inducing labor near term except that they lack its antidiuretic effect. There is some evidence that they might have a slight advantage over oxytocin in inducing labor in preterm patients with an unripe cervix. In direct comparisons between PGF_{2a} and oxytocin infusions, the success of the induction depended upon the original state of the cervix. At any Bishop's score, there was no statistical difference in the success rate whether the subjects received oxytocin or PGF_{2a}.

Previous studies referring to the intravenous administration of prostaglandins for the induction of labor have reported success rates that varied from 40 to 100 percent with dosages from 0.025 μg per kilogram per minute to 40 μg per minute.

Prostaglandins are clearly at a disadvantage to oxytocin in some areas, particularly in the incidence of gastrointestinal side effects. Some reports also mention cases of fetal distress secondary to hypertonus, in addition to patient vomiting, vein phlebitis, and a transient skin rash.

It has also been suggested that more bleeding occurs in the PGF_{2a} group. There is no doubt that the occurrence of uterine hypertonus is a major obstetric hazard that has resulted in a significantly higher cesarean section rate for the prostaglandin group.

Although PGF_{2a} appears as safe as oxytocin in some biochemical studies and in the resultant neonatal conditions, the range of safety in terms of uterine response does not appear to be as wide as that of oxytocin.

Clearly the advantage of prostaglandins over oxytocin for induction of labor is the availability and apparent safety of prostaglandins given by routes other than the intravenous.

In some European centers, the routine method for induction of labor is with the use of PGE_2 vaginal suppositories. The patient is usually admitted in the evening and receives 3 mg of PGE_2 between 8:00 PM and 11:00 PM. The following morning, if the patient is considered to be in strong labor, no further medication is given. If she is not considered to be in established labor, she is given another 3 mg of PGE_2 between 7:00 AM and 8:00 AM. After the second dose, no further prostaglandin is given. Since PGE_2 vaginal suppositories are not approved by the FDA for labor induction, they should only be utilized after approval by the hospital's institutional review board and according to strict protocols and after informed consent. The 3-mg E_2 prostaglandin suppositories may be obtained by cutting 20 mg prostaglandin E_2 suppositories (Prostin E_2, Upjohn Company, Kalamazoo, MI) into 3-mm chips. Assays performed in several institutions have confirmed the homogeneous distribution of PGE_2 throughout the wax-based suppository. One of the most common criticisms against the use of PGE_2 vaginal suppositories for labor induction is that it is not as controllable or as easily reversible as oxytocin. In the occasional occurrence of hyperstimulation, an intravenous bolus of a beta-mimetic tocolytic agent may be useful.

In order to achieve cervical ripening and induce labor in term patients with a low Bishop's score, PGE_2 suspended in a viscous gel can be instilled into the cervical canal (intracervical application).

The mode of action of the locally administered PGE_2 on cervical tissue is not known. It has been recognized that cervical dilation during labor is an active process involving changes in cervical composition. In the cervix immediately after delivery, there is a slight increase in water, a marked decline in collagen and glycoprotein, and a marked increase in glycosaminoglycans. PGE_2 reduces the cervical connective tissue stiffness and also has a direct relaxing effect on the smooth muscle of the nonpregnant uterine cervix.

The dose of intracervical PGE_2 gel varies from 0.5 mg to 1 mg. The gel is prepared for clinical use by mixing K-Y jelly with an ethanol solution of PGE_2 (Upjohn). The intracervical application of PGE_2 gel is usually performed via a semiflexible nylon catheter. The gel is placed at the level of the internal os, and after the application, a diaphragm is inserted and the patient is maintained in bed and the fetus monitored electronically by continuous external cardiotocography. Once active labor is established, a surgical amniotomy should be performed and an internal pressure catheter inserted for more adequate fetal monitoring. In patients who are not successfully induced, a considerable ripening of the cervix is obtained, and in those patients a repeat dose of intracervical gel may be applied.

Another method for induction of labor is with the use of buccal PGE_2. This has an advantage over oral administration in that the tablets can be removed in the event of untoward side effects. Usually 0.5 mg buccal tablets of PGE_2 are inserted and increased hourly until adequate uterine stimulation is achieved or until a maximum single dose of 3 mg is reached. There is ample evidence that PGE_2 is absorbed by the buccal route, and the mean total dose used is similar to the oral dose necessary to induce labor.

Oral PGE_2 Tablets

Studies from the United States and Europe have suggested that the efficiency of oral PGE_2 tablets is at least as good as that of intravenous oxytocin. Oral PGE_2 is superior to oxytocin in patients with low Bishop's scores. The usual regimen for oral PGE_2 is as follows:

1. Begin with 0.5 mg and repeat in 1 hour.
2. After 2 hours, increase dose to 1 mg if required.
3. After 3 hours, increase dose to 1.5 mg as required.
4. Labor should be evaluated on an hourly basis. Once good labor is established, the dose is usually decreased to 0.5 mg.
5. At each subsequent hour, the dose is determined by the quality of labor.
6. The maximum dose allowed is 1.5 mg per hour. The most common side effects with this regimen are nausea, vomiting, and/or diarrhea, with approximately 35 percent of patients experiencing some type of gastrointestinal tract disturbance. In approximately 5 percent of the patients the gastrointestinal tract symptoms may be a significant contributing factor in discontinuing the induction with oral PGE_2.

POSTPARTUM HEMORRHAGE AND PROSTAGLANDINS

The current treatment of postpartum hemorrhage (PPH) secondary to uterine atony usually includes massage of the uterine fundus, bimanual compression of the uterus, and the parenteral administration of oxytocin or ergotamine or both. When these less invasive measures fail, ligating the uterine or hypogastric arteries may help control intractable bleeding. Fortunately, a less frequent occurrence is the need for an emergency hysterectomy.

More recently, emphasis has been placed on the use of prostaglandins for the medical management of PPH.

In 1976, prostaglandins were introduced into the obstetric literature and intramyometrial PGF_{2a} was first used in patients with PPH. Several reports since then have described the successful use of different forms and doses of prostaglandins. Significant success has been noted after the intramuscular injection of 200 μg of 15-methyl

PGF_{2a}, although repeated injections are required for the successful control of postpartum uterine atony. This analogue of PGF_{2a} is a much more potent uterotonic agent with a much longer duration of action than the parent compound. Common adverse effects include flushing, nausea, vomiting, and diarrhea. Mild rises in temperature and modest hypertension can be seen. Its use in hypertensive and asthmatic patients can be dangerous. Patients with PPH and chorioamnionitis have a high failure rate with the use of 15-methyl PGF_{2a}.

We are currently using 15-methyl PGF_{2a} in the management of severe PPH caused by uterine atony that is unresponsive to conventional therapy. In cases in which persistent uterine atony is noted at the time of cesarean section, we inject 1 mg of PGF_{2a} into the myometrium and subsequently follow with 250 μg injected intramuscularly and repeated at 2-hour intervals for a total of four doses. Patients who fail to respond obviously require surgical intervention.

More recently we have had marked success in patients with PPH due to uterine atony who did not respond to the injection of 15-methyl PGF_{2a} but responded extremely well after the insertion of a PGE_2 suppository via the rectal route.

INDUCTION OF ABORTION WITH PROSTAGLANDINS

The abortifacient properties of PGE_2 and PGF_{2a} are now well established.

The extra-amniotic and intra-amniotic administration of prostaglandins into the uterus has been shown to be a valuable alternative to other methods of inducing midtrimester abortion.

The administration of intravenous PGE_2 and PGF_{2a} is an effective method of inducing abortion in almost all cases. Because of the severity of the side effects, intravenous therapy is currently not utilized. The three most common forms of administration are:

1. vaginal suppositories of PGE_2 placed adjacent to the cervix,
2. PGE_2 or PGF_{2a} in gel inserted into the cervical canal via a soft plastic catheter,
3. intra-amniotic administration of PGF_{2a} or its analogue 15-methyl PGF_{2a}.

These three forms of administration stimulate the myometrium of the gravid uterus to contract in a manner that is similar to that seen in the term uterus during labor. These myometrial contractions are sufficient to produce evacuation of the products of conception from the uterus in the majority of cases.

Unfortunately, these three approaches are also capable of stimulating the smooth muscle of the gastrointestinal tract. This activity may be responsible for the vomiting and/or diarrhea that is not uncommon when these agents are used to terminate pregnancy. Often, repeated doses of the prostaglandin may be required in order to effect the expulsion of the fetus.

Vaginal Suppository of PGE_2

Indications for the use of PGE_2 vaginal suppositories are (1) termination of the pregnancy from the 12th through the 20th gestational week, and (2) evacuation of the uterine contents in the management of missed abortion or intrauterine fetal death up to 28 weeks of gestational age. Contraindications include (1) hypersensitivity to PGE_2, (2) acute pelvic inflammatory disease, and (3) active cardiac, pulmonary, renal, or hepatic disease.

Dosage—Administration

A suppository of 20 mg of PGE_2 should be inserted high into the vagina, after which the patient should remain in the supine position for 10 minutes. Additional administration should be at 3- to 5-hour intervals until the abortion occurs. The maximum number of suppositories used should be between 10 and 12.

Adverse reactions that are commonly observed include nausea, vomiting, and diarrhea (Table 3).

The use of PGE_2 and PGF_{2a} administered by extra-amniotic instillation for the induction of abortion has been associated with some success during the termination of second trimester pregnancies. Using PGE_2 gel, 93 percent of patients are aborted in 36 hours, and the mean abortion time is usually around 19 hours.

A 14 F gauge Foley's catheter or a flexible nylon catheter is introduced through the cervix with the aid of a bivalve speculum so that the inflatable balloon or tip of the catheter is just within the internal os. The extra-amniotic catheter is linked via a small bore connecting the tube and a three-way tap to a syringe, which is used for making the prostaglandin injections. An initial test dose of 50 μg of PGE_2 or 250 μg of PGF_{2a} is given. If no adverse effects occur in half an hour, a fully effective dose of 200 μg of PGE_2 or 750 μg PGF_{2a} is injected, and this dose usually is repeated at 2-hour intervals. An alternate method can be to administer the prostaglandin by means of an automatic infusion pump. Vital signs should be measured at least every 2 hours and close observation for serious side effects maintained.

With this technique, 72 percent of patients abort within 24 hours and 94 percent within 48 hours. The mean duration time is less, and the success rate is higher when PGE_2 is utilized. On average, multigravid patients abort more quickly than primigravidas.

The most common side effects, vomiting and diarrhea, are low, and the incidence of infection is not significant, especially if prophylactic antibiotics (tetracyclines) are utilized.

TABLE 3 Adverse Effects of PGE_2

Vomiting	Dyspnea
Diarrhea	Weakness
Nausea	Blurred vision
Fever	Cardiac arrhythmia
Headache	Uterine rupture
Chills	Rash
Chest pain	Paresthesia

Intra-amniotic injection of PGF_{2a} or its analogue is another method of abortion, which achieved some popularity in the past. This method has some advantages over amnioinfusion of hypertonic saline: the abortion process is faster, there is no direct adverse effect on blood coagulation as there is with hypertonic saline, and an accidental intravenous injection is much less likely to be fatal. Some problems with the use of PGF_{2a} intra-amniotically are:

1. gastrointestinal side effects are common,
2. transient fetal survival,
3. many patients require more than one dose,
4. retained tissue, and
5. infection and bleeding.

In approximately 10 percent of the cases transient fetal survival occurs, presenting serious ethical problems. The addition of 80 g of urea instilled into the amniotic sac along with 5 mg (5,000 μg) of PGF_{2a} tends to solve this problem. The mean time to abortion is 17.5 hours, and 80 percent of subjects abort by 24 hours. Often patients who fail to abort from intra-amniotic prostaglandin infusion go on to abort after only one or two doses of PGE_2 vaginal suppositories, which is currently one of the more popular methods for the termination of second trimester pregnancies.

SUGGESTED READING

Hayshi RH, Castillo MS, Noah ML. Management of severe postpartum hemorrhage due to uterine atony using an analogue of prostaglandin F_{2a}. Obstet Gynecol 1981; 58(4):426–429.

Ogburn PL Jr, Brenner WE. Physiologic actions and effects of prostaglandins. Current concepts. Kalamazoo, MI: Upjohn Company, 1981.

Tagaki S, Yoshida T, Togo Y. The effects of intramyometrial injections of prostaglandin F_{2a} on severe postpartum hemorrhage. Prostaglandins 1976; 12:565–579.

Thiery M, Amy JJ. Perinatal effects of prostaglandins used for induction of labor. In: Karim SMM, ed. Obstetric and gynecological uses of prostaglandins. Baltimore, MD: University Park Press, 1976:31.

INTRAUTERINE FETAL DEMISE

ALVIN LANGER, M.D.
WILLIAM M. HOLLS III, M.D.

The management of intrauterine fetal demise involves the question of when and how to empty the uterus of the nonviable products of conception as well as the evaluation and management of subsequent pregnancies. Often the first is not a particular problem since, in over 90 percent of cases, spontaneous expulsion occurs within 3 weeks of fetal death. Management depends upon adequately explaining, if possible, the cause of the intrauterine death and determining the risk of repetition, as well as dealing with the concerns of the patient and/or couple.

ETIOLOGY AND DIAGNOSIS

A variety of etiologies of intrauterine fetal demise may be found. They are of utmost importance in managing subsequent pregnancies.

Contemporary diagnosis of the condition has been greatly simplified by real-time ultrasonography. No longer must the physician rely upon absence of fetal heart sounds, the patient's report of no fetal movement, and serial measurements that show either no growth or an actual decrease in uterine size. At the present time, with sonographic evidence of morphologic changes in the fetus, and particularly with absence of fetal cardiac activity seen during the scan, the diagnosis can be made based on a single examination and can be demonstrated conclusively to the gravida and her mate.

NATURAL COURSE OF THE DISORDER

Since spontaneous onset of uterine contractions and expulsion of the fetus and placenta occurs so frequently with these cases, there is a question of whether the physician should intervene early and whether such intervention would increase the risk to the gravida. If spontaneous labor occurs, accompanied by expulsion of the fetus and what appears to be the complete placenta, then no further immediate therapy is necessary. A gross evaluation of the morphology of the fetus and placenta should always be carried out in an attempt to explain the etiology, and the physician should attempt to obtain parental permission for autopsy in order to obtain the maximum information. If the intrauterine death has been recent, one may be able to evaluate the fetal karyotype by culture of the skin or fascia lata. In most instances, the attempt should be made using those tissues rather than fetal blood, from which recovery of viable cells is rare.

The mother's emotional response to the loss may complicate the decision-making process as to when and how to empty the uterus. Many women, realizing that their fetus is no longer alive, suffer a sense of revulsion and wish to terminate the pregnancy as soon as possible. Decisions must be made by the patient and her physician after discussion of the pros and cons of each alternative. If she is adamant about immediate management, or in the event that spontaneous labor does not begin within approximately 4 weeks, steps may be taken to evacuate the uterus.

Physical risks to the gravida from carrying the dead fetus are minimal immediately after fetal death. Retention of the products after rupture of the membranes may predispose to intrauterine, and subsequent disseminated, infection, and rupture of the membranes is considered to be an indication to proceed.

If retention of the nonviable products of conception is allowed to continue for more than 4 or 5 weeks, there is the risk of disseminated intravascular coagulation (DIC), which results from the infusion of tissue thromboplastin into the maternal circulation from the degenerating products of conception. This initiates the extrinsic cascade of coagulation, which is virtually never seen before 5 weeks post fetal demise; it is not an acute process, but a chronic one. Rarely does DIC result in significant maternal hemorrhage. Since this is the most significant maternal complication of intrauterine death, monitoring for the condition must be done. In the absence of ruptured membranes or infection, and with no evidence of a developing coagulopathy, there is no urgency to intervene, provided that the woman is comfortable with the delay.

SURGICAL EVACUATION

Depending upon uterine size, surgical removal by dilation and evacuation (D & E) may be the procedure of choice. There is varying opinion as to maximum uterine size at which this procedure is acceptable, usually up to 20 to 24 weeks of gestation. Beyond that time it should not be attempted because of the possible difficulty in removing the larger fetal parts, which may result in an increased risk of incomplete removal and/or hemorrhage. Although in the appropriately chosen case D & E appears to be the safest means of intervention, it should not be attempted by the inexperienced operator since risks may then become considerable.

An unfavorable cervix may considerably increase the risk of a D & E, and some form of ripening procedure is indicated. The cervix must be dilated enough to accommodate a 14-mm vacurrette and a large ovum forceps. Any attempt at forceful mechanical dilation to this degree may be difficult and is associated with the risk of cervical laceration, with possible incompetence and/or extension into the uterine corpus. Rather, dilation should be accomplished slowly by intracervical insertion of tents from the dried cold water seaweed, laminaria japonica, which are hydrophilic and can gradually soften and dilate the cervical os to as much as 3 cm, thereby giving easy access to the products of conception. Besides applying moderate radial force that dilates the cervix, laminaria extracts water from the large molecules of proteoglycan that make up most of the composition of the cervix. The removal of the water diminishes the tension between the proteoglycan molecules, which results in cervical softening.

As laminaria tents cannot be completely sterilized, bacterial spores may remain even after treatment with ethylene oxide, which gives rise to concern about the potential of infection. This may be avoided by the alternate use of synthetic osmotic dilators made up of a polyvinyl alcohol sponge impregnated with magnesium sulfate, which draws water into the sponge. The action of these sponges is more rapid than laminaria, and they can achieve the necessary cervical dilation in about 4 hours, compared to up to 24 hours as required with laminaria tents.

After cleansing the cervix with an antiseptic solution, the tents are inserted so that the upper end just passes through the internal os. It is important to utilize as many laminaria as can fit and to pack them tightly into the cervix. They may be held in place by gauze sponges that are placed in the vagina. By the middle of the second trimester, the cervix should accommodate several tents, and after about 16 hours, additional tents may be added or the original tents may be removed and replaced by a greater number of fresh tents. Although there may be slight cramping associated with the insertion of the tent, generally no anesthesia is necessary. Paracervical block may be utilized if requested. Complications of laminaria include displacement into either vagina or uterus. In the latter case, it is important to completely remove the laminaria from the uterus at the time of evacuation. Herniation and rupture of the membranes may also occur. This is not an indication to remove the tent, but management should continue as planned.

After satisfactory dilatation of the cervix, a vacuum suction is used to bring the products of conception into the lower part of the uterus, using a 14-mm vacuum canula. At that time, intravenous oxytocin is administered in order to initiate contractions; this makes the uterine wall firmer and less vulnerable to perforation. Large fetal parts are then removed using a large ovum forceps. Simultaneous real-time sonography may be used to lessen the chances of uterine perforation and to provide information as to any remaining products of conception. The procedure may be performed under general or paracervical block anesthesia with heavy sedation. Alternately, vacuum suction and ovum forceps are used to remove the fetal parts. At the end of the procedure, sharp curettage is performed to make certain that all products of conception are removed.

Complications of the procedure increase with gestational age and include hemorrhage, infection, uterine injury, and cervical incompetence.

Hysterotomy or hysterectomy are not usually acceptable or necessary procedures for removal of a dead fetus. They are rarely used and only when other medical indications require the procedure to be performed regardless of the fetal demise.

MEDICAL EVACUATION

Intravenous oxytocin is unlikely to be effective in the initiation of labor for delivery of a dead fetus except very late in pregnancy when the uterus contains an adequate number of oxytocin receptors. In later pregnancy, when cervical ripening has occurred, it is the method of choice, with induction of labor being similar to that with a live fetus. The maternal risks of induction, such as uterine rupture, are unchanged from the usual induction.

Numerous substances have been injected intra-amniotically to initiate uterine contractions; these include hypertonic saline, urea, and prostaglandin F2-alpha. Because of the availability of less invasive methods with fewer side effects, these techniques have largely fallen into disuse. They have been replaced by intravaginal administration of suppositories that contain prostaglandin E2.

Prostaglandins are 20-carbon compounds found in numerous body tissues, the highest concentration being in seminal fluid. They are also released from the amnion and decidua to act upon specific cellular receptors in the myometrium. They are formed by the action of the enzyme prostaglandin synthetase on the precursor arachidonic acid. Although the uterus is slightly less sensitive to prostaglandins early in pregnancy, prostaglandins that are administered by means of injection or vaginal suppositories can reliably produce uterine contractions and expulsion of the products of conception at virtually any stage of pregnancy. There is no sudden increase in responsiveness at the end of pregnancy as there is with oxytocin.

Among the advantages of removal of the products of conception by prostaglandin induction of uterine contractions is that the fetus can usually be removed intact for morphologic examination and perhaps genetic evaluation. The technique also has fewer complications than surgical procedures and is even safe for most women with medical disorders. Prostaglandins are contraindicated in women who have a hypersensitivity to prostaglandins, active pelvic inflammatory disease, a previous vertical scar in the uterine corpus, or placenta previa. In the patient with hypertension, diabetes, cardiovascular disease, asthma, peptic ulcers, renal disease, jaundice, or any uterine scar with a nonlongitudinal lie, prostaglandins should be used with caution.

In 1973, the Food and Drug Administration (FDA) approved the use of prostaglandins for treatment of intrauterine fetal death up to 28-weeks gestation. Their use for this indication was recommended in 1979 by the American College of Obstetricians and Gynecologists. Although their initial use was by intra-amniotic injection of prostaglandin F2-alpha, currently the use of prostaglandin E2 suppositories is more practical and equally effective. The suppositories do not involve an invasive procedure, and the E2 form is without some of the adverse side effects of prostaglandin F2-alpha, such as bronchoconstriction and hypertension. They are not generally used beyond 28 weeks. At that time, if the cervix is favorable, intravenous oxytocin is the treatment of choice, whereas, if it is unfavorable, expectant therapy may be continued until cervical ripening occurs.

In a patient in whom the cervix is not ripe, the onset of effective uterine contractions and expulsion of the fetus may be somewhat delayed, and the cervical resistance may lead to sacculation of the lower uterine segment or even annular detachment of the cervix. Prostaglandin E2 can be used to ripen the cervix. Either a quarter of a 20-mg suppository may be inserted into the vagina, and the insertion repeated at 4-hour intervals, or 2 mg of prostaglandin E2 gel may be introduced into the cervical canal via a polyethylene catheter. Since the gel is not marketed in the United States, it must be made by the hospital pharmacy by melting a 20-mg suppository and completely mixing it with 50 ml of a surgical lubricant. A 5-ml aliquot contains the necessary 2 mg of gel. Usually insertion at bedtime can result in ripening and successful induction the following morning. The patient should be observed in the hospital overnight and should be kept well hydrated with an electrolyte solution because of the vasodilatation that may be produced by the prostaglandin.

The method of action in cervical ripening does not depend upon uterine activity, but upon biochemical changes within the cervix. Although the exact mechanism of action is not known, it appears that dermatan and chondroitin sulfate, which are tightly bound to collagen fibers in the unripe cervix, are separated from the collagen, making it less rigid and ultimately degrading it.

After cervical ripening, the suppositories are inserted high into the posterior vaginal fornix. Since the prostaglandin is somewhat thermolabile, the suppositories should be kept refrigerated until ready for use. An additional 20-mg suppository may be inserted every 3 to 5 hours, depending upon the uterine response. Generally the fetus is expelled within 24 hours with a mean time of approximately 16 hours. Concurrent use of intravenous oxytocin is not recommended since it may increase the risk of uterine rupture or cervical laceration.

As prostaglandins are powerful stimulants of contraction of the smooth muscle of the alimentary tract, vomiting and diarrhea are common side effects. These side effects may be prevented to a large degree by administration of an antidiarrheal agent, such as diphenoxylate hydrochloride 5 mg orally, and an antiemetic, such as prochlorperazine 10 mg, about 1 hour prior to the insertion of the first suppository; this is repeated as necessary. Since prostaglandin E2 produces a transient pyrexia caused by a direct action on the hypothalamic thermoregulatory centers, acetaminophen 300-mg rectal suppositories are used to control fever in excess of 38° C. Demerol or paracervical block may be to used to alleviate pain.

After prostaglandin-induced fetal expulsion, there is a risk of placental retention. If the placenta is not spontaneously expelled, it may be possible to remove it using sponge forceps; however, a dilation and curettage (D & C) may be necessary in order to complete the procedure.

Other analogues of prostaglandin or methods of administration may be effective in emptying the uterus, but the vaginal suppositories are the simplest and do not have the increased risks of infection and hemorrhage that are associated with an invasive procedure. Oral prostaglandins are readily absorbed from the gastrointestinal tract, but are impractical because high doses are necessary and because there are significant gastrointestinal side effects, particularly with prostaglandin F2-alpha. The intramuscular injection of prostaglandin E2 or F2-alpha causes local irritation, and the medication is rapidly metabolized after absorption. However, a 15-methyl analogue of prostaglandin F2-alpha has increased potency and duration of action and does not cause local irritation. It is commercially available, but has been used mainly in the management of postpartum hemorrhage because of its high incidence of gastrointestinal stimulation and because it is a potent vasoconstrictor, which predisposes the patient to hypertension. Extra-amniotic administration of prostaglandin has been used mainly for cervical ripening, and the technique requires more expertise.

DISSEMINATED INTRAVASCULAR COAGULATION

Since the coagulopathy, which results from the gradual infusion of tissue thromboplastin from the degenerating fetus, takes some time to develop, it is not a consideration shortly after fetal death. However, when the diagnosis of fetal demise is made, a complete blood count and baseline coagulation studies, which include a platelet count, fibrin split products, fibrinogen level, prothrombin time, and activated partial thromboplastin time, should be obtained. As long as the patient retains the products of conception, monitoring should be repeated at least weekly. In the event that the laboratory studies ultimately show evidence of a coagulopathy, then immediate steps should be taken to interrupt the coagulation process, and the uterus should be emptied as soon as there is replacement of the coagulation factors. Prior to any evacuation of the uterus, there should be screening for a coagulation defect because the first sign that it has occurred may be a severe postpartum hemorrhage.

The initial changes seen in DIC are an increase in fibrin split products and a decrease in fibrinogen levels. Later there is an increase in prothrombin time (PT) and partial thromboplastin time (PTT). The platelet count may fall, but the fall is less marked than that of fibrinogen levels. Fibrinogen and platelet levels may not fall if the liver and bone marrow respond sufficiently to compensate for their consumption, and the only evidence of a coagulopathy may be an elevation of fibrin split products to greater than 10 mg per deciliter. This elevation indirectly confirms the diagnosis of DIC by detecting the secondary production of response fibrinolysins. During the process of intravascular coagulation, factors V and VIII are also reduced, but their measurement is difficult, and the prothrombin and activated partial thromboplastin time are used as determinants of decreases in those factors. A more sensitive test is measurement of antithrombin III, the major in vivo inhibitor of thrombin generation, which is consumed during intravascular coagulation. However, its measurement is much more difficult, and the simpler tests usually suffice.

The patient with intravascular coagulation may bleed from multiple sites and may be hypotensive because of blood loss. However, more common than fulminant cases are low grade disseminated intravascular coagulation cases in which the patient is able to adequately compensate and rarely bleeds dramatically. A low grade coagulopathy may not persist as long as the fetus remains in utero, but may resolve spontaneously after several weeks of anticoagulant therapy. It is preferable to empty the uterus when this entity is encountered without awaiting spontaneous resolution.

Management should be aggressive. If the patient is compensated, there is only a small risk of hemostatic failure, and the fetus should be delivered as expeditiously as possible. If she has decompensated, then it is imperative to minimize the risk of hemorrhage by restoring the coagulation factors to hemostatic levels. If she is in labor, blood component therapy is essential. Fibrinogen may be replaced using cryoprecipitate which is preferable to fresh frozen plasma, as fresh frozen plasma adds sufficient colloid, to predispose to circulatory overload. Ten units of cryoprecipitate can raise the fibrinogen level about 50 mg per deciliter, and the goal should be to bring the fibrinogen levels to the range of 200 to 300 mg per deciliter. Platelets usually do not decrease below a count of 60,000, and their administration is usually not necessary.

If the patient is not in labor, an intravenous infusion of 5,000 units of heparin is initiated, followed by 5,000 to 10,000 units every 12 hours, which can be modified by the response as measured by serial coagulation studies. When the fibrinogen is in the range of 200 to 300 mg per deciliter, the platelets are greater than 60,000, and the activated PTT is not greater than 2.5 times that of the control (which usually can be accomplished within 24 to 48 hours) then heparin is stopped. The evacuation is begun 6 hours after stopping the heparin since the effect of the heparin lasts only 4 hours.

A singleton pregnancy should then be evacuated, whereas a twin pregnancy should be continued until such time as delivery of the living twin is indicated. Heparin should not be given in doses sufficient to increase the activated partial thromboplastin time, since over a prolonged period of administration, it may predispose to osteoporosis.

Multiple Pregnancy

If one fetus of a twin pregnancy dies and the pregnancy is at term, then in the event of a coagulopathy either immediate prior-to-labor heparinization or intrapartum replacement of coagulation factors should be instituted. If the fetus is not mature, then heparinization and temporization (as previously described) may be necessary. The surviving twin may have a coagulopathy if there is an anastomosis between the placentas and resultant embolization of thromboplastic material from the dead into the living twin. Such a state of affairs is only encountered in monozygotic twins and can result in renal cortical necrosis or multicystic encephalomalacia in the surviving twin.

PSYCHOLOGIC SUPPORT

The patient should be allowed to grieve the loss of her child with the help of her physician and support of her family. In spite of the fact that prior to birth there is often close maternal bonding with the fetus, until recent years, the management of intrauterine fetal death has often been regarded as different from that of neonatal death. Frequently the mother was not shown the fetus or allowed to hold it, and there was no funeral; consequently, the mother was unable to go through an appropriate mourning period. Family and friends often attempt to minimize the loss by telling her that she can replace the fetus, and she may conclude that she is not entitled to grieve. Some mothers may feel guilt and may doubt their femininity for having failed to produce a living baby. Often when the etiology of the fetal demise cannot be determined, the mother may blame herself or other family members. When a diagnosis of the fetal demise has been proven, the parents often go through a stage of shock. The latter is followed by a period of searching for answers, which may be associated with guilt and anger. Eventually the fact that the pregnancy is unsuccessful is accepted, although this may occur some time after the fetal death. During the early stages, conflict between the parents may occur because of differences in their grieving processes.

The physician may help the parents cope with the grieving process by recognizing his or her own feelings and difficulty in discussing the subject. As far as possible, the patient should be allowed to express her anger and participate in the decision as to how and when the pregnancy is terminated. During the labor process, a support person is helpful, and enough medication to relieve pain without oversedation should be prescribed, if desired. The parents should be allowed to see and hold their baby if they wish and to arrange a funeral if this is desired. A request for an autopsy should be made at the earliest possible time after the diagnosis of fetal demise has been made. Any positive findings should be thoroughly discussed so as to alleviate any sense of guilt on the part of the parents. They should be given the option of whether they wish a private room. The nurses assigned to the mother should be skilled in handling perinatal death. Inappropriate references to a living baby must be avoided. Discussion of either sterilization or subsequent pregnancies is best avoided in the puerperium. Finally, support groups, if available locally, may be extremely beneficial to the parents in the ensuing weeks.

Abnormal grief, which may be characterized by no apparent reaction, by agitation, or by extreme anger and hostility may require psychiatric consultation.

MANAGEMENT OF SUBSEQUENT PREGNANCIES

In the management of subsequent pregnancies after a stillbirth, it is critical to identify, whenever possible, the cause of the stillbirth. No specific cause for fetal demise can be found in the majority of cases, although this is less likely if a thorough postmortem examination has been performed in conjunction with histopathologic studies of the placenta. It has been demonstrated that the autopsy findings fail to substantiate the presumptive diagnosis as to the cause of the fetal death in over 10 percent of cases.

More than half of the stillbirths occur in infants weighing greater than 1,500 g, which is well into the range of neonatal viability. Almost half of the stillbirths appear to be related to hypoxia, defined in part by evidence of intrauterine growth retardation, cord complications, maternal hypertension, placental insufficiency, and postmaturity. The single largest component of hypoxia related to stillbirth is intrauterine growth retardation, which is evident in about 26 percent of cases. Hypertension is noted in about 17 percent of hypoxia-related stillbirths. Only about 19 percent of stillbirths cannot be classified as to their etiology.

A study of 337 patients referred for antepartum fetal heart rate testing in a subsequent pregnancy revealed that 52 percent had a high-risk indication for testing in the current pregnancy as well as in the previous pregnancy, which terminated with a stillbirth. Hypertension was noted in 25 percent of the patients, diabetes mellitus in 21 percent, and intrauterine growth retardation in 9 percent. The etiology of the previous stillbirth was not defined, but the presence of such a high percentage of "chronic" utero-placental problems in subsequent pregnancies is significant.

With the availability of such information, the management of a subsequent pregnancy is strongly dependent on the recurrent risk factors for the associated pregnancy complications. Placental abruption has an approximately 9 percent recurrence risk, ten times the primary occurrence rate. Severe preeclampsia has an approximately 12 percent and eclampsia a 1 percent recurrence risk. The recurrence risk for chronic hypertension and diabetes must be considered to be 100 percent. Although not addressed in stillbirth studies due to the lower prevalence, other chronic medical problems such as systemic lupus erythematosus must also be considered to have a 100 percent recurrence.

In subsequent pregnancies, basic obstetrical management should not be ignored, and treatable risk factors should be addressed. These include chronic hypertension and social factors, such as alcohol and tobacco use, as well as analysis of the work and home environment, so as to remove stressful conditions. Though placental abruption is difficult to prevent, its association with cigarette smoking should increase the physicians efforts to have the patient discontinue this habit, particularly when the previous pregnancy was complicated by abruption. The presence of hypertension is also significant in that in one study the general risk for recurrent abruption was only 4 percent in patients without increased blood pressure, less than half the general recurrence risk.

The association of previous intrauterine demise with growth retardation in a subsequent pregnancy makes sonographic monitoring of any subsequent pregnancy mandatory. Sonographic studies must include complete assessment of all parameters of fetal growth, including head and abdominal circumference, long bone measurements, evaluation of placental size and grading, as well as assessment of amniotic fluid volume. Serial measurements of fetal growth should be plotted on a standard chart as acute changes in fetal mensuration are easier to appreciate from a graph. If the head or abdominal circumference deviate from previous growth percentiles, a cause must be sought, and treatment, which may include early delivery, should be instituted.

The mainstay of fetal assessment still remains antepartum fetal heart rate testing. Patients with previous stillbirth who are found to be hypertensive or who present with clinical intrauterine growth retardation are at significantly higher risk for a positive contraction stress test than are those without a prior stillbirth. In one study using aggressive antepartum fetal heart monitoring, there was no apparent increase in risk of a stillbirth in those patients with current risk factors and a previous stillbirth compared with those with the same risk factors and no stillbirth history. Those patients with a history of stillbirth were found to have a higher incidence of respiratory distress syndrome due to earlier intervention. Thus, general management plans can be determined for the subsequent pregnancy of a patient with a history of stillbirth. The latter should begin with a diligent search for the cause of the previous stillbirth. Prior to a subsequent pregnancy, the maternal medical condition should be assessed and all chronic diseases evaluated and treated. If she is diabetic, rigid control of blood sugar should be instituted before the next pregnancy. Adverse social habits such as smoking, alcohol and illicit drug use, and unsatisfactory dietary habits should be addressed, and an attempt should be made to eliminate them in any subsequent pregnancy. Once pregnant, the patient should be followed closely. Alterations in maternal homeostasis, whether caused by preexisting disease or pregnancy related problems, should be immediately addressed. Serial ultrasonographic studies should be used to elicit the fetal growth pattern, and antepartum fetal heart rate testing should be initiated early in the gestation, particularly in those patients at risk for uteroplacental insufficiency. Though it is psychologically impossible to ignore the history of stillbirth, iatrogenic prematurity must be avoided. However, a mild increase in the incidence of the respiratory distress syndrome, particularly in the hypertensive patient or intrauterine growth retarded fetus, may be acceptable in order to circumvent a further stillbirth. Biophysical and/or biochemical indications for intervention should be established and recorded. Preparation for delivery should include the availability of persons skilled in neonatal resuscitation.

During the pregnancy, the psychological needs of the patient and her family must not be ignored. The patient requires greater reassurance as to the health of the fetus during the pregnancy, and the obstetrician must be alert to an increase in stress at anniversaries of critical periods in the prior pregnancy. Any particular situation may be differently perceived by the patient. There is a tendency for the patient with a history of previous stillbirth not to demonstrate the degree of bonding to the unborn child that is usually observed in the mother-to-be. However, this usually resolves with a successful outcome of the pregnancy. It must be realized that sophisticated antepartum assessment is a two-edged sword. It may well not have the reassuring effect that would be hoped for in the patient who is still engaged in a protective mechanism of not relying on a successful outcome to the pregnancy until it is proven by delivery of a live, healthy baby. These problems require a sympathetic, caring, and technically competent obstetrician.

SUGGESTED READING

Hovatta O, Lipasti A, Rapola J, Karjalainen O. Causes of stillbirth: a clinicopathological study of 243 patients. Br J Obstet Gynecol 1983; 90:691–696.

LaFerla JJ, Good RS. Helping patients cope with pregnancy loss. Contemp Obstet Gynecol 1985; 25:107–115.

Morrison I, Olsen RN. Weight-specific stillbirths and associated causes of death: an analysis of 765 stillbirths. Am J Obstet Gynecol 1985; 152:975–980.

Stubblefield PG. Surgical techniques of uterine evacuation in first and second trimester abortion. Clin Obstet Gynecol 1986; 13:53–70.

BREECH PRESENTATION

J. PETER VAN DORSTEN, M.D.
RICHARD C. DICKSON, M.D.

Nothing in obstetrics has provoked more controversy in the last decade than the issue of proper management of breech presentation. Consumer advocates, bureaucrats, lawyers, and health care professionals have hotly debated the route of delivery for the breech fetus. Current practice has been forged more by emotion and sentiment than by scientific data. Nevertheless, today, 70 to 90 percent of all breeches are delivered by cesarean section. Accordingly, there may not be enough experience in residency programs to train future obstetricians adequately in the art of gentle vaginal breech delivery. Recent evidence suggests that a reduction in perinatal morbidity and mortality has not followed the rise in the cesarean delivery rate. Perhaps the abandonment of the vaginal breech delivery has been premature! In this chapter, we will review the history of breech presentation and the factors that have shaped our current practices.

Approximately 3 to 4 percent of all labors are complicated by breech presentation. In the premature setting, the likelihood of breech presentation becomes even greater: 7 percent at 32 weeks and 25 percent or more at less than 28 weeks. The frank breech (flexion at the hips and extension at the knees) accounts for 48 to 73 percent of all breeches. The complete breech (flexion at both the hips and the knees) constitutes 5 to 12 percent and the footling breech (extension at one or both hips), 12 to 38 percent. The more premature the fetus, the greater the likelihood of the footling presentation, which complicates the majority of labors with the very low birth weight breech (less than 1,500 g). This latter point becomes important because the risk of a prolapsed cord increases from 0.5 percent with the frank breech to 18 percent with the footling breech.

Factors predisposing to breech presentation relate to one of three causes: abnormal uterine shape, excessive fetal mobility, or interference in fetopelvic relationships. There are maternal factors such as age, parity, uterine or pelvic masses, and contracted pelvis. Fetal conditions may also predispose: polyhydramnios, congenital anomalies (e.g., anencephaly or hydrocephaly), multiple gestation, macrosomia, and prematurity. Placenta previa or premature rupture of the membranes is also associated with breech presentation.

The diagnosis of breech presentation is often suspected by abdominal examination in which the ballotable cephalic pole is appreciated in the uterine fundus. Leopold's maneuvers should be performed at each prenatal visit; if the typical cephalic pole is not appreciated at the pelvic inlet, a confirmatory vaginal examination should be performed near term. Today's patient does not like to be surprised by a breech presentation during labor. As we will discuss later in the chapter, multiple options are available to the patient with a breech presentation if the diagnosis is made in the antepartum period. Decisions cannot be carefully weighed when the diagnosis of breech presentation is made during labor. When breech presentation cannot be excluded by careful abdominal and vaginal examination near term, ultrasonography is indicated. The diagnosis must be suspected when there is an obstetric history of a previous breech presentation; 20 percent of patients with intrapartum breech presentations give such a prior history.

Nowhere in obstetrics does the obstetrician face such a dilemma as with an intrapartum breech presentation. So many variables must be quickly entertained: type of breech, possible hyperextension of the fetal head, presence of labor, status of the membranes, estimated fetal weight, estimated gestational age, cervical dilatation and effacement, station of the presenting part, presence of fetal anomalies (possibly incompatible with life), possibility of a coexisting placenta previa, possibility of a prolapsed cord, adequacy of the bony pelvis, and possibility of a twin configuration. And while this data analysis is under way, the medicolegal specter casts its shadow on the process. Certainly, the older literature supports and confirms the obstetrician's concern about the dilemma of breech presentation. A recent review speaks to a 16-fold increase in intrapartum fetal death, a 3- to 8-fold increase in intrapartum asphyxia, a 5- to 20-fold increase in risk of cord prolapse, a 13-fold increase in birth trauma, an 8.5 percent incidence of arrest of the aftercoming head, a 5.0 percent incidence of hyperextension of the fetal head (accompanied by a 21 percent risk of spinal cord injury with attempted vaginal breech delivery), a 6 to 18 percent risk of coexisting fetal anomalies, and a 16 to 30 percent incidence of prematurity. The older literature has suggested that there is increased morbidity and mortality in the breech delivered vaginally, even when the higher risk of prematurity and congenital anomalies is excluded. It has been suggested that this risk can be brought into proper alignment if cesarean section is the mode of delivery. No wonder the obstetrician has responded with a cesarean delivery rate that approaches 100 percent for intrapartum breech presentation. As the overall cesarean rate has doubled and tripled over the past decade, those done for breech presentations have accounted for 15 to 20 percent of the increase. Of all cesarean deliveries, breech presentation accounts for 25 to 30 percent.

Who has expressed concern about this trend toward almost universal cesarean delivery for breech presentation? Those who fund the more expensive procedure and hospitalization care. Those who are subjected to greater maternal morbidity and those who may be condemned to repeat cesarean should also care. Analysis of the literature gives us some indication of how we arrived at the present state of affairs, how steeped we are in the current practices, and how to manage the different scenarios encountered with breech presentation.

PRETERM BREECH PRESENTATION

The management plans for the preterm breech presentation have been colored by confusing and often conflicting data. In addition to the risks of malpresentation, the preterm fetus faces the risks inherent in premature delivery. To the practicing obstetrician with a sincere desire to do what is in the best interest of *both* patients, a review of the current literature often contributes to his or her confusion. In addition to drawing conflicting conclusions, careful review of the data collection or data management or both more often than not raises questions as to the validity of the conclusions. Much of the data is of pediatric origin, and important obstetric and medical factors are often ignored. The following is a discussion of our management plan of the preterm breech presentation, along with the rationale for our decisions.

The combination of prematurity and breech presentation is not an unusual event; in fact, in several studies the most common predisposing factor to breech presentation seemed to be prematurity. Approximately 20 to 30 percent of premature infants present in the breech position, with the percentage decreasing as the gestation advances. In the preterm infant, the frank breech is the most common, followed by the incomplete and footling breech. However, in infants weighing less than 2,000 g, two-thirds present in the non-frank position.

During labor, with continued descent of the breech fetus, the umbilical cord becomes more vulnerable. Furthermore, the irregular presenting part of the non-frank breech predisposes to cord prolapse. Cord accidents are more common in breech fetuses in general, and the preterm fetus appears less able than the term fetus to withstand potential acidosis. The circumferences of the abdomen, thorax, and shoulder are all smaller than the head circumference until approximately 36-weeks gestation. The soft parts may traverse the lower uterine segment and cervix without incident only to have the aftercoming head entrapped by the cervix. The subsequent trauma to the mother and fetus in efforts to effect delivery can be appreciable, even fatal in the case of the fetus. Furthermore, hypoxia alone may be sufficient to cause lifelong sequelae.

Prior to 36-weeks gestation, the germinal matrix lines the fetal intracranial ventricles. This loose stroma with its rich capillary network is vulnerable to subsequent intraventricular hemorrhage (IVH). Hypoxia and acidosis further the risk of advanced grades of IVH with potential hydrocephalus and psychomotor retardation. The true influence of vaginal breech delivery on IVH is complicated by the fact that IVH has been documented in utero prior to labor. It has also been shown that, in the low birth weight fetus greater than 29-weeks gestation, the incidence of IVH in the breech infant is approximately three times that experienced by vertex infants. This occurred even when all were delivered via cesarean delivery. Cesarean delivery, therefore, does not guarantee avoidance of IVH.

Recent studies indicate that certain preterm breeches may be delivered as safely by the vaginal as the abdominal route. When evaluating patients who present with the preterm breech, it should be remembered that these fetuses have a higher than expected rate of serious congenital anomalies, up to 6 to 18 percent. Ultrasonography may identify anomalies that would modify treatment.

Birth weight appears to be the most important determining factor in perinatal outcome of the preterm breech, followed closely by the type of breech. Ultrasound-derived estimated fetal weight and composition of the breech, therefore, constitute the cornerstones of our management.

MANAGEMENT OF LOW BIRTH WEIGHT INFANTS WITH BREECH PRESENTATION (1,500 to 2,500 g)

There is little evidence in the recent literature that supports routine abdominal delivery for breech infants over 1,500 g. However, the risk of cord compression may be unacceptably high in presentations other than the frank and the complete breech. The risk of prolapsed cord ranges up to 18 percent, and many such instances occur late in labor after commitment to vaginal delivery. We agree that the complete breech is similar to the frank breech in regard to cord prolapse. Footling breech presentations, however, are managed by cesarean once careful assessment has been made by ultrasonography to identify malformations incompatible with life.

In addition to the search for serious malformations, careful ultrasound assessment is made to ascertain estimated fetal weight. Prior to assigning the patient to a trial of labor, a minimum fetal weight of 2,000 g is mandatory. This assures a minimum weight of 1,500 g, allowing for the possibility of the intrinsic 20 percent error with ultrasound-derived estimation. In addition, attention is directed to the angle from the axis of the fetal spine to the base of the skull. It must be clear that the angle does not exceed 105 degrees; if not, the patient undergoes abdominal x-ray examinations for radiologic confirmation. Avoiding the deflexed head, or "stargazing breech," is just as important here as in the term infant. In the patient with adequate clinical pelvimetry, x-ray pelvimetry is deemed unnecessary in the low birth weight setting.

The fetus is monitored by electronic fetal monitoring. One must be prepared for prompt operative delivery if there is suspected fetal distress or an abnormal labor pattern. If membranes are ruptured, the direct electrode is applied. If membranes are intact, indirect fetal monitoring is usually sufficient. Advantages of artificial rupture of the membranes for application of the direct system may be negated by the risk of cord prolapse and loss of the possible benefit of the cushion effect provided by an intact amniotic sac. If spontaneous rupture of the membranes occurs, the patient should be examined immediately to detect prolapse of the umbilical cord.

The preterm fetus in general, and the breech fetus in particular, seem to be more susceptible to stress and to develop acidosis more quickly than their cephalic counterparts. As with cephalic presentation, fetal pH assessment may be used to further define a confusing heart rate pattern. Samples are obtained in the usual fashion from the presenting buttock between contractions and interpreted the same as scalp samples.

As time permits, conduction anesthesia is used as our method of choice when considering a vaginal breech delivery. Not only does the regional block provide excellent pain relief and muscle relaxation, but the strong bearing-down and expulsive reflexes are abolished as well. In addition, a controlled, calm atmosphere promotes patient compliance.

The patient is taken to the delivery room earlier than usual, accompanied by fetal monitoring at all times. Neonatal intensive care and anesthesia personnel have previously been notified and are in attendance. Even when epidural anesthesia is used, the possibility of a sudden event requiring general anesthesia and/or uterine relaxation remains.

The proper technique of breech delivery involves patience and constant monitoring. A minimum of two obstetricians must be in attendance; a third person is useful to guide the aftercoming fetal head into the pelvis, thus maintaining flexion and presenting the smallest fetal diameter to the pelvis. Ideally, membranes are not ruptured until the last possible moment to gain the potential advantage of the cushion effect and perhaps to minimize cord compression. A generous episiotomy is performed, generally in the midline. The breech is allowed to deliver spontaneously to the umbilicus, at which time support of the body becomes necessary. It has been shown that up to 3.5 minutes can elapse without compromising Apgar scores in the breech delivery, and efforts to accelerate delivery at this point can lead to deflexion of the head or development of a nuchal arm or both. Nuchal arm complications are difficult to reduce and may lead to excessive rates of brachial plexus injury.

It is crucial not to allow excessive elevation of the body above the horizontal plane, as significant stretching of the cervical vertebrae and spinal cord injury may result. A warm towel is wrapped around the fetus to facilitate manipulation and provide a supporting sling. As the scapulae emerge, gentle rotation will bring the respective shoulder anteriorly to aid in the delivery of each humerus. In most cases the aftercoming head may be assisted in delivery by the well-known Mauriceau-Smellie-Veit maneuver, with concurrent suprapubic pressure by an assistant. Frequently Piper's forceps are used in the low birth weight breech, since even moderate traction should be avoided in an effort to effect delivery. Although it has been suggested that all breeches benefit from routine use of Piper's forceps, we do not feel that the routine use of forceps in this weight group provides a distinct advantage.

Finally, after suctioning the oropharyngeal airway and handing the infant to the neonatal personnel, umbilical cord blood gas studies are carefully obtained. Separate arterial and venous samples are preferable. Not only do these parameters help the neonatal staff in treatment guidelines, but the values may serve as present and future evidence of the true metabolic condition of the fetus at birth. Apgar scores are known to correlate poorly with true metabolic status and prognosis in the low birth weight fetus.

As is obvious from the above discussion, we do not feel that *all* low birth weight breech infants above 1,500 g can be safely delivered vaginally. However, the corollary is also true, that the majority *can* be safely delivered vaginally by proper selection and adequate documentation of normal progress of labor.

MANAGEMENT OF VERY LOW BIRTH WEIGHT INFANTS WITH BREECH PRESENTATION (<1,500 g)

Decisions in this group (<1,500 g) are now becoming increasingly more complex as smaller infants become salvageable. The data regarding the best mode of delivery in this weight group are again conflicting and subject to differences in interpretation. At least one randomized trial to determine the "best" treatment was terminated, as it was discovered that almost half of the eligible patients were withdrawn by attending physicians in favor of cesarean delivery.

At the current state of knowledge and skills, we feel that infants with estimated weight by ultrasound examination between 750 and 2,000 g should be delivered abdominally. Although the survival rate in our nursery for 750 to 1,499 g infants is 89 percent, the rate drops to 32 percent (of 22 patients) in the 500 to 750 g group. The patient and her husband are counseled in detail regarding the outlook for any infant below 750 g, and we tend not to recommend cesarean delivery for those infants.

Incision

The type of uterine incision is also subject to discussion. The low vertical incision is popular, but potential consequences in subsequent pregnancies include "impaired uterus," uterine rupture, and iatrogenic premature delivery. Others feel that the low vertical incision is quite safe and necessary. The low transverse cervical incision may not provide room for safe delivery, especially in a thick, undeveloped lower uterine segment. An alternate incision has been recommended, described as "upward curved transverse" over the lower uterine segment designed to provide subsequent strength.

We individualize each patient at the time of surgery, preferring the low transverse curved incision in the presence of a well-defined lower uterine segment. In the absence of a well-defined lower uterine segment, the low vertical is the incision of choice.

In addition to types of incisions, different *methods* of delivery of the very low birth weight fetus have been described in efforts to promote as atraumatic a delivery as possible. An example is the "splint" technique, in which the surgeon's forearm is inserted into the uterus to "splint" the torso, while cupping the fetal head in the palm of the hand. Although this procedure seemed to work well, we cannot attest to its efficacy.

We consider continuous epidural analgesia to be the method of choice for cesarean delivery. General anesthesia has been implicated in a two- to threefold rate of neonatal depression over epidural. The problem occasionally encountered with conduction analgesia is lack of rectus muscle relaxation, but with an adequate level this is not a problem. The patient should be placed in a lateral tilt position to avoid hypotension.

TERM BREECH PRESENTATION

The management of the patient with a term breech presentation likewise remains controversial. Despite modern reports that vaginal breech delivery is safe in selected patients, most obstetricians have opted for cesarean delivery as the method of choice. Certainly, the physician can refer to older literature that supports this decision. When confronted with this information, the patient herself heartily accepts an increase in maternal morbidity and mortality inherent in this procedure to ensure the safety of her unborn child. However, the more recent literature supports the vaginal route of delivery when careful selection criteria are fulfilled and when the obstetrician is skilled in the technique of vaginal breech delivery. Collea's criteria have been well accepted: frank breech presentation, estimated fetal weight of 2,500 to 3,800 g, flexion of the fetal head, and adequate x-ray pelvimetry (Table 1). Collea employed these criteria in a randomized, prospective trial. Half of the patients in the vaginal trial group had inadequate pelvimetry measurements. However, 43 percent of patients in this group ultimately delivered vaginally, but there were two Erb's palsies reported. Of those patients randomized to cesarean delivery, maternal morbidity was reported in 36 percent and intraoperative complications in 9 percent.

A modification of Collea's criteria was applied to the non-frank breech presentation in another randomized prospective trial; the estimated fetal weight was expanded to 2,000 to 4,000 g. In patients randomized to vaginal delivery, 33 percent failed pelvimetry, but 44 percent ultimately delivered vaginally; of the three neonatal deaths, only one was felt to have been preventable. Again, in the patients in the cesarean delivery group, there were increased morbidity and longer hospital stays.

A retrospective study from Montreal looked at 600 term breech deliveries from 1963 to 1973. With an overall cesarean delivery of 22 percent in this group, there was an 18 percent incidence of birth trauma and asphyxia. On this basis, it was recommended that the cesarean rate should be higher. By 1978, the cesarean rate for term breech presentation had escalated to 94 percent. Interestingly, the risk of birth trauma and asphyxia was still 18 percent, although there was a trend toward decreased trauma.

In conclusion, there are a host of authors who have advocated a vaginal trial of labor for term breech presentation, provided that a strict protocol is followed. The recent literature suggests that fetal-neonatal complications are rare. If the following criteria are met, it would seem that a vaginal trial of labor is acceptable: (1) satisfactory pelvimetry measurements (Collea; see Table 1), (2) ultrasound or x-ray determination of flexion of the fetal head, (3) capability for electronic fetal monitoring, (4) adherence to a normal Friedman's curve, (5) familiarity with vaginal breech delivery (including the use of Piper's for-

TABLE 1 Critical X-ray Pelvimetry Measurements

Pelvic Dimension	*Cm*
Inlet	
Transverse	11.5
Anteroposterior	10.5
Midpelvis	
Transverse	10.0
Anteroposterior	11.5

From Collea JV, et al. The randomized management of term frank breech presentation: vaginal delivery vs. cesarean section. Am J Obstet Gynecol 1978; 131:186.

ceps), (6) competent assistance to maintain flexion of the fetal head and to assist the primary obstetrician during delivery, (7) immediate availability of general anesthesia (halothane to relax the lower uterine segment in the event of an entrapped head), and (8) availability of personnel who can resuscitate the neonate.

Several additional points need to be mentioned. We do not use oxytocin in the event of an arrest or protraction disorder; the literature has also cautioned against this practice. We expect the labor to progress without deviation from the normal Friedman's curve. If the slightest hint of abnormality is present, we would advocate a cesarean delivery. As mentioned previously, the issue of anesthesia is also controversial. Some have decried conduction anesthesia (epidural) because of interference with pushing, whereas others have recommended epidural as the anesthesia of choice because it prevents too rapid a delivery (with the potential for nuchal arms or an entrapped head). We are very satisfied with epidural anesthesia in the management of the term breech labor and delivery so long as the other criteria are met. We advocate the assisted breech delivery technique (with or without Piper's forceps to the aftercoming head), in which the fetus is allowed to deliver spontaneously to the umbilicus before any traction or manipulation is attempted. Basically, the same delivery techniques alluded to in the previous section on low birth weight and very low birth weight infants would also apply to the term breech delivery. The breech extraction is reserved for unusual cases of fetal distress. In the unlikely event of an entrapped head, the obstetrician might consider administration of a beta-sympathomimetic agent to aid in uterine relaxation; a bolus of terbutaline (0.25 mg) has been successfully used in such circumstances. The effect might be more rapid than 4 percent halothane general anesthesia, which can take 4 minutes or more to effect satisfactory relaxation.

External Cephalic Version

External cephalic version (ECV) was first described by Hippocrates in the fourth century AD Until the mid-1970s, however,the procedure had been relegated to antiguity. By that time, the management of breech presentation at term had been reduced to two schemes: routine cesarean delivery or selection algorithms for safe vaginal delivery. Neither approach attacks the primary problem, that of breech presentation itself. Historically, some have suggested that ECV is a simple, safe method for reducing the incidence of intrapartum breech presentation. Others have pointed out that successful versions would have converted spontaneously if left alone and that the unsuccessful ones would not have converted; they have reported the high incidence of spontaneous reversion to breech after successful ECV. There have been reports of fetal demise following ECV from cord accidents or placental abruption.

Careful analysis of the older literature suggests the following generalizations: ECV early in the third trimester is generally successful but spontaneous reversion to breech is common; ECV near term is rarely successful, but if successful, spontaneous reversion is uncommon; spontaneous conversion from breech to cephalic at term is uncommon. Fetal death has been generally confined to cases of unsuspected intrauterine growth retardation or to cases in which general anesthesia has been employed for relaxation (perhaps allowing too much force to be applied). Antepartum biophysical testing in terms of electronic fetal heart monitoring or ultrasonography to determine fetal well-being was not done in the older studies or reports.

In the early 1970s, Saling in West Berlin reported on a series of patients who had undergone ECV under tocolysis near term. He selected term patients so that in the unlikely event of fetal distress, the fetus presumably would be mature for immediate cesarean delivery. Aware of the dismal success rates by other investigators at term, he employed a beta-sympathomimetic agent to relax the uterus so as to minimize the amount of force necessary to accomplish ECV. Saling was successful in three-fourths of attempted versions without apparent maternal or fetal-neonatal ill-effects. As compared with a previous era when versions were not performed, he was able to reduce the percentage of intrapartum breech presentations. Soon after, two papers from Scandinavia corroborated Saling's results. However, the studies were neither randomized nor prospective in design. Skeptics still doubted the true place of ECV in the obstetric armamentarium.

In 1979, we embarked on a randomized, prospective trial to test the hypotheses that ECV would reduce the incidence of intrapartum breech presentation, that it would concomitantly reduce the cesarean delivery rate, and that within the scope of a small study, it was safe for the mother and the fetus-neonate. Only normal patients with a documented breech presentation at 37 to 39 weeks were included. A normal real-time ultrasound and a reactive nonstress test were prerequisites. After informed consent, the patients were randomized to either the control group (which was followed in the routine clinic to await delivery) or the study group (who underwent ECV). The procedure was performed in close proximity to the labor and delivery suite, where immediate cesarean delivery capabilities were present. In study patients, ritodrine hydrochloride was infused at 100 μg per minute by infusion pump for 10 to 15 minutes. Using ultrasound gel on the maternal abdomen and monitoring the fetus continuously with a Doppler ultrasound monitor, we used a two-man technique according to the following protocol: if the fetal head and back were on the same side of the maternal midline, a backflip was attempted; if the fetal spine crossed the maternal midline, a traditional forward roll was attempted. The first maneuver was to elevate the fetal buttocks from the maternal inlet. Then, with one operator manipulating the fetal head and the other the fetal buttocks, the fetus was turned 180 degrees. The mother's pain threshold and the fetal heart rate dictated how much rigor was employed; version was interrupted according to the mother's intolerance of the pain or deceleration of the fetal heart rate. No anesthesia or analgesia was used. Success was confirmed by ultrasound examination. After another reactive nonstress test, the patients were discharged to the routine clinic to await spontaneous labor. Patients were told to call if bleeding, rupture of membranes, or decreased fetal movement occurred. Full-dose Rh-immune globulin (300 μg) was given to Rh-negative patients.

Ultimately, 48 patients entered the study. ECV was successful in 68 percent (50 percent with nulliparas and 90 percent with multiparas). Significantly more study patients entered labor with a cephalic version presentation and significantly more delivered vaginally. If ECV was unsuccessful, no fetus spontaneously converted to cephalic prior to labor. Similarly, if ECV was successful, there was no case of spontaneous reversion to breech presentation. However, in the control group, several patients did convert spontaneously to cephalic version prior to labor, a fact suggested by the older literature. No untoward maternal or fetal-neonatal outcomes occurred. Factors that prejudiced success included nulliparity, maternal obesity, and engagement of the presenting part. There were no significant side effects from the tocolytic agent.

Based on these results, we felt confident that ECV under tocolysis at term significantly reduced the risk of both intrapartum breech presentation and also cesarean delivery. We were still concerned about the safety of the procedure. Fortunately, further research and observation have validated its efficacy and safety. The overall success rate ranges from 65 to 75 percent; with experience, the success rate with nulliparas still remains approximately 50 percent, whereas one can expect an 80 to 90 percent rate if the patient has had at least one term delivery. We have had no adverse outcome in over 500 attempted ECVs and have never had to do an emergency cesarean delivery; however, we still perform the procedure in the labor and delivery suite with an anesthesiologist physically present and with a delivery room available. There have been transient decelerations of the fetal heart rate, but it has always responded to desistence or a tincture of time.

In addition to nulliparity, obesity, and engagement of the presenting part, we have identified an anterior position of the fetal spine as undermining success. In fact, we now exclude patients with the following: (1) anterior position of the fetal spine, (2) inability to elevate the breech from the pelvis by abdominal manipulation (at the initial evaluation prior to administration of a tocolytic agent), and (3) inability to palpate the fetal head through the maternal abdomen (usually secondary to maternal obesity). Some investigators have touted subcutaneous terbutaline as a simple, effective tocolytic; in our institution, we have not found it to be as effective as intravenous ritodrine (100 μg per minute). In the patient with a contraindication to beta-sympathomimetics (e.g., diabetes mellitus), intravenous magnesium sulfate (4 g over 15 to 20 minutes) is an acceptable alternative.

With the success of antepartum ECV with term breech presentation, its use has expanded to other clinical settings: (1) intrapartum breech presentation and transverse lie, (2) breech second twin after vaginal delivery of the first (cephalic), (3) breech presentation in patients with a previous cesarean delivery approved for a trial of labor, (4) premature breech presentation when tocolysis has failed and cesarean delivery is the standard treatment.

We and others have achieved 50 percent success with intrapartum ECV in patients at term in early labor with intact membranes; the same protocol is followed as with antepartum ECV. The lower success rate is obviously a function of increased uterine tone and the generally lower station of the presenting part.

Phelan and others have reported their experience with intrapartum ECV in patients with a transverse lie. If the specific inclusion criteria were met (estimated fetal weight greater than 2,000 g, reactive nonstress test, intact membranes, and normal amniotic fluid), ECV was attempted in the delivery room with an anesthesiologist present. The procedure was successful in 10 of 12 patients and six of the 10 underwent a vaginal delivery without incident. Would antepartum ECV have been more effective in these patients?

The one regret we have about the early experience with ECV is that patients with a transverse lie were excluded. Nevertheless, such patients were followed prospectively with disturbing results. Though many had spontaneously converted to a longitudinal lie prior to labor, the cesarean delivery rate remained high (45 percent), with both perinatal and maternal morbidity and mortality (cord prolapse, neonatal death, and spontaneous uterine rupture). The authors recommended that patients with a persistent transverse lie at 39 weeks undergo ECV; with failure, a cesarean delivery should be strongly considered.

There are now a substantial number of patients, approved for a trial of labor after a previous cesarean delivery, who have undergone ECV without a problem. To our knowledge, there has not been a case of rupture or dehiscence of a uterine scar. If there is not a contraindication to labor, there should be none to ECV.

The role of ECV in the premature setting remains unclear and untested. In institutions where there is a policy of routine cesarean delivery for the low birth weight and very low birth weight breech, there is appeal to employment of ECV in patients with premature labor (with intact membranes) in whom tocolysis is unsuccessful. Perhaps ECV should be done in conjunction with the initial attempt at tocolysis with a beta-sympathomimetic agent or magnesium sulfate. It would seem that the success of ECV would be greater early in the tocolytic process than after it has been deemed unsuccessful. On the contrary, there is concern about the ability of the premature fetus to withstand the rigors of ECV, particularly in concert with the potential ill-effects of labor itself. The ultimate benefit of ECV in this setting must await randomized, prospective trials.

BREECH PRESENTATION IN TWINS

The obstetrician is confronted with a breech presentation in one or both twins in more that half of cases of twin gestation. Currently, cesarean delivery is the method of choice when the first twin (twin A) is in a noncephalic presentation, since there are no data supporting the safety of vaginal delivery in such circumstances, irrespective of the gestational age. There is no consensus as to the management of the second twin. Although the older literature suggests that more frequent use of cesarean section may improve the outcome of the second breech twin (twin B), the recent literature suggests that cesarean delivery may not always be warranted.

When managing a twin gestation, the obstetrician should perform an ultrasound examination to assess the fetal configuration, to estimate fetal weights, and to assess possible fetal anomalies. With the availability of ultrasonography, x-ray evaluation is unnecessary to assess fetal presentation. If twin B is discovered to be in a breech presentation, multiple options are open. Some have advocated routine cesarean, irrespective of gestational age. Others have advocated a sonographic estimation of fetal weight, accurate to within 20 percent (two standard deviations). If the fetal weight is 2,000 g or more, an intrapartum external version under sonographic guidance and with electronic fetal monitoring is attempted after vaginal delivery of a twin A. Upon failure, vaginal breech delivery may still be considered. The type of breech delivery (assisted or extraction) does not seem to be important. In this group in which vaginal breech delivery is being evaluated, pelvimetry also should be strongly considered. Several authors have suggested that a second twin breech should be accorded the same precautions as a singleton breech. Adequate pelvimetry measurements would seem to be a prerequisite.

If twin B is in a breech presentation and has a sonographic estimation of fetal weight less than 2,000 g, an intrapartum external version may still be attempted after vaginal delivery of twin A. With failure, most authors have advocated cesarean delivery; one study indicated that all of the neonatal deaths, all cases of neonatal intraventricular hemorrhage, and significantly more lower 5-minute Apgar scores were confined to the very low birth weight group (1,500 g or less) that delivered by the vaginal breech route. Recent data suggest that vaginal delivery of twin A followed by a cesarean delivery of twin B does not alter the perinatal outcome of the second twin. The current 20 percent error in sonographic estimation of fetal weight, excluding patients under 2,000 g, should prevent a vaginal breech delivery in the very low birth weight group. Cesarean delivery may be employed outright for both twins in this very low birth weight setting when twin B is in the breech presentation.

When vaginal delivery of twin B is anticipated, electronic monitoring should be undertaken as soon as possible. Several studies have shown that the interval between deliveries is unimportant as long as progress is being made, the fetal heart rate is normal, and there is no evidence of bleeding or cord prolapse. With the onset of fetal distress, cesarean delivery is the treatment of choice, as the effect of total breech extraction is uncertain.

Several additional points need to be made regarding the management of twins. Both twins should be electronically monitored on a continuous basis. This is technically easier if twin A is monitored via a scalp electrode and twin B via Doppler ultrasound apparatus. Many of the newer models allow for simultaneous monitoring on the same monitor. Possibly, much of the poorer delivery outcome of twin B can be ascribed to undetected fetal distress. Again, all of the above maneuvers require anesthesia, immediate capability for cesarean delivery, pediatric support, real-time ultrasound equipment, and requisite skills in external cephalic version and vaginal breech delivery.

SUGGESTED READING

Chervanak FA, Johnson RE, Youcha S, et al. Intrapartum management of twin gestation. Obstet Gynecol 1985; 65:119–124.

Collea JV, Rabin SC, Weghorst GR, Quilligan EJ. The randomized management of term rank breech presentation: vaginal delivery vs. cesarean section. Am J Obstet Gynecol 1978; 131:186–195.

Doyle LW, Rickards AL, Ford GW, et al. Outcome for the very low birthweight (500–1,499 g) singleton breech: benefit of caesarean section. Aust NZ J Obstet Gynaecol 1985; 25:259–265.

Effer SB, Saigal S, Rand C, et al. Effect of delivery method on outcomes in the very low-birth weight breech infant: Is the improved survival related to cesarean section or other perinatal care maneuvers? Am J Obstet Gynecol 1983; 145:123–128.

Gimovsky ML, Wallace RL, Schifrin BS, Paul RH. Randomized management of the nonfrank breech presentation at term: a preliminary report. Am J Obstet Gynecol 1983; 146:34–40.

Kauppila O, Gronroos M, Paavo A, et al. Management of low birth weight breech delivery: Should cesarean section be routine? Obstet Gynecol 1981; 57:289–294.

Kitchen W, Ford GW, Doyle LW, et al. Cesarean section or vaginal delivery at 24 to 28 weeks' gestation: comparison of survival and neonatal and two-year morbidity. Obstet Gynecol 1985; 66:149–157.

Main DM, Main EK, Maurer MM. Cesarean section versus vaginal delivery for the breech fetus weighing less than 1,500 grams. Am J Obstet Gynecol 1983; 146:580–584.

Myers AA, Gleicher N. Breech delivery: Why the dilemma? Am J Obstet Gynecol 1986; 155:6–10.

Seeds JW, Cefalo RC. Malpresentations. Clin Obstet Gynecol 1982; 25:145–156.

Van Dorsten JP, Schifrin BS, Wallace RL. Randomized control trial of external cephalic version with tocolysis in late pregnancy. AM J Obstet Gynecol 1981; 141:417–424.

THE FETUS

ERYTHROBLASTOSIS FETALIS

FREDRIC D. FRIGOLETTO Jr., M.D.
VANESSA A. BARSS, M.D.

Isoimmune hemolytic disease of the fetus results from placental transfer of maternal IgG antibodies directed against one or more fetal red blood cell antigens. Maternal-fetal Rh_o(D) incompatibility has been the most common cause of severe erythroblastosis leading to stillbirth; however, a small number of cases result from incompatibility of other red blood cell antigens, such as Kell, c, E, C, C^w, JK^a, S, M, k, and Fy^a. Although two-thirds of cases of hemolytic disease are due to ABO incompatibility between a blood group O mother and a group A or B fetus, this problem does not cause severe fetal erythroblastosis or stillbirth and does not warrant antenatal testing either by titer or amniocentesis. These infants usually have a weakly positive (Coombs') direct antiglobulin test and may require phototherapy or exchange transfusion after birth.

SCREENING

All pregnant women should have their blood screened for ABO and Rh type and for irregular antibodies at the first prenatal visit. Rh-negative unsensitized women should have antibody screening repeated at 28 and 36 weeks.

When an irregular antibody is present, it must be specifically identified to determine whether it is potentially harmful to the fetus. Anti-$Lewis^a$ (Le^a) and anti-$Lewis^b$ (Le^b) are antibodies detected fairly frequently. Both are of no clinical significance because they are usually IgM antibodies that do not cross the placenta. In addition, the Lewis antigens are not present on fetal red blood cells. "Nonspecific" antibodies usually are cold agglutinins that do not cause erythroblastosis. "Nonspecific" or "unidentified" antibodies are generally only saline-reacting and therefore do not cross the placenta.

When the patient has anti-Rh_o(D) antibodies or another antibody capable of causing erythroblastosis fetalis, titers must be obtained and repeated at 2- to 4-week intervals until 34 weeks, and then at 1- to 2-week intervals thereafter, provided the titer remains below the "critical titer level."

Ideally, antibody identification and serial titer determinations should be performed in a laboratory that has extensive experience with detection of erythroblastosis fetalis. Such a laboratory should have a well established protocol so that maximal reproducibility is achieved. In addition, the outcome of many pregnancies should be known so that a logical and reasonable correlation between titer and pregnancy outcome can be made. In this manner many laboratories have been able to establish the concept of a "critical titer" level, which is defined as the titer below which there have been no stillbirths or severely affected infants. Since test cells, technicians, and details of titration methods differ, titer results in one laboratory may differ from those of another, and therefore each laboratory must establish its own critical titer level according to its own experience.

Amniocentesis for amniotic fluid bilirubin determination (ΔOD_{450}) better defines the subgroup of fetuses who are severely affected. This procedure should be initiated when the critical titer is met or exceeded or in patients with a past history of severe erythroblastosis regardless of titer. Many mildly sensitized patients with low antibody titers may complete their pregnancies without requiring an invasive procedure. When amniocentesis is indicated, the time of the first amniotic tap can be as early as 18- to 20-weeks gestation, depending upon the titer and past history of erythroblastosis. The amniotic fluid specimen should be centrifuged and separated promptly in order to remove any contaminating blood cells. It should also be protected from light, which can break down the bilirubin pigments to be evaluated. The fluid is then filtered and the ΔOD_{450} is determined by spectrophotometric analysis and interpreted by the method of Liley. In the most severe cases lethal involvement can occur prior to 20-weeks gestation. In these rare situations identified by past obstetric history and laboratory results, other means of fetal surveillance, such as ultrasonography and fetal umbilical blood sampling, must be employed from early pregnancy.

Amniotic taps are usually repeated at 2-week intervals; serial determinations to observe the trend of the ΔOD_{450} values make possible a more reliable evaluation of fetal condition than a single tap alone. The interval between amniocenteses varies depending on the previous test result. An upper middle zone result would indicate repeat amniocentesis in 1 week or fetal blood sampling, whereas a very low result would permit an interval of up to 3 weeks, depending on assurance from other methods of surveillance.

Until recently the prescription for the interpretation of amniotic fluid ΔOD_{450} determinations was relatively simple, primarily because there were no established alternatives. Low values indicated minimal hemolysis and therefore minimally affected fetuses. Very high values indicated severely affected fetuses. Therefore, high ΔOD_{450} determinations were indications for intrauterine transfusion or delivery, depending on gestational age. Low to moderate values called for expectant management with repeated amniocentesis. Recently, Nicolaides has shown that an occasional fetus with a ΔOD_{450} in the low midzone of Liley's graph can be severely affected, as evidenced by hydrops and hematocrit readings obtained from percutaneous umbilical blood sampling (PUBS). This has made the decision-making process more complex. Because of these observations, it may not be sufficient to assess the fetal state with respect to erythroblastosis fetalis by amniotic fluid bilirubin measurements alone. Fetal state can be assessed more accurately when ultrasonography by sophisticated fetal ultrasonographers is used in conjunction with ΔOD_{450} values and PUBS. By using a battery of tests, both underdiagnosis and overdiagnosis of severity of hemolysis can be avoided. Whether or not the benefits and risks of direct fetal blood sampling should be applied to all fetuses suffering from this condition has not been ascertained. In our own setting we reserve percutaneous umbilical sampling for hematocrit determinations for ΔOD_{450} values in the top 30 percent of Liley's middle zone, unless other parameters indicate that invasive testing is warranted earlier. A legitimate question is whether or not one can manage the rhesus-sensitized patient without performing percutaneous umbilical blood sampling.

Between 1982 and 1986, patients identified as being at risk for severe isoimmune hemolytic disease of the fetus who were referred to the authors were followed by ΔOD_{450} determinations. When the ΔOD_{450} reached Liley's top zone, if the pregnancy was less than 32-weeks gestational age and the fetal lungs were immature as measured by the amniotic fluid lecithin:sphingomyelin ratio (L:S), the patients were offered the alternatives of expectant management or intrauterine fetal transfusion. Expectant management included ultrasound examinations every 24 to 72 hours by the same ultrasonographer, paying particular attention to placental thickness, collections of fluid in serous cavities, fetal skin thickness, and amniotic fluid volume.

Detailed consultative ultrasonography is the cornerstone of this alternative management protocol. It requires continuity of examiner from day to day and a systematic study with high-resolution equipment. Polyhydramnios and placental thickening are considered indirect signs of decompensation. Organomegaly, such as enlargement of the fetal liver or spleen, can be a chronic finding and does not in itself mandate intervention but simply close surveillance, such as every other day scanning. Some of the signs that we have noted to be associated with early decompensation include pericardial effusion or dilation of portions of the heart, particularly the right atrium. Very early signs of ascites, such as visualization of both sides of the bowel wall, indicate that the fetus will require delivery or intervention within 24 to 48 hours. If there is a suspicion of ascites, daily scans are required, and if ascites is confirmed, action is mandatory.

The biophysical profile is a crucial adjunct to the fetal sonographic examination. The biophysical evaluation supplemented by fetal heart rate monitoring serves to determine how well the fetus is compensating for its anemia. We have had no mortality or unexpected morbidity using this protocol with a limited number of patients. One of the patients managed expectantly had a fetus with a cord hematocrit of 9 ml per deciliter at birth despite reassuring nonstress tests and ultrasound examinations. This points out that indirect evaluation has its limitations. Beginning in mid-1986 we added transabdominal fetal blood sampling to the protocol as stated above to obtain direct information regarding fetal hematocrit levels. The actual protocol that is used at any given center depends on experience, expertise, and technical resources at that institution. It would appear that intrauterine cord blood sampling via maternal transabdominal puncture under ultrasound guidance to determine hematocrit and hemoglobin readings, coupled with sonographic surveillance of fetal well-being, may become the most accurate and safe approach.

Our present protocol includes the use of ΔOD_{450} determination, ultrasound surveillance, electronic fetal heart rate monitoring, and fetal umbilical blood sampling when the ΔOD_{450} falls in the top 30 percent of Liley's middle zone or in the presence of hydrops fetalis. The ultimate criterion in our protocol for performing intrauterine fetal transfusion is a fetal cord hematocrit below 25 ml per deciliter. We followed one fetus with repeated fetal hematocrits between 22 and 28 ml per deciliter for 8 weeks with a successful outcome, suggesting that the exact hematocrit criteria for transfusion are not established at this time.

TREATMENT

By means of the above protocol or variations thereof, the fetus who is severely compromised by erythroblastosis can be identified. The fetal gestational age and status of fetal lung maturity are variables that determine whether in utero treatment or delivery is in the best interest of the fetus. In general, we favor continuing the pregnancy if the fetus is less than 34 weeks, irrespective of the L:S ratio, because of other morbidity from prematurity. This decision must be individualized in each case.

A number of technical aspects of intravascular intrauterine transfusions should be discussed. The procedure has been described by a number of authors, each with his or her own variations. One group starts an intravenous infusion and the patient is premedicated with a narcotic, a tranquilizer, an antiemetic, a tocolytic agent, and an antibiotic. In contrast, our own protocol calls for none of these measures. There is as yet no series that allows for conclusions regarding outcomes based on any of these differences. There appears to be a high degree of agreement that the target vessel should be as close to the cord root as possible. When the placenta is in an anterior position, the cord can often be approached through the placenta without having to enter the amniotic cavity. Obviously the key to this technique is high-resolution ultrasonography performed by experienced ultrasonographers. One of the apparent advantages of intravascular over intraperitoneal transfusion is that the exact amount of blood that the fetus needs can be calculated. In addition, there is already strongly suggestive evidence indicating a markedly increased efficacy for intravascular over intraperitoneal transfusion in the hydropic fetus. There are a number of small uncontrolled series with hydropic fetuses, including our own, which support this conclusion. There is nothing at the present time, however, that allows one to conclude that the intravascular route is superior in the fetus who is not hydropic or who has resolved hydrops and is receiving a subsequent transfusion. As stated earlier, in these situations the consensus appears to be that the technically more feasible route is the procedure of choice. Other investigators have employed in utero exchange transfusion by direct intravascular injection. The benefits of exchange transfusion over intravascular transfusion alone have not been demonstrated. The theoretical benefits are based on tenuous assumptions regarding fetal blood volume, increased myocardial burden, and so forth. Studies have to be done comparing the results by the two methods in similar cases. These exchange procedures are more difficult and time-consuming than simple transfusion.

Following intrauterine transfusion, the transfused fetus should be followed to determine well-being and when to perform repeat transfusion. It is agreed that the most accurate way to assess fetal anemia is by fetal hematocrit. However, this is associated with a small (1 percent) but real risk of fetal loss. Consequently, investigators have been assessing ways of estimating the fetal hematocrit noninvasively. Recently Copel reported on umbilical velocity waveforms and their value in predicting the fetal hematocrit following transfusion. The results were disappointingly negative. At present we use some simple calculations that take into account the posttransfusion hematocrit, the blood volume (based on fetal size and expansion with growth), and the natural decay curve of the transfused red cells to determine the time of the follow-up fetal blood sampling. This, in conjunction with our protocol for noninvasive fetal surveillance in the erythoblastic fetus, has been the basis of our posttransfusion follow-up.

One final but important area for consideration is timing. At what gestational age is it "too late" to do an intrauterine transfusion? There are no absolute criteria that provide an answer; however, our own protocol favors prolonging these pregnancies to 36 weeks, other factors permitting. The final decision is determined by variables of a given case, which include fetal lung maturity, fetal state, and ease of procedure.

SUGGESTED READING

Bang J, Bock JE, Trolle D. Ultrasound-guided fetal intravenous transfusion for severe rhesus haemolytic disease. Br Med J 1982; 284:373–374.

Benacerraf B, Frigoletto FD. Sonographic sign for the detection of early fetal ascites in the management of severe isoimmune disease without intrauterine transfusion. Am J Obstet Gynecol 1985; 152:1039–1041.

Berkowitz RL, Chitkara U, Wilkins I, Lynch L, Mehalek KE. Technical aspects of intravascular intrauterine transfusions: Lessons learned from thirty-three procedures. Am J Obstet Gynecol 1987; 157:4–9.

Copel JA. Clinician scientist award paper. 7th Annual Meeting, American Gynecological and Obstetrical Society: Phoenix, AZ, September 9–12, 1987.

Daffos F, Capella-Paulousky MD, Forestier F. Fetal blood sampling during pregnancy with use of a needle guided by ultrasound: a study of 606 consecutive cases. Am J Obstet Gynecol 1985; 153:655–660.

de Crespigny LC, Robinson HP, Quinn M, Doyle L, Ross A, Cauchi M. Ultrasound-guided fetal blood transfusion for severe rhesus isoimmunization. Obstet Gynecol 1985; 66:529–532.

Frigoletto FD, Greene MF, Benacerraf BR, Barss VA, Saltzman DH. Ultrasonic fetal surveillance in the management of the isoimmunized pregnancy. N Engl J Med 1986; 315:430–432.

Grannum PA, Copel JA, Plaxe SC, Scioscia AL, Hobbins JC. In utero exchange transfusion by direct intravascular injection in severe erythroblastosis fetalis. N Engl J Med 1986; 314:1431–1434.

Liley AW. Liquor amnii analysis in the management of pregnancy complicated by rhesus sensitization. Am J Obstet Gynecol 1961; 82:1359–1370.

MacKenzie IZ, MacLean DA, Fry A, Evans SL. Midtrimester intrauterine exchange transfusion of the fetus. Am J Obstet Gynecol 1982; 143:555–559.

Nicolaides KH, Clewell WH, Rodeck CH. Measurement of human fetoplacental blood volume in erythroblastosis fetalis. Am J Obstet Gynecol 1987; 157:50–53.

Nicolaides KH, Rodeck CH, Mibashan RS, Kemp JR. Have Liley charts outlived their usefulness? Am J Obstet Gynecol 1986; 155:90–94.

Seeds JW, Bowes WA. Ultrasound-guided fetal intravascular transfusion in severe rhesus immunization. Am J Obstet Gynecol 1986; 154:1105–1107.

Torday JS, Carson L, Lawson EE. Saturated phosphatidylcholine in amniotic fluid and prediction of the respiratory distress syndrome. N Engl J Med 1979; 301:1013–1018.

Vintzileos AM, Campbell WA, Ingardia CJ, Nochimson DJ. The fetal biophysical profile and its predictive value. Obstet Gynecol 1983; 62:271–278.

FETAL HEART RATE MONITORING

WAYNE R. COHEN, M.D.

Technologic advances of the past two decades have resulted in unprecedented insights into fetal condition during pregnancy and labor. The ability to obtain reliable information about the state of fetal oxygenation from fetal heart rate monitoring and fetal capillary blood sampling has altered the practice of obstetrics dramatically. The interpretation of information from these new technologies is now considered a major prerequisite for the practice of obstetrics.

Obstetricians have sought information about the fetus from knowledge of the fetal heart rate since the middle of the 19th century; however, it was not until the 1970s when electronic fetal heart rate monitoring became generally available, that sophisticated insight could be achieved. Fetal heart rate monitoring is now used extensively for fetal evaluation during both the antepartum period and labor. Fetal capillary blood sampling to measure fetal pH and respiratory gases was first introduced in the 1960s. It has now achieved a place as primarily an adjunctive technology that can sometimes provide useful information when fetal heart rate patterns are abnormal.

FETAL OXYGENATION

Nutrients and respiratory gases are transferred between mother and fetus across the placental membranes. The diffusion of oxygen from maternal to fetal circulation is influenced by a number of factors. The most important of these relates to the adequacy of blood flow in both circulations. In this sense, oxygen transfer to the fetus is primarily a flow-dependent process, and the most commonly encountered clinical situations involving fetal oxygen deprivation are a consequence of reduced fetal (umbilical) or maternal (uterine) blood flow. Examples of clinical situations in which uterine blood flow diminishes include hypotension from maternal blood loss or the sympathetic blockade of conduction anesthesia, chronic or acute hypertension, and excessive uterine activity. Decrements in umbilical blood flow are most commonly a result of acute umbilical cord compression, although some disorders, including intrauterine growth retardation, are probably associated with chronically deficient umbilical flow.

Several features of the fetal cardiovascular system make it relatively resistant to oxygen deprivation. The placenta appears to have a large reserve, in that its ability to transport oxygen far exceeds the normal respiratory requirements of the fetus. Fetal blood has a higher affinity for oxygen than maternal blood; therefore fetal blood contains larger amounts of oxygen than maternal blood at the same partial pressure of oxygen. Thus, although fetal blood has a much lower Po_2 than maternal blood, the difference in oxygen affinity results in a relatively smaller gradient in oxygen content. An anatomic feature of the fetal circulation is of interest with regard to the distribution of blood oxygen. The fetal circulation contains several shunts that help to maintain maximal oxygenation of the heart and brain at the expense of the lower body.

The functional correlates of these biochemical and anatomic facets of the fetal circulation result in adequate delivery of oxygen to fetal tissues under most circumstances. In fact, despite the prevailing low oxygen tension in the fetus, the design of its circulation and its relatively high cardiac output result in oxygen consumption that is actually greater (per unit weight) than that of the mother.

During conditions of reduced oxygen availability, fetal homeostatic mechanisms that serve to maximize oxygen delivery and blood flow to vital organs are called into play. Under these conditions, the fetus is able to maintain its cardiac output relatively well and to redistribute this output to maintain blood flow to the central nervous system, myocardium, adrenal glands, and placenta at the expense of less physiologically vital tissues such as skeletal muscle, skin, and kidneys. Although oxygen supply to tissues during mild or moderate hypoxemia tends to be maintained relatively constantly, when hypoxemia becomes very severe, acidosis may develop, the ability of the myocardium to maintain cardiac output diminishes, and the mechanisms responsible for redistribution of systemic blood flow to vital organs may fail. The result is a reduction of tissue oxygen delivery.

The fetus generally responds to hypoxemia by a change in heart rate. Under most clinical circumstances, bradycardia develops. Tachycardia may be a response to hypoxemia that is very mild or slowly progressive or both. Although decreased fetal heart rate had long been considered an ominous feature, electronic fetal monitoring has taught us that this is not invariably so. In fact, hypoxic fetal bradycardias are part of the normal compensatory response to reduced oxygen availability, i.e., a decrease in fetal heart rate may be a response to hypoxemia but does not necessarily imply that the availability of oxygen to fetal tissues is seriously compromised.

The clinician must always bear in mind the impressive abilities of the fetus to adapt to at least modest degrees of deoxygenation. Certain features of fetal heart rate patterns to be described can be helpful to determine when normal compensatory mechanisms have begun to fail. The recognition of the potentially beneficial aspect of fetal bradycardia and the understanding of the fetus' ability often to maintain tissue oxygenation in the presence of hypoxemia are the cornerstones of the method of heart rate pattern interpretation to be elaborated here.

FETAL HEART RATE MONITORS

Electronic fetal monitors are devices that calculate the fetal heart rate electronically and measure uterine contractions. This information is printed out on a continuous two-channel strip chart recorder for on-line evaluation.

Heart rate is measured generally by one of two techniques. External monitors employ an ultrasound transducer that detects fetal heart motion and through a series of complex electronic filters translate this information into a trigger pulse for each beat. These pulses are counted electronically to determine the heart rate. Direct fetal monitoring employs a stainless steel electrode that is applied to the fetal scalp (or, in breech presentations, to the buttocks) and that detects fetal electrocardiographic (ECG) voltages. By identifying the R wave of the fetal ECG and measuring the interval between ventricular complexes, the monitor's cardiotachometer calculates a new rate for each heart beat. The rate is expressed as the number of beats per minute that would occur if the measured interval were present unchanged for 1 minute.

Fetal cardiac activity can also be detected by obtaining the fetal ECG from the maternal abdominal wall, or by the use of sensitive external microphones (phonocardioaphy). Both of these methods are used in a very limited fashion.

Uterine contractions can also be measured internally or externally. A device that is sensitive to changes in the contour of the mother's abdominal wall may be used to detect contractions. This tocodynamometer has the advantage of being noninvasive but has the drawback of not providing information about the absolute or relative intensity of contractions. More precise and complete information may be obtained by inserting a plastic fluid-filled catheter into the amniotic cavity during labor and connecting the catheter to a standard pressure transducer. By recording changes in intrauterine pressure, reliable information concerning the intensity as well as the frequency and duration of contractions may be obtained.

Baseline Heart Rate Patterns

Heart rate is normally between 110 to 150 beats per minute in the human fetus at term. Observation of a continuously recorded heart rate pattern reveals small irregularities or oscillations in the rate. These reflect the fact that heart rate normally changes slightly with almost every beat. This physiologic fact confers a visible irregularity termed *variability* on clinical monitor patterns. This beat-to-beat variability is a result of frequent variations in fetal autonomic nervous system impulses as they influence heart rate and cardiac output in response to various afferent signals, which probably relate to changes in venous return, metabolic demands, and other factors. Although a number of methods exist for the electronic quantitation of heart rate variability, visual assessment is used clinically and correlates well with fetal condition. Variability should be classified as absent, decreased, average, or increased. Sometimes reference is made to "long-term" variability. This term describes broad changes that occur with a frequency of three to six cycles per minute and really represent trends in short-term (beat-to-beat) variability. The latter is most important in the assessment of fetal condition.

The abnormalities in the fetal baseline heart rate that are encountered most commonly are persistent tachycardia or bradycardia or alterations in beat-to-beat variability. Less commonly one observes sinusoidal oscillations in the baseline, which may sometimes be of ominous portent.

Periodic Heart Rate Changes

In addition to observations of the baseline heart rate, periodic changes in the fetal heart rate pattern are of importance. Transient accelerations in the fetal heart rate pattern are seen frequently. By definition, these excursions in rate persist for at least 15 seconds and rise to at least 15 beats per minute above the baseline. Periodic accelerations are usually accompanied by fetal movements—or, during labor, by uterine contractions—and are considered signs of fetal health. In fact, their presence during antepartum fetal heart rate monitoring is considered to be the most reliable sign of fetal well-being.

Heart rate decelerations are common, and their identification and interpretation are important aspects of defining the mechanism of fetal asphyxial insults. The most widely applied system of nomenclature describes decelerations as *early, late*, *variable*, or *prolonged*.

Early decelerations are uncommon, symmetric, and uniform. They begin with the onset of the uterine contraction, reach a nadir at the peak of the contraction, and return to baseline at the same time as the contraction. Early decelerations rarely decrease more than 20 beats per minute below baseline and are most common in the second stage of labor. They result from a vagal discharge that is the consequence of transient cerebral hypoxemia resulting from fetal head compression during uterine contractions. Most data suggest that early decelerations defined in this way are not associated with any increased risk of fetal acidosis or other compromise. Therefore, they do not require intervention.

Late decelerations are recurrent bradycardias that begin at least 20 seconds after the onset of the contraction. They are generally repetitive and proportional in size to the amplitude and duration of the accompanying contraction. Late decelerations are always a response to fetal hypoxemia. Two physiologic mechanisms may produce them. When oxygen deprivation is relatively mild, late decelerations are mediated primarily through increased vagal tone, a consequence of chemoreceptor stimulation; but when hypoxemia is severe, direct myocardial depression occurs and contributes to the production of the deceleration. The judgments concerning the severity of the hypoxemia that accompanies late decelerations should be made primarily by an assessment of the baseline heart rate pattern between contractions. The size of the deceleration is not necessarily a direct indication of severity. Late decelerations that are accompanied by normal rate and normal beat-to-beat variability in the baseline are associated with less severe hypoxemia or acidosis than late decelerations that occur with absent variability and/or tachycardia between them. The presence of variability appears to be an important clinical index of fetal condition, particularly in the presence of recurrent decelerations. The presumed explanation for this is that variability is controlled primarily by fluctuations in autonomic (especially in parasympathetic) tone. The absence of variability suggests that the central nervous system centers that control variability are not functioning normally. Since the compensatory mechanisms involving redistribution of cardiac output and maximization of stroke volume during hypoxemia are also controlled to a large extent by the autonomic nervous system, the absence of variability may be an index of potential central nervous system injury.

Late decelerations that occur in the presence of good baseline variability are seen frequently in a previously normal fetus in response to an acute decrease in uterine blood flow, such as may accompany hypotension from conduction anesthesia. Late decelerations with an abnormal baseline are seen more commonly in fetuses with diminished reserve and evidence of chronic compromise. Thus, problems such as maternal diabetes mellitus, hypertension, cyanotic heart disease, or fetal intrauterine growth retardation may produce long-standing deficiencies in fetal oxygen transfer. Also, such fetuses may be considerably more vulnerable to stresses that would not perturb a normal fetus.

Variable decelerations are usually caused by umbilical cord compression. They are so named because they vary in shape and in their relationship to the onset of the contraction. This variation probably reflects a considerable change in the degree and rapidity of cord occlusion even in response to contractions of similar intensity. Although variable decelerations may occur at any time during labor, they are the most common pattern observed during the second stage. They may be accompanied by considerable compromise or may be innocuous, depending upon the frequency, severity, and duration of cord impingement. The degree of accompanying fetal compromise can usually be judged, as it can for late decelerations, by an assessment of the baseline heart rate condition. Diminished variability and developing tachycardia are ominous signs.

Occasionally, in the presence of severe recurrent variable decelerations with absent variability, one sees transient rebound accelerations immediately after the bradycardia has returned to the baseline. These "overshoot" patterns are emblematic of serious fetal compromise, but they should be interpreted in that way only when heart rate variability is virtually absent. Some investigators believe that the rate of return to baseline of a variable deceleration is a reflection of the severity of accompanying hypoxemia, but most evidence does not support this view. Accelerations that precede or follow variable decelerations in the presence of good beat-to-beat variability are not ominous signs.

Prolonged decelerations are defined as precipitate drops in the fetal heart rate that last for at least 2 minutes and that drop at least 30 beats per minute below the baseline. These patterns are heterogeneous with regard to configuration, timing, and etiology. They may sometimes represent prolonged cord compression or be a response to fetal manipulation such as vaginal examination or scalp blood sampling. Most importantly, they can represent a response to sudden or severe asphyxia such as may accompany uterine hypercontractility, placental abruption, or a maternal seizure or sudden hypotension. Most prolonged decelerations have not been associated with adverse fetal outcome, particularly when there is good variability, the provoking factor can be eliminated, and the fetal heart rate pattern was normal before the deceleration. Those fetuses most likely to suffer serious problems in the presence of prolonged decelerations have been previously compromised in some way.

Sometimes observed fetal heart rate decelerations are not easily classified into these traditional categories. A general operational principle is to classify decelerations by the company they keep. For example, when some decelerations can be identified with reasonable certainty as variable, it is most likely that any accompanying decelerations of ambiguous character are also variable. In fact, the nature of the deceleration is less important than judgments about the severity of its impact upon the fetus.

CLINICAL ASSESSMENT OF FETAL HEART RATE PATTERNS

Antepartum Monitoring

Fetal evaluation prior to the onset of labor is often necessary in high-risk pregnancies. This testing is instituted most commonly in the third trimester, when delivery in response to an abnormal test would result in a potentially viable newborn. The use of fetal heart rate monitoring and various kinds of ultrasound evaluation of the fetus are the most common surveillance tools. Occasionally, biochemical testing of amniotic fluid or maternal plasma is performed, and the technology for direct umbilical cord blood sampling is developing rapidly.

The screening test used most commonly is the nonstress test (NST), which involves an assessment of fetal heart rate changes in response to fetal body movements. The patient is placed in semi-Fowler's position or in a degree of left lateral tilt to minimize aortocaval compression. An external ultrasound fetal heart transducer and a uterine activity detector are placed on the mother's abdomen and connected to a standard fetal heart rate monitor. The fetal heart rate, uterine activity, and fetal movement activity are observed for a minimum of 20 minutes. If there are at least two fetal heart rate accelerations that accompany fetal movement (each acceleration at least 15 beats per minute in amplitude and lasting at least 15 seconds), and there are no decelerations, the test is considered *reactive* , consistent with fetal health. If there are no accelerations, the test is *nonreactive*. This suggests possible fetal compromise and requires further evaluation promptly. Equivocal tests that cannot be determined to be clearly reactive or nonreactive should be repeated within 24 hours. Other variants of the test have been described, including the *terminal* pattern, in which there is absence of fetal movements and no periodic changes in the heart rate, resulting in a very monotonously flat-appearing tracing. If even mild uterine contractions are present, late decelerations may be seen. The terminal pattern suggests severe fetal asphyxia.

When the NST is abnormal, further information may be obtained either from ultrasound evaluation or from another heart rate assessment called the *contraction stress test* (CST). During this evaluation, the patient is monitored in the same manner as for the NST, and the response of the fetal heart rate to uterine contractions is evaluated. A valid test requires three palpable uterine contractions within a 10-minute period. These contractions may sometimes be spontaneous or, more often, are induced by a slow intravenous infusion of oxytocin. Some advocate the use of maternal breast stimulation to produce contractions for this test.

A uterine contraction represents a potential hypoxic stress to the fetus because increasing intramyometrial pressures may impede or eliminate intervillous blood flow by compressing uterine arteries that traverse the myometrium. In a fetus with limited placental reserve, uterine contractions may provoke late decelerations.

The absence of late decelerations with three contractions in a 10-minute period is a negative test; a pattern with three late decelerations is a positive test. The presence of variable decelerations or of sporadic late decelerations may be explained sometimes on the basis of the clinical situation. Both require prompt follow-up evaluation.

Both the antepartum NST and CST have a strong negative predictive value, i.e., when the tests are normal they are excellent predictors of fetal health; however, both have high false-positive rates. This is especially true of the NST, which always requires confirmatory evidence before fetal jeopardy may be diagnosed. This evidence may involve a CST or, more commonly, an ultrasound biophysical profile evaluation.

Intrapartum Monitoring

External monitoring often is used early in labor or in situations in which rupture of the fetal membranes could be hazardous, such as with an unengaged presenting part. Although the newest generation ultrasound monitors use autocorrelation cardiotachometric methods and generally give accurate information concerning heart rate variability, direct monitoring provides the most reliable and accurate information regarding fetal heart rate patterns. It should be used whenever any abnormality is identified by external monitoring.

Clinical assessment of intrapartum heart rate patterns should involve a systematic evaluation of the baseline heart pattern between contractions (its rate and variability) and then a description of any periodic changes (accelerations or decelerations) that are present. The configurations of the decelerations are useful to deduce the mechanism of the fetal insult, i.e., whether it involves direct fetal hypoxemia or umbilical cord compression. The severity of a series of decelerations should be judged by the changes in the baseline that accompany the decelerations rather than by the size of the decelerations per se.

Sometimes baseline aberrations are seen in the absence of decelerations. Fetal tachycardia (sustained rates above 160 beats per minute) is commonly seen with maternal fever, chorioamnionitis, or fetal infection. Less frequent causes of tachycardia include fetal tachyarrhythmias, maternal thyrotoxicosis, and some drugs. Beta-adrenergic agonists, which are used often in obstetrics to suppress premature labor, may cause a rise in fetal heart rate. In the human fetus, heart rate is generally highest in early pregnancy and declines as term approaches; however, sustained rates above 170 beats per minute even early in the third trimester should prompt a search for other causes. Fetal hypoxia may cause fetal tachycardia. As noted previously, when this occurs it is usually in the context of slowly developing oxygen deprivation and most commonly in the absence of significant uterine contractions.

Persistent fetal bradycardia (less than 110 beats per minute) is seen occasionally with normal variability and accelerations and with no other ominous features. As such it may be a variant of normal. When persistent bradycardia occurs as a consequence of fetal hypoxemia, it is usually severe, and variability will be diminished. Some drugs (e.g., beta-blockers), reflex responses to umbilical cord compression, or persistent hypoglycemia may also produce fetal bradycardia.

Diminished baseline variability may occur as a solitary finding in response to many medications (narcotic analgesics, barbiturates, tranquilizers, anesthetics) or, rarely, may be a consequence of fetal anomalies or cardiac arrhythmias. Because vagal dominance in heart rate control increases as gestation progresses, premature babies tend to have less variability in their heart rate patterns than do their term counterparts. As indicated previously, fetal hypoxia alters heart rate variability. Sometimes, mild degrees of hypoxemia may result in exaggerated variability, but when the oxygen deprivation becomes significant clinically, variability will usually diminish. During active labor, late decelerations tend to occur before a diminution in variability when the fetus is exposed to an acute asphyxial insult.

The physiologic mechanism of sinusoidal heart rate patterns is not known. When it is persistent, this pattern has been accompanied by adverse outcome in several situations, including Rh sensitization and other causes of fetal anemia. The pattern has also been described in association with postmaturity syndrome, cardiovascular malformations, fetal infection, and toxemia. When sinusoidal patterns occur intermittently, they are less ominous. In general, fetal blood sampling is necessary to ascertain fetal condition in these situations, particularly if any of the above-named risk factors exist.

When recurrent heart rate decelerations exist in conjunction with normal baseline rate and variability, it may be inferred that the fetus is being stressed intermittently but that its compensatory cardiovascular mechanisms are probably functioning to maintain adequate oxygenation. In these situations, it is of vital importance to follow trends in the characteristics of the heart rate pattern and sometimes to obtain other information in order to make judgments about the need for intervention. The combination of recurrent decelerations and abnormal baseline (absent variability, tachycardia or bradycardia) is extremely ominous and almost always suggests serious degrees of hypoxia. Prompt intervention is usually justified in these circumstances.

INTRAUTERINE RESUSCITATION

Generally, abnormal fetal heart rate patterns do not

require urgent intervention and should be dealt with initially by attempts at intrauterine resuscitation. These consist of simple clinical efforts to improve and maximize fetal oxygenation. Because, as discussed previously, most encountered cases of fetal distress are a consequence of diminished blood flow, attempts to maximize uteroplacental and umbilical flow may sometimes be salutary in cases of fetal distress. For example, insofar as late decelerations reflect a deficiency of uterine perfusion, they may be improved by placing the mother in the left lateral position (to minimize aortocaval compression), reducing uterine contractility (if ecbolic agents are being used), correcting maternal hypotension (if present), and giving a rapid infusion or crystalloid solution to enhance blood volume. In addition, one can improve the oxygen availability for the fetus by giving the mother a high inspired oxygen concentration. This should be done promptly but will be maximally effective only if good uterine blood flow can be reestablished. When variable decelerations are noted, all of these maneuvers to encourage uterine perfusion should be carried out. In addition, the mother's position should be changed in order to attempt to relieve umbilical cord compression.

Recurrent severe variable decelerations sometimes result from umbilical cord prolapse. Vaginal examination should always be done when this pattern is observed. If overt cord prolapse is diagnosed, elevation of the presenting part may be used to reduce cord compression while preparations for abdominal delivery are accomplished. Monitoring helps define the urgency of that intervention. If the fetal heart rate is monitored after the presenting part has been elevated, delivery may be delayed if the heart rate pattern is normal or is recovering. When occult prolapse of the cord is suspected and recurrent variable decelerations do not respond to the usual resuscitative maneuvers, preparations for cesarean section should be made. The presenting part should be elevated manually. If no recovery in the heart rate pattern develops, prompt delivery must be undertaken; however, if improvement occurs, the fetus should be allowed to recover in utero and then be released to descend again. If the ominous pattern recurs, elevation may be reinstituted and a cesarean section carried out after fetal recovery. If the fetal heart rate remains normal after the presenting part has been released, the labor may often be allowed to continue and to eventuate in vaginal delivery.

Two new methods of treating fetal distress are now being studied, but their precise role in clinical management is still uncertain. Under certain circumstances, uterine contractions may be diminished by a rapid infusion of a beta-mimetic drug. This approach might be particularly useful in settings in which cesarean section cannot be accomplished immediately. The intrauterine instillation of saline via a transvaginal intrauterine catheter to replace amniotic fluid volume has been reported to have some value in the alleviation of variable decelerations.

IATROGENIC FETAL DISTRESS

All medical interventions carry some inherent risk, and obstetric procedures are no exception. The availability of continuous fetal heart rate monitoring has disclosed and explained many of the potential risks associated with common obstetric procedures. Monitoring has enabled us to have insights into the effect on the fetus of maternal position, excess uterine activity, and the potential of conduction anesthesia to provoke maternal hypotension.

The development of understanding of these problems has led to the use of electronic infusion pumps for the judicious administration of oxytocin, to the custom of adequate prehydration of patients expected to receive conduction anesthesia, and to avoidance of the supine position during labor.

FETAL BLOOD SAMPLING

The adaptive cardiovascular mechanisms that allow the fetus to maintain tissue oxygenation in the presence of reduced oxygen availability have been alluded to previously. Under conditions of severe or prolonged hypoxemia, these mechanisms eventually fail, and tissue hypoxia and acidosis develop. A sample of capillary blood may be obtained from the fetal presenting part during labor to assess fetal acid-base balance. Under conditions of severe hypoxemia, the fetus is deprived of its ability to perform oxidative metabolism, and glucose (the primary fetal metabolic substrate) can be oxidized only to the fixed organic acids pyruvate and lactate. This results in a metabolic acidosis, the nature and severity of which depend on the duration and intensity of the hypoxic insult. Relatively mild or transient decreases in uterine or umbilical blood flow result initially in a decrease in carbon dioxide transfer from fetus to mother, and consequently a primarily respiratory acidosis. More severe or persistent insults may produce a combined respiratory and metabolic acidosis.

Performance of blood sampling is not difficult and with proper technique, an adequate sample for measurement of fetal pH can be obtained in at least 85 percent of cases. The sampling site should avoid sutures or fontanelles as well as areas of caput succedaneum. It is important to verify that hemostasis in the scalp has occurred after the sample has been obtained.

Fetal scalp capillary pH during labor ranges between 7.25 and 7.40. In some fetuses a slow decline in fetal pH occurs during labor, which becomes more rapid during the second stage. This is a position-dependent event, and significant decreases in pH are less likely to occur in women who labor and deliver in the lateral position. Fetal pH below 7.20 suggests the presence of asphyxia, and values between 7.20 and 7.24 are suspicious and require repeat observation.

The obstetrician must be aware of the pitfalls in the measurement and interpretation of fetal pH values. Falsely low pH values (normal neonatal Apgar scores and low pH) may be the result of technical errors in blood collection or measurement, may be the consequence of maternal acidosis and passive transfer of hydrogen ions to the fetus, or may reflect a true asphyxial insult that has reversed prior to delivery. Falsely normal pH results are encountered also and are frequently the result of unfortunate timing of the sample, i.e., fetal acidosis may have developed subsequent to a blood sample taken in the absence of acidosis. In addition, low Apgar scores may be contributed to by many factors other than asphyxia, including fetal sepsis, trauma, and depressant medication.

The relationship between fetal pH and fetal heart rate patterns has been studied by several investigators, and some useful generalizations may be stated. Persistent fetal tachycardia or bradycardia in the absence of any other associated heart rate pattern abnormalities is rarely associated with significant acidosis. When tachycardia or bradycardia accompanies diminished variability or recurrent decelerations or both, it is more likely to reflect serious oxygen deprivation and acidosis. Late decelerations are always accompanied by at least a transient decrease in fetal oxygen availability but are associated with a low pH only about 50 percent of the time. Most of the late decelerations that produce progressive or severe acidosis are accompanied by decreased variability or tachycardia. Variable decelerations are the most difficult to assess. The degree of acidosis that accompanies them depends on their frequency and duration to an extent but primarily on their association with other heart rate abnormalities. As with late decelerations, the features of the baseline heart rate between variable decelerations are most important to determine the impact of the intermittent cord compression on fetal homeostasis. Variable decelerations are almost always accompanied by a degree of respiratory acidosis, which may resolve very shortly after the deceleration. More persistent or prolonged decelerations with baseline abnormalities are more likely to be associated with respiratory and metabolic acidosis, which resolves much more slowly. Therefore, timing is of particular importance in the presence of variable decelerations, and the blood sample should be taken immediately before the contraction in order to provide the most useful information. When the sample is measured during or immediately after a contraction, the obstetrician may be misled by the presence of a temporary respiratory acidosis.

Prolonged decelerations are usually accompanied by significant fetal hypoxemia but when a prolonged deceleration occurs after a previously normal heart rate pattern, significant acidosis is unlikely in the first several minutes.

The foregoing reinforces the now generally accepted clinical notion that baseline heart rate and variability are reflections of fetal oxygen reserve. The nature of the heart rate deceleration provides insight into the mechanism of the insult. On the basis of these principles, one can assess the impact of a series of decelerations by identifying the changes in baseline rate and variability that accompany them.

As is the case with most types of fetal testing, the presence of a normal fetal heart rate pattern is an extremely accurate indicator of fetal health. Abnormal heart rate patterns are much less precise in identifying abnormal fetal conditions and have a high false-positive rate. The ability to predict fetal jeopardy on the basis of abnormal heart rate patterns requires considerable experience and keen judgment. Clearly, the most important virtue of this technique is its ability to identify the healthy fetus and therefore to reduce the need for potentially hazardous intervention.

COMPLICATIONS OF FETAL MONITORING

Maternal Infection

Several retrospective studies have indicated an increased risk of maternal intrapartum or postpartum infection in patients who are monitored internally. However, the most comprehensive and best-controlled studies fail to show a significant influence on infection risks by fetal monitoring. Most likely, other factors (primarily duration of labor and of ruptured membranes) have such a considerable influence on the risk of infection that the effect of monitoring in this regard is minimal.

Although the adverse effects of internal monitoring are somewhat uncertain in this regard, it is sensible to take ordinary precautions to minimize the likelihood of infection, and reasonable aseptic technique should be used during the insertion of all monitoring devices into the uterus. Presumably, the intrauterine catheter or scalp electrode provides access to the fetus or uterine cavity for vaginal bacteria.

Neonatal Infection

Concerns have been raised about the possible production of neonatal infections by fetal scalp electrodes. Areas of scalp erythema and possibly cellulitis are seen occasionally after monitoring, probably in fewer than 1 percent of cases. The vast majority of these respond to local therapy (warm packs, drainage) and have no serious consequences. However, antibiotic treatment is necessary sometimes and serious, even lethal, infections have been reported. The use of a scalp electrode is relatively contraindicated in the presence of documented amnionitis and/or positive cervical cultures for herpes simplex virus or group B streptococci. Nevertheless, the potential benefits of the information to be obtained from internal fetal monitoring may justify its use in selected cases.

The potential for scalp infection at the site of fetal blood sampling punctures is also present, and appropriate precautions should be taken when this technique is used.

Other Complications

Rare cases of major fetal hemorrhage from scalp sampling sites have been reported, and if the incision is not placed properly, particularly in very small premature babies, perforation of the fetal skull with cerebrospinal fluid leaks is possible. Uterine perforation with the intrauterine catheter has occurred rarely, and sometimes the monitor may be unable to provide accurate information because of peculiarities in the fetal ECG. Of greatest concern are the complications of erroneous interpretation of monitoring data. This may unnecessarily increase the rate of cesarean or operative vaginal delivery.

EFFICACY OF FETAL MONITORING

The rapid dissemination of fetal monitoring techniques has been associated with considerable controversy over their effectiveness. Some critics have pointed out that the risks of monitoring are not inconsiderable. Maternal infection, fetal scalp abscess and soft tissue injury, and uterine perforation are all real risks, but occur rarely. In parallel with the increasing use of this technology, a trend toward a reinfusion of family-oriented obstetrics and a naturalization of the traditional hospital-based birth process occurred. Many argued that electronic fetal monitoring was intrusive and potentially dehumanizing. Of even greater concern was the observation that the introduction of monitoring was associated with a nationwide increase in cesarean section rates, which could in some circumstances be linked directly to the use of fetal monitoring.

Like all aspects of medical intervention, fetal monitoring must be judged by balancing its virtues against its medical risks and financial burden. Fortunately, serious infectious consequences of monitoring are exceedingly rare, and most patients do not find that the monitor interferes with their ability to use natural childbirth techniques, as long as they have been appropriately informed about such issues prior to labor. The cesarean section problem is real, but several institutions have demonstrated that when monitoring information is used in an appropriate and enlightened fashion, it has little or no influence on cesarean delivery frequency. Thus, in many respects, it is not the monitoring equipment per se but rather the individuals who have used monitoring inappropriately who are responsible for some of its adverse effects.

Even if one were to accept that the real risks of properly used fetal monitoring are minimal, a benefit would have to be demonstrated in order to justify its use. The medical literature does not provide satisfactory data in this respect. Most retrospective analyses of fetal monitoring suggest that some benefit can be accrued from its use. All have found that the intrapartum fetal death rate may be reduced by the use of fetal monitoring. However, since intrapartum death is uncommon and a relatively small contributor to overall perinatal mortality, many have been unconvinced that this is a suitable justification for universal monitoring. At least six randomized clinical trials of fetal monitoring have been performed, most of which have failed to provide proof of its efficacy. The conclusions of many studies are vitiated because of inadequate sample sizes or flaws in experimental design.

Despite the continuing polemics, electronic fetal monitoring is used by the vast majority of obstetricians, particularly in high-risk patients. Its utility in the low-risk patient is more controversial but has many advocates. Monitoring should be employed only by physicians who are trained intensively in its application and interpretation. A clear understanding of the capabilities and limitations of this sophisticated technology is necessary in order for it to be advantageous.

SUGGESTED READING

Cohen WR. Invasive electronic and biochemical fetal monitoring. In: Iffy L, Charles D, eds. Operative perinatology. New York: Macmillan, 1984:489.

Hon EH. Electronic evaluation of the fetal heart rate. VI. Fetal distress—a working hypothesis. Am J Obstet Gynecol 1962; 83:333.

Parer JT. Handbook of fetal heart rate monitoring. Philadelphia: WB Saunders, 1983.

Schifrin BS, Dame L. Fetal heart rate patterns. Prediction of Apgar score. JAMA 1972; 219:1322.

FETAL THERAPY

JOHN W. SEEDS, M.D.

The direct or indirect treatment of illness or malformation of the unborn with the intention of promoting the health and survival of the infant is a relatively recent development. The concept of the fetus as an independent patient evolved as the technical ability to evaluate fetal condition developed. In the last 30 years, techniques such as ultrasonography, amniocentesis, and fetal blood sampling have allowed the prenatal diagnosis of fetal illnesses or conditions.

As amniocentesis was developed to evaluate the severity of fetal hemolytic disease from maternal isoimmunization in the late 1950s, fetal treatment followed closely in the form of intrauterine transfusions. Real-time ultrasonography, introduced in the mid 1970s, fetoscopy in 1971, and direct percutaneous fetal umbilical venous blood sampling in 1983 are other fairly recent techniques that constitute the basis for contemporary prenatal diagnosis, and therefore they are the diagnostic techniques upon which modern fetal therapy is built.

Fetal therapy may be divided into two broad categories. Medical therapy describes the administration of a drug to the mother not to treat a maternal condition but with the intention of benefit to the fetus. A wide variety of agents cross the placental diffusion barrier because of low molecular weight (less than 1,000 daltons) or nonpolar chemical characteristics, and they often achieve equal or near equal concentration in fetal as compared with maternal serum. The second main category of fetal therapy is that of surgical intervention and includes the aspiration drainage of fluid accumulations within the fetus, the placement of in-dwelling diversion drainage catheters, or even the removal of part or all of a fetus through a laparotomy-hysterotomy procedure with performance of a fetal surgical intervention, and the replacement of the fetus.

In the case of any fetal therapy, issues of efficacy and safety are of paramount importance in patient selection and counseling. But because of the sequestered environment of the fetus and the interposition of another individual between the therapist and the patient, efficacy can be difficult to evaluate, and safety considerations must include the welfare of the mother as well as that of the baby. The decision to treat or not to treat a fetal condition becomes the consideration of three alternatives—treatment, nontreatment, or delivery. The patient and the physician must consider each of these in terms of prognosis and risk. Gestational age is important in the consideration of delivery. Although delivery prior to 24 weeks excludes fetal survival, it is one of the mother's options in the case of early diagnosis of a serious fetal illness or malformation. After 32-weeks gestation, most fetal conditions are more safely treated in the neonatal intensive care setting, although there are exceptions. Fetal hydrops secondary to supraventricular tachyarrhythmia even at advanced gestational age might benefit from therapeutic attempts to resolve the arrhythmia and reverse the hydrops prior to delivery. Finally, treatment of a fetal condition should be compatible with the future health and well-being of the fetus. It would be inappropriate, for example, to consider treating a fetal bladder obstruction in the case of an anencephalic.

The decision to treat or not to treat a fetal condition, therefore, requires first the most accurate diagnostic information available, including the nature and extent of the primary disorder and the exclusion, if possible, of any other malformations or conditions that would alter or impair the final outcome. The decision requires consideration of the prognosis of the specific condition, including likely outcome given no treatment as well as estimated outcome given treatment. Finally, the decision requires careful consideration of advantages or disadvantages of in utero treatment as compared with early delivery and neonatal treatment. These factors are usually if not always best evaluated by a team that includes a perinatologist, ultrasonographer, neonatologist, and pediatric surgeon. It is probable that only such a team of specialists can adequately sort out the complex questions involved in such a decision and formulate a logical plan of therapy to present to the parents. In the final analysis, it is the parents' decision to accept or reject such a care plan after careful counseling.

We will review in detail a variety of fetal conditions that have been treated in utero.

MEDICAL (INDIRECT) FETAL THERAPY

The medical treatment of a fetal condition is affected by placental transfer kinetics and maternal and fetal metabolism of the pharmacologic agent. Placental transfer is accomplished by one of three possible mechanisms: passive diffusion, active transport, and pinocytosis. Most pharmacologic agents gain entry to the fetal circulation by passive diffusion. Passive diffusion is a function of the concentration gradient between the mother and the fetal serum, the molecular weight of the substance, and the polarity of the molecule. Agents with a molecular weight over 1,000 daltons generally do not cross the placenta and relatively polar molecules generally do not cross. It is unlikely that any agent will achieve a higher concentration in the fetal circulation than in the mother's; in fact, the more likely situation is that there will always be a somewhat lower level in the fetus than in the mother.

The physiology of pregnancy can affect the efficacy of administration of a drug to the mother for a fetal condition. Decreased enteric absorption, increased renal clearance, or increased hepatic metabolism can result in the need to increase dosage in order to achieve and maintain the desired maternal plasma concentration. The normal maternal blood volume expansion in pregnancy can also result in the need for higher than expected drug dosage in order to achieve the desired plasma level. Table 1 summarizes categories of fetal conditions that might be treated medically.

Cardiotropic Therapy

Fetal supraventricular tachyarrhythmia is a rare complication of pregnancy that can result from a variety of electrical malfunctions within the fetal conduction system. In general, such arrhythmias do not become clinically apparent prior to the third trimester, and unless fetal ventricular rate is over 200 beats per minute, they do not represent a significant danger to the fetus. If fetal ventricular rate exceeds 200 beats per minute, ventricular filling is impaired, cardiac output falls, and fetal venous hypertension may develop, with hydrops fetalis a likely result. Hydrops fetalis involves skin edema and effusions of two of three serous cavities, including the peritoneal, pericardial, or pleural (Fig. 1). The diagnosis is made both from auscultation of the fetal tachycardia at the time of a prenatal visit and sonographic examination with real-time visualization of the cardiac activity. Occasionally the patient will be seen because of decreased fetal movement or increased fundal growth that is later found to be secondary to polyhydramnios. M-mode echocardiography is useful in evaluating the cardiac activity and confirming the atrial origin of the problem (Fig. 2). Pharmacologic treatment is directed at either eliminating the source of the tachyarrhythmia or reducing ventricular response in order to promote cardiac output.

Digoxin has been the first-line drug in the treatment of fetal tachyarrhythmias. Digoxin may be given by mouth in a standard loading protocol; however, it is often necessary to augment the loading dose even to the extent of repeating the loading sequence in order to reach therapeutic levels. The goal is not to produce supertherapeutic drug levels in the mother, but more drug is often required to reach the usual therapeutic level. If digoxin alone fails to reduce ventricular rate, other agents have been reported to be useful in conjunction with digoxin, including propranolol, procainamide, and quinidine. If hydrops fetalis is noted on ultrasound examination, fetal cardiotropic therapy may be considered even at an advanced gestational age to attempt to reverse the pathologic process in utero because the effusions and edema of the lungs can complicate survival of even the mature fetus.

TABLE 1 Fetal Therapy

MEDICAL (INDIRECT)	
TREATMENT	INDICATION
Digoxin	Supraventricular tachycardia
Propranolol	SVT
Procainamide	SVT
Quinidine	SVT
Promethazine	Rh isoimmunization
Corticosteroid	Rh disease, prematurity
Antibiotics	Sepsis
Plasmapheresis	Rh disease, immunologic thrombocytopenic purpura
Diet	Phenylketonuria
SURGICAL (DIRECT)	
Fetal transfusion	Severe isoimmunization
Intraperitoneal	
Intravascular	
Acute aspiration	Large perinephric cyst Large ovarian cyst Pleural effusion
Diversion catheter	Bladder obstruction
Open surgery	Diaphragmatic hernia Obstructive uropathy

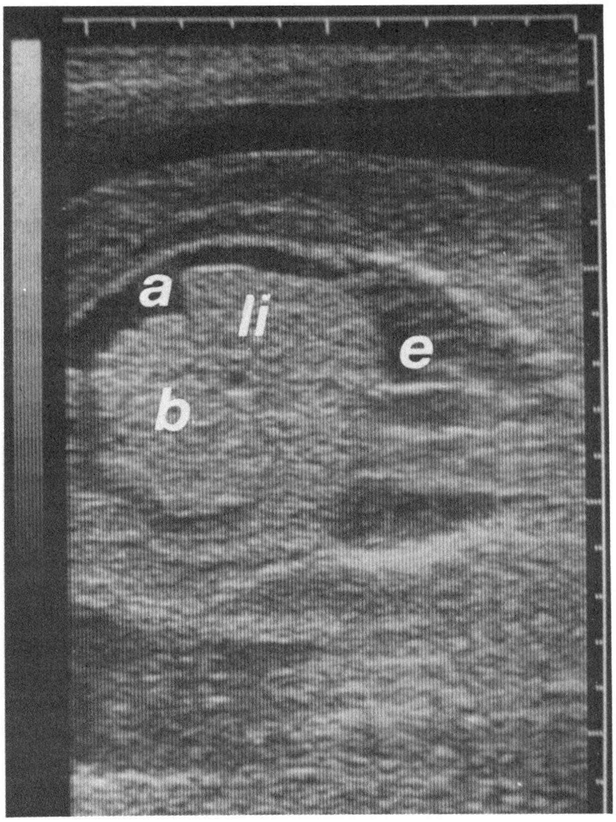

Figure 1 This longitudinal sonogram of the trunk of a fetus with hydrops demonstrates the ascites (a), and the pleural effusion (e) typical of the condition. The fetal liver (li), bowel (b), and skin edema are also seen.

Immunologic Suppression

Severe fetal hemolytic anemia can result from Rh isoimmunization as well as from maternal-fetal antigenic incompatibility with a large family of uncommon red cell antigens. Conventional care includes periodic monitoring of fetal condition with both ultrasonography and amniocentesis. The optical density of amniotic fluid is determined with a scanning spectrophotometer at 450 mμ wavelength of light and is a measure of the bilirubin concentration. Serial optical density studies identify the fetus with severe hemolysis, and either delivery or transfusion may be considered (see further on).

Since the basis of the hemolytic condition is immunologic, it has been suggested that adrenocortical steroids may be useful in treatment. Many steroids have been shown to cross the placenta, including beta-methasone and cortisol. In fact, optical density studies after treatment for other indications such as prematurity have shown a drop in amniotic fluid light absorption at 450 mμ, but the clinical efficacy of long-term therapy has not been shown. Promethazine (Phenergan) has also been reported to benefit severe isoimmunization in high doses (300 mg per day) by some investigators but not by all. Observed benefits included fewer intrauterine transfusions in treated pregnancies when compared with previously untreated siblings. Investigations showing no benefit might have resulted because of the use of too low a dose. Further studies are needed. These high doses are likely to result in toxic side effects such as somnolence in the mother and must be continuously maintained throughout pregnancy.

The fetal thrombocytopenia associated with maternal immunologic thrombocytopenic purpura has in some cases also appeared to benefit from maternal steroid therapy, but

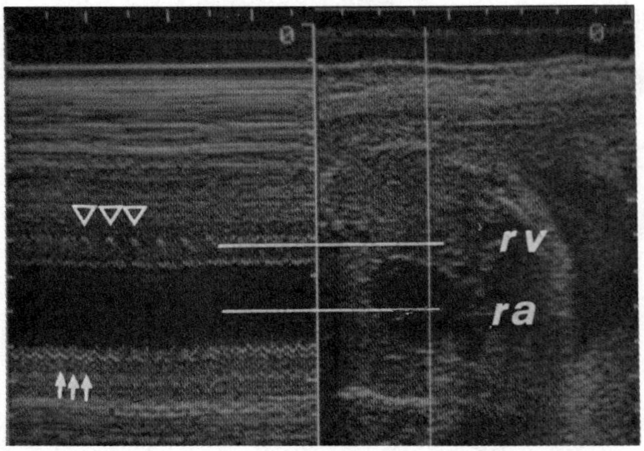

Figure 2 The wavy lines on the left side of this M-mode fetal echocardiogram follow movements of the left ventricle, indicated by open triangles, and the right atrium, indicated by arrows. In this case of atrial flutter with partial conduction block, dilatation of the right atrium (ra) is apparent (rv = right ventricle).

documented fetal benefit is unpredictable and inconsistent. A rise in maternal platelet count has not always indicated a rise in fetal platelet count.

Maternal plasmapheresis has been anecdotally reported to benefit both Rh isoimmunization and immunologic thrombocytopenic purpura, but no evidence from larger series of patients supports this. Twice to three times weekly pheresis of 2,500 to 5,000 ml of plasma has been used.

Antibiotic Therapy

Amnionitis and neonatal sepsis are significant risks in the case of prolonged premature rupture of membranes. Although the danger of fetal infection justifies intensive neonatal evaluation and often prophylactic therapy pending culture results, most neonates deal successfully with bacteremia in the case of many pathogens. The exception is beta streptococcus. Neonatal sepsis and death can occur with such striking and relentless speed that when vaginal or amniotic fluid cultures show the presence of beta streptococcus, treatment of the mother with appropriate antibiotic agents is wise. The first choice for beta streptococcus alone is penicillin, although ampicillin is often selected in practice.

It has been clearly shown that both penicillin and ampicillin cross the placenta well and achieve effective levels in fetal tissues. It appears that the best neonatal outcomes result when the antibiotic therapy is begun prior to delivery.

Adrenocorticoids and Lung Maturity

Since the first studies almost 20 years ago showing unusually mature lung function in animals born prematurely after prenatal steroid administration, the use of steroid therapy to promote lung function in patients facing the imminent birth of a premature infant has gained wide acceptance.

Certain criteria describe those patients most likely to benefit from steroid administration. These include gestational age between 28 and 32 weeks, delivery likely within 7 days, and delivery not likely within 24 hours. Debate continues concerning the efficacy of treatment prior to 28 weeks and after 32 weeks, the utility of pretreatment amniotic fluid maturity studies, the use of steroid treatment in the presence of premature rupture of membranes, and apparent racial differences in response to steroid therapy.

It should be clearly understood also that predelivery steroid therapy does not under any circumstance eliminate the danger of respiratory distress in the individual case. Such therapy has only been shown in large studies to reduce the incidence at a given gestational age by from one-third to one-half.

It should also be understood that although no apparent side effects have been found in humans, reduced brain growth has been described in primates exposed in utero to steroids in high doses for somewhat extended periods. The assumption of not yet identified long-term risks should continue to encourage conservative use of steroid therapy with emphasis on those candidates who are members of the group most likely to benefit.

Several specific pharmacologic agents have been shown to be associated with benefit, including betamethasone, cortisol, and dexamethasone. It appears that in order to show a clinical response, the infant must remain undelivered for at least 24 hours. It is not known how long after administration the benefit is sustained. Although the interpretation of some data suggests that the advantage is lost after 1 week, the data are incomplete and may be misleading.

Maternal Dietary Restrictions

Screening newborns for phenylketonuria is standard practice and has been for many years. The practice is responsible for the early identification and prevention of developmental brain damage in such infants that would have resulted from high serum levels of phenylalanine. Treatment with a low phenylalanine diet may be discontinued in late adolescence without danger to the affected individual, even though serum phenylalanine levels will rise to high levels. However, pregnancy in such a patient subjects the fetus to sufficiently high levels of amino acid that mental retardation is reported to result and increases in frequency with each trimester before a low phenylalanine diet is begun. Best results are seen when the therapeutic diet is begun prior to conception.

FETAL SURGICAL THERAPY

The treatment of a human fetal condition by direct fetal intervention is less than 25 years old, although animal fetal surgical models have been known for over 50 years. Beginning with guinea pigs in the 1920s, lambs in the 1930s, and dogs and other animals in the 1950s, animal fetal surgical models provided vital information about a variety of disease processes and malformations. These included intestinal atresia, coarctation of the aorta, and diaphragmatic hernia. Intrauterine transfusion was the first clinically practical and successful direct human fetal treatment, and it stood as the only accepted fetal surgical procedure until the early 1980s, when a variety of other interventions were reported, including treatments for hydrocephalus and obstructive uropathies.

Intrauterine Transfusion

In 1963 Liley reported the first successful intrauterine fetal blood transfusion using a technique that became the standard of care therapy for severe Rh isoimmunization. He described the placement of a transfusion needle into the peritoneal cavity of the fetus and the injection of tightly packed, washed, compatible red cells.

The early technique involved the location of the fetus with fluoroscopy prior to the placement of the needle. Each transfusion resulted in about a 2.2-rads dose of absorbed radiation to the fetus, and only about a 50 percent correct needle placement occurred with each attempt. Procedure-related fetal mortality was about 10 percent with the first procedure and 5 percent with each transfusion after the first. Mortality was often attributed to operative trauma (40 to 50 percent), including liver laceration or bleeding. If hydrops fetalis was present at the time of the first transfusion or was noted between the first and the second transfusions, neonatal survival dropped to only 25 percent. Furthermore, if intrauterine transfusion was necessary prior to 25 weeks, survival was as low as 9 percent. Overall, survival of infants needing intrauterine transfusion varied from 25 to 70 percent. Recent investigators have reported higher survival rates of infants with hydrops at the time of transfusion by adding intraperitoneal diuretic and digoxin to the blood transfused. Furthermore, after the introduction of real-time ultrasound to guide visually the intraperitoneal transfusion needle in the late 1970s, the incidence of fetal trauma was dramatically reduced and procedure-related risk cut to near zero.

It is of historical interest that in 1964 an alternative approach to treatment of the same disease was reported. A laparotomy incision, hysterotomy, and exteriorization of a lower limb of the human fetus with cannulation of the femoral vessels and a direct exchange transfusion was described. Afterward, the limb was returned to the amniotic cavity and the uterus and abdomen repaired. Further reports described complete fetal removal and cannulation of a fetal jugular vein. Limited practical success and the evolution of the Liley method severely limited development of human fetal exteriorization.

Fetoscopy with fetoscopic fetal blood sampling became available in the late 1970s and offered the opportunity to determine directly the extent of fetal hemolysis and possibly perform intravascular transfusion of donor red cells. This approach to direct transfusion of the fetus did not require radiation, laparotomy, or hysterotomy but instead the transabdominal placement of a 2.4×3 mm fiberoptic fetoscope and the visualization of the umbilical vein with puncture and aspiration of fetal blood using a 25-gauge needle through a side channel. Probably because of the large size of the fetoscopic trocar and associated uterine trauma, the reported pregnancy loss rate was 4.5 to 5.0 percent with fetoscopy, but the several advantages made this method arguably superior to intraperitoneal transfusion. The fetal hematologic condition could be directly evaluated. Donor blood could be directly transfused, avoiding the inconsistency of absorption from the peritoneal cavity. The technical difficulty, prerequisite skill and experience, and rare practical availability of the procedure served to prevent fetoscopic transfusions from replacing the Liley technique. In addition, fetoscopy is technically impractical past 26-weeks gestation.

Most recently (1982), percutaneous umbilical vein puncture and aspiration of fetal blood using an ultrasonically guided narrow-gauge needle have been reported and adapted to intrauterine transfusion. Donor blood may be directly infused into the fetal circulation. The technique is accomplished with ultrasonography on the sterile field, using a 20- to 25-gauge 10- to 17-cm long needle with stylette. The needle is guided to the umbilical vein either at its insertion on the placenta or the infant, or to a free loop of cord in the amniotic cavity (Fig. 3). Another potential aspiration and transfusion site is the umbilical vein

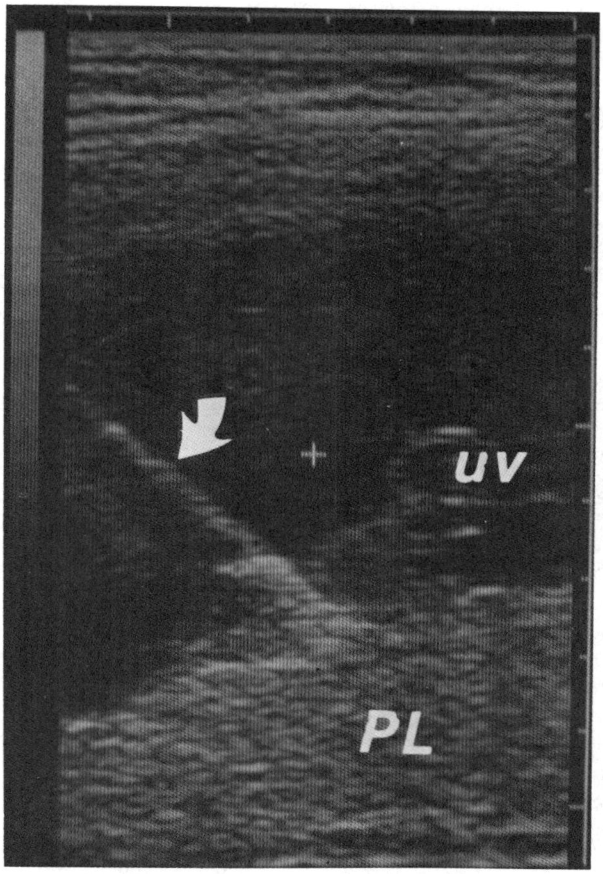

Figure 3 The arrow overlays amniotic fluid and indicates the aspiration needle tracking to the umbilical vein (uv) at the insertion site on the placenta (PL).

within the fetal liver. Complications have been rare, and the pregnancy loss rate associated with this procedure has been similar to the loss rate associated with amniocentesis. The reported pregnancy loss rate after cord blood sampling in gestation of less than 24 weeks is 0.8 percent. Observed cord bleeding after puncture ceases in less than 2 minutes in 98 percent of cases. Particularly in the case of the fetus with hydrops fetalis, direct intravascular transfusion appears to be superior to the intraperitoneal alternative. The complete reversal of hydrops fetalis in utero after intravascular transfusions have been observed.

The fetal intravascular transfusion has been done both as an isovolumetric exchange in small aliquots or direct injection of donor blood with no withdrawal. Both methods have been successful. Often in the case of the isovolumetric exchange, withdrawal through the narrow-gauge needle becomes difficult or impossible because of clot formation at the tip.

Despite the published safety record of percutaneous umbilical vein sampling, complications can and do occur. Fetal movement during aspiration, transfusion with a needle crossing the amniotic cavity, or using the umbilicus or umbilical vein within the liver suggest the obvious danger of laceration of the vein with serious consequences very likely. For this reason, a fetal intramuscular or intravascular injection of either pancuronium bromide or curare prior to aspiration may be used if the puncture site appears vulnerable to fetal movement. Also, during blood injection, displacement of the needle tip could lead to perivenous injection with possible umbilical vein occlusion. Fetal heart rate should be monitored during the transfusion to guard against this. The patient and the team should be prepared to deliver the infant at any time that irreversible compromise is detected. Neonatal management of the delivered infant who is paralyzed by pancuronium is not difficult if the neonatal team is prepared for such an event.

The technical ability to perform direct intravascular transfusion as early as 18 weeks now indicates the value of amniotic fluid optical density studies much earlier than previously believed useful. Therefore, in the case of a mother with a previously affected infant or a high antibody titer, amniocentesis may be useful at 18 to 20 weeks. Furthermore, if the father is a heterozygote, early fetal blood sampling to determine fetal blood type and Rh status may eliminate the need for serial amniocentesis in some cases.

Drainage of Obstructed Fetal Systems

A congenital malformation causing obstruction to the normal flow of a fetal fluid may be diagnosed as a result of either secondary clinical complications of the pregnancy, such as abnormal uterine growth related to polyhydramnios or oligohydramnios, or as a result of ultrasonography performed for these or other indications. The abnormal accumulation of a fetal fluid above the obstruction enables sonographic visualization, because any homogeneous fluid produces a striking anechoic (black) appearance on ultrasound, contrasted with adjacent echogenic (white or gray) fetal soft tissue (Fig. 4).

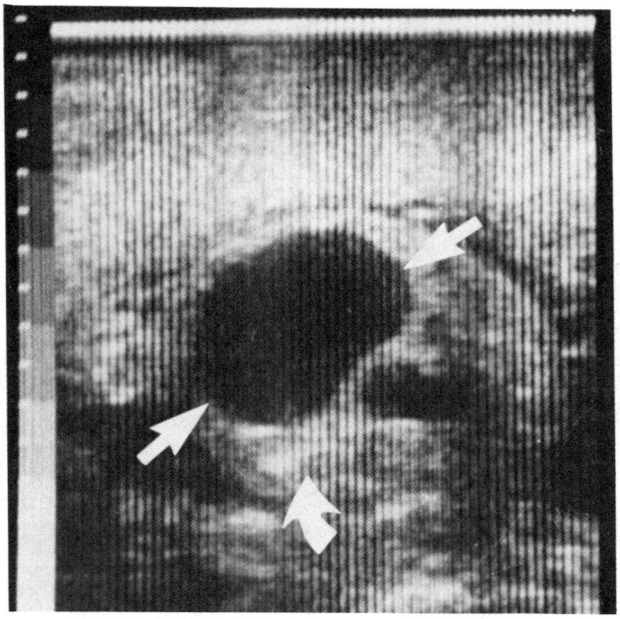

Figure 4 The echo-free (anechoic) visual nature of this perinephric urinoma (straight arrows) is in striking contrast to the surrounding echogenic fetal soft tissue.

There is the inevitable temptation to intervene in the case of any fetal malformation detected with ultrasound examination if a feasible technique for intervention is available. This is the "if we can see it, let's do something" phenomenon. A large number of such malformations, however, are stable, do not cause any direct or indirect complication of the pregnancy, and result in no predictable neonatal loss of life or health if left alone. If the malformation directly threatens a vital fetal system, for example the brain, or secondarily leads to conditions that threaten the pregnancy at a previable gestational age, such as polyhydramnios prior to 32 weeks, then in the absence of associated malformations that themselves alter neonatal outcome, intervention might be considered.

The parents considering such intervention should understand that although every effort has been made to exclude other associated and potentially compromising malformations or conditions, it is impossible to absolutely exclude all such possibilities. In every case, intervention must be considered without absolute guarantees of outcome. Furthermore, it has proved impossible to predict absolutely the presence of permanent organ system damage in, for example, the kidneys with obstructive uropathy, and the lungs with severe oligohydramnios. Intervention must be considered without absolute knowledge of fetal renal or pulmonary function.

Reported interventions have included single needle aspiration of fluid, serial aspiration, placement of continuous in-dwelling diversion catheters, and, in very limited numbers, open laparotomy-hysterotomy procedures with exteriorization of the fetus and surgical repair of palliation of the fetal condition. Many of these procedures are reported to and cataloged by the International Registry of Fetal Surgery, maintained at the University of Manitoba,

Canada. In summary, we will draw on the accumulated data of this registry. We will consider these various approaches individually, by type of procedure rather than by organ system.

Acute Aspiration Drainage

Acute needle aspiration of a fluid accumulation within the fetus is relatively simple. The detection of the problem in the first place implies the presence of a distinct fluid mass within a discrete space that is visible on ultrasound examination (Fig. 5). Using aseptic technique with ultrasound on the sterile field by covering the transducer with a sterile bag allows the operator to guide a narrow-gauge needle to the fluid mass visually. If necessary, a pancuronium injection arrests fetal movement, and mild sedation is all that is necessary to provide maternal comfort. It is desirable to avoid the placenta if possible. Care must be taken to avoid damage to the fetal liver and/or bowel if possible. Renal cysts may be approached from the fetal flank and bladders from the flank or anterior midline above the pubis. The needle may be guided either in a coplanar fashion so that it enters the maternal skin just behind the heel of the transducer and tracks within the scan plane itself, or it may enter the skin adjacent to the transducer and track in a transplanar fashion, where only the shaft is seen as it crosses the scan plane.

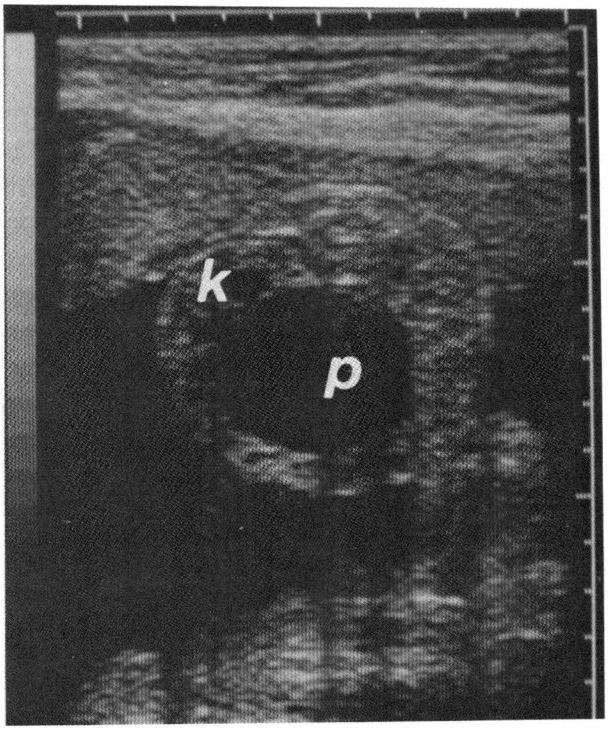

Figure 5 This transverse midabdominal scan of a fetus with an obstruction of the ureteropelvic junction illustrates a severely dilated renal pelvis (p) and the severe caliectasis of the kidney (k).

Central Nervous System

Blockage of the aqueduct of Sylvius, the foramina of the posterior fossa, or a Chiari type II malformation of the fetal posterior fossa associated with spina bifida results in fetal hydrocephalus. The formerly poor prognosis for severe hydrocephalus overt at birth, with survival of less than 20 percent and normal neurobehavioral development in fewer than 10 percent, suggested that when severe fetal hydrocephalus was discovered, prenatal decompression might be helpful. The neurosurgical axiom that the sooner the intraventricular pressure is relieved the better was simply carried into the womb. The expanded lateral ventricles are easily seen with ultrasound as a result of the anechoic (black) cerebrospinal fluid contrasted with the surrounding brain and the more ventral midbrain (Fig. 6). These fluid chambers offer large targets, and the simplest intervention is needle aspiration of fluid. Reaccumulation is rapid, however, and repeated craniocenteses are required. The predictable risks of infection, fetal and maternal trauma, and possible rupture of membranes or initiation of labor prevented broad acceptance of serial craniocentesis in the care of fetal hydrocephalus. Furthermore, greatly improved outcome in more recently reported series of congenital hydrocephalus overt at birth suggests that clear benefit from fetal intervention is now more difficult to show.

Nonimmune Hydrops Fetalis, Fetal Hydrothorax, Fetal Ascites

Hydrops fetalis may be defined as fetal skin edema plus effusions in two of the three serous cavities (the peri-

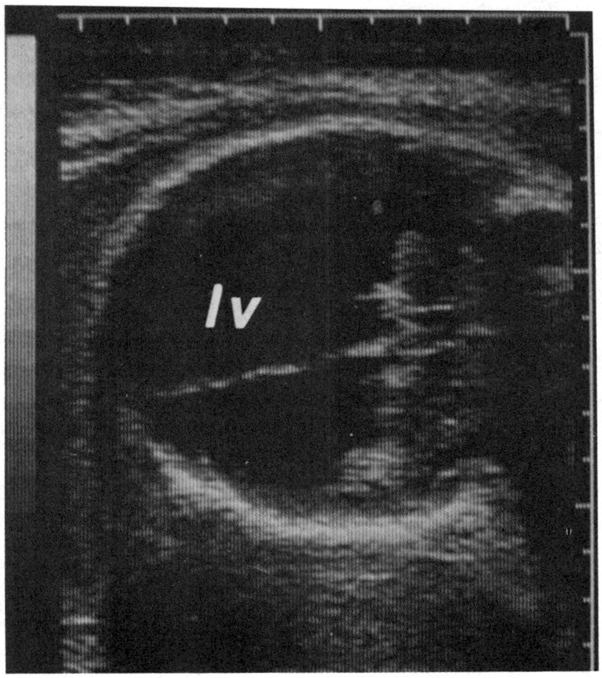

Figure 6 The severely dilated lateral ventricles (lv) are easily seen in this coronal view of the fetal cranium.

toneal, pleural, or pericardial cavity). Hydrops that is not the result of fetal-maternal antigenic incompatibility is termed nonimmune hydrops. This condition can result from a wide variety of malfunctions or malformations, including cardiac defects, chromosomal abnormalities, umbilical venous thrombosis, and other malformations or conditions including infection that may secondarily result in fetal portal and/or umbilical venous hypertension and hydrops.

Often nonimmune hydrops presents a balanced appearance, with mild or severe effusions of the affected cavities being relatively equal in a given case. In many patients, however, there is an unbalanced appearance, with either the pleural (Fig. 7) or the peritoneal (Fig. 8) effusions drastically worse than the others. The imbalance is possibly a reflection of the primary etiology. Consideration of intervention in such cases is based on two possible benefits to the fetus or the mother. Aspiration of the accumulated fluid allows further diagnostic testing, including karyotyping from cultured fetal cells within the effusion, chemical analysis both for electrolytes and immunoglobulins, antibody testing for specific infectious antigenic stimulation, and direct viral or bacterial fluid culture. In addition, aspiration of the fluid allows evaluation of the relationship between the condition and secondary effects such as polyhydramnios or preterm labor or both.

Congenital fetal hydrothorax often has been referred to as "congenital chylothorax," since it was most often not diagnosed until after birth and after feedings. When aspirated, the fluid was typically chylous. In utero, however, the pleural effusions are not chylous but instead are serous in character, and the condition is therefore more properly termed "congenital hydrothorax." The condition can present at or near term, in which case the appropriate intervention is delivery at a facility prepared for immediate neonatal ventilatory support and thoracentesis. Not infrequently, however, the condition can occur earlier, often between 28 and 32 weeks, with polyhydramnios and associated preterm labor. Probably because of increased intrathoracic pressure, ascites is often seen, and fetal edema can also be noted. The increased intrathoracic pressure also alters fetal swallowing and leads to the polyhydramnios and through it to preterm labor. Neonatal survival of the infant born at this premature gestational age with hydrops and hydrothorax is very poor, since ventilation of the compressed and possibly edematous lungs is difficult if not impossible. Aspiration of the thoracic fluid (Fig. 9) offers the diagnositic opportunities outlined earlier, and possibly the chance to alter amniotic fluid dynamics and prolong pregnancy as well as promote fetal lung development. Three such cases have been reported, with successful aspiration or drainage and neonatal survival in one patient. It has been shown that amniotic fluid volume does appear to respond to chest decompression at least transiently, supporting the existence of a dynamic relationship between the intrathoracic pressure and amniotic fluid hydrodynamics.

Aspiration of fetal ascitic fluid for diagnostic and possible therapeutic purposes has also been reported, but with no survivors. The spectrum of etiologies in cases characterized by severe ascites is much more complex than that

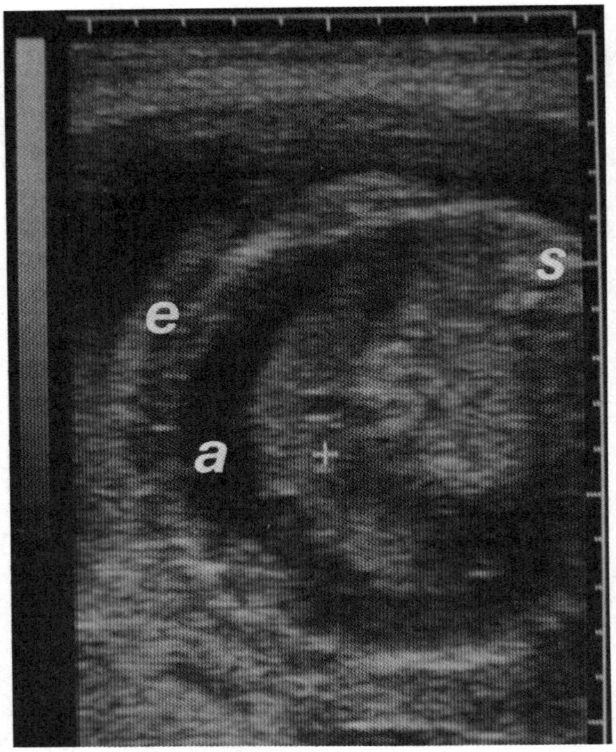

Figure 8 This transverse midabdominal view of a hydropic fetus demonstrates ascites (a) and skin edema (e); the fetal spine (s) and the fetal liver (+) are also visible.

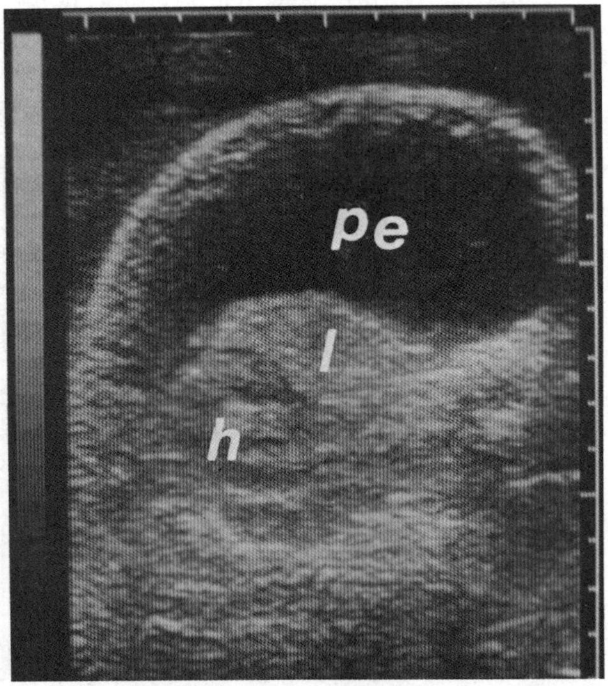

Figure 7 The severe asymmetric pleural effusion (pe) is easily seen in this transverse scan of the fetal chest. The right lung (l) and heart (h) are also visible.

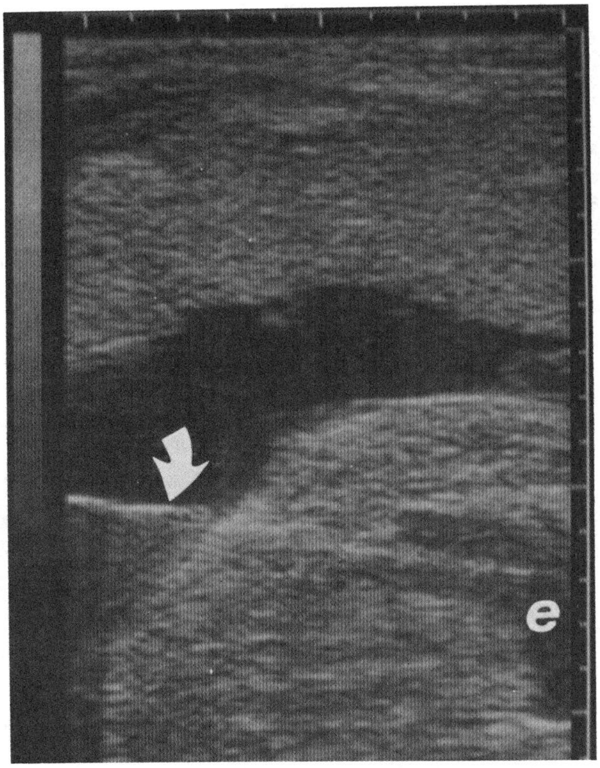

Figure 9 The needle (arrow) draining a fetal pleural effusion (e).

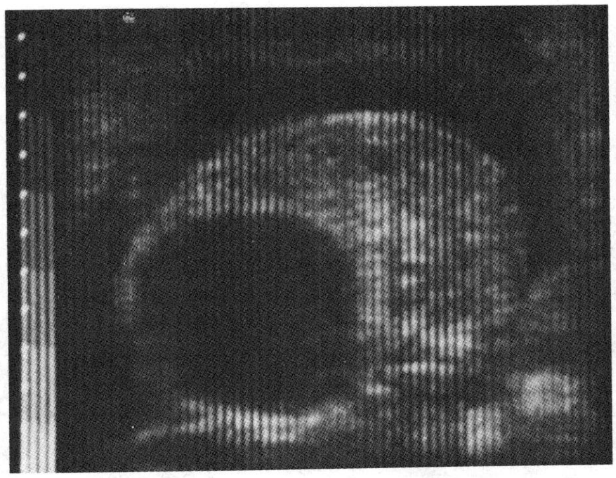

Figure 10 This transverse fetal abdominal scan clearly illustrates the discrete, symmetric, echo-free appearance of the typical perinephric urinoma associated with fetal ureteropelvic junction obstruction.

associated with hydrothorax, and although simple aspiration of ascitic fluid does offer diagnostic opportunities, the physiologic impact on amniotic fluid hydrodynamics and finally on fetal survival of antenatal drainage of fetal ascites is less clear than in the case of hydrothorax.

Obstructive Uropathy

Congenital obstruction of the urinary tract may occur at any of several points, including the ureteropelvic junction, the ureterovesicular junction, or the urethra. The urinary tract is the second most common system affected by congenital malformation and is the origin of over 50 percent of congenital abdominal masses. The obstruction may be partial or complete, with stenosis or atresia, or, in the case of urethra, result from posterior valves.

Ureteropelvic junction obstruction is usually unilateral, with a normal contralateral kidney. In the case of complete obstruction, the result may be severe hydronephrosis with caliectasis (see Fig. 5) or the formation of a retroperitoneal perinephric cyst or urinoma (Fig. 10). In the usual unilateral case, there is normal bladder filling and normal amniotic fluid volume. In some cases there may be polyhydramnios if the perinephric cyst becomes large enough to cause extrinsic proximal bowel compression and obstruction. Examples of needle aspiration of unilateral lesions are reported, but in most cases, the affected kidney may be salvaged with immediate neonatal decompression, and prenatal intervention is not recommended unless there are consequential effects such as polyhydramnios and/or preterm labor that justify consideration of drainage. Acute aspiration offers only short-term benefit but allows analysis of urine and documentation of refilling rate. Continuous diversion catheterization might then be considered if benefits are sufficient to balance the risks.

Ureterovesical junction obstruction is less common and is often associated with an ectopic ureter and ureterocele of the bladder wall. Probably since only a part of one kidney is affected (Fig. 11), the impact is usually less severe, and clinically significant renal cysts of sufficient size to justify intervention are rare.

Bladder outlet obstruction causes enlargement of the bladder and usually bilateral hydroureter and hydronephrosis. Severe oligohydramnios is typical after 20-weeks gestation, since amniotic fluid after that time is dependent on fetal urine for maintenance (Fig. 12). In the case of this classic presentation, consideration of intervention is justified since long-term development in such a case makes neonatal survival unlikely. Pulmonary hypoplasia with a wet lung weight of less than 1.8 percent of the total neonatal body weight is the most common cause of death. Acute needle aspiration is not a long-term solution, although urinalysis, karyotype, and observation of refilling rate do offer information upon which a decision regarding in-dwelling diversion catheterization might be based. In the case of a fetus in whom after aspiration drainage the urine obtained is of good quality, the karyotype is normal, and the bladder has refilled fairly rapidly, long-term diversion carries some likelihood of successful benefit (see next section). In the absence of these features, further intervention may be of little value.

Other Masses

A variety of other rare cystic masses might benefit from aspiration drainage if consequential clinical events appear to threaten the pregnancy and appear to be associ-

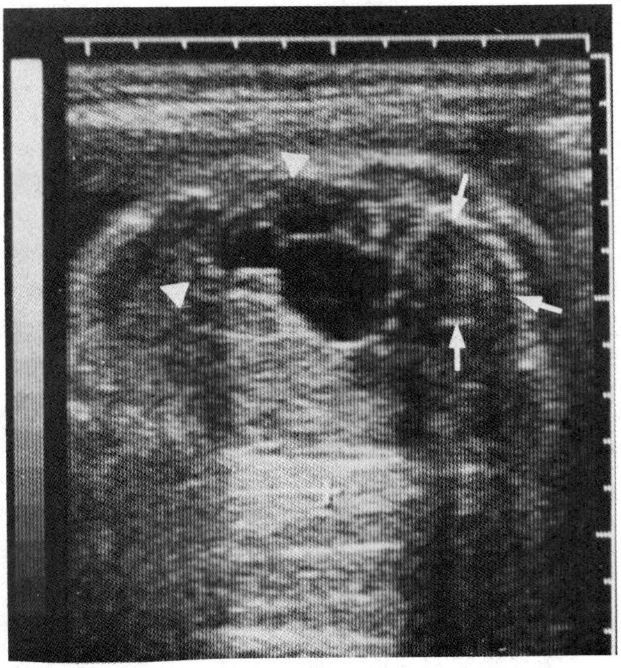

Figure 11 The hydronephrosis of the upper pole of this kidney (closed triangles) should be compared with the normal appearance of the lower pole (arrows). This kidney proved to have a duplicate collecting system and obstruction of only the upper pole.

ated with the mass. Ovarian cysts, mesenteric cysts, and thoracic lymphatic cysts all have been reported to cause or be associated with polyhydramnios, and needle aspiration might therefore benefit the clinical situation and warrant careful consideration. It is clear that the simple observation by sonography of such a mass unaccompanied by life- or health-threatening implications does not justify needle aspiration but instead serial observation and reconsideration if conditions change or simply appropriate preparation for birth.

Diversion Catheterization

Continuous in-dwelling diversion catheterization in the human fetus was first reported in 1981 in the case of fetal hydrocephalus, and in 1982 in the case of a bladder outlet obstruction. Such intervention was undertaken on the basis of historical data showing a very poor prognosis for both conditions in the untreated case and animal models in sheep and primates that suggested benefit from in utero decompression of both conditions.

The catheterization technique in the case of both malformations is fairly similar. Diversion catheters are designed to bypass the obstruction and divert fluid from the lateral ventricles or the bladder to the sterile amniotic cavity (Fig. 13). There are basically two catheter delivery systems available. In the case of one, a small-bore double pigtail catheter is slipped over the outside of an operative needle that is then advanced under sonographic guidance into the obstructed bladder, and then the catheter is pushed off the needle as the needle is removed. In practice, this system proves very difficult because the frictional resistance to advancement of the catheter against maternal and fetal tissue is great. The alternative is a narrow Silastic tubing that is slipped through the internal lumen of a 13-gauge thin-walled cannula needle placed into the affected organ under sonographic guidance. As the catheters are advanced, the cannula is removed. Certainly, catheter placement through the lumen of the needle is easier, although the 13-gauge needle is a significant intrusion into both the uterus and the fetus. Ruptured membranes or even amniotic fluid leakage into the maternal peritoneal cavity may occur. The double pigtail catheter may, alternatively, be placed in the fetus through the lumen of the 13-gauge cannula.

Fetal Hydrocephalus

As recently as the mid-1970s, neurosurgical reports showed that as few as 14 percent of infants with congenital hydrocephalus overt at birth could expect normal neurologically intact survival. Only half of the survivors were expected to have an IQ over 80. With the untreated outcome so bleak, it was natural to consider antenatal treatment.

Animal models in both sheep and primates showed that in utero treatment of congenital hydrocephalus increased survival and arrested ventriculomegaly. Neurobehavioral development was more difficult to assess. Clinical trials were undertaken using the Denver Hydrocephalus Shunt in the human case. Severe, symmetric, progressive hydrocephalus in the absence of associated

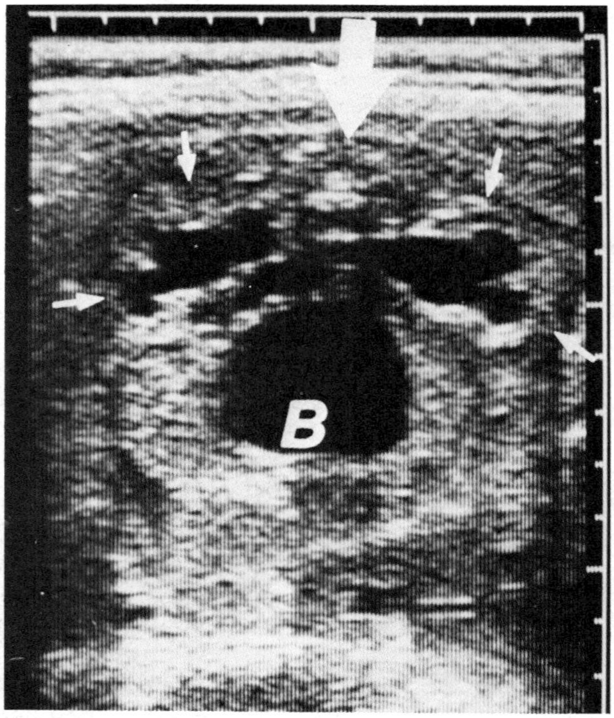

Figure 12 The hydronephrosis (arrows) and the enlarged fetal bladder (B), along with severe oligohydramnios, are typical of posterior urethral valves.

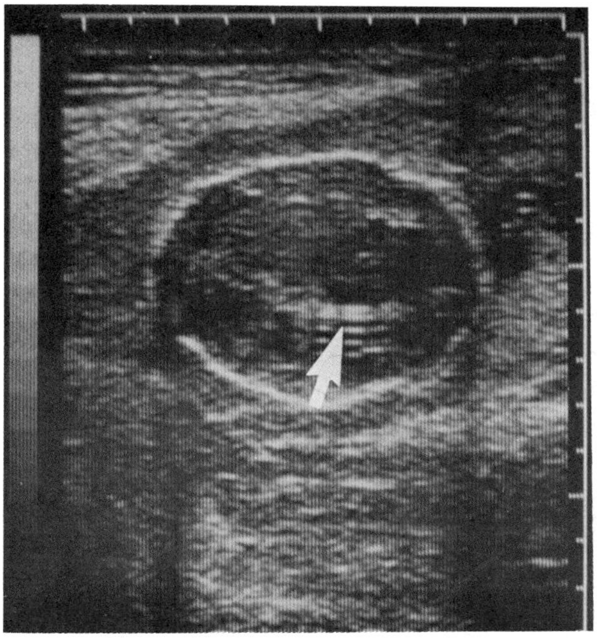

Figure 13 The arrow in this occipitofrontal scan of a fetal cranium indicates the internal portion of a fetal ventriculoamniotic diversion catheter.

defects at less than 30-weeks gestational age identified the desired candidate.

Between 1981 and 1986, 43 cases of fetal treatment were reported to the International Registry. There were six deaths associated with treatment. A large number of cases did not satisfy the criteria in that the primary malformation was not simple symmetric hydrocephalus, or there were serious associated malformations that had been missed. Among those 21 infants finally shown to have isolated aqueductal stenosis, two-thirds survived with no deficit or only a mild disability. Although this outcome compares favorably with historical conventional therapeutic results, contemporary neurosurgical reports recommending serial monitoring of cranial growth and advanced delivery and neonatal neurosurgical care show excellent outcomes, with intact survival the rule. In view of the delicate nature of the surgery, the difficulty in properly selecting candidates, and the improved outcome with conventional care, fetal treatment of congenital hydrocephalus has largely ceased.

Bladder Outlet Obstruction

Bladder obstruction can result from urethral atresia, posterior urethral valves, or anomaly complexes including caudal regression and persistent cloaca. The ultimate prognosis for the infant is quite different for each of these because the developmental impact on the urinary tract and the lungs is quite different. Experiments in sheep reported in the early 1970s strongly suggested that ureteral ligation in the first half of pregnancy resulted in cystic dysplastic changes in the fetal kidneys that were irreversible. The kidneys were large, the parenchyma was replaced with cysts of variable size, and little function remained. Ligation after the midpoint in gestation caused instead a central radial hydronephrosis without the dysplastic changes. These experiments were analogous to the distinction in insult in the human fetus between urethral atresia causing obstruction from the earliest point in the development and urethral valves that cause obstruction at variable times, most often after the midpoint in pregnancy. Other investigators repeating this work in the early 1980s confirmed the distinctly different renal response to obstruction in the first and second half of pregnancy again in sheep and also showed the secondary impact of the oligohydramnios on the development of fetal pulmonary hypoplasia and the potential reversibility of some of the effects if the obstruction were relieved.

During the past 5 years, efforts have concentrated on developing methods for distinguishing the fetus who has already suffered irreversible renal damage from the fetus who has not, and on predicting the presence or absence of pulmonary hypoplasia before the placement of an indwelling diversion catheter. Visually, the enlarged, cystic dysplastic kidneys appear different from normal kidneys, and such an appearance is strong evidence for renal nonfunction (Fig. 14). The absence of such an appearance, however, is not proof of normal function. Urine electrolytes and osmolarity seem to correlate with recoverable renal function, and if the urine is hypotonic, good renal function is implied, whereas if the urine is isotonic, poor function is suggested. Poor bladder filling after drainage or poor output with chronic catheterization is further evi-

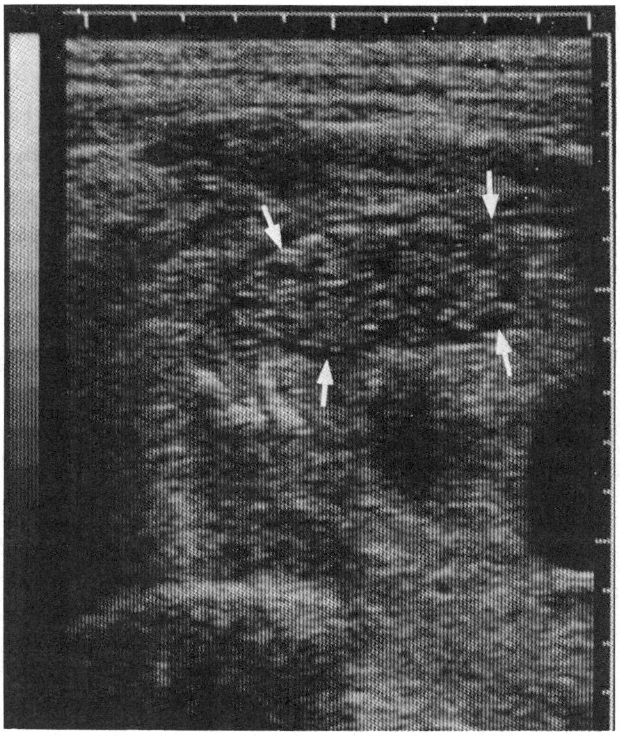

Figure 14 The fetal kidney highlighted here by arrows is large and contains numerous small cortical cysts of variable size. This is the typical late appearance of a cystic dysplastic kidney.

dence of poor function. Evidence of poor renal function may not preclude survival, however, as neonatal transplantation may still offer the infant the opportunity to survive.

Pulmonary hypoplasia is the most frequent cause of death. Since pulmonary hypoplasia may be defined on a mass basis, it appears logical that comparison of fetal chest or lung dimensions with normals should identify the fetus with undeveloped lungs. Studies attempting to confirm such a relationship have shown a rough correlation between chest dimensions and pulmonary hypoplasia, but successes have come only in those cases in which the dimensional anomaly was found shortly before birth. As yet no system has proved its value in predicting pulmonary function many weeks in advance, when such information would be useful in considering intervention.

In summary, the infants most likely to benefit from antenatal diversion of bladder outlet obstruction are those with posterior urethral valves that result in bladder distention, oligohydramnios, and central hydronephrosis (Fig. 15). The presence of amniotic fluid is evidence that complete obstruction is not present. After 32 weeks, delivery and neonatal intervention are more attractive alternatives.

Discrimination between atresia, persistent cloaca, and posterior urethral valves is not perfect. Although the symmetric, discrete outline of the simple bladder obstruction (Fig. 16) differs from the irregular, segmental appearance that is typical of the cloacal mass (Fig. 17), the distinction by sonography alone occasionally is difficult, and drainage or catheterization can be helpful in discriminating one from the other.

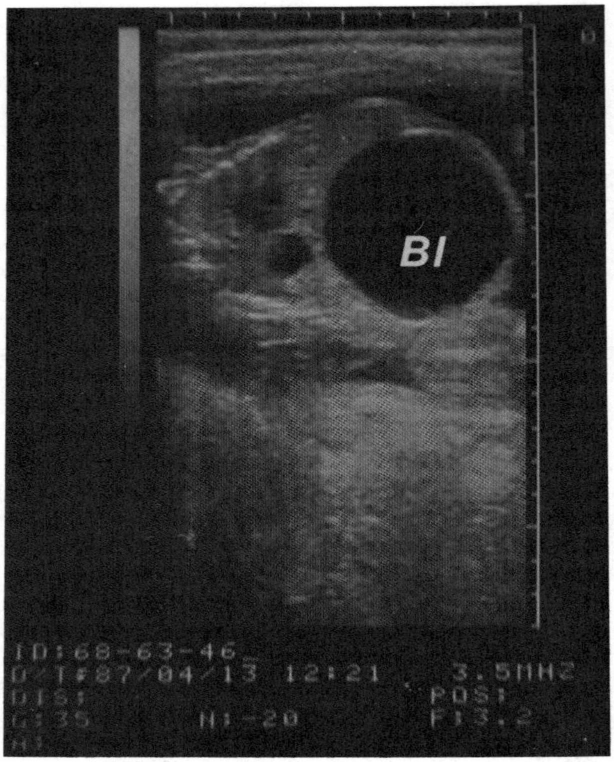

Figure 16 Compare the discrete, symmetric outline of this obstructed fetal bladder (Bl) with the appearance of the persistent cloaca in Figure 17.

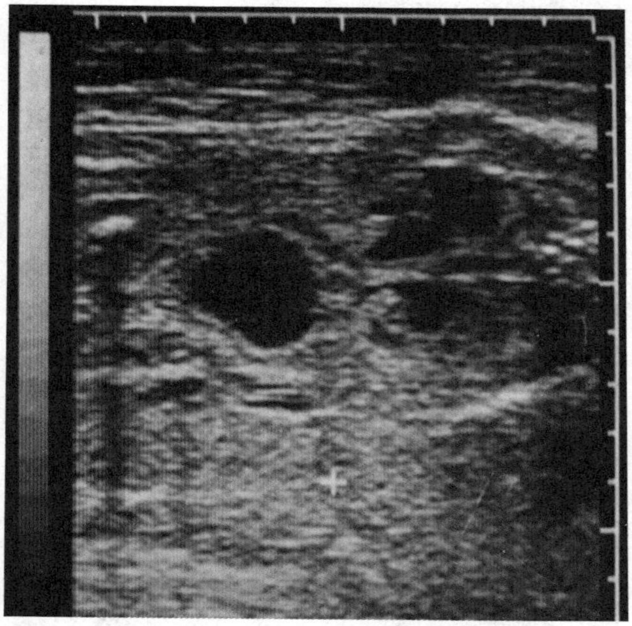

Figure 15 Posterior urethral valves produce a picture similar to this coronal view showing severe oligohydramnios, bilateral hydronephrosis, and bladder enlargement. The greater portion of this bladder is in front of the plane of this scan.

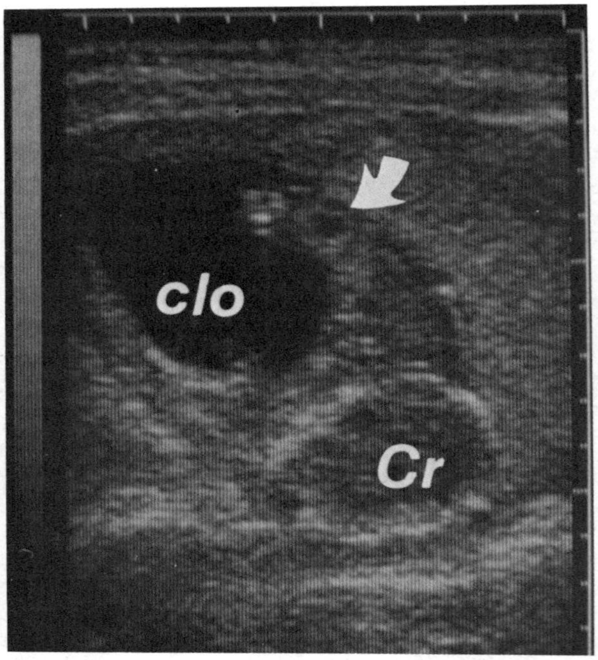

Figure 17 A caudal regression (Cr), persistent cloaca complex produces this type of appearance. There is severe oligohydramnios, an irregular fetal abdominal mass representing the cloaca (clo), and a mildly hydronephrotic kidney (arrow).

In any case, the patient must usually consider the alternatives of treatment, nontreatment, or delivery without absolute exclusion of undetected associated malformations, without absolute knowledge of final renal or pulmonary function, and with the knowledge that such intervention might be complicated by infection, premature rupture of membranes, or premature labor.

The survival rate of treated fetal bladder obstruction reported to the International Registry is 40 percent. The infants reported were found to suffer from a variety of lesions that precluded survival in some cases. About 15 percent of infants showed chromosomal abnormalities, thus underlining the importance of a karyotype early in the evaluation of an infant with bladder obstruction.

Open Fetal Surgery

The open approach using laparotomy and hysterotomy to remove the fetus, perform the surgery, and then return him or her to the uterus has been performed on only a very few human infants. Both obstructive uropathy and diaphragmatic hernias have been approached in this way. Only one infant (with obstructive uropathy) has survived, although in most cases the procedure was performed and pregnancy sustained after repair of the uterus. The failure to survive in the case of diaphragmatic hernia treated in this manner may result from early and irreversible insult to lung development in the case of the malformation sufficiently large to be detectable early in gestation.

The open approach raises several serious questions. Such a hysterotomy inevitably is performed in the muscular fundus of the uterus and leaves the mother clinically less functional. Cesarean births are strongly recommended following such surgery. Infertility may occur subsequently, and, although rare, uterine rupture can follow such a procedure. Without clear and reliable methods for selecting the infant who is likely to benefit and survive, and with less intrusive alternatives such as catheter diversion available for at least the case of bladder obstruction, the open method for fetal intervention is not likely to gain wide popularity.

SUGGESTED READING

Beck AD. The effect of intrauterine urinary obstruction upon the development of the fetal kidney. J Urol 1971; 105:784–789.

Glick PL, Harrison MR, Golbus MS, et al. Management of the fetus with congenital hydronephrosis II. Prognostic criteria and selection for treatment. J Pediatr Surg 1985; 20:376–387.

Manning FA. International fetal surgery registry, 59. Winnipeg, Manitoba: Emily Street, R3E 0W3.

Seeds JW, Bowes WA. Ultrasound-guided fetal intravascular transfusion in severe Rhesus immunization. Am J Obstet Gynecol 1986; 155:818–819.

THE BREAST

LACTATION

DOUGLAS D. GLOVER, B.S. Pharm., M.D.

Today's society with two wage-earner families is in sharp contrast to the norm that formerly existed in America wherein women were expected to fulfill the role of housewife and mother whilst the support of the family was the sole responsibility of the husband. Today, the decision of whether to breast-feed frequently depends upon the duration of the mother's leave of absence from her employment. The situation is difficult for the career woman at a management level, who could be superseded if her absence from work is prolonged. Therefore, the working woman must consider her priorities and take into account whether she is to invest time in her career or solely in the care and emotional growth of her child.

Many women find the decision stressful, particularly if cessation of their employment would mean financial sacrifice or change in the family lifestyle. Some women work because they need the money, whereas others do so for the emotional and intellectual satisfaction. On the other hand, for some women, staying at home with the new baby provides a great deal of personal satisfaction. The obstetrician should assist the gravid patient in attaining the decision that is most beneficial to both.

The attitude of the husband is of the utmost importance; specifically, is he supportive of breast-feeding and the time his wife must dedicate to their child. Some husbands resent having to share their wife's attention, and marital discord may ensue. Some men insist that breast-feeding is essential for the infant, and under these circumstances, the decision to nurse may be based on a husband's demands. Without proper motivation, a woman can indeed fail at breast-feeding, and thus, it is important that the physician take time to discuss all aspects of lactation with gravid patients.

PREPARATION FOR LACTATION

As women wear nylon and other synthetic materials next to their skin, the hard protective layer of epidermis gets worn off. As a result, the nipple does not stand up well to the stress of nursing, and small fissures are common. Since these may become so painful that continued nursing is a torture, nursing may be abandoned; therefore, prevention constitutes a cardinal duty. The pregnant woman should be advised, when discussing lactation, to wash the nipples daily, and then rub them briskly with a rough towel for a few minutes, and, in the summertime months, to expose the nipples to direct sunlight and get them tanned. Unfortunately, the sun lamp does not do this as effectively as the sun, and its utility in this regard is doubtful. There would be no problem with cracked nipples if women were able to expose their breasts as they do their faces.

Early in the third trimester, the gravid woman should be advised on breast care. Nipple dryness may lead to cracking and fissuring of the nipples. As soap and detergents contribute to dryness, the patient should be advised to use these sparingly when bathing the breasts and should be cautioned never to apply alcohol or perfumed preparations. The nipples should be washed daily with soap and warm water in order to remove encrustations of dried secretion. Lanolin may be applied as a lubricant, albeit to some the odor is objectionable; safflower oil is a satisfactory alternative for relieving nipple dryness and itching.

Preparation of the breasts for lactation should commence about the sixth month of gestation. If the nipples are flat or inverted, they should be gently drawn out by the finger and thumb for a short time each day. It is generally recognized that an important predisposing cause of acute mastitis is the stagnation of the milk in the mammary ducts. Due emphasis on the importance of getting the milk to flow freely once the baby is nursing must be made prior to delivery, and the mother should be taught how to express the milk by hand. This method has two components: the first is a downward movement in which the hands compress the whole breast from its margin to the areola, a maneuver that should be repeated several times a day; and the second is a repeated compression by the thumb and forefinger in order to empty the lacteal sinuses.

There is not unanimity concerning the effectiveness of nipple preparation techniques in preventing discomfort. Some consider these exercises unimportant, and it is a fact that many women successfully nurse their babies without any formal preparation and without experiencing any problems. On the other hand, there is evidence that supports the effectiveness of nipple care in reducing the tenderness and pain a mother may experience with initiation of lactation. In addition to the procedures mentioned, sucking of the breasts during lovemaking may be equally effective in preparation of the breasts for future lactation. How these preparatory exercises reduce nipple tenderness and breast pain has not been completely delineated. Proponents of these procedures speculate that discomfort is diminished by physical preparation of the breasts, whereas others suggest the effect is largely psychological. Most concur that these procedures cause no harm and make lactation easier for the majority of women.

LACTATION

In the initial 3 to 4 days of the puerperium, the breasts produce only colostrum, which undergoes a gradual transition to mature milk over a period of 3 weeks. During pregnancy, both estrogen and progesterone stimulate mammary alveolar gland development. After delivery, prolactin from the anterior pituitary brings about the change from colostrum to milk. The continued production of milk depends on the suckling infant. In the absence of suckling, the breasts engorge, and milk production ceases.

On the second day or shortly thereafter, the breasts become engorged and swollen; this may be associated with pain and a low-grade fever. Some deny that the initiation of lactation produces a temperature elevation, but, over the years, many women have noted a fever the day the milk comes in, which is often referred to as milk fever. This is not to be confused with the use of the same term by some individuals to denote mastitis. The temperature returns to normal within 24 hours. If the engorging breasts are overly painful, an ice bag may help, as does a baby with a good sucking reflex.

Some pediatricians prescribe glucose and water for the baby until the maternal breast starts to secrete milk. It is preferable to put the baby to the breast than to let hours pass because infant stimulation of the breast is much better than time in initiating the production of milk. The first day, the neonate is able to nurse only a few minutes before falling asleep; the next day, it may nurse for about 3 minutes every 4 hours, and by the fifth day, the infant may be nursing for about 20 minutes at 4 hour intervals. It should be emphasized that early and prolonged contact between the mother and her baby is necessary to the development of mother-infant bonding and the subsequent growth of the infant. In the human, the critical period for ideal bonding takes place in the first 12 hours after birth. Elimination of impediments to early bonding not only influence the future behavior of the child, but contribute to the success of lactation.

On occasion, the obstetrician is confronted by a woman who has such fear of breast-feeding that lactation may indeed be delayed. Apprehension over her ability to successfully breast-feed may cause diminished milk yield. Chlorpromazine, given in a dose of 25 mg 2 or 3 times daily for a day or two, may relax the mother, relieve the anxiety, and thereby increase milk production. The amount of the drug that appears in the colostrum is small and is without risk to the infant.

When a fissure occurs, it should be treated at once with the greatest of care. Immediately after nursing, the nipple is washed with sterile water, thoroughly dried, and painted with tincture of benzoin. When the benzoin has completely dried, sterile gauze is applied, and the breasts are supported. However, in many cases, they need not be supported if the milk flow is adequate and the breasts have been well prepared. If the breast becomes engorged and the baby does not relieve the engorgment, the breast should be emptied either by use of a hand pump or by manual expression. The hands should be washed, and the milk should be collected in a sterile container, if it is to be used. Plastic containers have an advantage over glass in that immunoglobulins and leukocytes adhere to glass and are therefore lost to the baby.

An alternative to pumping the affected breast is to empty it atraumatically by putting the baby to the opposite breast first and, after the initial milk let-down, transferring the baby to the fissured breast. In this way, nursing may be accomplished with less pain. The pain may be further reduced by the use of a nipple shield.

Giving birth to a low-birth-weight infant who requires a prolonged hospital stay may necessitate the storage and transportation of milk to the baby from the mother already at home. Career women who plan to breast-feed after they return to work may lack refrigeration for expressed milk at the workplace. Such individuals have concern about the safety of milk storage for interval feeding. Proper collection and storage techniques minimize the risk of milk contamination and prevent serious illness in infants. It is well known that the risk of microbial contamination of milk from improperly sterilized pumping devices is greater than from the mother's breast. The organisms found in expressed breast milk represent normal skin flora and not neonatal pathogens. The need to discard the initial 5 ml of milk, previously thought necessary in order to reduce bacterial contamination, has not been confirmed and is no longer recommended. The presence of naturally occurring antimicrobial properties in human milk prohibits bacterial proliferation, which abrogates the need for refrigeration for as long as 6 hours (Table 1). Likewise, unsterilized milk may be refrigerated for as long as 24 hours prior to use, and transportation of the milk from the mother to the infant is safe.

A woman with a prior history of successful lactation may elect to start breast-feeding a preterm infant of several weeks of age when it arrives home from the hospital. In a mother who has been physiologically prepared by the previous pregnancy, lactation may be reestablished after an interval by a process call relactation. Although initial milk production may be less than optimal in many cases,

TABLE 1 Protective Factors in Human Milk

Cellular Factors	*Soluble Factors*
Macrophages	Immunoglobulins, sIgA, IgA, IgG, IgM
Neutrophils	Lactoferrin
B-lymphocytes	Lysozyme
T-lymphocytes	Lactoperoxidase
Non-T, non-B lymphocytes	Xanthine oxidase
	Complement
	Epidermal growth factor
	Bifidus factor
	B_{12}-binding protein

it will be sufficient to meet the nutritional requirement of the infant in about a month. A commercial product, the Lact-Aid System*, is available to supplement the mother's milk during the first weeks of nursing. In this method, the infant suckles both the breast and the nursing trainer simultaneously; the milk from the Lact-Aid trainer serves as an incentive for continued nursing. About 50 percent of nursing mothers who utilize this technique are able to discontinue use of the trainer after 4 to 6 weeks.

Relactation is another feeding option for the woman who must prematurely wean her child on account of illness or hospitalization of her child. The development of a milk allergy is also an indication of relactation. Although rare, acrodermatitis enteropathica or Danbolt-Closs syndrome, is a disease caused by zinc deficiency, for which one treatment is maternal breast milk. Oral administration of zinc sulfate is also effective in the treatment of this entity, but relactation is an alternative method that should be made available to the mother.

NUTRITION DURING LACTATION

During pregnancy, a woman stores between 2 kg and 4 kg of extra tissue in preparation for lactation. At the end of the first trimester, the weight of the breasts have increased by 60 g; their weight triples over the next 8 weeks, and by term, the additional mammary tissue has increased by 400 g. This accounts for about 10 percent of the total body storage. It has been estimated that it takes 940 kcal to produce a liter of milk, and the daily caloric requirement of the lactating woman is about 600 kcal more than is required during pregnancy. The recommended daily allowances (RDA) for lactation are shown in Table 2. It should be noted that consideration must be given to the metabolic rate of the lactating mother and duly adjusted for her age.

This increase in the nutritional requirements for lactation reflects the need to preserve the health of the mother. It is well known that women who live on inadequate diets produce adequate milk for the growth and development of their progeny. "Hunger winter" was the ultimate contemporary experiment in a developed country that confirmed this fact. For a 6-month period during the winter of 1944–1945, the urban population of northwestern Holland existed on severely restricted rations. Pregnant and lactating women who received a daily allowance of between 700 and 1,400 kcal were able to initiate and sustain lactation, albeit with decreased milk volume. It has been

* Lact-Aid International Inc., P.O. Box 1066, Athens, TN 37303

TABLE 2 Recommended Daily Dietary Allowances

	Age			
	11-14 Years	*15-18 Years*	*19-22 Years*	*23-50 Years*
Body Characteristics				
Weight in kg	46	55	55	55
Weight in pounds	101	120	120	120
Height in cm	157	163	163	163
Height in inches	62	64	64	64
Nutrients				
Protein in g	46	46	44	44
Vitamin A (RE)*	800	800	800	800
Vitamin D (μg)†	15	15	12.5	10
Vitamin E activity (mgα tocopherol equivalent)††	13	13	13	13
Vitamin C (mg)	90	100	100	100
Thiamin (mg)	1.6	1.6	1.6	1.5
Riboflavin (mg)	1.8	1.8	1.8	1.7
Niacin (mg NE)§	20	19	19	18
Vitamin B_6	2.3	2.5	2.5	2.5
Folacin (μg)	500	500	500	500
Vitamin B_{12} (μg)	4.0	4.0	4.0	4.0
Calcium (mg)	1600	1600	1600	1600
Phosphorus (mg)	1600	1600	1600	1600
Magnesium (mg)	450	450	450	450
Iron (mg)	18	18	18	18
Zinc (mg)	25	25	25	26
Iodine (μg)	200	200	200	200
Energy in kcal	2700	2600	2600	2500

* Retinol equivalents. 1 retinol equivalent = 1 μg retinol or 6 μgβ carotine
† As calciferol. 10 μg calciferol = 400 UI of vitamin D
‡ Alpha-tocopherol equivalents. 1 mg d-alpha-tocopherol = 1α-TE
§ 1 NE (niacin equivalent) = 1 mg niacin or 60 mg of dietary tryptophan
Reprinted with permission from Recommended dietary allowances. 9th ed. Washington, DC: National Academy Press, 1980.

reported that the composition of the milk showed no significant deviation from the norm in its chemical constituents. The latter is in accord with a recent report from Guatemala, which confirmed that dietary supplementation increased milk volume as well as infant weight gain in lactating mothers whose milk production had been maintained at the expense of maternal storage.

The production efficiency of the mammary glands has been variously estimated to range from 60 to 90 percent. In undernourished populations, the protein content of breast milk remains stable at 0.8 to 0.9 g per deciliter, even as milk volume declines. Protein supplementation results in an increased milk yield without any alteration in the protein content. The concentration of protein is higher in colostrum than in the milk secreted by mothers of term or preterm infants. Whereas a portion of the protein fraction of human milk is derived from maternal plasma, other proteins are synthesized in the mammary gland. Alpha-lactalbumin, one of the major whey proteins in breast milk, originates in the alveolar cell. On the other hand, the immunoglobulins, are dervied from the maternal circulation. Secretory immunoglobulin A (IgA) is part of the enteric immune response of the mother and protects the infant from bacterial and viral infections. Overall, IgA comprises about 75 percent of the proteins in colostrum.

Water constitutes between 87 and 95 percent of the milk volume and is independent of fluid intake. The antidiuretic effect of prolactin conserves water in order to complement fluid intake and to ensure adequate milk volume. Appropriate water consumption by the lactating mother is important for the prevention of constipation rather than as an adjunct to lactation.

The lipid fraction of human milk is the primary source of calories for the nursing infant. The fat content of breast milk ranges from 2.1 to 3.3 percent and varies in a diurnal manner with a peak level at 10 AM and the nadir between 6 and 10 PM. Triglycerides comprise 81 percent of the fatty acid content. Unlike the content of protein and lactose, which is unaffected by dietary intake, the lipid content is responsive to diet and approximates to the composition of subcutaneous fat when the caloric intake is reduced. The amount of linoleic acid increases when the maternal diet is high in polyunsaturated fats, whereas a diet high in carbohydrate increases the saturated fatty acid content of milk (Table 3).

As previously stated, nutritional deprivation leads to a reduction in both the volume and lipid content of breast milk. Malnutrition may decrease the lipid content to less than 1 percent and compromise the growth of the infant. The lactating woman must have adequate nutrition and avoid fad diets. Breast-feeding is not the time for weight reduction, which must be deferred until the nursing infant has been weaned.

NUTRITIONAL SUPPLEMENTS

The lactating woman requires 1,600 mg of calcium a day, which is not readily achieved without ingesting milk or milk products. It should be noted that some dietary calcium is lost through the kidneys and into the intestine. Absorption from the gut is somewhat dependent upon body reserves. Nearly 2 decades ago, it was shown that in 3 months the lactating woman may lose as much as 2 percent of her skeletal calcium. A woman who is unable to consume milk products because of an allergy may compensate for this deficiency by eating a diet high in legumes, greens, spinach, and Swiss chard in addition to fish and liver. Although most nuts have a limited calcium content, Brazil nuts and almonds are exceptions and serve as additional sources of calcium.

Iron is important in order to replenish iron stores that have been depleted by pregnancy and parturition. The iron content of milk is relatively independent of the iron content of the diet and is not enhanced by oral administration of elemental iron. As the neonate has ample iron stores, iron-deficiency anemia is rarely observed in the breast-fed infant during the first 6 months of life.

Although thiamin deficiency can occur in nursing infants, it is rare in the United States. It occurs primarily in those countries in which rice is the major component of the diet. Beriberi in infants has been reported in breast-fed babies of mothers on thiamin-deficient diets. Likewise, the pyridoxine content of milk is reduced if the maternal dietary content is less than 2.5 mg a day.

Megaloblastic anemia, caused by vitamin B_{12} deficiency, occurs in India in women who adhere to a vegetarian diet. Strict vegetarians should receive vitamin B_{12} supplementation during lactation.

The ascorbic acid content of the tissues of the newborn is the highest it will be at any stage in its life. Maternal consumption of drinks high in ascorbic acid 30 minutes before breast-feeding can significantly increase the amount of vitamin C ingested by her infant. The daily dietary allowance recommended for lactating women by the Food and Nutrition Board of the National Research Council is 100 mg. Although no adverse effects from excessive vitamin intake have been documented, the risk does exist and must be taken into account when counseling the breast-feeding mother as to her dietary requirements.

In regard to the fat-soluble vitamins, the content of

TABLE 3 Chemical Composition of Human Milk: Lipids and Carbohydrate

Constituent	*Colostrum*	*Transitional Milk*	*Mature Milk*
Cholesterol	31 (24–45) mg/dl	29 (14–44) mg/dl	13 (7–19) mg/dl
Fat	3.2 (0.9–8.2) g/dl	3.7 (1.6–7.1) g/dl	3.3 (0.5–9.0) g/dl
Lactose	5.7 (1.1–7.9) g/dl	6.8 (5.7–8.4) g/dl	7.1 (5.8–8.4) g/dl

vitamins A and D in breast milk is low (Table 4). Vitamin A deficiency in breast-fed infants is rare. Historically, the coupling of these two fat-soluble vitamins was related to their common source, cod liver oil. There is little need for vitamin A supplementation of the lactating woman's diet. On the other hand, administration of vitamin D to the nursing infant is important. Infants who have dark skin and limited exposure to sun light are at risk of developing rickets unless they receive vitamin D supplementation. Although vitamin E deficiency is rarely encountered, even in malnourished individuals, it may occur in an infant who has anomalous fat absorption or in a low-birth-weight infant who has been placed on an unfortified formula. The vitamin E content of breast milk is high, and additional vitamin E is probably unnecessary for the mother on a well-balanced diet. Most prenatal formulations contain 30 U of alpha-tocopherol, which supplies 100 percent of the daily requirement. Dietary supplementation of the fat-soluble vitamins should be directed to maternal need in contradistinction to the breast-fed infant, in that administration of the fat-soluble vitamins does not enhance the lacteal content.

Although the zinc content of human milk is less than bovine milk, the bioavailability of this element is greater in breast milk (Table 5). The zinc-binding ligand of human milk has been identified by chromatography as prostaglandin E. Acrodermatitis enteropathica is a rare autosomal recessive trait, which may occur in artificially fed infants about the third week of life or in breast-fed babies after weaning. This entity is characterized by extremely low plasma zinc and arachidonic acid levels. Breast milk is important in the treatment of this disease in that zinc from the zinc-prostaglandin complex is more readily available in human lacteal secretions.

The fluoride content of milk is low. Milk and milk products decrease the bioavailability of sodium fluoride in adults. It is doubtful that the small amount of fluoride found in breast milk contributes significantly to the infant's requirement or that supplementation of the nursing mother's diet would be beneficial.

The iodine content of human milk exceeds the plasma concentration, and excessive iodine ingestion by lactating women is to be avoided. This is particularly true in respect

TABLE 4 Chemical Composition of Human Milk: Vitamins

Constituent	*Colostrum*	*Transitional Milk*	*Mature Milk*
Vitamin A	161 (75–305) μg/dl	88 (58–183) μg/dl	61 (15–226) μg/dl
Carotenoids	137 (41–385) μg/dl	38 (23–63) μg/dl	25 (2–77) μg/dl
Thiamin			
Total	2 (0.5–27) μg/dl	6 (2–10) μg/dl	14 (8–23) μg/dl
Free	0.4 (0.1–0.9) μg/dl	0.8 (0.2–1.9) μg/dl	5.3 (1.2–15.8) μg/dl
Cyanocobalamin	0.04 (0.0–0.15) μg/dl	0.3 (0.0–0.7) μg/dl	Trace
Pyridoxine			18 (10–22) μg/dl
Folic acid	0.05 (0.0–0.15) μg/dl	0.02 (0.01–0.02) μg/dl	0.22 (0.14–0.36) μg/dl
Ascorbic acid	7.2 (4.7–10.4) mg/dl	7.1 (4.5–9.0) mg/dl	3.7 (0.4–7.7) mg/dl
Tocopherol	1.48 (0.25–2.9) mg/dl	1.32 (0.48–3.0) mg/dl	0.24 (0.1–0.48) mg/dl
Vitamin D			(0.4–10) USP units/dl
Niacin	75 (50–145) μg/dl	175 (60–360) μg/dl	183 (66–330) μg/dl
Vitamin K			50 (0–200) Dam-Glavind units
Pantothenic acid	183 (29–302) μg/dl	288 (135–412) μg/dl	246 (86–584) μg/dl

TABLE 5 Chemical Composition of Human Milk: Electrolytes

Constituent	*Colostrum*	*Transitional Milk*	*Mature Milk*
Aluminum			Trace
Barium			Trace
Boron			Trace
Calcium	23 (13–34) mg/dl	26 (21–33) mg/dl	34 (17–61) mg/dl
Chlorine	78 (20–233) mg/dl	48 (17–116) mg/dl	38 (9–73) mg/dl
Chromium			Trace
Copper	0.04 (0.02–0.05) mg/dl	0.05 (0.04–0.07) mg/dl	0.03 (0.01–0.07) mg/dl
Iodine	12.2 μg/dl	2.4 μg/dl	(4.5–9.0) μg/dl
Iron	0.04 (0.02–0.05) mg/dl	0.04 (0.02–0.05) mg/dl	0.36 (0.29–0.45) mg/dl
Magnesium	4 (3–8) mg/dl	4 (2–5) mg/dl	4 (2–6) mg/dl
Manganese	Trace		Trace
Phosphorus			
Total P	16 (8–25) mg/dl	20 (10–32) mg/dl	16 (12–19) mg/dl
Inorganic P			5.13 (1.5–8.77) mg/dl
Lipid P	2 mg/dl	3 (2–4) mg/dl	3 (2–4) mg/dl
Potassium	74 (66–87) mg/dl	64 (53–77) mg/dl	52 (27–81) mg/dl
Sodium	50 (26–136) mg/dl	29 (19–54) mg/dl	17 (6–44) mg/dl
Zinc	0.55 (0.07–0.98) mg/dl	0.38 (0.03–0.58) mg/dl	0.118 (0.017–0.302) mg/dl

to radioactive preparations. Iodine-containing expectorants should also be avoided by breast-feeding mothers.

THE COMPOSITION OF HUMAN BREAST MILK

Human milk is unique in that it is a nearly complete food for an infant. The American Academy of Pediatrics only recommends dietary supplementation of the nursing infant's diet with vitamin K at birth and vitamin D and fluoride in the first 4 to 6 months after birth. The iron stores of the neonate are such that iron-deficiency anemia is rare before 4 to 6 months of age. Although the iron content of the lacteal secretions is low, about half is bioavailable; this is in contrast to the limited availability of iron from other sources.

Initially high, the protein content of colostrum falls rapidly during the first week and is followed by a more gradual decline through the transition to mature milk. The casein content of human milk is approximately one-seventh of that found in bovine milk, which probably accounts for the lower calcium and phosphorus concentration in human milk. Whey protein represents about 65 percent of the total protein in mature milk. These soluble proteins include the immunoglobulins, lactoferrin and lysozyme, as well as other minor proteins that play a role in protecting the newborn child from infection. Breast milk also contains about 25 percent nonprotein nitrogen as compared to about 5 percent in bovine milk. Table 6 summarizes the nitrogenous composition of human milk.

The fact that colostrum is important in protecting the offspring of domestic animals from disease has been recognized since antiquity. Infectious diarrhea is a leading cause of infant mortality in the third world and a frequent contributor to infant morbidity in the United States. There is ample evidence to confirm that the breast-fed infant is less susceptible to certain mucosal infections than its artificially fed counterpart, largely because of the protective components in the protein fraction of human milk (see Table 1).

The predominant lacteal immunoglobulin is secretory immunoglobulin A (sIgA). Plasma cells and, to a lesser extent, neutrophils, which are located at the basal membrane of the alveoli, produce IgA; this is converted to sIgA in the secretory cell. Secretory IgA represents about 97 percent of the colostral protein on the first day post partum, and then it rapidly declines to 25 percent by the

TABLE 6 Chemical Composition of Human Milk: Nitrogenous Substances

Constituent	*Colostrum*	*Transitional Milk*	*Mature Milk*
Protein			
Total	5.5 (1.4–21.5) g/dl	1.6 (1.1–2.7) g/dl	1.1 (0.7–2.0) g/dl
Casein	2.0 (0.7–5.17) g/dl	0.9 (0.4–1.8) g/dl	0.3 (0.1–0.6) g/dl
Lactalbumin		0.8 (0.7–0.8) g/dl	0.3 (0.1–0.6) g/dl
Lactoglobulin	3.5 (0.4–13.2) g/dl	0.4 (0.2–1.3) g/dl	0.172 g/dl
Whey	1.7 g/dl		0.7 (0.4–1.0) g/dl
Amino Acids			
Arginine	75 (62–96) mg/dl	64 (48–89) mg/dl	45 (28–64) mg/dl
Alanine			35 mg/dl
Aspartic acid			116 mg/dl
Cystine		55 mg/dl	41 mg/dl
Glutamic acid			230 mg/dl
Glycine			0 mg/dl
Histidine	41 (35–46) mg/dl	38 (29–45) mg/dl	23 (16–34) mg/dl
Isoleucine	100 (88–115) mg/dl	97 (73–121) mg/dl	68 (46–102) mg/dl
Leucine	169 (145–214) mg/dl	151 (112–197) mg/dl	108 (72–159) mg/dl
Lysine	114 (95–139) mg/dl	113 (86–148) mg/dl	76 (53–104) mg/dl
Methionine	26 (19–36) mg/dl	24 (16–34) mg/dl	14 (9–21) mg/dl
Phenylalanine	70 (60–84) mg/dl	63 (48–74) mg/dl	41 (30–58) mg/dl
Proline			80 mg/dl
Serine			69 mg/dl
Threonine	84 (75–104) mg/dl	79 (61–96) mg/dl	54 (40–76) mg/dl
Tryptophan	32 (25–42) mg/dl	28 (23–33) mg/dl	18 (13–26) mg/dl
Tryosine		125 mg/dl	78 mg/dl
Valine	118 (98–149) mg/dl	105 (77–136) mg/dl	71 (48–114) mg/dl
Urea		23.3 mg/dl	37 (26–49) mg/dl
Creatine			3.1 (0–12.4) mg/dl
Creatinine			3.0 (2.0–5.1) mg/dl
Uric acid			6.6 (3.9–12.3) mg/dl
Nitrogen			
Protein N	424 mg/dl	251 mg/dl	188 mg/dl
Casein N	188 mg/dl	110 mg/dl	63 mg/dl
Lactalbumin N		126 mg/dl	47 mg/dl
Lactoglobulin N		78 mg/dl	31 mg/dl
Whey N	267 mg/dl		94 mg/dl
Nonprotein N	91 (51–127 mg/dl	84 (48–140) mg/dl	32 (17–60) mg/dl
Amino acid N		4 (4–5) mg/dl	5.0 (2.8–11.3) mg/dl

fourth day from dilution as a result of the increase in the volume of the mammary secretion. It has been estimated that the breast-fed infant consumes 1 g of sIgA per day. Unlike immunoglobulin G (IgG) that readily crosses the placenta, there is no transfer of either IgA or immunoglobulin M (IgM) from the mother to the fetus. Although the mechanism for the manufacture of IgA is in place at birth and the synthesis of IgM begins soon after, IgA is a mucosal immunoglobulin that is produced in the lungs and gut of the infant only after antigen exposure and is therefore the slowest immunoglobulin to be generated. The importance of an abundance of IgA in the lacteal secretions is readily apparent. About 30 percent of ingested IgA is not absorbed; it descends through the intestine unchanged and is therefore able to protect the mucosal surface of the entire gut until the neonate begins to form its own. The purpose of IgA is not to kill bacteria, but to mediate an orderly process of mucosal colonization with nonpathogenic microorganisms, thereby prohibiting attachment of enteric pathogens. The decline in colostral content of IgA coincides with the infant's capability to produce its own antibodies.

The maximum concentration of IgM is present in colostrum and then declines as lactation progresses. However, the levels of IgM are consistently lower than those of IgA. Likewise, the colostral content of IgA is 20 to 30 times that of IgG, although the IgG level remains stable as lactation is established. The importance of these two immunoglobulins in human milk is not fully understood.

Lactoferrin is a soluble lacteal protein that has an iron-binding capacity analogous in function to transferrin in serum. Iron is essential in the replication process of bacteria. The low iron content of human milk assures a dearth of unbound iron in the fecal content. The ability of lactoferrin to bind fecal iron deprives microorganisms of an element necessary for their growth and expression of virulence. Furthermore, it has been suggested that the association of IgA with lactoferrin may enhance the latter's antibacterial activity.

Lysozyme is a peptide that is known to have enzymatic activity against cell wall components of gram-negative bacteria and, in conjunction with complement, may cause lysis of *Enterobacteriaceae*. This cationic peptide is stable throughout the length of the infant gut. The concentration in lacteal secretions is 3,000 times that found in bovine milk. Although its specific function has not been determined, there is a suggestion that it plays a role in the development of the intestinal microflora.

Lactoperoxidase and xantine oxidase are two minor inhibitory systems in the protein fraction of milk, which may contribute to host defense mechanism. The antimicrobial action of lactoperoxidase appears to be related to the formation of the radical hypothiocyanate. This oxygen-containing radical is formed at low pH in the presence of hydrogen peroxide and thiocyanate and exerts its action on the bacterial cell wall. On the other hand, xanthine oxidase functions largely as a producer of peroxide, which is necessary to activate the lactoperoxidase system.

In addition to these soluble factors, human lacteal secretions contain cellular components. It has been estimated that the neonate ingests 100 million leukocytes per day, predominantly in the form of macrophages. Although the relative cellular concentration is greater in colostrum, the number delivered to the infant remains constant throughout lactation. The larger volume of milk ingested compensates for the lower concentration of cells in mature milk.

Probably 90 percent of the cellular fraction represents macrophages that function in milk as they do in other tissue. The ability of the macrophage in lacteal secretions to phagocytize *Cryptococcus neoformans, Candida albicans,* and *E. scherichia coli* is well known, although complement activation is required for the latter. Macrophages have the ability to produce complement components, as well as soluble lysozyme and lactoferrin, which contribute to the host defense mechanism. In addition, macrophages serve as transport vehicles, which carry IgA to the neonatal intestine where release occurs during phagocytosis.

In the formation of milk, fat enters the alveolar lumen in droplet form by the process of reverse pinocytosis, and each globule is encased in a thin covering derived from the lipid membrane. Phagocytosis is less efficient in liquid suspension than when the microorganism to be phagocytized is attached to a solid structure. The propensity of *E. coli* for attachment to the membranous cover of the fat droplet enhances the process of phagocytosis in the gut lumen.

Lymphocytes comprise about 10 percent of the cells found in human milk. Approximately 50 percent of colostral lymphocytes are thymus-drived cells (T cells), whereas 34 percent are B-lymphocytes, and the remainder of non-T, non-B subpopulations. As lactation progresses, the T-cell concentration declines to about 20 percent at 6 months. Precursor cells, located in Peyer's patches of the ileum and in the lymphoid tissue of the bronchi, form B cells, which migrate to the mammary gland, a process that is enhanced in pregnancy. Although less is known of the formation of T cells, their origin is probably similar to that of B cells. Antigens, such as rubella virus, enhance the T-cell proliferation response in milk, whereas the response to the antigen of *E. coli* is limited to the mucosal surfaces of the gut.

For many years, it has been an established fact that infectious diarrhea is less common in breast-fed infants. It is recognized that the intestinal microflora of breast-fed babies consists largely of a gram-positive anaerobe, *Bifidobacterium bifidum*, whereas gram-negative facultative anaerobic bacteria, some of which are known to be enteropathogens, predominate in the gut of formula-fed infants. The high lactose content of breast milk is thought to produce a "starter effect," along with other factors, which are responsible for the predominance of *Bifidobacteria* in the gut of the breast-fed baby. Differences in the lipid composition of these milks may contribute to the disparity in the intestinal microflora. Breast milk has a higher triglyceride content, which may actually enhance the growth of *Bifidobacteria*, whereas the fatty acid and monoglyceride content of bovine milk inhibit the growth of these gram-positive anaerobic bacteria, although not intestinal pathogens.

No consideration of the contribution of human milk to the host defense mechanism could be complete without mention of acquired immunodeficiency syndrome (AIDS). It has been suggested that between 1 and 2 million Americans are infected with the human immune virus (HIV) virus. The seroprevalence rates today in the maternity units of some metropolitan hospitals in the United States exceed 2.5 percent. It is predicted that by 1991, there will be more than a quarter of a million Americans with AIDS, which will include the offspring of lactating women. The predilection of the HIV virus for T4-lymphocytes, which are excreted in the lacteal secretions, is the probable mode of transmission of the virus to the infant. There are now documented cases of seroconversion of nursing infants whose mothers, following a blood transfusion, became seropositive during lactation. It is important that the woman at risk for acquiring this syndrome be identified and be apprised of the risk to her breast-fed child. The importance of the advice regarding prophylaxis given by her obstetrician in such cases cannot be overemphasized.

SUGGESTED READING

Larson BL, ed. A comprehensive treatise. IV. New York: Academic Press, 1978.

Lawrence RA. Breastfeeding: a guide for the medical profession. 2nd ed. St. Louis: CV Mosby, 1984.

Report of the Surgeon General's workshop on breastfeeding and human lactation. Washington, DC: U.S. Department of Health and Human Services, 1984.

MASTITIS

DOUGLAS D. GLOVER, B.S. Pharm., M.D.

Over the years, a confusing terminology has been employed for inflammation of the breast in association with lactation. The term "acute puerperal mastitis" alludes to the abrupt onset of subjective symptoms, whereas "epidemic mastitis" is an appellative that suggests a nosocomial etiology. "Sporadic puerperal mastitis," also known as "nonepidemic mastitis," suggests a random occurrence and implies a dissimilarity from the epidemic mastitis. Epidemic mastitis does, however, occur occasionally in a sporadic manner as mastitis, found in women who have had their babies at home, and it may not appear until many weeks after delivery, negating the idea that this infection is the result of institutional care. Mastitis is a nonspecific term and refers to any inflammatory lesion of the breast. Since the majority of cases of acute mastitis arise during lactation, the terms "puerperal mastitis" and "lactational mastitis" are both employed with respect to this condition. Despite the confusion in terminology, milk stasis is of fundamental importance in the pathogenesis of mastitis (Table 1).

TABLE 1 Characteristics of the Forms of Mastitis

Breast Infections	
Sporadic form of mastitis	Epidemic form of mastitis
Poor nursing technique	Hospital-acquired
Breast engorgement	Mammary adenitis
Nipple trauma	Pus expressed from nipple
Interlobular connective tissue cellulitis	Fissure usually absent
	Insidious onset
Onset 2 to 3 weeks post partum	Protracted course

This painful entity is encountered in 2.5 percent of lactating women, and nearly 5 percent of these individuals develop a breast abscess. A small investment in time by the physician in furnishing advice to the woman who plans to nurse may yield bountiful rewards by preventing the evolution of the condition and substantially reducing the morbidity of the inflammatory process. The sporadic form of mastitis involves the interlobular connective tissue that emanates in mammary cellulitis. Milk stasis due to breast engorgement frequently precedes the onset of symptoms. Some consider this form of mastitis to be due to a poor nursing technique and, in fact, engorgement after a missed feeding with fissuring due to nipple trauma is frequently observed in women with sporadic mastitis. Entry of pathogenic microorganisms into the mammary duct system is via a fissure, and the stage is thereby set for the evolution of mammary cellulitis.

Most patients experience a sudden onset of symptoms, such as breast tenderness, chills, and fever. The febrile response frequently exceeds 101°F and may be as high as 105°F. Anorexia, cephalalgia, and general malaise may suggest a flu-like syndrome. Influenza symptoms in the absence of respiratory complaints, however, should lead the physician to suspect the presence of sporadic mastitis.

Epidemic mastitis is another form of mammary inflammation in which introduction of the pathogenic microorganisms involves the ductal system as well as the periductal lymphatics, and it progresses to mammary adenitis. Nipple fissure with associated nipple pain is less common with this form, and its onset is usually insidious in nature. Although the symptoms are similar to sporadic mastitis, they are often less severe, but in some instances pus can be expressed from the breast. As the nomenclature implies, epidemic mastitis may be hospital-acquired, although characteristically it has its onset 2 to 3 weeks post partum when the patient is at home.

Staphylococcus aureus and *Staphylococcus epidermidis* are the bacteria commonly encountered in both forms of mastitis. *Staphylococcus aureus* is found in all puerperal breast abscesses. The infection usually involves only one breast, and when bilateral mastitis is encountered, group B beta-hemolytic streptococci are generally the causative organisms. The various pathogenic microorganisms found in puerperal mastitis are enumerated in Table 2. Although septicemia may occur, it is rare in patients with sporadic mastitis. Abscess formation is observed in 2 to 8 percent of these cases; however, prompt drainage reduces the risk of septicemia.

As previously stated, poor nursing technique may lead to the development of mastitis. In a study of 53 mastitis cases, it was noted that of six women who had experienced mastitis, two had previously developed an abscess while breast-feeding. In addition, one of the women had previously had three episodes of mastitis. That certain women have recurrent mastitis lends support to the contention that a faulty lactation technique may be the reason.

It is a matter of conjecture that diminished mammary blood supply precedes abscess formation, as abscess formation is rare in the woman who maintains lactation. Mammary blood flow in the lactating patient is 400 to 500 times the volume of milk produced, but it rapidly declines when nursing ceases. Compromised perfusion of the tissue may lead to an ineffectual concentration of antibiotic at the site of infection, and in the presence of milk stasis an abscess evolves. Treatment delay beyond 24 hours leads to tissue ischemia, whereas prompt therapy with antimicrobial agents reduces the risk of abscess. Only the presence of an abscess requires discontinuance of lactation.

Both the epidemic and sporadic forms of mastitis can progress to abscess formation. It must be emphasized that the ligaments of Cooper support the mammary parenchyma and act as a temporary barrier to the spread of the infectious process. Fluctuation that normally accompanies abscess formation may be masked by the supporting structures that preserve the breast architecture. Although many abscesses are relatively superficial and present as subareolar masses, an abscess may be more extensive than its outward appearance implies and extend deep into the interlobular tissue. In some instances, a retromammary collection may form a deep abscess that is difficult to define. In such instances, radiologic assistance may be a useful adjunct in establishing the diagnosis. Over the years, mammography has been employed, but this technique has certain drawbacks. Breast compression is necessary with mammography, and this may be painful for the patient. The mammographic findings are nonspecific, and it may not be possible to distinguish an abscess from a carcinoma or an area of fibrocystic disease. The abscess cavity on mammography may resemble a cyst unless a gas-producing microorganism is present. On the other hand, the ultrasonographic appearances of abscesses are more complicated and may vary from being hypoechoic and having clean, smooth walls that resemble a cyst to having shaggy walls and variable amounts of debris (the latter characteristics are diagnostic of an abscess). On ultrasonography, some pressure on the breast is required, but in general the patient experiences less pain from this investigation than from mammography. Last, since deep abscesses are hot, thermography may be of diagnostic value. Prompt treatment with antibiotics will prevent progression of the infection in the majority of cases, particularly if therapy is started during the appearance of the initial symptoms. Once an abscess has formed, prompt surgical intervention is mandatory.

An occasional woman with early mastitis will experience breast pain but no fever. In such instances, the physical examination may contribute little to establishing the diagnosis. In the past, it has been the experience of many that milk cultures contribute little to either the diagnosis or the management of mastitis and that microbiologic correlation with presenting symptoms is lacking. However, in a recent study of 213 such women, it was possible to classify breast pathology into three distinct groups, which were termed milk stasis, noninfectious inflammation, and infectious mastitis (Table 3). Milk samples from the women were collected after preparing the breasts with a chlorhexidine solution that was allowed to dry. Leukocyte counts were made on expressed milk samples and cultures obtained for sensitivity testing. The nature and duration of the symptoms and physical findings were recorded in each case. Those women whose milk cultures were either sterile or contaminated by the skin ecosystem and who had leukocyte counts of less than 10^6 per milliliter were classified as having milk stasis. Women with similar culture results but with leukocyte counts in excess of 10^6 per milliliter were diagnosed as having noninfectious inflammation, whereas those cases in which the bacterial count exceeded 10^3 per milliliter and the leukocyte count was over 10^6 per milliliter were considered to have infectious mastitis.

Management consisted of emptying the breasts by continued nursing, augmented by manual expression and, in some cases, by mechanical suction. Antimicrobial therapy was reserved for women with bacterial counts in excess of 10^3 per milliliter of milk. With such treatment, most of the lactating women with milk stasis became asymptomatic in less than 3 days, whereas the remainder experienced either a recurrence of symptoms or a decline in milk volume. In the group of individuals with noninfectious inflammation, however, the duration of symptoms was considerably longer, and the condition progressed to infectious mastitis in about half of the cases. The benefits of continued lactation were confirmed by the fact that the duration of symptoms was significantly reduced in those whose breasts were emptied, and the prognosis for continued lactation was markedly improved. Likewise, in individuals with infectious mastitis, only 15 percent of those

TABLE 2 Bacterial Isolates in Order of Frequency

Staphylococcus aureus
Staphylococcus epidermidis
Group B beta-hemolytic streptococci
Group A beta-hemolytic streptococci
Streptococcus faecalis
Escherichia coli
Haemophilus influenzae
Serattia marcescens
Klebsiella pneumoniae

TABLE 3 Classification of Patients with Inflammatory Breast Symptoms

Milk Stasis	*Noninfectious inflammation*	*Infectious mastitis*
Bacteria count $<10^3$ Leukocyte count $<10^6$	Bacteria count $<10^3$ Leukocyte count $>10^6$	Bacteria count $>10^3$ Leukocyte count $>10^6$

not treated had a good outcome as compared to 50 percent of those who had their breasts emptied. When antimicrobial therapy was combined with emptying of the breast, a good prognosis was achieved in 96 percent of cases. Abscess formation occurred only in the group with infectious mastitis for an incidence of 11 percent of those treated conservatively without antibiotic therapy. This is in accord with the fact that prior to the availability of antibiotic agents, not all breast infections progressed to abscess formation.

The penicillins are the treatment of choice for mastitis. Oral penicillin in a dosage of 250 mg four times a day may be prescribed or, if the patient is allergic to penicillin, erythromycin, 250 mg four times a day, can be ordered. If the physician suspects the infection is caused by an organism resistant to penicillin, a pencillinase-stable penicillin such as oxacillin, dicloxacillin, or nafcillin may be used. These penicillins are highly effective against both the penicillinase-producing and nonpenicillinase-producing strains of staphylococci. It must be remembered that more than 90 percent of hospital-acquired staphylococci and 70 percent of community-acquired staphylococci are resistant to penicillin. The earlier treatment is instituted, the more rapid the response to therapy, since abscesses are the result of delayed therapy. Complete resolution of the infection without the risk of abscess formation is reasonable to expect provided antibiotic therapy combined with emptying of the breast is commenced within 24 hours of the onset of symptoms.

Defervescence is likewise prompt after the initiation of therapy. Antipyretic agents, such as aspirin or acetaminophen in a dosage of 650 mg every 4 hours are satisfactory for the control of even a high fever. Few doses of such agents should be required. In the majority of cases, the patient will become afebrile and the pain will subside within 24 to 36 hours. Failure for this to occur is suggestive of a purulent collection and necessitates further evaluation.

Breast-feeding is contraindicated only in the presence of an abscess or when pus can be expressed from the nipple. In cases of infectious mastitis, antibody production in the mammary gland serves to reduce the risk of infection to the nursing infant. If it is necessary to discontinue breast-feeding, the affected breast should be gently expressed. The use of mechanical expression in a fissured nipple is less painful than an infant suckling. The mother should be encouraged in this practice by her physician. Even in such cases, lactation can be continued from the unaffected breast, and once the symptoms have abated, full nursing can be safely resumed.

Most cases of mastitis can be effectively managed at home without admission to the hospital. The laboratory can be useful to the clinician in those cases in which the indication for use of an antibiotic is unclear or concern exists regarding penicillinase-producing organisms. In the case of the afebrile patient with mild breast symptoms, one can defer antibiotic therapy while awaiting the bacterial count, provided the patient's symptoms remain benign. The patient who presents with evidence of florid mastitis, however, should be immediately treated with pencillinase-resistant penicillin and be advised to maintain close contact with her physician.

SUGGESTED READING

Devereux WP. Acute Puerperal mastitis: evaluation of its management. Am J Obstet Gynecol 1970; 108:78–81.

Gibberd GF. Sporadic and epidemic puerperal breast infections. Am J Obstet Gynecol 1953; 65:1038–1041.

Marshall BR, Hepper JK, Zirbel CC. Sporadic puerperal mastitis—an infection that need not interrupt lactation. JAMA 1975; 233:1377–1379.

Thomsen AC, Hansen KB, Moller BR. Leukocyte counts and microbiologic cultivation in diagnosis of puerperal mastitis. Am J Obstet Gynecol 1983; 146:938–941.

Thomsen AC, Espersen T, Maigaard S. Course and treatment of milk stasis, noninfectious inflammation of the breast and infectious mastitis in nursing women. Am J Obstet Gynecol 1984; 149:492–495.

DRUG EXCRETION IN HUMAN MILK

DOUGLAS D. GLOVER, B.S. Pharm., M.D.

The reversal of the trend that advocated artificial feeding has stimulated interest in the risk of drug and environmental pollutant exposure to the nursing infant through breast milk. Six of every ten American women now breast-feed their progeny, and most are aware that a child may be the unintended recipient of maternally administered medications. When prescribing therapy to lactating mothers, due attention must be given to the effect the medication may have on milk production as well as on the infant. Overall, no more than 1 percent of any drug administered to the mother is transferred to the child via her milk. Although it is true that most drugs ingested do not have a deleterious effect on the infant, the potential for harm does exist and may be a cause for concern.

Some physicians recommend weaning the infant when drugs are prescribed for a nursing mother. Although the risk of drug exposure is thereby reduced, this may not be in the best interest of the child. Only recently have accurate analytic methods been available to quantitate the content of drugs and their metabolites in human milk. The techniques previously used were relatively insensitive and potentially susceptible to confounding materials. Current methodology can detect compounds at nanogram and picogram levels in a 0.1-ml sample. In the past, data on drug concentration were derived predominantly from animal sources or from anecdotal case reports. Differences in the pH of the blood and milk that exist among various animals and humans as well as the presence of species-specific milk proteins render data from other than human sources of limited value to the clinician.

In order for a pharmaceutical agent to enter milk, it must first cross the capillary endothelium, traverse the extracellular space, and pass through two biologic membranes as well as the alveolar interstitial space before becoming incorporated in the lacteal secretions in the alveolar lumen. It is necessary that the drug be nonionized, lipid-soluble, and have a sufficiently low molecular weight to cross the lipid barrier. Most drug transfer occurs by passive diffusion across a concentration gradient from a higher to a lower concentration. Some of the larger drug molecules are transferred by facilitated diffusion. Active transport, an energy-requiring process, transfers the drug from a site of lower concentration to one of higher concentration. This process is largely reserved for the egress of glucose, amino acids, calcium, and magnesium. Electron microscopy has demonstrated the existence of small, water-filled pores in the biologic membrane through which ionized, lipid-insoluble drug with a molecular weight of less than 200 daltons may enter milk. Additionally, a drug may directly enter the milk by way of intercellular clefts, but the amount of drug so transferred is small and of no clinical consequence.

The pH of the lacteal secretions varies over a wide range, from as low as 6.35 to as high as 7.65. In general, the pH of breast milk is lower than that of maternal plasma. The nonionized drug fraction reaches equilibrium across the biologic membrane so that the concentration in the milk is equal to that in the plasma. Weak acid drugs, such as the penicillins, are highly ionized at plasma pH and the concentration in milk is low. Likewise, as the plasma level of the drug declines, back diffusion from the mammary lumen may occur, and this may further lower the drug concentration in the milk. On the other hand, a weak basic drug is largely nonionized at plasma pH and, upon egress to the milk with its lower pH, it will become highly polar, which leads to "ion trapping" in the lacteal secretions.

The milk:plasma ratio of a medicinal compound is determined by two physiochemical properties of the agent: the relative extent of drug ionization in the milk compared with that in the plasma and the relative degree of protein binding in the two biologic fluids. As previously stated, a weak basic drug will become highly polar upon entry into the mammary secretions, and this results in continual diffusion of the agent across the biologic membrane until equilibrium of the nonpolar substances is achieved. In such a case, the concentration of the drug in the alveolar lumen is greater than that in the plasma, and the milk:plasma ratio exceeds unity. On the other hand, a weak acid drug that is highly polar in the plasma allows for only the nonionized fraction to diffuse across the lipid membrane, and consequently the drug concentration in the milk will be low and the milk:plasma ratio less than unity.

Another characteristic important in determining drug concentration in the milk is the drug's lipid solubility. Even if it is nonionized, its passage through the lipid barrier will be gradual if its lipid solubility is low. For example, sulfisoxazole, which is a weak acid, is 86 percent protein-bound in maternal plasma. The free drug fraction is small and lipid solubility is limited, resulting in low concentrations in the aqueous fraction of the milk. In fact, the lipid solubility of the N^1 acetyl metabolite of sulfisoxazole is greater than the solubility of the parent drug, and the metabolite readily diffuses into the milk to appear in the lipid fraction. Most drugs cross the biologic membranes to enter the fat droplets of milk. The fat globules, which are surrounded by a thin membrane, enter the milk by a process known as reverse pinocytosis and are suspended in the aqueous phase to form an oil-in-water emulsion. Since the fat content of colostrum is low, drug transfer in the early puerperium is low, and this lowers the neonate's exposure to fat-soluble drugs.

The amount of drug ingested by an infant may be diminished if he or she nurses at those times when the plasma drug level is minimal. In general, the peak plasma concentration of a drug occurs about 1 to 2 hours after oral administration. Milk is not produced or stored in the breast between feedings but is formed at the time of suckling by the infant. The plasma concentration of a drug at the time of nursing, therefore, determines the content of the medicinal agent that appears in the ingested milk. The lipid content of breast milk varies in a diurnal pattern, attaining a peak at midmorning and a nadir between 6 PM and 10 PM. Administration of the first daily dose of a lipophilic compound after the 10 AM feeding and timing the later doses to be given after the feedings during the day will substantially reduce the amount of drug consumed by the infant.

Since the appearance of the initial article by Sapeika in 1947, there have been more than 40 publications dealing with the transmammary excretion of drugs. Through the years, a number of drugs have been identified that are considered by many to be best avoided or used with due caution by the lactating woman (Table 1). There is no consensus, because the recommendations were often based on theoretic suppositions and anecdotal case reports that were frequently unsupported by critical pharmacokinetic data. As previously stated, many of the older assays lacked specificity and sensitivity, so that the results were often incomplete and discordant. Yet, despite the availability of superior laboratory technology in recent years, the content of many pharmaceutical agents in human milk has not been determined, and consequently there is a significant lack of knowledge pertaining to drug exposure by the breast-fed infant. The pharmacokinetic data that are available are summarized in order to assist the clinician treating a lactating patient to make therapeutic decisions based on fact rather than surmise.

BROMIDES

Drowsiness and skin rash have been reported in nursing infants whose mothers had taken bromide compounds. In an era that is now history, bromides were promoted for the relief of nervous tension and were available as both prescription pharmaceuticals and products for over-the-counter sale. The highly advertised proprietary preparation of Dr. Miles Nervine was an example of the latter. The 1970 edition of *Remington's Pharmaceutical Sciences* listed nine bromide compounds that were available in the United States. By the end of the decade, each of the nine products had been removed from the market or had been reformulated, as was the case with Miles Nervine. The bromide content in milk is only of historic interest, since these compounds are no longer available in the United States.

IODIDES

Iodides, like other halides, are concentrated in breast milk and transmitted in considerable quantities to the nursing infant. Over 50 years ago, it was reported that 15 percent of a 600-mg dose of potassium iodide administered to a lactating woman was found in the milk. More recently, a review of 49 cases of congenital goiter revealed 14 infant deaths due to tracheal compression when the mothers had received iodides for bronchial asthma. Four of these infants had cardiomegaly. Additionally, transient hypothyroidism has been identified in babies exposed to iodine absorbed from a povidone-iodine perineal preparation used at the time of parturition. These reports confirm the sensitivity of the fetus to iodides as well as of the neonate who is exposed to these agents via the mammary secretions.

In general, the short-term administration of iodides appears to pose a minimal risk to the nursing infant, and a 10-day course of iodides for use prior to thyroid surgery can be safely prescribed for the breast-feeding patient.

TABLE 1 Drugs Commonly Considered to be Contraindicated in Lactation

Bromides	Iodides
Aspirin	Antithyroid drugs
Lithium carbonate	Radioactive pharmaceuticals
Chloramphenicol	Isoniazid
Tetracyclines	Metronidazole
Barbiturates	Phenytoin
Ergot alkaloids	Anticancer drugs

ASPIRIN

Caution in the use of aspirin by the lactating mother is recommended because salicylate intoxication or coagulopathy may occur in the suckling child. There is one case report of acidosis and dyspnea in a 2-week-old breast-fed infant following maternal daily ingestion of 2,400 mg of aspirin. Serum salicylate levels in the child were reported to be 24 mg per deciliter. To date, there have been four prospective studies of the transmammary excretion of aspirin. In one report, a single maternal dose of 650 mg of aspirin yielded peak salicylate levels of 17.3 to 48.3 mg per deciliter in the milk, and between 14.5 and 18.8 mg per deciliter of the drug was recovered from the urine of the infants. In another study, nursing mothers received 20 mg per kilogram of the drug and a total of 1 mg per kilogram was recovered from the milk during the ensuing 48 hours, and between 0.18 and 0.36 percent of the maternal dose was recovered from the infant's urine. A third communication details four women who received 0.6 to 4 g of aspirin in divided doses at 4-hour intervals. The drug content of the milk ranged from 0.02 to 1 mg per deciliter. A final study reports peak milk salicylate concentrations to be 0.33 mg per deciliter after 454 mg of aspirin had been administered to the mother. With the exception of the first study, the data suggest that the casual use of aspirin by the lactating woman is probably safe. It would, however, be advisable for infants of mothers who require prolonged salicylate therapy to be monitored for evidence of platelet dysfunction.

ANTITHYROID DRUGS

More than 40 years ago, propylthiouracil levels in breast milk were found to be three times those in maternal plasma. Thereafter, mothers taking this compound were advised not to nurse their infants, since the drug may lead to goiter or agranulocytosis in the child. Information on other antithyroid agents is limited. Two recent studies, however, have failed to demonstrate that these drugs have a detrimental effect on breast-fed infants. In one study, labeled thiouracil was measured in milk during the 24 hours after drug ingestion, and it was shown that only 0.077 percent of the administered dose was present in the milk collected. In another study, nine lactating women received 400 mg of propylthiouracil and the mean serum level at 1.5 hours reached 7.7 μg per milliliter, which was ten times the milk concentration. One breast-fed infant whose mother received propylthiouracil throughout a 5-month period of observation exhibited no alteration in thyroid function. Although conclusions regarding safety cannot be made from such a small patient sample, the use of propylthiouracil by lactating mothers is probably safe provided the thyroid function of the suckling infant is closely monitored.

LITHIUM CARBONATE

The first publication that warned that a mother receiving lithium therapy should not breast-feed was a report of toxicity in an infant within hours of birth. Cyanosis, hypotonia, and hypothermia were the initial signs of drug intoxication. Although the infant improved on conservative therapy, toxicity recurred when the baby was put to the breast. At 5 days of age, the maternal serum lithium level was 1.5 mEq per liter, as compared with 0.6 mEq per liter in the infant, and the content of lithium in the lacteal secretions was equivalent to the plasma concentration in the infant.

The pharmacodynamics of lithium carbonate appears to be altered in the lactating woman and the neonate compared with other women. During the first week of extrauterine life, serum levels of lithium in the infant equal the concentration in the milk and are approximately half the maternal serum level. In the subsequent 7 weeks of life, the maternal serum levels decline to one-third of those in the milk, and the ratio of the drug in the milk compared with in the infant's serum is about 0.2.

In another communication, a breast-feeding patient required a progressive increase in lithium dosage during the puerperium. The dosage of lithium required increased from 400 mg at the time of parturition, to 600 mg daily during the subsequent week, to 800 mg daily by the 18th day. Despite the 50 percent increase in maternal dose, the infant's serum drug level declined during the initial 2 weeks and remained relatively constant during the third and fourth weeks of life, even though the lithium concentration in the milk had doubled. No evidence of lithium intoxication was seen during 2 months of observation, and the infant's development was normal. It appears that the early neonatal period is the time of greatest risk to the breast-fed infant. Breast-feeding is a viable option for the child of a woman receiving lithium therapy, although close supervision is required during the early weeks of life.

RADIOACTIVE PHARMACEUTICALS

A lactating woman may require a diagnostic procedure that utilizes a radioactive drug. In such instances, lactation is interrupted. Uptake of radioactive iodine by the thyroid of the breast-fed infant has been computed, and the maternal to placental ratio of iodine-131 has been shown to be 65. Resumption of breast-feeding is permissible several days after the use of radioactive materials. Table 2 lists the time interval that is recommended to protect the infant from any ill effects.

CHLORAMPHENICOL

Chloramphenicol is a lipid-soluble antibiotic that is less than 50 percent protein-bound in maternal plasma and therefore readily crosses the alveolar cell to enter the mammary secretions. In the bacterial cell it reversibly binds to the 50 S subunit ribosome to inhibit protein synthesis. Chloramphenicol can interfere with mitochondrial protein synthesis in the human cell and, since this activity is greatest in the initial month of life, the potential for toxicity is enhanced in the neonate. Likewise, neonatal hepatic immaturity permits drug accumulation to toxic levels that may lead to either the gray baby syndrome or reversible bone-marrow depression. If the serum concentration in the infant reaches ten times that required to inhibit bacterial protein synthesis, the potential for toxicity is enhanced by interference with electron transport in the mitochondria.

Pharmacokinetic studies have demonstrated that a lactating woman who ingests 1.5 g of chloramphenicol a day will excrete 40 mg of the drug in her milk, an amount sufficient to be toxic to a child of less than 2 weeks of age and in the therapeutic range for a 3-week-old infant. An additional fact to be taken into account when treating a nursing mother with chloramphenicol is that antibacterial therapy with bacteriocidal agents may be compromised in the infant by the presence of a bacteriostatic agent in the milk. This could have disastrous effects if the child requires therapy for such severe infections as pneumonia or meningitis.

ANTITUBERCULAR DRUGS

Because of the nature of tuberculosis, antitubercular agents are employed for long-term therapy. The suckling infant, therefore, may be exposed to these drugs through the duration of lactation. However, little information is available to aid the clinician in making decisions as to whether or not the mother should breast-feed her baby or the extent of the risk of the ingested drug to the nursing infant.

Of the antitubercular drugs studied, isoniazid appears in the highest concentration in human milk, achieving a peak level of 16 mg per liter at 3 hours. Approximately

TABLE 2 Recommended Interval Before Resumption of Lactation After Administration of Radioisotopes

Radioisotope	*Interval in Days Before Resumption of Lactation*
^{131}I	2–10 days (depends on dose size)
^{67}G	14
^{99m}Tc	2

20 percent of the therapeutic dose for an infant is consumed via the mammary secretions. Hepatotoxicity has been attributed to the acetyl metabolite, which reaches a peak level of 3.76 mg per liter 5 hours after the drug has been administered to the mother. Although the toxicity appears to be due to acetylisoniazide, the concentration of the metabolite necessary for this to occur is unknown.

Rifampin, *p*-aminosalicylic acid, ethionamide, and streptomycin have antibacterial activity and may alter the intestinal microflora of the nursing infant. Although aminoglycosides are excreted in breast milk, they are poorly absorbed from the child's gut, and thus the potential for systemic toxicity is small. Nevertheless, the risk to the infant of infectious diarrhea or pseudomembranous enterocolitis due to changes in the gut flora must be taken into account when the physician counsels the patient on the risks of breast-feeding during antitubercular therapy.

Table 3 summarizes the available data on infant exposure to antitubercular drugs via maternal milk. A limited number of women participated in the studies; consequently the number of samples that were analyzed was small, but available information suggests the risk of toxic reaction is low. This is consistent with the sparsity of adverse reactions reported. Because of hepatic immaturity in the neonate, the potential for toxicity is at a maximum in the first weeks of life.

THE TETRACYCLINES

The introduction in recent years of less toxic antimicrobial agents has led to a dramatic decline in the use of tetracyclines. Awareness of the true prevalence of *Chlamydia trachomatis* infections may lead to a reversal of this trend, and consequently exposure of the infant to these drugs via breast milk is a distinct possibility.

Tetracycline levels in the alveolar secretions have been shown to be about 70 percent of those in the maternal serum. When a lactating woman receives 250 mg of tetracycline four times a day, the milk contains between 1 and 2 μg of the drug per milliliter. The highest level recorded in human milk is 4 μg per milliliter when a patient received the drug in a dosage of 500 mg four times a day. Consumption of 600 ml of milk a day by an infant weighing 3,000 g could result in the neonate's receiving 1/25 of the standard therapeutic dose of 20 mg per kilogram.

Although reports in the literature have demonstrated a 40 percent reduction in bone growth of the fibula of premature infants receiving tetracycline, retarded osteogenesis has not been recorded in infants exposed to tetracycline in breast milk. Tetracycline is largely bound to calcium, and the complex so formed reduces tetracycline absorption from the gut. Short-term administration of this antibiotic to the lactating mother is probably safe, and the risk to the suckling infant is minimal. Until confirmation of drug safety has been documented, the possibility of dental discoloration, enamel hypoplasia, and decrease in linear skeletal growth rate in the infant must be considered whenever tetracyclines are prescribed for the treatment of chlamydial infections in the lactating patient.

METRONIDAZOLE

Our concerns about infant exposure to metronidazole via breast milk are the result of reports of mutagenicity and teratogenicity that are known to occur in laboratory animals. Although these effects have been produced in animals by prolonged exposure to large amounts of the drug, neither effect has been observed in children whose mothers received metronidazole during pregnancy or lactation.

The milk content of metronidazole has been determined at steady state from women on an oral dosage of 200 mg three times a day. The metronidazole content in the lacteal secretions was approximately 5 μg per milliliter. Extrapolation from this data to the 250-mg dose available in the United States suggests that the infant would receive 40 mg of the drug during a 7-day course of treatment.

A group of investigators treated 15 lactating women for endometritis with oral metronidazole. The content of the drug and its hydroxy metabolite was measured simultaneously in the maternal and infant plasma as well as in the milk. Four of the 15 mothers received 1,200 mg and 11 received 600 mg of metronidazole a day in divided doses. The concentration of the drug in the milk was found to be comparable to that in the plasma in those women who received the 600-mg regimen. The plasma levels in the infants whose mothers received the higher dosage were comparable to the level required during therapy for a neonate. If we take into account the fact that the antibiotic activity of the hydroxy metabolite is 30 percent of that of

TABLE 3 Estimated Amount of Drug Ingested via Mother's Milk

Drug Usual Adult Dose	*Adult Dose In Milk per 24 hr (%)*	*Amount Ingested by Infant (mg)*	*Amount Ingested mg/kg of Body Weight**	*Usual Therapeutic Dose for Infants (mg/kg)*	*Therapeutic Dose*
Isoniazid, 300 mg	0.75–2.3	2.2–6.9	0.64–2.0	10	6.4–20
Rifampin, 600 mg	0.05	0.30	0.085	15	0.57
Streptomycin sulfate, 1.0 g	0.5	5	1.4	15	9.5
Kanamycin sulfate, 1.0 g	0.05	0.5	0.14	15	0.95
Cycloserine, 1.0 g	0.6	6.0	1.7	15	11.3
Ethambutol hydrochloride, 15 mg/kg	unknown	1.8–3.0	0.51–0.86	15	3.4–5.7

* Assumes a body weight of 3.5 kg. (Reproduced with permission from Snider DE, Powell KE. Should women taking antituberculosis drugs breast-feed? Arch Intern Med 1984; 144:589–590.

the parent compound and consider the functional immaturity of the newborn's kidney, there is a potential risk of metronidazole toxicity in the neonate.

No information is available on the exposure an infant receives when the mother is treated with an oral or parenteral dose of 500 mg, which is now frequently prescribed in therapeutic regimens. Only one report has appeared regarding the amount of drug excreted in the milk after a single 2-g dose used for the treatment of vaginal trichomoniasis. Three lactating patients were prescribed such a dose and the metronidazole content of their milk determined. The amount of drug excreted in the 48 hours subsequent to drug administration was estimated to be 25 mg. If a bottle feeding is substituted for the initial 24 hours, the infant's consumption will be reduced to 4 mg on the second day.

BARBITURATES

Prohibiting the use of barbiturates by lactating women was largely based on anecdotal communications that were, unfortunately, either unsubstantiated by analytic methods or accompanied solely by qualitative data. The concern about transmission of barbituric acid derivatives via milk evolved from animal studies that demonstrated an increased mortality rate as well as growth retardation in litters fed with milk containing barbiturates. However, the amount of drug that was administered to the mothers in these studies exceeded the usual dosage required for hypnotic and anticonvulsive therapy.

The results of human investigation are both variable and confusing. In a study in the 1930s that employed a qualitative analytic method, phenobarbital was confirmed to be present on the first day of treatment. Two of the 11 infants whose mothers were given phenobarbital for sleep were somnolent and difficult to rouse. An infant death has been recorded in whom the plasma level of phenobarbital was 8.3 μg per milliliter, and this was considered to be a contributory factor in the child's demise.

The results of a study of epileptic women who were given phenobarbital in the dose customarily used for seizure control were different. The drug content of the milk was found to be minimal, and no ill effects were observed in the infants. This is in accord with the observations of another investigator who reported the barbiturate content of milk to be only 1.5 percent of the maternal plasma concentration. The phenobarbital in the milk of this group of epileptics who received up to 200 mg a day averaged 0.9 μg per milliliter, and this low concentration resulted in no toxicity in the breast-fed infants.

The high fat solubility of barbiturates enhances their excretion in human milk. The risk of toxicity to the nursing infant is minimal provided that the maternal dose does not exceed the accepted therapeutic amount. The potential for drug intoxication is greater in the early weeks of life when the infant has both renal and hepatic immaturity. Short-term administration of low doses of the drug should pose no risk to the breast-fed infant.

PHENYTOIN

Transmammary passage of phenytoin occurs, although the plasma levels in the nursing infant are low. In a report of 38 breast-fed infants exposed to the drug, no adverse effects were recorded. One case of methemoglobinemia associated with drowsiness and ecchymosis has been reported in a child when the maternal seizures were controlled with a product containing both phenobarbital and phenytoin. Although the relationship of the reaction to phenytoin was not established, the infant's symptoms disappeared on cessation of lactation.

ERGOT PREPARATIONS

Death from ergotism in nursing infants was first reported with the Ukranian rye smut disaster earlier this century. Vomiting, loss of weight, and a thready pulse are evidence of ergot intoxication. Confirmation of the cause of these symptoms has been verified in the breast-feeding child by administering fluid extract of ergot to the lactating woman. Ergotamine derivatives are concentrated in the milk and excreted in large quantities. Ergot alkaloids have been used in the obstetric suite for many years to reduce blood loss at parturition. These have also been used for the treatment of vascular headaches. Unfortunately, minimal data are available to confirm either the safety of these compounds or their potential adverse effects on the infant when they are prescribed for the lactating woman. Other modalities of therapy are available for each of the entities for which these products are prescribed, and until there is proof that these drugs are safe, one should be cautious in prescribing them for the lactating woman.

As previously stated, weak basic, lipid-soluble drugs with low protein binding as well as the heavy metals are concentrated in breast milk and appear in concentrations that exceed the maternal plasma levels. Although the infant is frequently exposed to these agents, only a few have been shown to have a detrimental effect. The risk of toxicity is greatest in early neonatal life before hepatic and renal maturation have occurred. A list of the medicinal agents and environmental pollutants that are known to be excreted in high concentration in the milk is given in Table 4.

RECREATIONAL DRUGS

The use of psychedelic drugs can not only adversely affect the health of the mother, but also alter the pattern of maternal behavior and her ability to care for her child. Like other alkaloids, morphine and heroin are concentrated in the milk and attain higher levels than observed in maternal plasma. Nevertheless, morphine and the other opiates do not constitute a risk to the nursing infant as long as the dosage used is consistent with regimens appropriate for pain relief. Marijuana has a high lipid solubility and, as a result, is concentrated in the milk and excreted for several days after its use by the mother has ceased.

TABLE 4 Drugs and Other Substances Excreted in Breast Milk in Quantities of Unity or Greater

Drug	*Milk:Plasma Ratio*
Atenolol	3.0
Carbamazepine[1]	1.9 + 1.6
Casanthranol (Peri-colace; Dilose Plus)[4]	No quantitative data
Cascara sagrada	No quantitative data
Cimetidine[2]	4.6 – 11.76
Clemastine	2.0
Codeine	2.16
Cycloserine	0.3–1.18
Digoxin	0.45 – 1.0
Erythromycin[2]	0.5 – 3.0
Ethambutol	1.0
Haloperidol	0.5 – 1.0
Iodine-131[1]	65
Isoniazid[1]	>1
Kanamycin[3]	0.4 – 1.0
Kepone[1]	No quantitative data
Lincomycin[3]	0.15 – 2.25
Meprobamate[1,3]	2 – 4
Mercury[1]	No quantitative data
Methadone	0.3 – 1.89
Methenamine	1.08
Meperidine	1.2
Metronidazole[2]	1.0
Methotrexate[2]	0.08 – 1.0
Methimazole[1]	1.16
Metoprolol	3.0 – 3.7
Nadolol	4.6
Perphenazine	1.0
Phenyton	1.23–2.11
Polybromated Biphenyl (PBB)[2]	No quantitative data
Polychlorinated biphenyl[1]	No quantitative data
Procainamide	4.3 – 2.4
Propranolol	0.05 – 1.65
Ranitidine[2]	6.8 – 23.8
^{90}Sr[1]	1.0
Streptomycine[2]	1.1 – 1.3
Sulfanilamide[1,3]	1.0
Tapazole	>1
^{99m}Tc[1]	3 – 5.2
Terbutaline	1.4 – 2.9
Tetrachlorethylene[1]	No data
Tetracycline[3]	0.2 – 1.4
Timolol[2]	0.25 – 1.73
Trimethoprim[1,3]	3.7

[1] Drugs or pollutants known to exert toxic effects.
[2] Drugs or pollutants with high potential for toxicity, although intoxication has not been reported.
[3] Drugs that may alter gut flora.
[4] Anecdotal reports of toxicity only; no quantitative data available.

TABLE 5 Drugs that May Reduce Milk Production

Bromocriptine	Ergot compounds
Levodopa	Clomiphene
Diethylstilbestrol	Nicotine
Progestogens	

Delta-9-tetrahydrocannabinol has been shown to attain a concentration in the milk that is ten times that in the maternal plasma. Although there are limited data from human studies, endocrinologic and behavioral changes have been demonstrated in suckling rodents. Our department has recently had an infant death caused by starvation following several days of neglect because of maternal drug addiction and overdose. Women who are at risk for drug abuse require support and education regarding the deleterious effects these agents can have on their family.

DRUGS THAT REDUCE MILK PRODUCTION

To a large extent, the blood supply to the breast controls the volume of milk produced, and any substance that reduces mammary vascularity can adversely affect infant nutrition. The vasculature of the chest wall is responsive to sympathomimetic agents, and vasoconstrictor drugs should not be used during lactation. The nicotine content of cigarettes can decrease milk volume if consumption exceeds a pack a day. The additive effect of passive smoking likewise should not be overlooked. Dexbrompheniramine, an antihistamine commonly found in over-the-counter cold preparations as well as some prescription products, reduces mammary blood flow and may produce excessive crying, irritability, and sleep disturbance in the nursing infant. Other drugs that reduce milk volume are listed in Table 5, and it is preferable that the physician avoid using these agents during lactation.

Most drugs used by the lactating woman appear in the breast milk. The mammary gland is an organ of excretion and participates in the clearance of drugs from the body. Some agents are excreted in large quantities in milk, whereas others are found in negligible amounts. Unfortunately, the effect a therapeutic modality may have on a breast-fed infant cannot be equated with the quantity of drug to which it is exposed, because a modest amount of one agent may have a more profound effect than several times that amount of another. In an attempt to overcome the frustration caused by the lack of scientific knowledge, clinicians have devised lists of drugs that endeavor to categorize pharmaceutical agents by their presumed safety. The futility of these canons has been demonstrated in this chapter. Improvement in patient education, particularly in regard to the avoidance of self-medication with over-the-counter drugs, may provide protection for the nursing infant and reduce both the consumption of drugs by the mother and the possibility of drug to drug interaction when several agents are administered concomitantly.

SUGGESTED READING

Briggs GG, Freeman RK, Yaffe SJ, eds. Drugs in pregnancy and lactation. 2nd ed. Baltimore: Williams & Wilkins, 1986.
Wilson JT, Brown RD, Cherek DR, et al. Drug excretion in human breast milk. Clin Pharmacokinet 1980; 5:1–66.

MALIGNANT DISEASE

MALIGNANT DISEASE IN PREGNANCY

HUGH R. K. BARBER, M.D.

Cancer-complicating pregnancy, is uncommon, but does occur with an average frequency of 1 in 1,000 births. The problem had special relevance at one time when the controversy surrounding the question of whether abortion was therapeutic in women with cancer (or was instead an unnecessary interference) made a difficult decision for the clinician faced with this problem. Each hospital had an Abortion Committee as well as a Tumor Board, and in order to perform an abortion, it was necessary to show that the mother's life was jeopardized by the continuance of the pregnancy. The conflicting reports in the literature made the decision difficult for Abortion Committees. There were as many papers stating that pregnancy had no deleterious effects as those that reported on the dangers of cancer-complicating pregnancy. However, with today's liberalized abortion laws, women are free to have an elective abortion whenever a diagnosis of cancer is made. The Abortion Committee no longer has to deal with the decision to abort or not. Faced with a life-threatening disease, there are women and their families who ask very direct and specific questions about whether the pregnancy can have an adverse effect on the cancer and vice versa. If these women elect to continue the pregnancy, they seek help from a physician who is experienced in managing cancer-complicating pregnancy. This clinical dilemma may be the one occasion when a joint decision must be reached among the obstetrician, surgeon, medical oncologist, social workers, clergy, and other involved specialists.

The introduction of new concepts in preventative medicine, the enlightened use of antibiotics, and the establishment of blood banks has brought about a sharp decline in such killers of pregnant women as heart disease, toxemia, hemorrhage, and infectious diseases; whereas cancer has assumed an increasingly important role in maternal mortality studies.

Mortality from cancer for the five leading sites and in the major age groups for women is as follows: under 15 years—leukemia, cancer of the brain and central nervous system, kidney, bone, and connective tissue; 15 to 34 years—leukemia, Hodgkin's disease, and cancer of the breast, brain and central nervous system, and uterus; 35 to 54 years—cancer of the breast, lung, colon and rectum, uterus, and ovary. Since women are delaying childbearing until they have established themselves as executives or in their profession, a great number are having their children after age 35. At the same time, the incidence of certain cancers, such as cancer of the breast, ovary, and endometrium, is more frequent under age 40 than has heretofore been recognized. Therefore, it is anticipated that more cancer-complicating pregnancy will be encountered.

The majority of malignant diseases that are associated with pregnancy are breast cancers, lymphomas, malignant melanomas, and gynecologic and bone cancers. This association represents a major physiologic process for the maintenance of the race, a major pathologic process that accounts for numerous deaths, and a struggle that leads to biologic immortality or destruction. In cancer-complicating pregnancy, there is the combination of a controlled growth (pregnancy) and an uncontrolled growth (cancer) in the same host, which provides a setting that is stimulating and likely to be rewarding in answering important questions relative to both the pregnancy and the cancer.

The opinions expressed in the literature of the effects of pregnancy on malignant process range from those who feel that pregnancy increases resistance to cancer to the other extreme expressed by those who state that pregnancy has a stimulating effect. The lack of agreement makes it difficult, if not impossible, for the average physician to plan treatment. Unfortunately, decisions are based all too often on emotion rather than on recorded, objective, scientific data of which there are little available.

Cancer-complicating pregnancy is best divided into pelvic and extrapelvic malignancy. Barber and Brunschwig reported on gynecologic cancer-complicating pregnancy. Boronow, in a very thorough and comprehensive article, reviewed extrapelvic malignancy and pregnancy. This division is followed in this chapter and pelvic cancer-complicating pregnancy will be discussed first.

PELVIC CANCER-COMPLICATING PREGNANCY

Pelvic cancer-complicating pregnancy is most often treated by surgery. The rationale for this is based upon the following arguments:

1. The preferred treatment for any cancer is to excise it widely when this can be done without an inordinate risk of morbidity or mortality.
2. Surgery provides an all-embracing approach in the shortest period of time.
3. When cancer and pregnancy coexist, the principle of eradication of cancer is still valid.

In the past 25 years, there has been an improvement in therapy for cancer in general. It follows that more women may become pregnant during treatment of cancer or during subsequent follow-up. The impact of greater emphasis on cancer detection remains to be evaluated, but early reports indicate that the discovery of cancer in pregnancy has increased due, in no small measure, to diligent screening programs. It is important to establish a firm histologic diagnosis. Decidua changes in pelvic organs should be recognized so that these changes do not confuse the clinical and histologic diagnosis. Having established the diagnosis, the philosophy must be to treat the cancer and ignore the pregnancy. However, in certain instances, therapy may result in the interruption of pregnancy. Since there is no direct attack on the fetus in the management of cancer of the pelvis, and since this approach is medically sound, this therapy is accepted but not necessarily condoned by conventional religion.

Holleb and Farrow grouped their patients with cancer into the three categories: (1) simultaneous with pregnancy, (2) post partum, and (3) subsequent pregnancy. This provides an orderly approach to the overall problem of cancer-complicating pregnancy.

The pregnant state is divided into the standard three trimesters plus a fourth postpartum period, which extends for 4 to 6 months depending upon the protocol of a given institution. There are now well-established guidelines for treatment in each trimester, and principles should be adapted to patients on an individual basis. There is an increasing body of evidence appearing in the current literature that favors primary surgery as the preferred method of treatment for gynecologic cancer-complicating pregnancy. Radiation therapy has its optimum effect in well-oxygenated tissue that is undergoing rapid growth. As soon as the pregnancy is damaged by radiation, involution follows and creates an anoxic type of tissue. This is a poor setting in which to achieve a good radiation effect.

These questions constantly arise: Does pregnancy affect prognosis? What effect does cancer have on the fetus? What would treatment do to the fetus? These questions are discussed as each organ system affected by pregnancy is reviewed.

The cancers that are included in the pelvic group are cancers of the vulva, vagina, cervix, endometrium, ovary, and rectum.

Cancer of the Vulva

Cancer of the vulva accounts for only 1 percent of all cancers and 3 or 4 percent of gynecologic cancers. It is a disease of the aged. It is rare in the young and extremely rare in association with pregnancy. When it does occur, patients are surprisingly young.

With the current sexual revolution and the start of intercourse at much earlier ages than previously recorded, the incidence of abnormal vulvar cytology and histology is increasing. Vulvar carcinoma in situ (VIN) is increasing, and this may be caused by a variety of reasons such as increasing numbers of infection from the herpesvirus 2, human papilloma virus, and unnamed viruses. Condyloma acuminata, which are frequent in the 20 and 30 age group, are increasingly occurring and are present in 7 to 31 percent of cases of vulvar carcinoma in situ. Human papilloma virus has become the prime suspect in vulvar neoplasms. In addition, whatever the initial treatment, the incidence of recurrences is increasing, and intraepithelial lesions are not uncommon. In addition to the viral problems that contribute to increased in situ microinvasion and an anticipated increase in invasive cancers, the problem of cigarette smoking undoubtedly plays a role. There are a great number of carcinogens in cigarettes, and heavy smokers are known to have an increased incidence of bladder cancer. Therefore, it is conceivable that if urine that contains these carcinogens bathes the vulva, this may contribute to the increase in premalignant and malignant vulvar lesions. Currently, in situ lesions and marked condyloma are being identified with increasing frequency in pregnant patients.

Barclay, in a review of the literature, found only 31 women with vulvar cancer that was associated with pregnancy. Of these cases, only two were actually diagnosed and treated during pregnancy, with another two being treated following termination of pregnancy. Lutz et al in 1977 reported five vulvar cancers associated with pregnancy, of which three were diagnosed and treated during pregnancy and two within 6 months post partum. The author reported on three other cases of vulvar cancer associated with pregnancy. Two were diagnosed prior to pregnancy and one in the fifth month of pregnancy. The patients were surprisingly young. The average age in the series reported by the author was 27.3 years; an age range of 25 to 35 is reported in the literature.

Patients with in situ condyloma and small microinvasive cancers, which have been proved by biopsy and histologic study, can be successfully treated during pregnancy by laser therapy. Since these lesions are often multifocal and multicentric, laser surgery is ideally suited to controlling preinvasive and small, early microinvasive lesions without mutilating the vulva. It is to be emphasized that microinvasion of greater than 1 cm in diameter or 5 mm in depth should be considered for more aggressive treatment. It is acceptable during the pregnancy to treat the patient with a unilateral vulvectomy and ipsilateral groin lymphadenectomy, if this is deemed necessary.

Regardless of the pregnancy, more established and advanced disease should be treated by the previously mentioned procedure or by radical vulvectomy and bilateral groin lymphadenectomy. The author's plan of management for a pregnant patient with diagnosed cancer of the vulva is as follows:

1. First trimester: Radical vulvectomy, bilateral superficial node dissection. A deep node dissection is only carried out if the highest node is positive (so-called

Cloquet node) or if the lowest external iliac node (or several positive nodes) are present in the groin.
2. Second trimester: Same treatment as for the first trimester. However, it may be technically impossible to do an adequate node dissection. If so, a radical vulvectomy should be done and node dissection delayed until after delivery.
3. Third trimester: If the lesion is small and unlikely to interfere with vaginal delivery, this method of delivery should be permitted. Radical vulvectomy and node dissection should be carried out in the immediate postpartum period (2 to 4 weeks).
4. Post partum: The conventional operation of radical vulvectomy and lymph node dissection should be carried out. At this point, it must be pointed out that among all patients with invasive cancer of the vulva, there has been a trend to scale down the procedure and even to treat the deep node area with radiation.
5. Subsequent pregnancy: The patient should only have a cesarean section if obstetrically indicated.

Following radical vulvectomy, vaginal delivery should be allowed if there is suitable care of the introitus and a timely episiotomy in order to avoid scar tissue from tearing. If there is a significant vaginal stenosis or fibrosis, abdominal delivery is advisable. Should labor occur before the wound is healed, or if there has been a degree of dehiscence, then elective cesarean section is advisable. Pregnancy has no adverse effect on the prognosis, and termination is not indicated in such patients.

Cancer of the Vagina

Cancer of the vagina is extremely rare, comprising less than 1 percent of all genital cancers. The ratio of cancer of the cervix to vaginal cancer is roughly 50 to 1. It is often difficult to tell if the tumor arises primarily in the vaginal epithelium or extends to it from a primary locus in the cervix. When both are involved, the cervix is considered the primary locus.

Cancer of the vagina has been found mainly in women over the age of 50 years. The average age was 61 for white women and 58 years for black women.

Collins and Barclay reported 10 vaginal carcinomas associated with pregnancy, which were collected from the literature. Lutz and his associates reported one such case. Among those reported with a follow-up, the prognosis was poor.

Carcinoma in situ of the vagina is appearing more frequently than heretofore reported. This is probably related to the same suspected epidemiologic and etiologic factors as reported for the vulva. These patients can either be carefully followed throughout their pregnancy or treated with laser therapy.

The lack of collected experience in managing vaginal cancer-complicating pregnancy makes it difficult to establish a plan for therapy. However, management in general should be similar to that for a patient who is not pregnant. If the fetus is viable, delivery by a high vertical cesarean section should be performed, and therapy should be started as if the pregnant patient were not recently pregnant. If the infant is not viable or near viable age, treatment should be started with external radiation therapy followed by intracavitary radium or cesium application. The application must take into consideration the location of the lesion. In the rare instance that the patient does not spontaneously abort following the external therapy, the uterus should be emptied before the cesium application is carried out. If the lesion is early (stage I) and located in the upper part of the vagina, it can be managed by radical hysterectomy, vaginectomy, and pelvic node dissection.

Herbst, Ulfelder, and Poskanzer reported 7 girls, 15 to 22 years of age, with adenocarcinoma of the vagina (clear cell of müllerian type) between 1966 and 1969. The results of the study revealed a significant association between the treatment of their mothers with diethylstilbestrol (DES) during pregnancy and the latter development of adenocarcinoma in their daughters. The incidence for the development of clear cell carcinoma of the vagina and cervix is probably less than 0.1 percent in the female fetus of a mother who took stilbestrol. However, about 80 to 90 percent of these patients develop adenosis of the vagina or have a congenital anomaly of the cervix and/or vagina. From these observations, it has been suggested that DES acts as a teratogen rather than as a primary carcinogen.

Should adenocarcinoma be diagnosed during pregnancy in a DES-exposed patient, management should be the same as in the nonpregnant state, that is, radical hysterectomy, vaginectomy, and pelvic node dissection with the construction of a vagina. If the diagnosis is made at viability, a cesarean section should be carried out and then followed immediately by the treatment previously outlined.

Kistner, Gorbach, and Smith reviewed the world literature up to 1957 and found only 106 cases of invasive cervical cancer-complicating pregnancy in which the duration of pregnancy, stage of disease, and 5-year results were available for study, and to these, they added 30 more cases from three Boston hospitals. Kinch in 1961 added 105 cases of cancer of the cervix not reported in Kistner's series. Kinch's cases were diagnosed during pregnancy or within 6 months post partum over a 20-year period from 1933 to 1953. Lutz and co-workers in 1977 reported 30 cases of invasive cancer of the cervix.

The average incidence from large centers is 1 in 2,500 pregnancies, whereas the incidence of carcinoma in situ during pregnancy is 1 in 750. With increased screening programs and wide-spread availability of cervical smears at antepartum clinics, an increase is anticipated in the incidence of carcinoma in situ and in the detection of invasive cancers at a very early state.

Often the diagnosis is delayed in pregnancy. The youth of the patient and the accompanying pregnancy undoubtedly play a role in the reluctance on the part of responsible physicians to examine them at the first sign of abnormal bleeding. This emphasizes the importance of investigating excessive discharge and vaginal bleeding during pregnancy. Speculum examination is indicated in all pregnant women, particularly those with symptoms and most particularly those with any bleeding. Wide screening by cytologic studies should be carried out during pregnancy. The experience of Schmitz, Isaacs, and Featherston along these lines, in which 25 cases of cancer of the cervix were detected by the use of smears in 10,369 pregnant women, bears this out.

Consensus in the literature is that cancer of the cervix diagnosed in the latter part of pregnancy or immediately post partum has a grave prognosis. This is probably a function of the stage of disease rather than of the gestational age at the time of diagnosis. Creasman, Rutledge, and Fletcher found no difference in survival of women diagnosed during any of the three trimesters or in the post partum, when the stage of disease was correctly identified.

Approximately 10 to 15 abnormal smears are reported per 1,000 pregnancies in the average, large, antenatal clinic, and these should be followed carefully. Colposcopic assessment may be readily performed and should be carried out by somebody who is experienced in colposcopy. Fortunately, during pregnancy, the endocervix rolls out, and the ectocervix is displaced so that it is easy to get a good view of the ectocervix and the lower endocervical canal. It is important to exclude invasive carcinoma; this is usually done with colposcopic-directed biopsy, with the bleeding controlled easily by the use of Monsel's solution. If no invasion is present, the patient can be followed by being examined colposcopically in each trimester. If there is no change, there is no need for any treatment. However, any change should be followed by biopsy examination. There is no contraindication for these patients to deliver vaginally, and cesarean section is only required for an obstetrical complication. There is practically no indication for a cone biopsy during pregnancy as this procedure is fraught with danger because of possible abortion and infection as well as hemorrhage. Microinvasion can be observed carefully during pregnancy, and if there is any change, biopsy should be carried out.

Although surgery is the preferred method of treatment for invasive cancer of the cervix in pregnancy, radiation therapy is chosen by many physicians. The surgical treatment of clinical invasive cancer of the cervix in pregnancy is as follows:

1. First trimester and early part of second trimester: Radical hysterectomy and pelvic node dissection with the fetus in utero.
2. Late second trimester: Wait for viability of the fetus and then do a classic cesarean section followed immediately by radical hysterectomy and pelvic node dissection.
3. Third trimester: Classic cesarean section followed immediately by radical hysterectomy and pelvic node dissection.
4. Post partum: Radical hysterectomy and pelvic node dissection should be performed.

Radiation therapy of invasive carcinoma of the cervix in pregnancy is managed as follows:

1. Nonviable fetus, first and second trimesters: Treatment is given as if the pregnancy was not present. External therapy is given to the pelvis. Spontaneous evacuation is preferred to intervention.
2. Viable fetus, third trimester: Classic cesarean section immediately followed by external therapy and, on the completion of this, a cesium implant.
3. Post partum: Radiate as in the nonpregnant patient. Give external therapy first, followed by intravaginal and intrauterine radiation.

It is interesting to note the high frequency of occurrence of squamous differentiation in tumors discovered in pregnancy. Glucksman and Cherry noted a similar high frequency. This may be related to the hormonal milieu present during pregnancy.

Microinvasive disease requires a careful assessment and, perhaps, a cone biopsy in order to exclude invasion. For patients who have a lesion that is less than a centimeter in diameter and in whom invasion is less than 3 mm, the cone biopsy suffices as therapy, but requires reevaluation following delivery. However, if there are multiple foci of invasion, or if there is involvement of vascular lymphatic spaces and the penetration is greater than 3 mm, the patient must be treated as though she has invasive disease, and the previously mentioned protocol or either surgery or radiation should be carried out.

In the presence of untreated invasive cancer of the cervix, vaginal delivery is fraught with danger. Hemorrhage, sepsis, and cervical laceration may result. Whether malignant cells are spread by vaginal delivery is controversial. However, the complications that may arise give a strong impetus to carrying out a cesarean section in the presence of anything but a small invasive lesion.

Cancer of the Endometrium

Endometrial cancer-complicating pregnancy is extremely rare. Sandstrom, Welch, and Green reported one case and found six others reported in the literature. Four of the seven tumors were adenoacanthoma. Follow-up on four of the six previously reported patients indicates that three are well more than 5 years after diagnosis. Barber and Brunschwig reported one case that was discovered after curettage for a spontaneous abortion. Karlen and associates in 1972 reported that eight cases have been in the literature, two of which were incidental findings in conjunction with abortions, the one spontaneous, the other therapeutic. Of the other six, four were over the age of 35 years. The treatment is total hysterectomy, bilateral salpingo-oophorectomy, node sampling, as well as supplementary radiation therapy in high-risk patients with poor prognostic features.

Cancer of the Ovary

Cancer of the ovary accounts for approximately 5 percent of all cancers among women. Deaths from this disease have slowly increased over the last 40 years, and the rate is now 2.5 times that of the 1930 rate. In 1987, more than 18,000 cases of ovarian cancer and more than

11,000 deaths are anticipated. Cancer of the ovary is now the leading cause of death from gynecologic cancer. Common epithelial ovarian cancer is usually seen over age 40, but there are an increasing number of these tumors seen under age 40. Germ cell tumors of the ovary are seen most commonly from birth to age 20. Gonadal stromal tumors are usually seen during the child-bearing years. Germ cell and gonadal stromal tumors are more often unilateral than common epithelial ovarian cancer; therefore, if the tumors are confined to the ovary, a unilateral salpingo-oophorectomy may be an acceptable treatment.

Ovarian tumors are said to occur once in every 1,000 pregnancies: 1 in 10 of these are normal physiologic corporal lutea. Ovarian cancer occurs in about 1 in every 18,000 pregnancies. In the nonpregnant state, about 20 percent of ovarian tumors are malignant, whereas in the pregnant state, the rate drops to 5 percent. There is no explanation for this at the present time. Beral suggested that pregnancy may actually protect against the development of ovarian cancers, pointing out that ovarian cancers are rare in populations that do not practice birth control. Therefore, incessant ovulation is considered an epidemiologic factor.

Chung and Birnbaum found that fewer than 40 cases of ovarian cancer-complicating pregnancy had been reported between 1963 and 1972 and added an additional 10 cases during, and 4 after, pregnancy. Beischer and colleagues recorded 164 ovarian tumors that were diagnosed during pregnancy or in the puerperium at Royal Woman's Hospital in Melbourne during the years 1947 until 1969. More than 50 percent were either adult cystic teratomas or mucinous cystadenomas and only 4 (2.4 percent) were malignant. He commented on the difficulty of establishing a definite diagnosis during pregnancy and concluded that the size of the tumor was not a reliable criteria of malignancy. The various favorable pathologic types (adult cystic teratoma and mucinous cystadenoma) reflected an overall 5-year survival rate for ovarian neoplasia in pregnancy of 76 percent, as compared to a general figure for all age groups of 25 percent.

Novak, Lambron, and Woodruff reported on 100 cases of malignant ovarian neoplasia associated with gestation. There were 45 common epithelial ovarian tumors, 14 gonadal stromal tumors, 33 germ cell tumors, 2 sarcomas, 2 metastatic Krukenberg's-type tumors, and 4 metastates of which 2 were unclassifiable. The absolute 5-year survival in these 100 cases was 76 percent. The excellent salvage is a reflection of the favorable prognosis with these tumors.

The signs and symptoms of ovarian neoplasms are not basically different from those in the nonpregnant state. The presenting symptoms, such as torsion, rupture, hemorrhage, or infection, may be a complication of the tumor.

The pelvic findings are an important part in the decision of whether to operate immediately or to observe the patient until the second trimester. The unilateral, seemingly well encapsulated, freely movable mass of uniform consistency that is less than 10 cm in diameter can be kept under observation until the second trimester. If the mass decreases in size, presumably it represented a corpus luteum cyst. However, progressive growth requires exploration without further delay. On the other hand, a hard, nobby, fixed mass of variegated consistency, bilateral masses, or signs of ascitic fluid are indications for surgical intervention despite the trimester of pregnancy.

Fortunately, most malignancies in pregnancy are diagnosed at an early stage (stage I) because the patient seeks medical advice prior to the occurrence of symptoms related to the tumor and is examined at her antepartum visit. The survival rate is much the same as in the nonpregnant patient and is determined by the type of tumor and its staging. If the tumor is diagnosed in the third trimester, surgery may be delayed until the fetus is viable, but to delay beyond that is not justifiable.

At all cesarean sections, routine inspection of tubes and ovaries is mandatory. The management of ovarian cancer-complicating pregnancy is as follows:

1. Treat as in the nonpregnant state.
2. Undertake exploratory laparotomy.
3. Aspirate fluid from the pelvis and the abdomen for cytologic assessment.
4. If tumor is low grade, unilateral, and encapsulated, an unilateral salpingo-oophorectomy is performed, the opposite ovary is biopsied, and if negative, the treatment is considered to be adequate, and pregnancy is allowed to go to term.
5. If the tumor has extended beyond the ovary, undertake aspiration for cytology, total hysterectomy, bilateral salpingo-oophorectomy, appendectomy, omentectomy, and chemotherapy as indicated.

Cancer of the Rectum

Rectal cancer-complicating pregnancy is not strictly a gynecologic cancer, but a pelvic cancer.

Incidence of cancer of the rectum associated with pregnancy is extremely low as reported by McLean (1 in 50,000 cases). Less than 200 cases have been reported in the literature. Symptoms related to cancer may be overshadowed by those produced by pregnancy. Cancer of the rectum and/or colon is a rare complication of pregnancy; however, it should be included in the differential diagnosis of a patient with colonic symptoms. Rectal bleeding, abdominal pain, changing bowel habits, weight loss, palpable abdominal mass, and/or persistent nausea and vomiting in late pregnancy should alert the obstetrician to the possibility of a bowel lesion. Consideration of colonic cancer is particularly important in a patient with known factors that predispose to malignant change. Lesions have been discovered during all trimesters with equal frequency, as well as during labor, and a few patients have had obvious predisposing factors such as ultrasensitive colitis, familial polyposis, Gardner's syndrome, and vellous tumors. Too often these symptoms related to the gastrointestinal tract are dismissed as side effects of pregnancy, which are produced by hormonal changes in an enlarging uterus, or to hemorrhoids, with the result that obstruction or perforation of the colon ultimately discloses the correct diagnosis. Consequently, the prognosis for carcinoma of the colon during pregnancy has generally been poor.

Unless the symptoms improve, thorough investigation should be carried out. Harm to the fetus during barium studies must be equated against the fatal outcome that results from failure to diagnose cancer of the bowel in an early stage. The role of colonoscopy as a modality of management in these cases has not been reported, but would negate the danger to the fetus from radiation exposure. Once the diagnosis has been established, it is important to proceed with treatment. The suggested plan of management is as follows:

1. First and second trimesters: An abdominal perineal resection or an anterior resection is carried out depending upon the position of the lesion. The pregnancy usually does not have to be interrupted unless there are technical difficulties, and this situation is extremely rare. In most instances, the pregnancy is allowed to proceed unless the cancer has invaded the uterus.
2. Late second and third trimesters: If possible, management should be delayed until the fetus is viable. However, complications related to the cancer may require prompt treatment. Cesarean section is usually required in order to facilitate the technical aspects of the bowel operation. An abdominal, perineal, or anterior resection is the treatment of choice. If there is any evidence of local spread, total hysterectomy and bilateral salpingo-oophorectomy may be required as well. In the presence of large bowel carcinoma, there is increasing evidence to indicate that bilateral oophorectomy should be carried out in order to remove the ovary as a major site for later metastasis.

To date, the prognosis for pregnant women with colon cancer has been dismal. However, Barber and Brunschwig reported on a pregnancy that had occurred after an abdominal perineal resection (APR), the patient was still alive more than 20 years later. In general, the overall survival rate is comparable to the survival rate of nonpregnant women with rectal cancer. The stage of disease is the most important consideration.

EXTRAPELVIC MALIGNANCY IN PREGNANCY

In 1964, Boronow wrote a comprehensive review on extrapelvic malignancy in pregnancy. It has served as a model for numerous articles on this subject since that time.

The obstetrician feels secure in managing the pregnant patient with pelvic cancer. However, he is less secure in management and control if the patient has an extrapelvic malignancy. If castration or termination of pregnancy is indicated, the obstetrician is the technician, and all too often, the patient is then managed either by a medical or hematologic oncologist or by a surgeon who undertakes a radical approach to melanoma, breast, or gastrointestinal cancer; thus, the obstetrician becomes a bystander. This is neither ideal management nor in the best interest of the patient. The obstetrician is best qualified to serve as the primary care physician and to control and coordinate the care of the patient. If specialists are called in, they all should act as consultants and not as the physician-in-charge. The obstetrician must continue as the responsible physician, and all orders and treatment should be controlled by him or her. The obstetrician has a particular relationship with the patient since it has usually been going on for several weeks if not months.

Breast Cancer

Breast cancer, the most frequent cancer in women, is also the second leading cause of cancer deaths, which now number more than 37,000 yearly in the United States. About 15 percent of the cases occur in women younger than 41 years of age; about 3 percent occur during pregnancy, complicating approximately one in every 3,000 pregnancies. Breast cancer has had considerable public attention because of its frequency, the controversy about management, and the importance of the breast as a body and sexual image for the woman.

There is a familial incidence of breast cancer so that the risk of developing the disease increases by 5 to 10 times if a first degree relative has it. It is the leading site of mortality from cancer in women between 39 and 44 years of age. When women delay their first pregnancy until the age of 35 or more, the risk of breast cancer triples compared to those women who initially conceive prior to the age of 20. With changes in contraceptive practices and more women delaying their pregnancies and starting a family into their thirties, an increase in the incidence of this cancer-complicating pregnancy is likely. The dilemma for treatment is acute. Therapeutic abortion does not appear to improve the chances of a cure, even though this potentially lethal disease is hormone sensitive. Hormone receptor studies are not available in any significant series, but may in the future give an indication as to which pregnancies should be terminated in view of a positive receptor status.

The diagnosis is often difficult, as physiologic changes continue throughout the pregnancy, with alterations in vascularity, lymphatic permeation, and hormonal milieu. The breast is difficult to examine clinically, and physicians are reluctant to do mammograms during pregnancy. However, if there is any suspicion of a change in the breast, the approach to diagnosis should be the same as it is in the nonpregnant patient.

Management of breast cancer-associated pregnancy can be a severe test for the clinician. Widely different views are held by surgeons, obstetricians, and radiotherapists about its treatment and prognosis. In addition, nonclinical religious, psychologic, and socioeconomic considerations can influence the choice of management. Breast cancer with pregnancy is a clinical problem that demands skill and good judgment.

In the United States, 3 percent of newly diagnosed breast cancers are accompanied by pregnancy, the concurrence favoring women in the fourth decade of life. This has relevance at present because many women are now delivering their first babies after age 35.

Holleb and Farrow grouped patients into the following groups: simultaneous pregnancy, post partum, subsequent pregnancy.

The overall 5-year survival for these three major groups is 33 percent, 29 percent, and 52 percent respectively and 21 percent, 15 percent, and 30 percent when there are positive nodes. It should be noted that the frequency of positive nodes (70 percent of the cases) is somewhat higher than in the usual nonpregnant group. The outlook for such patients is less favorable than that of the nonpregnant, nonlactating woman, probably because the stage of the disease is more advanced when it is discovered. The most significant factor in the poor prognosis is physician and patient delay in diagnosis and therapy. If age and stage of disease are taken into account, pregnancy itself seems to have a negligible influence on prognosis. Modified radical mastectomy can be expected to be almost as curative for pregnant patients with operable cancers as for others and presents little chance of fetal loss. The decision of whether to perform a lumpectomy and to delay radiation until the pregnancy is terminated is controversial. It may take more time and the accumulation of a greater series of patients to answer the question of whether cancer of the breast should be treated in a pregnant patient in the same manner as in the nonpregnant patient.

The important questions in regard to pregnancy and lactating women with proven cancer of the breast are: How should the pregnant woman with breast cancer be treated? Is waiting for the termination of pregnancy indicated or even desirable before mastectomy is performed? Does accepted treatment by today's standards alter the life expectancy of women? If the woman is pregnant at the time of diagnosis or subsequent to mastectomy, is termination of pregnancy indicated? Should the surgeon plan to castrate women with treated breast cancer surgically for therapeutic reasons or primarily to prevent future pregnancies?

Some of these questions have already been answered. The consensus of opinion from the literature is that patients that present with early breast cancer in the first trimester should be treated in the same manner as the nonpregnant patient. However, this raises a question of whether lumpectomy followed by radiation therapy at a later point can be chosen or whether the fetus can be protected adequately during therapy of the breast. Once a mastectomy is carried out, there is no harm in allowing the pregnancy to continue. If elected, termination would then be based on social, economic, and psychological decisions. However, in several centers, patients with operable tumors and positive nodes receive adjuvant chemotherapy. If this regimen is followed, there must be an argument for aborting the fetus if the disease is treated in the first trimester because of the teratogenic risk of these drugs.

There does not seem to be any special risk in treating patients with breast cancer in the second half of pregnancy rather than waiting for the postpartum period. A modest delay in therapy to allow for delivery probably has no deleterious effects.

Patients with stage III and IV cancer have such a poor prognosis that a uniform plan of therapy is difficult to outline. After frank discussion with the patient, the patient may make the decision to accept treatment, knowing that there is a risk of teratogenesis; while others may elect termination of the pregnancy followed by aggressive therapy. There may be a place for prophylactic castration in the treatment of disseminated disease, but its role is yet to be defined.

Subsequent pregnancy is permissible if a 3-year interval elapses following treatment. This can identify patients who have a virulent tumor with early recurrence, whereas waiting beyond this time identifies patients who have a much better prognosis. If there is no sign of recurrence, there is no evidence to suggest that the pregnancy would alter the prognosis.

Breast feeding is a debatable issue; most surgeons suggest that this should be discouraged. Lactation, with subsequent engorgement of the other breast, would be inadvisable if a second occult primary were present.

Melanoma

Melanomas, or malignant melanomas, are carcinomas that generally originate from preexisting pigmented moles. The cancer is derived from the melanocyte, the cell concerned with melanin pigment formation, and the cancer cells usually maintain their function of pigment production. The melanocyte is embryologically derived from neural crest cells and migrates to sites in the skin, eye, central nervous system, and occasionally elsewhere during fetal development. The majority of melanomas arrive de novo from melanocytes and perhaps one third arise from nevi, many of which are congenital.

With a peak incidence in the third and fourth decades of life, melanoma is concentrated among women in their reproductive years. There is controversy on the effect of pregnancy on melanoma. In one updated report, the author reversed his opinion and showed a significant improvement in the prognosis of melanoma in some patients with associated pregnancy. Although some authors advise termination of pregnancy, there seems to be a consensus of opinion in the literature that termination of pregnancy is not considered therapeutic.

It has been suggested that melanoma may be induced or exacerbated by pregnancy. The assumption is based on the following observations: melanocyte-stimulating hormone (MSH) levels increase after the second month of pregnancy which results in increased pigmentation. Metastic spread would appear to be more rapid in pregnancy, but stage for stage, there may be no significant difference in the prognosis for the patient. At puberty, obvious pigmentation occurs in moles, genitalia, and elsewhere. There is also increased pigmentation in pregnancy as evidenced in the nipples, areolas, vulva, and linea nigra; in occasional changes in preexisting nevi, and in cases of chloasma. MSH of the pituitary has been quantitative and notably increases after the second month of pregnancy. Furthermore, Bischitz and Snell have demonstrated an estrogen role in the control of melanocytes when they studied guinea pig skin in ovarectomized animals given estrogen; however, they did not advance any specific conclusion.

In 1951, Pack and Scharnagel reported a poor prognosis in 32 cases of melanoma in pregnancy. In 1958, Shockett and Fortner demonstrated that pregnancy and lactation did not stimulate either the local development or metastatic spread of transplantable hamster melanoma. Rather growth of the local tumor appeared inhibited or evidenced a statistical significant difference in measured weight. In 1960, Fortner and Pack, who reported on 115 cases of melanoma in pregnancy, and 330 controls, found that the growth rate of regional nodes appeared to be more rapid in pregnant patients, but that stage for stage, there was little to support the prevailing opinion then that the outcome was influenced by pregnancy. In 1976, Shiu and co-workers reported that there was no statistical difference in survival rates for 5 years, free of disease, for stage I melanoma between nulliparous, parous, nonpregnant, and pregnant women. However, for stage II melanomas, a significant lower survival rate was observed for pregnant and parous women who had experienced activational lesion in a previous pregnancy as compared to that of nulliparous patients and other patients in the parous group. Their conclusion strongly suggests an adverse influence of pregnancy on women with stage II melanoma. It is obvious that melanoma remains one of the most erratic cancers, and there is no conclusive evidence of either a beneficial or a deleterious effect of pregnancy on its clinical course. It has been reported that women who had a pregnancy before the melanoma developed survived longer than women without a previous pregnancy. The explanation advanced is that exposure to fetal antigen might protect against the dissemination of melanoma cells that bear similar fetal antigens. However, these findings were not confirmed by Elwood and Coldman in Vancouver. This is presented to show that here is a great deal of controversy surrounding melanoma-complicating pregnancy.

The management is the same as in the nonpregnant patient. En bloc excision with regional node dissection is the treatment usually chosen. In order to insure adequate incision, the area of excision must be so wide that a skin graft is required to close the defect. There is a great deal of enthusiasm for the use of chemotherapy and immunotherapy in the management of melanoma.

Nevi on the feet, hands, and genitals should be excised, particularly in the pregnant patient. In our present state of knowledge, it can be stated that termination of pregnancy is not considered therapeutic.

Thyroid Cancer

The incidence of thyroid cancer is low. Even though it occurs most often in young women, it is not a common cancer, and firm conclusions regarding its relationship to pregnancy are difficult to make. It is a difficult cancer to prognosticate because of its erratic biologic behavior. In arriving at a clear decision on the management, clinical judgment of the responsible physician is often taxed. The disease frequently affects the young, even teenagers, and thus exposes a number of women to the possibility of this cancer-complicating pregnancy. Recently much has been written in both the medical and nonmedical literature about the occurrence of thyroid neoplasia after radiation therapy. This discussion is centered on the issue of the development of thyroid cancer after treatment for benign conditions, particularly during infancy and childhood. Currently, there is a great deal of discussion about the potential hazards of fallout radiation and the possible dangers of radioactive iodine use in the diagnosis and treatment of patients with thyroid disorders. The recent disaster at Chernobyl has again focused a great deal of attention on this problem. The prenatal history should explore the possibility of exposure to radiation.

Despite a common cell of origin, the disease is characterized by a wide variety of pathologic patterns that, in turn, on subdivision display further variety. The disease has a marked different lethality in the old and in the young. The young do well and have an overall 10-year survival rate, without evidence of disease, of 78.3 percent.

Thyroid cancer-complicating pregnancy is not often seen. When it does occur, there is a great deal of controversy concerning whether it is stimulated by the pregnancy. However, thyroid stimulating hormone (TSH) is elevated in pregnancy. The amount of free thyroxin is decreased so greatly by estrogen-binding globulins that the feedback mechanism to the pituitary is decreased. The protein-bound iodine (PBI) is elevated. About 10 percent of thyroid malignancies are functional and may respond to TSH stimulation. Reports indicate that those who have experience in this field maintain that pregnancy does not promote this tumor. Furthermore, pregnancy that is subsequent to treatment for thyroid carcinoma is believed neither to cause recurrence in those who have been successfully treated earlier nor to accelerate the tumor's growth in women who have not been cured. The most common type, papillary, is the most favorable, and the second most common, follicular, also has a favorable course. These two account for two-thirds or more of thyroid malignancy. One large series of papillary tumors in young adults revealed 73.3 percent living without evidence of disease at 10 years.

The management is similar to that in the nonpregnant state. Total thyroidectomy and unilateral and/or bilateral dissection of lymph nodes in the neck is the treatment usually chosen. Thyroid, in doses of 180 to 240 mg, is given daily in order to control the output of TSH. Radioactive iodine is contraindicated in pregnancy.

Although papillary and follicular cancer have a favorable prognosis, undifferentiated tumors are a highly lethal group, and they range from the giant and spindle cell varieties to the small cell varieties. Abortion has not been found to be therapeutic at this point.

Hodgkin's Disease

Hodgkin's disease is the most common of the lymphoma group and constitutes about 40 percent of malignant melanoma. It commonly affects young people and is now being cured and controlled for long periods with irradiation and chemotherapy. The disease is caused by neoplastic proliferation of lymphoreticular portions of the reticuloendothelial system that involves lymph nodes, bone marrow, spleen or liver. The majority present with tumor in the lymph nodes. There have been many recent advances in the management of Hodgkin's disease. The staging and comprehensive treatment are difficult to achieve during pregnancy without risk to the fetus. Evaluating the abdomen is the obvious handicap. The liver-spleen scan and staging laparotomy should be avoided during pregnancy. Lymphangiography presents the same problem, but it may be carried out, followed by a single abdominal film, 24 hours after the injection of dye.

Most young women treated for this disease wish to maintain a normal lifestyle, marry, and have children. The mutogenicity of irradiation and chemotherapy with the possibility of long-term damage to the gonadal tissue is well recognized. However, little is known regarding the magnitude of risk of fetal mortality and infant morbidity that may result from damaged gonadal tissue.

In those patients treated for Hodgkin's disease, if the disease remains active for 2 years after the start of treatment, the prognosis is poor. However, if the patient has remained free of disease for 3 or more years, the prognosis is good. Therefore, the patient should be told to wait for 3 years after treatment of her Hodgkin's before attempting pregnancy. This delay serves to identify those that do not respond or who have a recurrence. When exacerbations occur in association with pregnancy, the patient is most vulnerable during the postpartum period. Among 32 term deliveries, there are at least two documented cases of Hodgkin's disease in infants of mothers with Hodgkin's disease.

The surgical approach to Hodgkin's disease has changed radically in the last few years. The patient usually has an exploratory laparotomy, splenectomy, lymph node sampling, and often the ovaries are moved laterally out of all radiation fields.

When the patient is pregnant and found to have widespread Hodgkin's disease, the pregnancy usually has to be interrupted in order to give the maximum and optimal therapy so as to cure the disease. It is accepted that the pregnant patient, except in highly selected instances, should be treated as in the nonpregnant state.

A protocol that encompasses a variety of situations provides an outline for the responsible physician to make a judgment on managing the patient with lymphoma-complicating pregnancy. This includes the following: Women in the child-bearing age should not begin therapy for Hodgkin's disease unless a pregnancy test is negative, effective contraception should be used during therapy, and pregnancy should be avoided for at least 3 years following successful therapy. If the woman is pregnant at the time of diagnosis, desires the pregnancy, and the disease is not immediately life endangering, a staging laparotomy should be avoided before 12 weeks and beyond 18 weeks of gestation in order to minimize fetal jeopardy caused by technical difficulties that may be encountered. Treatment can be delayed until viability, if the patient and her family recognize the fact that she is at risk and in some danger of developing a more aggressive disease.

Both chemotherapy and irradiation are used to treat Hodgkin's disease, and both are potentially harmful to the growing fetus. Therefore, if therapy can be delayed without detriment to the patient, it should be postponed until after the fetus is viable and delivery is possible. McKean and associates investigated the results of pregnancy after treatment for Hodgkin's disease and found only 52 percent resulted in normal live births. Twenty-seven percent were either premature, stillborn, or spontaneously aborted, and 15 percent of live births had malformations. As usual, there is controversy; in sibling controls, however, Holmes and Holmes demonstrated no significant difference in spontaneous abortion or abnormal offspring in the subsequent pregnancy of patients treated for Hodgkin's disease.

Burkitt's lymphoma has been reported during pregnancy and lactation. The disease usually shows a predilection for the jaws, central nervous system, endocrine glands, gonads, and abdominal viscera; enlargement of the breast has been prominent in the gravid state, and the disease may run a rapidly fatal course. However, the disease does respond, usually to an alkylating agent, and this may be combined with radiation to selected areas.

Acute Leukemia

Leukemia is a cancer of the blood-forming tissues, striking both sexes and all ages. Although often thought of as primarily a childhood disease, leukemia strikes many more adults than children. Acute lymphatic leukemia accounts for 2,000 cases of leukemias among children, whereas in adults, the most common types are acute granulocytic and chronic lymphocytic leukemias. Modern treatment has dramatically changed the survival rate of those with acute lymphatic leukemia.

Leukemia can be expected to complicate less than 1 in 75,000 pregnancies. There are really too few cases to make a judgment, but at this point in time, there is no evidence that indicates pregnancy has a deleterious effect on leukemia, and therefore, termination of pregnancy has not proved to be therapeutic.

Leukemia does present a problem in pregnancy in that there is a greater susceptibility to infection, hemorrhage, and spontaneous abortion.

The management is the same as in the nonpregnant patient. Although abortion is not considered therapeutic, if the leukemia occurs during the first trimester, abortion is usually advised since the rate of spontaneous abortion is high in the first trimester and fetal malformations are common; this is especially the case when aggressive chemotherapy is used. Acute leukemia can be treated in second and third trimesters with little effect on the pregnancy or fetus. If the fetus is viable and amniocentesis reveals fetal lung maturity, delivery should be expedited before definitive therapy for leukemia is started. In patients cured of acute leukemia, the potential for subsequent pregnancies exists with little likelihood of increase in fetal malformations. The long-term effects of chemotherapy on infants exposed in utero are not completely known.

Chronic Leukemia

Chronic leukemia is very rare in pregnancy, and the incidence is difficult to establish. There are so few documented cases in the literature that it is difficult to make a definite statement. In most series, the average age is about 65, and the disease is more common in men than in women. Therefore, it is unlikely to be found associated with pregnancy.

Coincidence of a myeloproliferative disease in pregnancy is unusual. Pregnancy has no adverse effect on the course of the mother's hematologic disease. However, myeloproliferative disease, especially if uncontrolled, can result in increased fetal prematurity and mortality. Treatment of the pregnant patient should be conservative, and whenever possible, chemotherapy should be avoided until at least after the first trimester.

Gastrointestinal Tract Tumors

A significant number of cases of cancer of the stomach that are associated with pregnancy have been reported. Almost all are of the advanced stage of disease with secondary metastases to the ovaries. Most of these women have delivered healthy children, but have later died from the advanced stage of their disease. A high index of suspicion and early diagnosis is the key to successful management of these patients. Progressive increase in symptoms over and above that seen in pregnancy, especially if accompanied by pain, requires careful investigation. Fortunately, the incidence of cancer of the stomach in the United States has dropped dramatically in the last 15 years.

Liver tumors have been reported as a result of the use of contraceptive pills. The number of such cases of hepatic adenoma reported in the literature is increasing, and there are at least four that have complicated pregnancy. All patients were symptomatic during pregnancy, and two were admitted with rupture of the adenoma. One subsequently died. Increased growth and vascularity of adenoma during pregnancy is highly likely. The potential for the development of lethal complications is considerable. Surgery is the method of choice for management. Pregnancy is contraindicated in the presence of a nonresected liver adenoma or in one that has been partially resected.

Central Nervous System Tumors

The tumors of the central nervous system that are most commonly adversely affected by pregnancy are pituitary adenomas, craniopharyngiomas, and meningiomas. Pituitary tumors may or may not be associated with endocrinopathy.

Malignant brain tumors have a true population incidence of 4.5 cases per 100,000, with a slightly higher frequency in men than in women. The age distribution of patients with brain tumor is biphasic, with the first peak between the ages of 6 and 9 years and accounted for by cerebellar astrocytomas, meduloblastomas, and ependymomas. The second peak appears in patients between 40 and 60 years of age, the principal lesion being malignant gliomas, meningiomas, and adenomas. In the United States, it is projected that about 9 to 10 thousand patients will die from brain tumors in the coming year. Fortunately, malignant brain tumors that are complicated by pregnancy are extremely rare.

Pregnant women with malignant brain tumors are usually misdiagnosed because many of the early symptoms are identical to the complaints encountered in normal pregnancy. Pregnancy is normally associated with an enlarged pituitary gland, mainly as a result of hyperplasia of the acidophilic cells concerned with prolactin secretion, and existent pituitary tumors may also increase rapidly in size in pregnancy. The resulting symptoms include headache and visual disturbances, primarily decreased visual disturbances, primarily decreased visual acuity, and diminished visual fields.

Early diagnosis offers the patient maximum chance of salvage from an otherwise fatal or disabling outcome. A high index of suspicion in patients with headache, visual disturbance, or other cerebral symptoms that do not improve should suggest a work-up. A diagnosis may be established by complete physical and neurologic examination, CT scan, electroencephalography, by testing visual acuity and visual fields, and by angiography, if indicated.

Meningiomas predominate in women and have been reported to enlarge rapidly with pregnancy. They have been found to have estrogen receptors and, therefore, may be associated with hormone sensitivity. Meningiomas that are asymptomatic or do not enlarge probably can be observed until viability of the baby.

The treatment of malignant brain tumor during pregnancy is the same as in the nonpregnant patient. Surgical excision with or without radiation therapy is usually chosen.

Vaginal delivery is preferred, and cesarean section is reserved for obstetric indications or when instantaneous delivery is necessary. The increase in intra-abdominal pressure associated with bearing-down efforts in the second stage of labor markedly elevates cerebral spinal fluid pressure. This should be minimized by the use of outlet forceps. If the fetus has reached viability, delivery should be offered prior to surgical intervention or radiation therapy for the brain tumor.

Pituitary adenomas have recently received considerable attention in the literature. These are often microadenomas. During pregnancy, there is a physiologic enlargement of the pituitary, and an asymptomatic patient with a small pituitary tumor when not pregnant may develop acute neurologic symptoms during pregnancy. Therefore, the question arises of whether to treat the patients with a known prior-to-pregnancy adenoma, or not. Some patients became pregnant, and it is only at that time that the tumor becomes apparent. Since it is not possible to predict which tumors may enlarge and cause symptoms during pregnancy, it is probably safer to treat all patients with pituitary tumors before pregnancy is attempted.

Pheochromocytomas

Pheochromocytomas are extremely rare, but very dangerous during pregnancy, with a 50 percent maternal and fetal mortality. Pheochromocytoma is a catecholamine-secreting tumor, which consists of neuroectoderm- or neurocrest-derived cells that affects 1 in 200,000 members of the general population and is responsible for 0.1 percent of all cases of diastolic hypertension. The presentation of pheochromocytoma in pregnancy is rare, but well described, with approximately 150 cases reported in the literature. The majority of these tumors occur sporadically; approximately 5 percent are familial, and they are usually bilateral. Alpha-blocker control with phenoxybenzamine is required, and surgical removal is attempted only after localizing the tumor. It is preferable to do this in the postpartum period.

If a pheochromocytoma is diagnosed during early pregnancy, phenoxybenzamine should be started and a therapeutic termination carried out; next, attempts should be made to localize the tumor using the radiologic technique that had been associated with its diagnosis, and then the tumor should be removed surgically. Should the diagnosis not be made until the second or third trimester, the pregnancy should be allowed to continue under phenoxybenzamine control and with careful monitoring, until induction or cesarean section is indicated. If progress is satisfactory, localizing investigations can be postponed until after delivery.

Sarcoma

Sarcoma-complicating pregnancy is very rare. The management of the patient who is pregnant with a sarcoma depends on the type of lesion, anatomic location, stage of disease, and age of the gestation. The question is asked whether pregnancy can have an adverse effect on the growth rate of the tumor.

Cantin and McNeer reported on 57 women who were pregnant simultaneously with or subsequent to the treatment of a variety of soft tissue tumors and compared their 5- and 10- year survival rates to both those of premenopausal women without pregnancy and postmenopausal women. The study's conclusion was that the survival rate compared favorably with rates for nonpregnant women of reproductive age.

Pack and Ariel enumerate a list of soft tissue tumors that may be influenced by hormonal factors. One is angiosarcoma. Cystosarcoma phylloides, or more specifically giant intracanalicular myxoma, arise from fibroadenomas, most frequently in women of multiparity and suppressed lactation. Desmoids frequently arise or recur during pregnancy. They should be treated as in the nonpregnant state.

Fetal and Placental Transmission of Malignancy

Metastases to the fetus and/or placenta stir a great deal of interest and considerable controversy. When cancer complicates pregnancy, it is common for the afflicted woman and her family to ask whether the cancer can spread to the baby, and if so, whether it can have a delayed effect on the baby relative to the later development of cancer. Fortunately this is extremely rare. Probably fewer than 40 cases of metastatic disease of the placenta have been reported. The most common primary tumors are melanoma, breast tumors, and members of the leukemia-lymphoma group. The reason why the placenta appears to be resistant to metastasis is unclear, but this may be a property that is peculiar to the placenta. One of the most well-documented and often quoted cases was that of Holland in which a melanoma metastasized to both the placenta and the fetus. This may rarely occur with other tumors, such as adenocarcinoma of the rectum.

Metastasis from the mother to the fetus is indeed rare. There are about two dozen cases reported in the literature. Accepted criteria include maternal and placental invasion, and the occurrence of the same cancer in the baby within 1 year of birth. Beyond 1 year, the concepts of viral transmission, genetic transmission, or altered immunity are considered as factors in the development of the cancer.

Despite the fact that the incidence is rare, routine gross and microscopic examination of the placenta of women who have or have had cancers is desirable, as is careful examination of the infant, particularly if the maternal tumor was melanoma, leukemia, or lymphoma.

RADIOTHERAPY AND ANTINEOPLASTIC THERAPY

Surgery and radiation are effective forms of treatment for localized cancer. Chemotherapy, the treatment of cancer by means of drugs and hormones, can be used for disseminated as well as localized tumors. The treatment of cancer with drugs is a relatively new development that dates from 1945 when nitrogen mustard was found to be effective against lymphomas. Since that time, many drugs have been added to the therapeutic armamentarium.

A major goal of current chemotherapy is to achieve cures by the prompt and vigorous treatment of these malignancies. Combinations of antineoplastic drugs have been used with success, particularly when each drug acts on the cancer cell in a different way. Progress has been made by using the different drugs simultaneously as well as in sequence.

If employed only in the second and third trimester of pregnancy, a single drug chemotherapy gives rise to few problems. Various problems may arise from use of anticancer drugs in the first trimester; however, Nicholson reported that the risk is small if a single drug is used.

There are little data available on the use of newer combinations of drugs or agents during pregnancy. DeVita and co-workers observed ten women who became pregnant after therapy with nitrogen mustard, oncovin, procarbozine, and prednisone (MOPP); all gave birth to normal children. However, the physician must be cautious concerning the side effects of newer agents, especially in combination, and particularly prior to organogenesis.

The delayed consequences of chemotherapy remain controversial, and it may be some time before enough data are accumulated to make a positive statement. In women who have had chemotherapy, the fetus in future pregnancies may be at risk. In 96 later pregnancies in women who had chemotherapy, approximately 16 percent terminated in abortion and 3 percent in stillbirth. Three of the pregnancies resulted in the birth of infants with significant general malformations.

Exposure of the developing embryo to ionizing radiation may cause abortion, malformation, or possibly leukemia in the infant. Animal and atomic bomb studies clearly demonstrate the teratogenic and carcinogenic effects of radiation. Radiation injuries sustained late in fetal life are less harmful than those sustained early, when organogenesis and differentiation are more active and when each cell destroyed would have contributed a relatively greater part to the whole organism. Some abortions are not a direct effect of radiation, but may be indirectly produced by hormonal imbalance brought about by therapeutic radiation of the mother. Fetal structures, particularly the central nervous system, the eye, and the mesenchymal tissues, appear to be more radiosensitive than the same structures in adults. This is probably on account of more rapid growth rate and greater metabolic activity in the fetus. It is strongly suggested that pregnant women be given no radiation exposure during the first 16 weeks of pregnancy.

Cancers in pregnancy are uncommon, but do occur, with an average frequency of 1 in 1,000 births. This gives rise to opposing emotional reactions in these women; they are happy that they are pregnant, but usually devastated when they hear that they have cancer.

A major reason for suspecting that pregancy adversely affects the clinical course of cancer is the immunologic tolerance that characterizes both conditions. As Gleicher and associates pointed out, normal pregnancy and cancer are the only two biologic conditions in which an antigenic tissue is tolerated by a seemingly intact system.

It may be stated that the mechanisms that insure the survival of the fetus during pregnancy presumably also favor the progress of the neoplasia.

The management requires individualization with careful thought as to whether termination is necessary or whether continuing with the pregnancy is possible prior to definitive treatment. The physician's aim is to cure the cancer and deliver a live infant while insuring that both mother and child are healthy and not compromised. This is one occasion when a joint decision is probably best reached by concensus among the obstetrician, the surgical and medical oncologists, and other disciplines.

The life-threatening cancer should be managed both in the case of diagnosis and treatment as in the nonpregnant state. An early, small cancer gives a better prognosis than a more advanced cancer. The same holds for the nonpregnant patient. It has been reported that pregnant patients with the same stage cancer as nonpregnant patients have the same chance for survival. However, all too often in the pregnant state the cancer is more adanced than is found in the nonpregnant patient. The disease must be evaluated and treated in full light of its exact location and stage, in conjunction with an understanding of the natural history, within the context of the pregnancy with a potentially viable, unborn infant.

Concern that maternal cancer may metastasize to the fetus is not justified because in the accumulated series in the literature it is a rare occurrence. Infrequency of fetal involvement has lead to speculation about biologic protective mechanisms that may exist for the placenta and fetus and the role circulatory separation in the placenta or immunologic responses of the fetus may play. The association of cancer in pregnancy represents a major physiologic process for the maintenance of the race and a major pathologic process that accounts for numerous deaths. It presents a controlled growth and an uncontrolled growth in the same host. Whether studies of patients with cancer-complicating pregnancy can shed light on the mechanism and behavior of cancer remains to be seen.

SUGGESTED READING

Barber HRK, Brunschwig A. Gynecologic cancer, complicating pregnancy. Am J Obstet Gynecol 1962; 85:156–164.

Barber HRK. Malignant disease in the pregnant woman. In: Coppleson M, ed. Gynecologic oncology. New York: Churchill Livingstone, 1981:795.

Boronow RC. Extrapelvic malignancy and pregnancy. Obstet Gynecol Surg 1964; 19:1–29.

Nicholson HO. Cytotoxic drugs in pregnancy. Review of reported cases. J Obstet Gynaecol Br Commonw 1968; 75:307–312.

Gleicher N, Siegel I. Common denominators of pregnancy and malignancy. In: Gleicher N, ed. Reproductive immunology. New York: Alan R Liss, 1981:339.

CHORIOCARCINOMA—GESTATIONAL TROPHOBLASTIC NEOPLASIA

WELDON CHAFE, M.D., F.R.C.S.(C), F.A.C.O.G.
LINDA S. MORGAN, M.D., F.A.C.O.G.

Molar pregnancy and choriocarcinoma have been known as disease entities since the time of Hippocrates (400 B.C.), but it is only in this century that we have come to realize that these diseases represent a spectrum of neoplasia developing from the fetal chorion. This spectrum is now referred to as gestational trophoblastic neoplasia (GTN). A variety of terms continue to be used to classify the disease: hydatid mole, hydatidiform pregnancy, partial mole, incomplete mole, invasive mole, chorioepithelioma, chorioadenoma destruens, and choriocarcinoma. The terminology can be confusing to clinicians and pathologists involved in the care of these patients. Gestational trophoblastic disease develops from embryonic structures within the female genital tract and possesses the ability to metastasize widely and cause the death of the host.

Interest in the malignant aspects of the disease over the last 30 years has given rise to the modern era of chemotherapy. Choriocarcinoma was the first solid tumor with a complete cure reported after use of methotrexate chemotherapy by Li, Hertz, and Spence in 1956. Another unique feature of the disease is that it is capable of producing a hormone (human chorionic gonadotrophin, hCG) specific to the developing trophoblast. This hormone serves as a tumor marker and provides the basis for monitoring and making therapeutic decisions in the management of this disease. Regional trophoblastic centers have been established to study this disease. The expertise developed in these centers provides many of the guidelines used in managing patients with trophoblastic neoplasia today.

Nongestational choriocarcinoma usually appears in the younger, premenarchal patient and arises primarily in the ovary, although it may be seen in the mediastinum, sacrococcygeal region, base of the skull, neck, or brain. This disease is nonpregnancy-related and is managed by both surgery, if applicable, and multiple agent chemotherapy as utilized for germ cell ovarian tumors. Monitoring of this disease is done with serum hCG, but other tumor markers such as alpha-fetoprotein and carcinoembryonic antigen may also be elevated. Ovarian choriocarcinomas are usually one component of a mixed germ cell tumor. The hCG assays do not distinguish between gestational and nongestational choriocarcinoma.

This chapter deals with GTN as a spectrum of disease that ranges from hydatidiform mole to metastatic choriocarcinoma. This group of diseases develops from malignant transformation of the trophoblast. The incidence in North America is about one in 1,500 to 2,000 pregnancies, with higher incidences reported in subgroups of the overall population.

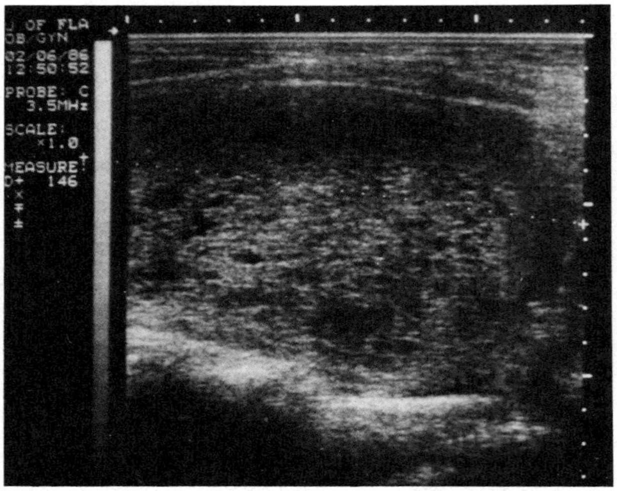

Figure 1 Sonographic snowstorm appearance of an intrauterine molar pregnancy.

HYDATIDIFORM MOLE

The spectrum of disease known as GTN begins with the well-recognized hydatidiform mole. Once the diagnosis of molar pregnancy is made, the patient's management should be directed by centers that have experience and possess the background knowledge of the clinical behavior of this disease so that treatment and follow-up can be instituted immediately. The primary care physician should be able to diagnose, perform the initial evaluation, effect pregnancy termination, and institute appropriate follow-up of an uncomplicated molar pregnancy. Once the necessity for additional treatment has been determined, referral of the patient to a regional center is recommended.

The patient with a molar gestation usually presents with bleeding in the first or early second trimester of pregnancy. On physical examination, one may see expulsion of the pathognomonic vesicles through the cervical os, but usually the clinical appearance is that of a threatened abortion. The diagnosis should be entertained in any woman with abnormal bleeding and a positive pregnancy test. Other factors increasing the suspicion would be absent fetal heart tones, a uterus large for dates (roughly 50 percent of cases), lower abdominal pain, hyperemesis gravidarum, pregnancy-induced hypertension before the second half of pregnancy, and the development of theca lutean ovarian cysts (unilateral or bilateral) in early pregnancy. In the differential diagnosis, one must rule out such problems as multiple pregnancy, threatened abortion, ectopic pregnancy, incorrect gestational dates, uterine anomalies, or pelvic neoplasm.

Ultrasonography should be performed if a molar pregnancy is considered. It is simple, noninvasive, and reliable, and the multiple intrauterine echoes (''snowstorm appearance'') are characteristic of molar pregnancy (Fig. 1). Radiologic techniques of amniography are more universally available, especially in many developing nations. The procedure involves invasive percutaneous needle entry into the pregnant uterus and is not without significant risk. If needle aspiration of the pregnant uterus yields amniotic fluid, no radiopaque dye is injected, and a normal pregnancy is felt to exist. A follow-up sonogram at this time would be worthwhile, since a molar pregnancy with a coexisting normal pregnancy may be present. If no amniotic fluid is aspirated, a radiopaque dye is injected, and x-ray films of the abdomen and pelvis are taken. The characteristic radiologic honeycomb pattern is seen as the dye disperses around the hydatid vesicles. Expulsion of vesicles is seen on physical examination of the cervical os in about 50 percent of patients presenting with hydatid pregnancy and makes diagnosis relatively easy. Most molar pregnancies are detected in early pregnancy by diagnostic ultrasonography.

THERAPY

Once the diagnosis of GTN has been made, the patient should be admitted to the hospital for preoperative evaluation and stabilization. Baseline parameters of hematocrit, chest x-ray films, quantitative beta-hCG, and coagulation studies as well as renal and liver profiles should be obtained. Attention should be given to pain relief, blood transfusions (if indicated), and fluid and electrolyte management. One must identify associated problems such as hyperthyroidism, toxemia, or coagulation disorders that can complicate the initial presentation and mandate more aggressive medical management.

Pregnancy termination is carried out in an operating room after cervical dilation. A large-bore suction curette is the instrument of choice. Oxytocin is administered via an intravenous drip through at least an 18-gauge catheter upon completion of the cervical dilation and on initiation of the suction evacuation. This is done to facilitate uterine contraction and decrease operative blood loss. Once suction evacuation is complete, gentle sharp curettage of the endometrial cavity is carried out and any tissue obtained is submitted separately for pathologic examination.

Hysterectomy as a primary method of treatment may be used to terminate a molar pregnancy in patients who desire sterilization and are good surgical candidates. Follow-up as outlined below should be carried out, because malignant sequelae can occur in these patients. When hysterectomy is used as the primary treatment, there is only a 3 percent chance that the patient will need subsequent treatment; this is well below the 15 to 20 percent malignant sequelae expected after other methods of termination. If chemotherapy is necessary in a patient treated by hysterectomy, fewer courses are needed to induce disease remission, as indicated by negative beta-hCG titers.

Techniques of induction using oxytocin and prostaglandin, the use of hypertonic solutions (urea, glucose, saline), and hysterotomy are not recommended as alternative methods of termination. They are dangerous and expose the patient not only to treatment complications but also to a higher risk of malignant sequelae from the molar pregnancy. The routine use of recurettage at planned intervals after suction evacuation is not recommended. The therapeutic efficacy of the suction evacuation is well attested to by the usual small amount of tissue obtained on the gentle curettage after such suction techniques. Continued bleeding usually signifies the presence of an invasive mole that requires treatment by chemotherapy or, in some situations, hysterectomy. This usually is confirmed by serial beta-hCG titers.

Potential complications of evacuation include those of hemorrhage, perforation, sepsis, and trophoblastic embolization with acute pulmonary insufficiency. These become more common as the duration and size of the gestation increase. Pulmonary insufficiency has been reported to occur in about 10 percent of molar gestations and up to 25 percent of those patients with a uterus greater than 16–weeks gestational size. Approximately 1 percent of women with molar pregnancies die from pulmonary complications during or shortly after evaluation of a molar gestation. This syndrome has generally been ascribed to massive intravascular deportation of trophoblastic tissue through the pulmonary vasculature. Most current investigations indicate that the most frequent cause of pulmonary compromise is pulmonary edema due to cardiac dysfunction and overvigorous fluid and blood administration. These women, although anemic by laboratory parameters, often have blood volume expansion that is 25 to 50 percent above nonpregnant levels and are not necessarily volume-depleted. If an associated preeclampsia is present, vigorous fluid therapy would be less well tolerated because of the inverse relationship that exists between the left ventricular stroke work index and systemic vascular resistance.

The symptoms of acute pulmonary insufficiency can occur at the time of evacuation and up to 12 hours after evacuation. The risk of these patients requiring cytotoxic chemotherapy is increased, but the frequency of true pulmonary metastasis is no greater than that of other patients with molar pregnancies.

Once uterine evacuation has been completed, perioperative observation is essential along with the concomitant administration of intravenous oxytocic agents to ensure continued uterine contraction and prevent postevacuation hemorrhage. In the absence of bleeding and pulmonary complications, the patient can be discharged within 24 hours. Specific instructions at the time of discharge would include information on activities, in particular contraception, and details of follow-up surveillance.

CONTRACEPTION AND FOLLOW-UP

Current recommendations for contraception in patients following evacuation of a molar pregnancy include the use of oral contraceptive pills. Avoidance of pregnancy in the follow-up period is essential, since a rising hCG titer from a new pregnancy cannot be differentiated from malignant sequelae of the antecedent molar pregnancy. At present a tendency exists to utilize barrier methods of contraception in Europe and hormonal contraception in North America. There are suggestions in the literature that hormonal contraception delays the return of hCG titers to nondetectable levels and leads to an increase in the incidence of trophoblastic sequelae. This question is currently being investigated in a prospective randomized fashion by the Gynecology Oncology Group, and it is hoped that a definitive answer will be available soon. Currently, one must individualize according to the wishes of the patient after appropriate counseling has been given.

The estrogen present in oral contraceptive pills (minimum of 50–μg dose) is essential to achieve posterior pituitary gonadotropin suppression, in particular, suppression of luteinizing hormone (LH) secretion, which can give false-positive titer results with hCG. Both hCG and LH are glycoproteins consisting of two dissimilar noncovalently linked polypeptide subunits. These subunits have been designated alpha and beta and are without biologic activity as individual free subunits. The alpha subunits of these hormones are identical in that they contain amino acid residues in identical sequences. The beta subunit, which confers both immunologic and biologic specificities, has similar amino acid contents and sequences. The beta subunit of hCG differs from LH by containing an additional 30 amino acid residue that is distinctive. This carboxy terminal sequence confers distinctive immunologic properties on the hCG in the radioimmunoassay that is used to measure the beta subunit. This identifies it as being separate and distinct from the LH beta subunit. The similarity in their structures accounts for the well-known cross-reaction between hCG and LH in both biologic and nonspecific radioimmunoassays. The beta-hCG specific radioimmunoassay is currently utilized in the follow-up management of patients with molar pregnancies. It is also a sensitive indicator of therapy response in patients needing adjunctive therapy.

The development of regional trophoblastic disease centers has given rise to reference laboratories with expertise in measuring the beta subunit of hCG. It is essential that appropriate serum monitoring of beta hCG be started after termination of a molar pregnancy to detect the presence of persistent disease or malignant sequelae. The quantitation of such results, in our experience, is best obtained from those reference laboratories that employ systems of checks and cross-checks with the standardization of the specific beta-hCG radioimmunoassay.

The biologic and immunologic assays of urine and serum for hCG are neither sensitive nor specific enough to provide optimal patient management. One must employ the use of beta-specific radioimmunoassay of hCG to appropriately follow these patients. This serum assay should be obtained prior to and after uterine evacuation. Levels should then be determined on a weekly basis until three negative titers have been recorded. Then titers should be done on a monthly basis for 1 year, with contraception being continued during this time. Titers normally would be expected to return to nondetectable levels by 12 weeks, indicating spontaneous remission of the disease. This occurs in about 80 percent of patients with molar pregnancies. After 1 year of negative follow-up, contraception may be discontinued in those desiring further pregnancies. Early ultrasonographic evaluation of uterine contents in subsequent pregnancies is recommended, since molar pregnancy recurs in about 1 percent of future pregnancies. Upon successful completion of a pregnancy, serum beta-hCG levels should be obtained during the 4- to 8-week postpartum visit to ensure that GTN is not present.

As part of the follow-up for molar pregnancy (Table 1), physical examination, including a pelvic examination, should be carried out every other week until remission and then at 3-month intervals for 1 year. The vagina is a common area for the occurrence of metastatic lesions. If vaginal lesions are detected, they should not be biopsied, since vaginal metastases communicate with a dilated arteriovenous vascular network created in the pelvis by invasive trophoblastic lesions, and biopsy can lead to exsanguinating hemorrhage.

Theca lutean cysts may be detected on pelvic examination in up to one-third of these patients with molar pregnancy and should be managed expectantly, with involution occurring spontaneously. Complications similar to those of ovarian hyperstimulation, with abdominal distention and ascites, may necessitate hospital admission and aggressive fluid and electrolyte management in the follow-up period. The occurrence of rupture, hemorrhage, or infection usually necessitates surgery.

A chest x-ray film is obtained on initial presentation and repeated if the follow-up titer plateaus or starts to rise. If metastatic disease is detected during the follow-up period, histologic diagnosis is not necessary, since biopsy of these lesions may result in severe bleeding. The level of hCG provides a reliable indicator of tumor burden.

In the event that abnormal hCG regression postmolar pregnancy is detected in the follow-up course (i.e., rising or plateauing of titers) investigations to rule out metastatic disease should be done and the patient started on chemotherapy. One problem area identified has been that of persistent bleeding following evacuation of a molar pregnancy. This has been thought to represent incomplete evacuation of trophoblastic tissue. If suction evacuation and curettage have been thoroughly done as the initial treatment, continued bleeding usually represents persistent disease in the myometrium. This has previously been referred to as invasive mole or chorioadenoma destruens and, although it was originally used to define a distinct entity, it is now felt to be part of the spectrum of GTN. Management in this situation includes investigations to rule out metastatic disease and treatment with chemotherapy.

Questions frequently arise when a diagnosis of hydropic changes is seen on histologic study of aborted products of conception, especially missed abortions. Currently we review the pathology with a gynecologic pathologist and have the patient return for a qualitative hCG test at 4 weeks. If results are positive, quantitative assays are obtained to rule out the development of malignant GTN.

TABLE 1 Molar Pregnancy Management

Early suction evacuation
hCG (beta) determination weekly until negative × three
Then monthly × 1 year
Contraception × 1 year
Chest x-ray on initial presentation
Repeat if hCG regression is abnormal
Physical examination every 2–3 weeks until remission
Chemotherapy if
hCG regression abnormal (plateau or rising)
Metastases
Persistent postevacuation bleeding

MALIGNANT GESTATIONAL TROPHOBLASTIC NEOPLASIA

Hammond and his colleagues at the Southeastern Regional Center for Trophoblastic Disease at Duke University have proposed a categorization of malignant GTN based on risk factors in patients with persistent disease and those with metastases at initial presentation or following molar pregnancy. Their categorization eliminates many of the cumbersome terms used to describe this spectrum of disease. This classification refers to nonmetastatic and metastatic GTN. Metastatic disease is further categorized into good and poor outcome groups based on known prognostic factors (Table 2).

Malignant trophoblastic neoplasia develops in 15 to 20 percent of patients who present with molar pregnancy. Risk factors associated with the development of malignant trophoblastic neoplasia include observations such as uterus large for dates at initial presentation, ovarian enlargement, excessive bleeding after evacuation, acute pulmonary complications, and a prior history of molar pregnancy. The

TABLE 2 Duke Classification of Malignant Gestational Trophoblastic Neoplasia

Nonmetastatic disease: No identifiable disease outside the uterus
Metastatic disease: Any disease outside the uterus
Good prognosis metastatic disease
Poor prognosis metastatic disease

disease in the vast majority of women with malignant GTN is confined to the uterus, but it is essential that all these women undergo a series of investigations for metastases. These tests (Table 3) separate those patients with nonmetastatic disease from those with metastases. If metastases are found, a low- or high-risk group can be assigned and appropriate cytotoxic chemotherapy and occasionally radiation therapy instituted.

The radiologic and laboratory investigations not only detect the presence of metastases but also allow one to estimate tumor burden. At the University of Florida School of Medicine, neoplastic sequelae to molar pregnancy are investigated with chest x-ray films, pelvic ultrasonography, and computerized tomography of the brain and liver. Hematologic investigations, coagulation studies, and both renal and liver functions are assessed during the investigation and prior to treatment. Other optional studies may be needed, depending on the patient's symptoms or previous clinical course. Anti-hCG antibodies tagged with radionucleotides are being utilized in a few centers to help detect metastases in patients with resistant disease in the hope that surgical excision may eradicate the occult persistent focus.

Patients found not to have metastases by the above investigations are presumed to have nonmetastatic GTN (diagnosis by exclusion) and should be treated with single-agent chemotherapy. The indications for therapy in this group may include patients with abnormal beta-hCG regression curves (i.e., rising or plateauing of titers) and patients with abnormal bleeding not explained by the onset of regular menses. Once persistent trophoblastic neoplasia or metastatic GTN has been diagnosed, it is extremely important that these patients be entrusted to the care of a gynecologic oncologist or other individuals with clinical expertise and knowledge of the disease process that allow them to direct the therapy.

TABLE 3 Investigations in Patients with Malignant Gestational Trophoblastic Neoplasia

Full history and physical examination
Blood tests
Serum beta-hCG titer
CBC, WBC, differential count, platelets
Coagulation profile
Renal and liver profiles
Thyroid studies
Blood type, Rh
Radiologic Studies
Chest x-ray film
Brain scan (nuclear, CT, or MRI)
Liver scan (nuclear, CT, or MRI)
Pelvic ultrasound study
Other studies (optional)
Lumbar puncture for beta-hCG in cerebrospinal fluid
Whole lung tomography, CT, or MRI scan
Intravenous pyelogram
Selective arteriograms
Radionucleotide anti-hCG scan
Surgical excision

NONMETASTATIC GESTATIONAL TROPHOBLASTIC NEOPLASIA (PERSISTENT MOLE, CHORIOADENOMA DESTRUENS, INVASIVE MOLE, CHORIOCARCINOMA)

Patients with nonmetastatic disease as identified by the above criteria need to be treated with chemotherapy. Single-agent drug therapy is effective in producing disease remission in nearly 100 percent of these patients. Multiagent therapy or surgery or both are reserved for patients in this group who fail to respond to single-agent treatment. Regimens (Table 4) currently in use employ drugs such as methotrexate, actinomycin D (dactinomycin), and VP16-213 (etoposide) as single agents. Methotrexate has been the drug most widely used in treating this disease. Methotrexate, 0.4 mg per kilogram (up to 25 mg maximum) given intravenously, intramuscularly, or by mouth on days 1 to 5 has been utilized since the late 1950s. Goldstein's group in Boston has added folinic acid rescue to decrease the toxicity from methotrexate alone. Their regimen uses methotrexate, 1 mg per kilogram intramuscularly or intravenously on days 1, 3, 5, and 7, with folinic acid rescue (0.1 mg per kilogram intramuscularly or intravenously) on days 2, 4, 6, and 8. Patients receiving methotrexate are encouraged to have liberal fluid intake in order to maintain a good urine output. Urine pH should be greater than 6.5. Bicarbonate administration may be necessary because methotrexate metabolites may precipitate in the renal tubules, producing renal damage in the patient with a low urine output and acidic urine. Avoidance of aspirin products and acetaminophen is encouraged in order to prevent cross-potentiation of renal and hepatic toxicities sometimes seen in patients on methotrexate.

Actinomycin D has been given in a 5-day regimen (10 to 12 μg per kilogram intravenously on days 1 through 5), and in more recent reports "pulse" actinomycin D (1.25 mg per kilogram, intravenous push) every 2 weeks has proven effective and convenient in treating nonmetastatic GTN.

TABLE 4 Single-Agent Chemotherapy

Methotrexate 0.4 mg/kg IM or IV (25 mg maximum dose) days 1–5 (Repeat every 7 days if possible)
Methotrexate, 1 mg/kg IM or IV on days 1, 3, 5, 7 Folinic acid, 0.1 mg/kg IM or IV on days 2, 4, 6, 8 (Repeat every 7 days if possible)
Actinomycin D, 10–12 μg/kg IV days 1–5 (Repeat every 7 days if possible)
Actinomycin D, 1.25 mg/kg IV day 1 ("pulse") (Repeat every 2 weeks)
a. VP16-213: 200 mg/m^2 PO days 1–5 (Repeat every 7 days if possible) b. VP16-213: 100 mg/m^2 IV days 1–5 (Repeat every 7 days if possible)

Treatment cycles utilizing methotrexate and actinomycin D are repeated at 7- to 11-day intervals until at least one course of therapy has been administered after achieving a negative beta-hCG titer. The interval allows for recovery of normal tissue (e.g., bone marrow, gastrointestinal tract, renal parenchyma) from the toxicity of treatment and optimizes the therapeutic effect on the increased mitotic index seen in the neoplastic trophoblast. Giving one additional course of chemotherapy after obtaining a negative titer has been shown to decrease the relapse rate to below 5 percent. Patients who relapse should be treated with the single agent not previously used to induce remission.

Both actinomycin and methotrexate have a high therapeutic efficacy, but use of actinomycin D is attended by less systemic toxicity. In the presence of abnormal liver and renal function, actinomycin D is the drug of choice because its toxicity is predominantly gastrointestinal and hematologic. Some authors have reported excellent results and lower toxicity by alternating courses of methotrexate and actinomycin. If a resistant focus of disease develops during therapy with one agent, a switch to the other usually results in prompt response.

VP16-213 use has been reported in the recent literature as both a single agent to treat nonmetastatic gestational trophoblastic neoplasia and in combination protocols for metastatic disease. Therapeutic efficacy (comparable to methotrexate and actinomycin D) as a single agent has been demonstrated with both oral and intravenous administration of the drug; however, the major complication of total alopecia is disturbing to some patients. Other side effects seen are nausea, vomiting, mild bone marrow suppression, and posttreatment amenorrhea. A recent 1987 Gynecology Oncology Group report by Homesley on the weekly scheduling of methotrexate (40 mg per square meter of body surface) has, as well, shown therapeutic efficacy with minimal toxicity. Newer protocols are being investigated in the management of nonmetastatic gestational trophoblastic disease. The goal is to decrease toxicity and improve cost-effectiveness, with preservation of the excellent clinical results (nearly 100 percent) already obtained with current regimens of treatment.

After treatment, follow-up is important. Once three negative beta-hCG titers have been obtained, weekly surveillance can be changed to monthly titers for a year. Then, if the patient desires pregnancy, contraception may be discontinued. Postpartum follow-up hCG titers are necessary as well as semiannual titers for 5 years because late recurrences are seen occasionally.

METASTATIC GESTATIONAL TROPHOBLASTIC NEOPLASIA (CHORIOCARCINOMA)

Once trophoblastic neoplasia has metastasized beyond the uterus, a diagnosis of choriocarcinoma is made. The presence of metastatic disease denotes a poorer prognostic situation in oncology patients in general. In patients with metastatic trophoblastic disease, the National Cancer Institute (NCI) has devised two well-defined prognostic groups based on the location of the metastasis, tumor burden, length of time from the antecedent pregnancy, and treatment with prior chemotherapy (Table 5).

Other patients with high-risk disease who do not meet the NCI prognostic criteria include those with a history of an antecedent term pregnancy, a histologic diagnosis of choriocarcinoma, or a placental site trophoblastic tumor.

The placental site trophoblastic tumor has been reported to have a variable clinical behavior, with metastasis usually portending a fatal outcome. Metastatic disease appears to be resistant to chemotherapy. Most reported patients, however, are clinically well after treatment with either curettage or hysterectomy.

Bagshawe in Great Britain has developed a system that assigns patients to low-, medium-, or high-risk groups by scoring prognostic factors of age, parity, antecedent pregnancy, interval, hCG titer, ABO blood group, metastases (number, site, and size), lymphocytic infiltration, immune status, and prior chemotherapy. The risk level in Bagshawe's system is derived from a relative assessment of each factor and not from any absolute value of any one factor. The lower the assessed score, the better the prognosis.

A modification of Bagshawe's scoring system was accepted by the World Health Organization in 1983 with low-, medium-, and high-risk categories being identified to enable universal reporting of treatment results. Many investigators have found the scoring systems of risk categorization to be cumbersome. In North America, the combination of hCG titer, investigative documentation of

TABLE 5 Metastatic Trophoblastic Neoplasia: National Cancer Institute Prognostic Criteria

	Good Prognosis	*Poor Prognosis*
β-hCG (serum)	< 40,000 mIU/ml	> 40,000 mIU/ml
hCG (urine)	< 100,000 IU/24 hr	> 100,000 IU/24 hr
Antecedent pregnancy	< 4 months	> 4 months
Prior chemotherapy	No	Yes
Metastases	Lung, vagina	Brain and/or liver

metastases, duration of time from antecedent pregnancy, and prior use of chemotherapy, as advocated by Goldstein and Hammond, has proven the most workable and useful in assigning prognostic groups and determining initial therapy.

DOCUMENTATION OF METASTASIS

Treatment in the patient with metastatic GTN depends on the location of metastatic disease. Once the baseline studies (see Table 3) have been obtained, an accurate delineation of the location of disease helps in the assignment of prognostic group and treatment protocol.

The lung is the most common site of metastases, and these lesions are usually detected on chest x-ray films. If metastatic disease is detected on the chest film at any time during the follow-up period, chemotherapy is indicated. Following lesions by serial x-ray study does not necessarily give an idea of disease response, since chest x-ray films have reportedly been positive for up to 2 years as a result of nonmalignant scarring around the focal tumor sites. Monitoring of disease response is done with quantitative beta-hCG titers, and if the lung is the only identified site of metastatic disease, single-agent therapy is usually adequate. The computerized tomographic scanner is more accurate than chest x-ray examination and will detect micrometastases when chest films have been reported as normal.

The female genital tract has proven to be the second most frequent area of metastasis, and lesions have been described in the vagina, on the vulva, and in the ovary. Multiagent chemotherapy is usually necessary to effect cure in patients with these lesions.

Brain metastases are uncommon but portend a poor prognosis. Choriocarcinoma is the most common gynecologic tumor to metastasize to the brain. Spread occurs hematogenously and may be occult or result in hemorrhage or thrombosis with infarction or form neoplastic aneurysms. Patients with cerebral metastases initially present with symptoms of headache, nausea, weakness, loss of consciousness, seizures, or parasthesias, suggesting a space-occupying lesion. Bagshawe's group reported that 4 percent of their patients with cerebral disease were asymptomatic.

Diagnosis of brain metastasis is most accurate by computed tomographic scan; radionucleotide scanning has only a 70 to 80 percent accuracy rate. Isolated brain metastases rarely occur. Steroids are often necessary to help decrease cerebral edema, and a combination of whole brain radiation and multiagent chemotherapy offers the best opportunity for cure. The radiation dose of 3,000 cGy (rads) has been arrived at empirically, and there is no evidence to indicate that radiation without chemotherapy would be tumoricidal in patients with central nervous system metastases. Intrathecal chemotherapy has been advocated in those patients without evidence of raised intracranial pressure because of the impermeability of the blood-brain barrier to cytotoxic chemotherapeutic agents.

Patients with documented central nervous system metastases should be managed in regional trophoblastic disease centers where the experience in managing these patients is concentrated. A salvage rate of 50 to 65 percent has been reported from centers utilizing a combination of aggressive cytotoxic chemotherapy and radiation.

Hepatic metastases are seen in about 30 percent of poor prognosis patients, and survival rates of 10 to 30 percent have been reported. Disease is usually detected when the patient presents with right upper quadrant pain secondary to subcapsular hemorrhage. Asymptomatic liver disease may be detected in the patient with evidence of other metastases by computed tomographic scan (most reliable) or by nuclear liver scan.

Therapy of liver metastases is with multiagent chemotherapy. Radiation (2,000 cGy in 10 fractions) is usually given for hemostasis in patients with subcapsular bleeding and is not tumoricidal at this dose. Hepatic toxicity can be severe from combination therapy and excessive radiation. Other hemostatic measures may include laparotomy and liver resection as a salvage procedure. Invasive embolization of hepatic artery branches may control hemorrhage enough to allow the cytotoxic chemotherapy to exert its effect.

Other sites of metastases include the gastrointestinal tract, usually manifested by gastrointestinal bleeding, and the kidneys or urinary tract, which may be indicated by urinary bleeding or obstruction. Rare sites reported include the spleen, bone, and skin, and all are indicative of the hematogenous route of spread of this disease. These lesions usually respond to chemotherapy, but other therapeutic modalities of surgery or radiation may be necessary to control hemorrhagic presentations of the metastatic disease.

THERAPY OF METASTATIC GESTATIONAL TROPHOBLASTIC NEOPLASIA

Good Prognosis

Patients with good prognosis metastatic trophoblastic disease can be treated with single-agent chemotherapy as outlined above (see Table 4) for nonmetastatic GTN. Patients who present with an antecedent term pregnancy, a histologic diagnosis of choriocarcinoma, or any of the factors indicative of poor prognosis disease (see Table 5) need multiagent chemotherapy. Most (80 percent) of the patients with metastatic GTN fall into the good prognosis category, and cure can be expected in 100 percent of these patients with single-agent chemotherapy. Methotrexate is still considered the drug of choice, with 20 to 25 mg given intramuscularly daily for 5 days and repeated after a 7- to 9-day window, if toxicity allows, until at least one course of treatment has been given past a negative hCG titer. Close monitoring of titers is essential to detect development of drug-resistant disease, as evidenced by plateauing or rising titers. This would mandate switching agents, usually to actinomycin D, and if resistance continues to be evident, combination multiagent therapy should be started.

Once the patient has received one course of therapy past a negative titer, observation of titers is done weekly until three negative titers have been obtained. Then monthly titers are drawn for 1 year, with effective contraception being employed.

Poor Prognosis

Multiagent chemotherapy protocols have been utilized for poor prognosis disease since the late 1970s. MAC (methotrexate, actinomycin D, and chlorambucil or cyclophosphamide) has been the therapy of choice for these patients (Table 6). The regimen is given over 5 days and repeated at 9- to 14-day intervals, as toxicity allows. These intervals are essential because tumor regrowth becomes significant if there are long treatment gaps, and improved cell kill is achieved by frequent exposure of the trophoblastic tumor to cytotoxic agents. Treatment is carried out until three courses of therapy have been delivered past the first negative hCG titer. Follow-up after treatment is imperative. Beta-hCG titers are done weekly until completion of the three courses of chemotherapy past the first negative hCG titer and then monthly for a year, with every other month titers being obtained for at least another year.

TABLE 6 MAC Protocol

Methotrexate	10–15 mg IM daily × 5
Actinomycin D	350–500 μg IV daily × 5
Chlorambucil	8–10 mg P.O. daily × 5
or	
Cyclophosphamide	200–250 mg IV daily × 5
Repeat therapy after 9–14 days as toxicity allows	

Bagshawe's group has treated their high-risk (poor prognosis) group of patients with a seven-agent protocol called CHAMOCA. This has been modified by many individuals because of the severe toxicity seen in the original protocol. The Duke modification is given below (Table 7). In their early experience, they reported less toxicity with this regimen than with the MAC protocol. Taking into account the rapid doubling time of trophoblastic tumors, the regimen is repeated every 9 to 11 days, as toxicity allows. In a recent presentation to the Society of Gynecologic Oncologists by the Gynecology Oncology Group, a prospective randomized comparison of MAC versus the modified Bagshawe regimen in poor prognosis metastatic gestational trophoblastic disease demonstrated the standard MAC regimen to be significantly more effective and less toxic that the modified Bagshawe regimen.

Many patients with poor prognosis disease have been treated previously with chemotherapy and have disease that is resistant to chemotherapy, usually also having accumulated significant toxicity (both general systemic and marrow reserves); this is a poor prognosis situation made poorer by previous therapy. It is imperative that people in centers with trophoblastic disease experience care for these patients. Specialized care, such as life-support measures and total parenteral nutrition, is often required to sustain these patients. Hospitalization is usually long, and life-threatening sepsis is seen in over 50 percent of these patients during subsequent treatment. Lurain, from the John I. Brewer Trophoblastic Disease Center in Chicago and Surwitt and Hammond, at Duke University, reported significantly improved survival (82 to 94 percent) in patients with poor prognosis disease referred for ther-

TABLE 7 Modified Bagshawe Chemotherapy

Day	*Hour*	*Treatment*
1	0600	Hydroxyurea 500 mg p.o.
	1200	Hydroxyurea 500 mg p.o
	1800	Hydroxyurea 500 mg p.o.
	1900	Actinomycin D 200 μg IV
	2400	Hydroxyurea 500 mg p.o.
2	0700	Vincristine 1 mg/m² IV
	1900	Methotrexate 100 mg/m² IV
		Methotrexate 200 mg/m² infused over 12 hr
		Actinomycin D 200 μg IV
3	1900	Actinomycin D 200 μg IV
		Cyclophosphamide 500 mg/m² IV
		Folinic acid 14 mg IM
4	0100	Folinic acid 14 mg IM
	0700	Folinic acid 14 mg IM
	1300	Folinic acid 14 mg IM
	1900	Folinic acid 14 mg IM
		Actinomycin D 500 μg IV
5	0100	Folinic acid 14 mg IM
	1900	Actinomycin D 500 μg IV
6	No treatment	
7	No treatment	
8	1900	Cyclophosphamide 500 mg/m² IV
		Doxyrubicin 30 mg/m² IV

From DiSaia PJ, Creasman WT, eds. Clinical gynecologic oncology. St. Louis: CV Mosby, 1984:209.

apy at initial diagnosis compared with those referred after prior chemotherapy failure (50 to 59 percent), since drug resistance frequently developed. This, again, illustrates that the disease should be managed in regional centers by people with experience in treating trophoblastic neoplasia. Although the prognosis for patients with poor prognostic metastatic GTN is not as good as for patients with nonmetastatic and good prognosis metastatic GTN, there has been a marked improvement in recent years, with a noticeable decrease in the number of deaths both from disease and toxicity of treatment.

Disease that is resistant to MAC and modified Bagshawe regimens has been treated with a variety of protocols of cytotoxic agents. Two newer drugs, cis-platinum and VP16-213, have been utilized in combination protocols as salvage therapy with encouraging results. Two newer drug regimens, EMA-CO (VP16-213, actinomycin D, methotrexate with folinic acid rescue, vincristine, and cyclophosphamide) and modified Einhorn (vinblastine, bleomycin, and cis-platinum) have shown encouraging results with both initial treatment and recurrent disease. Clinical studies continue in the development of less toxic treatment of poor prognosis disease as well as in the development of salvage regimens in patients who have failed initial therapy.

Recurrence

Recurrence does occur for all categories of GTN, so even after successful treatment, it is important to follow these patients and continue monitoring their beta-hCG titers. Nonmetastatic GTN and good prognosis GTN have 100 percent reported cure rates. A 2 percent recurrence rate of nonmetastatic GTN has been reported and a 5 to 6 percent recurrence figure for the good prognosis metastatic group. These recurrences are curable with the use of a different single agent or utilization of combination drug regimens, but detection must be immediate to optimize success.

Poor prognosis metastatic GTN has a recurrence rate of 21 percent, with only 60 percent of these patients responding to subsequent therapy. These figures, from Duke University, have shown improvement in recent years with the earlier referral of patients to the Southeastern Regional Center for Trophoblastic Disease.

The idea of treating after negative titers are obtained was advocated by Brewer from the Center at Northwestern University. Theoretically, small foci of persistent disease can exist in tumor sanctuaries at negative hCG titers (less than 5 mIU per milliliter), and this can give rise to recurrent disease. Current recommendations are to give at least one additional course of chemotherapy after achieving a negative titer in nonmetastatic and good prognosis metastatic disease and at least three courses of therapy for poor prognosis metastatic disease. Some centers recommend continuing single-agent methotrexate or actinomycin D at monthly intervals for 6 months in this highest-risk group.

All these patients need to be monitored closely, with patient examination carried out frequently and beta-hCG titers obtained on a monthly basis for 1 year in those with "lower" risk disease and for at least 2 years in those with poor prognosis disease. Following the 2-year anniversary of successful treatment, titers should be obtained at 6-month intervals in patients with poor prognosis disease. Titers should be obtained 6 weeks after any succeeding pregnancy regardless of its outcome.

Subsequent Pregnancies

If the beta-hCG titer promptly returns to normal after a molar pregnancy and remains there for 6 months, the risk of malignant GTN is about one in 500. The risk of another molar pregnancy in subsequent pregnancies is about one in 60. If the patient had two previous molar pregnancies, the risk of a third is about one in six. In patients with recurrent molar pregnancies, there is a higher risk of developing malignant trophoblastic sequelae.

Once contraception has been discontinued and pregnancy confirmed, early ultrasound examination should be performed to diagnose a normal intrauterine pregnancy. Follow-up after delivery requires histologic evaluation of the placenta and a beta-hCG titer 6 weeks post partum. In patients who have received chemotherapy for malignant GTN, there has been no increase in the incidence of congenital malformations reported, and chances for a successful pregnancy are high. There has been a higher than expected incidence of placenta accreta in subsequent pregnancies.

The period of contraception required varies from 6 to 12 months after uncomplicated molar pregnancy and up to 2 years for those with poor prognosis metastatic GTN. Most investigators are currently recommending 12 months of contraception after chemotherapeutic treatment of nonmetastatic and good prognosis patients because animal studies have shown that it takes up to 8 to 10 months for complete excretion of methotrexate and its metabolites. This 1-year time period may allow damaged oocytes to be eliminated and permit further excretion of potentially teratogenic metabolites of cytotoxic agents. Caution, however, is needed for the use of newer chemotherapeutic agents, since the long-term follow-up of patients treated with these drugs is not complete. These agents may be gonadotoxic as well as teratogenic and should be used with caution as first-line therapy.

SUGGESTED READING

Bagshawe FD. Choriocarcinoma: the clinical biology of the trophoblast and its tumor. Baltimore: Williams & Wilkins, 1969.

DiSaia PJ, Creasman WT. Gestational trophoblastic neoplasia. In: DiSaia PJ, Creasman WT, eds. Clinical gynecologic oncology. St. Louis: CV Mosby, 1984:192.

Gestational trophoblastic neoplasia. In: DiSaia PJ, Creasman WT, eds. Clinical gynecologic oncology. St Louis: CV Mosby, 1984.

Goldstein DP, Berkowitz RS. Gestational trophoblastic neoplasms: clinical principles of diagnosis and management. Philadelphia: WB Saunders, 1982.

Osborne RF, Fraser RC. Gestational trophoblastic neoplasia. In: Allen HH, Nisker JA. Cancer in pregnancy: therapeutic guidelines. Mount Kisco, NY: Futura, 1986.

CURRENT MEDICOLEGAL ISSUES

MAX BORTEN, M.D., J.D.

Medicolegal issues that affect the practice of obstetrics are complex and often controversial. Unfortunately, they only surface and attract national attention when we find ourselves in the midst of a so-called medical malpractice crisis. Repeatedly, this generates evaluations, debates, and calls for action, yet identification of the cause appears as elusive as the solution. Meanwhile, we witness a continuous rise in the frequency of claims as well as the size of awards and settlements.

No consensus has emerged concerning the medical malpractice problem. Debate has avoided factual issues and has been based on rhetoric, speculation, and long-cherished misconceptions. Physicians and lawyers have yet to establish a constructive dialogue. Mistrust and accusations undermine most prospective solutions. Trial lawyers believe medical carelessness is the leading cause of malpractice claims, whereas physicians believe that a larger pool of available lawyers is the source of the increment of patients seeking legal redress. Meanwhile, insurance companies, which are in the business of forecasting the uncertain, believe the uncertitude of predicting future claims is sufficiently great that they need protection and, as a result, they are forced to charge higher premiums. The net result is a paradoxical standstill accompanied by a continuous increase in the cost of practicing medicine.

Although all groups expect some miraculous change, physicians must continue to care for patients. As a consequence, physicians are certain to be held responsible for their actions. Whereas the subjects that follow do not pretend to be a treatise on medical malpractice, they delve into areas that affect the daily practice of obstetrics. As such, they deserve to be the subject of debates and discussions that may eventually evolve into a better understanding among the professions.

INFORMED CONSENT

Some physicians believe the whole idea of informed consent to be a fictional concept created by and for the members of the legal system. In support of their contentions, they charge that patients do not understand, cannot understand, and do not want to understand everything done to them. These physicians further point out that the law of informed consent is an attempt to redefine the doctor-patient relationship in a detrimental way. The fallaciousness of such arguments is obvious. The doctrine of informed consent is not meant to transform the physician-patient relationship but rather to fortify interactions between them. The essence of the art of medicine still lies in a strong physician-patient rapport with mutual respect and understanding. Most practicing physicians understand that a well-informed patient is a better patient than one who is misinformed or not informed at all.

Obtaining informed consent ought to be viewed not merely as the signing of a document to protect a physician from legal liability. In law, a fiduciary relationship is said to exist between the physician and the patient. This implies a mutual sense of trust and confidence, with each party owing the other a positive obligation to disclose all relevant facts. To that effect, informed consent represents a dynamic process of information exchange and decision making based on mutual respect and participation of patients and health professionals.

Ordinarily, a surgical procedure cannot be undertaken unless the patient has first given full consent. To undertake any operation without appropriate consent from the patient risks liability for medical negligence or battery or both. Although some exceptions to this principle exist, such as special emergency situations in which consent is considered implied, the burden is on the physician to justify proceeding without prior adequate consent.

In 1914, Justice Cardozo declared that "Every human being of adult years and sound mind has a right to determine what shall be done with his own body, and a surgeon who performs an operation without his patient's consent commits an assault for which he is liable in damages." Over the years, this holding has been interpreted as the basis for the doctrine of informed consent. This doctrine imposes on the physician a duty to obtain a patient's consent after providing enough information to allow him or her to make an intelligent decision. What constitutes enough information is a matter of individual interpretation. Overall, the quality of information usually prevails over the quantity. Factors to be taken into account by the physician include (1) the measure of duty involved, (2) the scope of disclosure, and (3) the standards of disclosure current for the particular condition.

The doctrine of informed consent is based on the supposition that a properly informed patient will weigh the risks against the benefits of the proposed treatment and compare them with the risk-benefit ratio of alternative treatments. This requires the patient to be informed about the diagnosis, contemplated treatment, risks inherent in such treatment, alternative methods of therapy, and the expected prognosis with and without treatment. The process of obtaining informed consent should be more of a dialogue than a monologue. The patient should not only be told but also must be permitted to comprehend what is being considered. The patient should be encouraged to ask questions and have ample time alloted for these to be thoroughly answered.

A physician's duty as it relates to disclosure is determined by the standards of the medical profession. This requires that disclosure made to patients conform to the general practice of the specialty. Because it is widely recognized that full disclosure of risks may be harmful to some patients, the physician may exercise the privilege of withholding disclosure. This privilege is subordinate to the duty to disclose and requires adequate substantiation. The privilege to withhold disclosure is not applicable just because a physician considers that knowledge about a particular risk might cause the patient to refuse permission for a procedure that the physician feels is necessary. Circumspection is in order when applying this principle.

As stated, a physician owes the patient a duty to disclose in a reasonable manner all significant medical information that he or she possesses, or reasonably should possess, to allow the patient to make an intelligent decision as to whether or not to undergo the proposed treatment. The medical and legal communities have been wrestling with the definition of what significant medical information represents. Since the early 1970s, a new approach has been gaining acceptance. The courts have defined the extent of information to be shared with the patient as that information which is material for a particular patient to know in order to make an informed decision. Materiality, as defined by some courts, is the significance a reasonable person would attach to the disclosed risk or risks in deciding whether or not to submit to a particular surgical procedure or treatment.

The inherent difficulties of its definition and application make informed consent the subject of continued debate and litigation. Undoubtedly, further refinement of the informed consent doctrine will be forthcoming. Until then, physicians should attempt to involve patients in the decision-making process to the full extent of their abilities and interest. The right of self-determination is an inalienable right each patient possesses that is not subject to usurpation.

RECORD DOCUMENTATION

Good practice requires the physician to document the patient's status on the hospital chart. This includes a detailed admission history and physical examination, probable diagnosis, plan of management, and consent to therapy. During hospitalization, facts relating to the patient's clinical condition, variations in diagnosis, and management plans must also be recorded. Notwithstanding the emphasis placed in the teaching of medical students, the completeness of the medical notes is usually inversely proportional to the length of time a physician has been in practice. Such custom is less than adequate. It has been proved time and time again that a skimpy, inaccurate, illegible, or otherwise poorly maintained record may support an unjustifiable malpractice claim. To the contrary, a medical record that accurately reflects the thought processes of the attending physician becomes a meaningful medicolegal document favoring the physician by denoting care and exercise of judgement.

A medical record should be limited to observations pertaining to the diagnosis and treatment of the patient. The writings should distinguish between information related by the patient, history given by a relative, data obtained from consultant opinions, and the physician's own objective findings. A complete record clearly documents the impression of the treating physician, what treatment plans have been instituted, and what was told to the patient. All entries must include date, time, and signature of the examining physician. Delay in making a notation risks error or omission of pertinent information.

Statements that are contradictory or contrary to facts have no place in the medical record. Although a diversity of opinions substantiated by thought processes can be included as an expression of a particular physician's judgment, the medical record is not the appropriate location for philosophical arguments. Following discussion among the medical team, the record should reflect the decision, obtained by consensus, taken by the physician in charge of the patient's care. In an academic environment, it is the responsibility of supervisory physicians to read, correct, and countersign notes written by house staff and students. This reflects that they are overseeing the care being rendered by those they are supervising.

Office record-keeping requires no less attention to detail than appropriate hospital recording. In a medical malpractice suit, the plaintiff's counsel will examine both sets of records for statements that can help to establish the cause of the alleged injury and determine liability. The plaintiff's counsel will also evaluate records from physicians providing care following an alleged medical malpractice. Thus, subsequent treating practitioners must refrain from including unnecessary references or subjective opinions regarding the quality of care rendered by other physicians. Physicians should especially refrain from comments in the medical record that place blame on or assess liability of other practitioners for adverse patient outcomes.

PREVENTIVE RISK MANAGEMENT

It is generally accepted that most surgical procedures are accompanied by certain unavoidable risks. Even when adequate informed consent has been obtained prior to surgery, occurrence of complications during the surgical procedure requires certain actions to be taken by the surgeon. The patient must be fully advised of such an occurrence. A frank and forthright discussion about the possible cause(s) should take place with the patient and her family (if they are included in her care) soon after recovery from anesthesia.

The patient should be informed of the complications and their probable causes and mechanisms. An open discussion concerning the diagnosis, therapeutic choices, the risks and benefits of each, as well as the prognosis must take place. Documentation of this exchange is critical. Failure to make such notes may prove injurious at a later stage. Detailed records of all relevant facts reflect good care and caring (see Record Documentation). All notations must contain the date, time, and signature of the inscriber.

There are times when the services of a consultant are required. It is advisable to clearly document the problem for which a consultant is being called and the rationale for the request. Likewise, it is important to state if the consultation is limited to evaluation and recommendation for treatment, or if the consultant also is expected to care for the affected patient. In the latter case, the attending physician should further specify if treatment is to be established in conjunction with the primary clinician or to become the full responsibility of the consultant. Abdication of responsibility for care to another physician requires the patient's specific acknowledgment and consent. Such transfer of responsibility should be clearly documented in the medical record and the nursing staff fully apprised of the change.

When it is anticipated that a consultant will be involved in the care of a patient, the primary physician must tell the patient beforehand about the issues that require resolution and the reasons why other physicians are necessary. Common courtesy and professional respect require the primary caretaker to introduce the consultant to the patient. To avoid conflicting messages and confusing information, the record must clearly identify who is in charge of the patient's care.

Although it is not mandatory to follow the consultant's recommendations, the primary physician should have substantive arguments as to why he or she chooses not to do so. Documentation of the reasons for choosing an alternative plan of management must be established. The rationale for a particular plan of action should be explained, elaborating the logic of the decisions. An honest error in judgment usually proves supportable if adequate and appropriate diagnostic methods were used to arrive at that decision.

When dictating a discharge summary, objectivity is essential. The discharging physician should refrain from including in the report conjectural statements or opinions that could be interpreted as self-serving. The discharge summary should be limited to a factual account of the events that transpired during the course of hospitalization. It should incorporate only information that can be found in the medical records. Missing reports at the time of discharge should be properly noted; when appended as addenda, they should be properly dated to show they were added afterward.

Preventive risk management is more than just reporting the occurrence of a complication. The mishap should be analyzed in depth by the physician, risk manager, and defense counsel if one has been appointed. This is best done as soon as feasible after the complication has surfaced, which ensures that recollection of events is still fresh in the minds of the participants. Forthrightness and honesty with the risk manager or legal counsel concerning the most likely causes of the complication are crucial and can prove to be the physician's best defense.

MEDICAL RECORD REQUEST

Not long ago, the receipt of a request for a copy of a medical record from an attorney was a source of anxiety for the treating physician. At present, it is not unusual for a doctor to receive several such requests in a single year. Of course, not all of them, if any, result in a full legal action. Because it is difficult to know the intention of each request, they must all be handled with caution and attention given to detail.

When confronted with a request from a patient or her legal representative for medical records or information, it is imperative that the physician obtain the patient's written consent for disclosure. Information relating to a patient's health is always obtained in a confidential capacity. In general, a physician is not lawfully permitted to disclose such information without the specific authorization of the patient. Unless the woman formally consents, she has the unlimited privilege to refuse and to prevent anyone else from disclosing all communications between herself and her physician. This restrictive principle does not hold, however, if the physician recognizes that there is a serious danger to the patient or to others. Under such circumstances, the physician may actually have an overriding obligation to disclose information in order to prevent harm.

Although the patient's medical records are actually the property of the treating physician, the patient has unlimited access to the information contained in them. Thus, the physician has an obligation to grant the patient or her authorized agent the opportunity to evaluate the contents of her medical record. This obligation derives from the confidence and trust inherent in the fiduciary nature of the doctor-patient relationship. In some states, the right to gain access to their own medical records is granted to patients by statute. A physician risks a charge of concealing information fraudulently by refusing or obstructing access to records to a patient or her authorized attorney.

Soon after the records are provided to the patient or representative, the physician should contact his or her insurance carrier. It is the obligation of the physician's medical liability insurance carrier to provide the services of competent counsel in the event a suit is filed or anticipated. Major hospitals have in-house counsel or risk management units to assist physicians in the preparation and evaluation of legal materials. It is advisable to avail oneself of these services well in advance of trial participation in order to review details of the particular case while such details are still fresh. Issues concerning the case should be freely discussed with the reassurance that all discussions will be held in strict confidence within the context of the attorney-client relationship; this is analogous to the privileged nature of the doctor-patient communications previously discussed.

Patients' records or information that is going to be provided to a patient or her legal representative must be reviewed by the treating physician. Medical records, related reports, correspondence, and billing information should be segregated from the rest of the office materials. This will ensure against loss or misplacement of this important material. Care must be exercised not to make any changes even if it is clear that there has been an erroneous entry made or information has never been entered. It is essential to keep in mind that no matter how fine the care or blameless the physician, it is impossible to mount a satisfactory defense when alteration of the medical record is proved.

No less important is to refrain from making additions or new entries in the medical records. This is a fruitless exercise because such notations are usually viewed as self-serving. Nevertheless, if important information concerning the case is recalled or surfaces, contact your legal counsel about how to handle and document this new material.

Once the physician has contacted the hospital's risk management officer or insurance company's appointed counsel, it is prudent to refrain from discussing the case or any of its details with anyone but these people. The desire to talk and to vent one's frustrations about the case is understandable, but it should be resisted. This attitude applies to one's colleagues or other personnel, even if they are principals in the case. Such actions may disseminate undesirable information and may cause more harm than good. Furthermore, the plaintiff's counsel may attempt to introduce such discussions to give the appearance of collusion. Any inquiries or communications should be referred directly to the defense counsel handling the case. The defendant physician should avoid any correspondence or direct contact with the patient or her attorney unless his or her own counsel is informed or invited to be present.

CREDENTIALING OF PHYSICIANS

The practice of medicine involves the representation by a physician to the public at large that he or she possesses the required knowledge and necessary skills that can aid in the prevention, diagnosis, and treatment of diseases affecting human beings. States, which as institutions are charged with the protection of their citizens, have instituted the process of licensing of professionals to protect the public and to foster professionalism. To that effect, they require an applicant to have completed in a satisfactory manner a prescribed course of studies and passed a variety of state-approved examinations. In addition, most states are now demanding evidence of continuing medical education for periodic renewal of a physician's license to practice.

State relicensure regulations are designed to provide a mechanism by which the continuous quality of medical care can be assessed. Such regulations need not be uniform among states. Differences are acceptable as long as they do not impose arbitrary or unreasonable demands upon a particular health care provider. The opportunity to practice medicine is not an absolute vested right. Instead, it is a conditional right given to an individual that is subordinate to the police power of the state to protect and preserve public health. The hospital credentialing process is another method employed by the state in assuring quality medical care in an institutional setting.

The last decade has witnessed an increasing number of regulations, statutes, and court opinions dealing with the credentialing of physicians. This serves to emphasize the importance of credentials committees in determining the competence and skill of physicians working within hospitals. What was considered in the past as a necessary evil to comply with accreditation standards and regulations has become at present one of the most important risk management functions performed by a hospital medical staff. Hospitals and individual members of the credentials committee may ultimately be held responsible for failing to properly investigate new applicants or those applying for reappointment. Thus, familiarity of each practitioner with the delineation of privileges process of each institution is of paramount importance.

As previously stated, hospitals have a legal obligation to monitor the quality of care rendered in their institutions. Such duty has been extended to require a hospital to apply due care in conferring on and renewing staff privileges for self-employed physicians who may not be hospital employees or its agents. Thus, the hospital has a positive requirement to ensure that all who apply to practice within its walls are qualified and competent before privileges are granted. Furthermore, it must also ensure that physicians remain competent for as long as they continue practicing within the institution's confines.

The law, with due consideration to interstate variations, carefully delineates the liability exposure of hospitals and physicians within the context of the credentialing process. Failure to adhere to such a credentialing process may expose the institution and the treating physician to liability in a medical malpractice suit brought by an injured patient. Liability theories utilized by a plaintiff's attorney include vicarious liability exposure under the respondeat superior doctrine; direct theory of liability exposure in which the hospital would be considered a joint tort feasor in conjunction with the defendant physician; and negligent supervision, which on nonagency principles differs from the aforementioned doctrine of respondeat superior or of agency.

Under the respondeat superior doctrine the exposure of the hospital is premised on a master-servant relationship between the hospital and the defendant physician. Under this theory, recovery against the hospital can be transferred to the defendant physician as a result of the right of indemnification the hospital possesses against the culpable party—in this circumstance, the defendant physician.

Under the direct theory of liability exposure, the hospital and the defendant physician would be considered joint tort feasors. Upon a judgment in favor of the plaintiff, the hospital would be entitled only to contribution by the defendant physician instead of complete indemnification, as is the case under the vicarious liability theory. Failure of the hospital to fulfill its credentialing requirements is usually measured under the direct liability exposure theory.

Recently, a minority of courts have imposed a duty on the chairman of the hospital department to protect patients from an increased risk of substandard treatment by an underqualified staff physician. Because duty is measured by the scope of risk that negligent conduct foreseeably entails, any patient treated by these physicians is considered to be a foreseeable victim of less than adequate care. Thus, the chairman's duty is to use reasonable care in the hiring of a staff physician who might increase the risk of danger to patients cared for in the unit. Notwithstanding the fact that this is a minority opinion, in the future it is reasonable to expect greater scrutiny of the chairman's responsibilities in the credentialing process.

Hospitals have a legal obligation to monitor the health care rendered in their institutions. Therefore, exercise of reasonable care in conferring staff privileges also extends to the renewal process of existing appointments. As a result of such quality assurance surveillance, the institutions can curtail or revoke staff privileges of physicians whose performance is substandard. The Health Care Quality Improvement Act of 1986 makes hospitals responsible for establishing vigorous peer review processes to monitor the quality of care provided. Simultaneously, the aforementioned Act grants immunity to those participating in peer review activities whenever their actions are in good faith, fair, and in accordance with due process.

Due process requires hospitals to establish a mechanism to permit physicians to redress their grievances. This includes the opportunity to answer the charges that sustain the constraining measures. With respect to staff appointments and renewals, minimal due process requires the opportunity for a formal hearing preceded by appropriate notice, a written statement of the charges or reasons for the denial of appointment or reappointment, the right to call witnesses on behalf of the physician, the right to cross-examine the hospital's witnesses, and the right to have a written statement summarizing the decision and the basis for the decision as formulated by the hearing committee.

Sometimes conflicting considerations are inherent in the credentialing process. Hospitals are mandated to assure that only competent and qualified physicians are accorded privileges to render care in accordance with their training and experience. Physicians are also assured a reasonable, fair, and impartial process when applying for staff privileges or reappointment. Attempts to establish an unusually high standard of patient care may infringe upon the professional goals of a particular physician. Nonetheless, it is possible to achieve a proper balance. Above all, for the protection of all parties, adequate documentation and substantiation of the credentialing process are imperative.

WRONGFUL LIFE

For the past 25 years the courts have been confronted with an increasing amount of litigation aimed at the interpretation of rights of specific individuals. Concurrent with the recognition and expansion of the constitutional rights of children, the previously unknown cause of action known as wrongful life emerged. This is an action filed by the child in which it is alleged that the physician failed to adequately inform and/or advise his or her parents concerning foreseeable fetal risks from genetic or other congenital defects. The physician's negligence to inform the parents of the possibility of their bearing a defective child is alleged to have prevented them from exercising their decision to avoid conception or birth, resulting in the birth of a wrongful child. Wrongful life must be distinguished from the generally accepted wrongful birth cause of action, which is the parental claim based on the loss and expenses incurred with the birth of a defective child that could have been prevented.

The claim for wrongful life is not that the physician's negligence was the proximate cause of the impairment but rather that the physician's failure to adequately counsel the parents led to the birth of a defective child. Consequently, if the impaired child had not been born, he or she would not have had to experience the suffering caused by the impairment. The claim essentially alleges that the defective infant would be better off never having been born. The allegation was without precedent and prompted statements by the courts such as: "Whether it is better never to have been born at all than to have been born with even gross deficiencies is a mystery more properly to be left to the philosophers and the theologians...."

Until recently, courts found such assertions conceptually in conflict and precluded recovery. Legal arguments advanced by the courts to deny claims for wrongful life included: (1) no legal duty was owed by the physician to the infant (plaintiff) because the child was not a legal being at the time the physician's negligent act is claimed to have occurred; (2) the prevailing public policy favoring life at any level rather than nonexistence precluded the courts from finding birth as a legally cognizable injury; (3) the court's inability to measure damages as a result of having to compare the difference between a life with defects against the void of nonexistence; and (4) extending the liability to include these types of cases would open the floodgates of litigation.

Early changes in such a drastic position adopted by the courts can be traced to the late 1960s. In a complete reversal, a California Court of Appeals decided that it was not contrary to public policy to allow a woman to recover damages against a physician who unsuccessfully performed a sterilization. Recognition of a cause of action for wrongful birth by parents was thus established. Parents were granted the right to sue for special damages, including emotional pain and suffering and out-of-pocket expenses incurred during pregnancy and delivery.

In the early 1970s, acceptance of contraception and legalization of abortion gave couples parental autonomy over their own procreativity. The courts found that regardless of the motivation, couples have a legally protected right to determine whether they will have a child. Violation of such a fundamental right as not to procreate was to be considered injurious and worthy of redress. Public policy considerations could not be used to deny recovery of damages proximately caused by the physician's negligent creation of such injury. It is essential to note that proven negligence is still required for such a cause of action to exist.

Recognition of a cause of action for wrongful life was based on the lack of concern by the courts with the fact that had the defendant not been negligent, the defective child may never have come into existence at all. The concept that any type of life was better than no life at all was beginning to face scrutiny. The reality facing the courts was that the child (plaintiff) exists and suffers as a result of the physician's negligence. Recognition of the defective child's entitlement to legal rights and privileges accorded to other members of society lends support to the child's claim. Thus, the afflicted child was given the right to sue the negligent physician irrespective of whether the parents were available and willing to assert such rights. The courts reasoned that the afflicted child's need for medical care and other rehabilitation costs will not miraculously disappear when the infant reaches majority, and thus damages are not dependent on whether the medical expenses are incurred at the time when the parents remain legally responsible for providing such care but should be granted to the child.

Obstetricians are primary care providers who are required to provide current state-of-the-art obstetric care. Advancement and refinement of prenatal genetic diagnosis expands the duty obstetricians owe to their pregnant patients. Failure to adequately advise and counsel patients concerning the ability to accurately identify chromosomal abnormalities during the prenatal period clearly reflects a breach of such duty. As a consequence, practitioners may incur liability not only to the pregnant patient but to her afflicted infant as well.

Drawing a parallel from history, which led the courts to recognize wrongful birth as a valid cause of action, it is reasonable to expect in the not too distant future a continuous decrease in reluctance by the courts to accept claims for wrongful life. Greater flexibility and recognition for this type of claim appear to be the trends among the courts. As for the physician, strict adherence to the prevailing standard of care seems to be the best measure to avoid liability.

COURT-ORDERED OBSTETRIC INTERVENTIONS

Conflicts in the intrapartum management of pregnancy have been surfacing with increasing frequency. A pregnant woman's refusal to accept a blood transfusion for religious reasons and a mother's denial of consent for a cesarean delivery in the event of acute fetal distress or placenta previa are just two examples of the many difficult situations that have arisen recently. To aggravate matters further, the physician's decisions about therapy have been complicated by the recently emerging concept of fetal rights. In reality, the issue confronting today's obstetricians is: What should a physician do when faced with situations in which there is a conflict between maternal and fetal rights?

Not long ago, the overriding principle guiding medical care was the physician's attempt to do his or her utmost for the benefit of the patient. In obstetrics, this meant that the mother's safety and rights always prevailed when treatment decisions were made. Fetal well-being was considered important, but seldom to the extent that it overshadowed concern for the mother's welfare. This situation was even recognized by the courts when in Roe v. Wade (410 U.S. 113, 1973), fetal interests were considered secondary to the wishes of the mother up to the point of viability; thereafter, preservation of the mother's life still remained the prevailing concern.

In recent years we have seen a trend away from the aforementioned principle. What was once considered by a physician as simply a moral obligation to safeguard the unborn infant has been slowly transformed by the concept of fetal rights. Perhaps it is appropriate to question the origin of fetal rights and whether they have emerged at the expense of maternal rights. If that is the case, is it reasonable to further ask if those maternal rights were abrogated or simply usurped?

Implicit in a pregnant woman's decision to carry a fetus to term is the moral obligation to act responsibly during pregnancy. How the extent of such a moral obligation can be determined and by which standards such evaluations should be made are at the core of this debate. To impose on the patient what her attending physician believes to be or ought to be her moral obligation is fraught with a wide range of consequences. To transform a moral obligation into a legal one is even more dangerous.

The emergence of the fetal rights concept has been interpreted by physicians as creating a moral dilemma when a pregnant patient chooses a treatment that will result in a less than desirable fetal outcome. Acceptance of the existence of fetal rights negates this controversy as a moral or ethical dilemma. Instead, it becomes a conflict between two parties with opposing interests. As a consequence, it seems unwise and perhaps unethical for a physician confronting such a conflict to attempt to protect both parties.

Proponents of court-ordered intervention cite the state's obligation, as parens patriae, to intervene in order to ensure that a child receives the necessary medical treatment. Opponents argue, on the contrary, that a woman should not be deprived of the right to control her own life just because she is pregnant. Although expansion of the concept of fetal rights has been the trend recently, to what extent the law allows the state or other third parties to control the behavior of pregnant women by asserting concern for the well-being of the unborn fetus remains unclear. The complete spectrum of implications associated with court-ordered obstetric interventions is just beginning to unfold.

In the absence of legislation on this point, physicians have sought guidance from the courts. In some instances the courts have granted permission to proceed against the mother's wishes. We must recognize that these court-ordered interventions are based on dubious legal grounds. Any legal recognition of the fetus that would diminish a woman's autonomy and infringe on her protected rights to privacy and equality is open to questions of constitutionality. Furthermore, the decisions have usually emanated from lower court judges and carry little, if any, precedential value.

Would the state be justified in prohibiting the ingestion of alcohol or smoking of tobacco by a pregnant woman in order to protect the well-being of her fetus? Could a cervical cerclage be ordered to maintain a gestation that risks prematurity because of an incompetent cervix? As progress is made in intrauterine fetal surgery, can we expect the courts to decide who is to have and when such a procedure should be performed? In addition to the moral implications of court-ordered obstetric interventions, physicians must also attempt to understand the legal implications that may result in expansion rather than limitations of their liability. Attempts by physicians to make decisions without judicial guidance may lead to serious consequences. It has been suggested that in order to salvage a previously normal full-term infant who is experiencing acute fetal distress, surgical intervention can be accomplished without the mother's consent. This is very disturbing. Obstetricians should be aware that the performance of any type of invasive intervention without the patient's consent is unacceptable conduct. When such action is taken in defiance of a patient's explicit wishes, a physician risks legal action in both civil and criminal courts. To be oblivious to a woman's right to decide what can be done to her body is to ignore the long-established concept of informed consent. That such action is taken for the sake of the unborn infant provides no justification to proceed and should not be relied on as a defense for such action.

The legal questions concerning fetal status or maternal rights to refuse treatment remain to be answered by the courts and the legislatures. What could be done if the patient refuses to obey the court's order is pure conjecture. The courts would be hard-pressed to enforce a contempt of court motion in a patient in active labor; nor is it easy to envision physically restraining a pregnant patient and forcing her to have some type of anesthesia to undergo a cesarean section.

In the meantime, physicians ought to explore the reasons why a pregnant patient would refuse a recommended therapy to benefit her yet-to-be-born infant. It is an established fact that a physician's ability to help a patient is in direct proportion to the patient's faith and trust in the care provider. The absence of such rapport or a breakdown of communication in an already tenuous physician-patient relationship may prompt the patient to reject the advice of her physician. It seems illogical that a patient would obey a judge, who has little or no medical experience, after refusing her physician's advice. In such a case, however, it is reasonable to assume that the jurist attained the trusted, authority figure status the attending physician failed to achieve.

On the other hand, serious thought must be given to an alternate approach. Instead of seeking court permission to perform a surgical procedure against the patient's will, efforts should be directed to restore the physician-patient relationship. After all, the patient is not rebelling against the profession of medicine, but rather implying a lack of confidence in the person making the recommendation for surgery. If she had rejected her basic belief in medicine, she would not have sought medical care in the first place. To reassume the role of authority figure, a physician must first lay the necessary foundation. Calling in a consultant or even the chief of the service may assuage a reluctant patient. Although involving another physician in such circumstances may negatively affect a physician's self-image, in the long run it may prove to be most beneficial for the patient as well as for the physician.

CONCLUSION

The subject as described here represents the medicolegal areas in obstetrics considered to be evolving at present. Unlike medical advances, variations in the law occur with greater procrastination and their application varies from state to state. Nonetheless, when changes in the current law do take place, they must be viewed as doctrinary and their effect as much broader than it appears at first glance. A sequence of decisions in any region of the country ought to be analyzed and evaluated as a potential trend, soon to be followed elsewhere. Minor variations in the doctrine of informed consent, or acceptance of fetal rights or the physician-hospital relationship, among others, may profoundly affect the practice of obstetrics for the foreseeable future. Obstetricians may benefit from a better understanding of these subject areas.

SUGGESTED READING

Fineberg KS, Peters JD, Willson JR, Kroll DA. Obstetrics/gynecology and the law. Ann Arbor:Health Administration Press, 1984.

Louisell DW, Williams H. Medical malpractice. New York:Mathew Bender, 1986.

Rozovsky FA. Consent to treatment: a practical guide. Boston:Little, Brown, 1984.

Southwick AF. The law of hospital and health care administration. Ann Arbor:Health Administration Press, 1978.

INDEX

The letter f following a page number indicates a figure; the letter t following a page number indicates a table.

E

F

Fetal alcohol syndrome, 5

I

N

O

R

S